MOLECULAR BIOLOGY
INTELLIGENCE
UNIT

Nucleic Acid Sensors and Antiviral Immunity

Suryaprakash Sambhara, DVM, PhD
Influenza Division
National Center for Immunization and Respiratory Diseases
Centers for Disease Control and Prevention
Atlanta, Georgia, USA

Takashi Fujita, PhD
Laboratory of Molecular Genetics
Institute for Virus Research
and
Laboratory of Molecular Cell Biology
Graduate School of Biostudies
Kyoto University
Kyoto, Japan

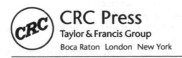

CRC Press
Taylor & Francis Group
Boca Raton London New York

CRC Press is an imprint of the
Taylor & Francis Group, an **informa** business

NUCLEIC ACID SENSORS
AND ANTIVIRAL IMMUNITY

Molecular Biology Intelligence Unit

First published 2013 by Landes Bioscience Publishers

Published 2018 by CRC Press
Taylor & Francis Group
6000 Broken Sound Parkway NW, Suite 300
Boca Raton, FL 33487-2742

© 2013 by Taylor & Francis Group, LLC
CRC Press is an imprint of Taylor & Francis Group, an Informa business

First issued in paperback 2019

No claim to original U.S. Government works

ISBN 13: 978-0-367-44590-4 (pbk)
ISBN 13: 978-1-58706-658-0 (hbk)

The chapters in this book are available in the Madame Curie Bioscience Database.

While the authors, editors and publisher believe that drug selection and dosage and the specifications and usage of equipment and devices, as set forth in this book, are in accord with current recommendations and practice at the time of publication, they make no warranty, expressed or implied, with respect to material described in this book. In view of the ongoing research, equipment development, changes in governmental regulations and the rapid accumulation of information relating to the biomedical sciences, the reader is urged to carefully review and evaluate the information provided herein.

Library of Congress Cataloging-in-Publication Data

Nucleic acid sensors and antiviral immunity / [edited by] Suryaprakash Sambhara, Takashi Fujita.
    p. ; cm. -- (Molecular biology intelligence unit)
Includes bibliographical references and index.
ISBN 978-1-58706-658-0 (alk. paper)
I. Sambhara, Suryaprakash, 1955- II. Fujita, Takashi, 1954- III. Series: Molecular biology intelligence unit (Unnumbered : 2003)
[DNLM: 1. Nucleic Acids--metabolism. 2. Antigens, Viral--immunology. 3. Immunity, Innate. 4. Signal Transduction--immunology. 5. Toll-Like Receptors--immunology. QU 58]

616.07'9--dc23

2012033875

Dedication

To all who contributed to our knowledge in innate immunity

About the Editors...

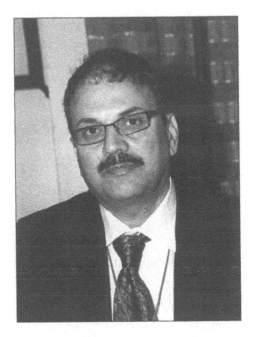

SURYAPRAKASH SAMBHARA is Chief of Immunology Section, Influenza Division at the Centers for Disease Control and Prevention, Atlanta and Adjunct Professor at the Georgia State University and Purdue University. His main research interests include innate immunity, viral immunology, vaccine development and human immunology. He is a scientific advisory board member of PATH and provides scientific advice to several national and international organizations. Suryaprakash Sambhara received his academic degrees DVM and MVSc from the College of Veterinary Science, Tirupati India, MS from the University of Wyoming, USA and PhD in immunology from the University of Toronto, Canada.

About the Editors...

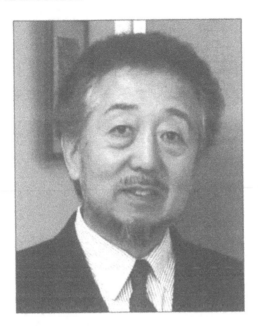

TAKASHI FUJITA is Professor of Molecular Genetics in Institute for Virus Research, Kyoto University Japan. He obtained his PhD from Waseda University, Tokyo 1982 on studies on interferon priming. He joined Dr. T. Taniguchi's laboratory at Cancer Institute, then later at Osaka University as a postdoctoral fellow until 1990, where he worked on interferon-β gene and identified virus-inducible enhancer element and cloned IRF-1. He joined Prof. D. Baltimore's laboratory as a postdoctoral fellow at Whitehead Institute and Rockefeller University until 1993 and worked on transcriptional regulation by NF-κB. He started his own laboratory in Tokyo Metropolitan Institute for Medical Sciences in 1993. His group discovered IRF-3 as a key regulator for interferon genes. In 2004, his group including Dr. M. Yoneyama, discovered RIG-I and related sensors for viral RNA. In 2005, his group moved to Kyoto University.

CONTENTS

Foreword...xix

Preface...xxi

1. Antiviral Responses in Invertebrates..1
   Jean-Luc Imler and Jules A. Hoffmann
   Introduction 1
   Apoptosis and the Control of DNA Virus Infections 2
   RNA Interference Confers Sequence-Specific Antiviral Immunity.....5
   The Antiviral Inducible Response 7
   A Phylogenetic Perspective on RNA Sensing in Invertebrates..........9
   Conclusion...12

2. Overview of TLRs 19
   Bruce Beutler
   Introduction 19
   C3H/HeJ and C57BL/10ScCr: Two Independent Lines
     of LPS-Refractory Mice 20
   CD14 and Its Crucial Role in LPS Sensing.....................................21
   Positional Cloning of the *Lps* Locus, and the Discovery of TLR4 21
   Discovery of MD-2 22
   XA21 in Rice, and Toll in the Fly: the Importance
     of LRR Proteins 22
   How Many Mammalian TLRs Are There, and What Do They
     Each Detect? 23
   The Need for Accessory Proteins in TLR Function........................ 26
   Signaling Pathways Activated by Mammalian TLRs 29
   The Overall Importance of TLRs.. 30
   Conclusion...32

3. Nucleic Acid-Sensing TLR Signaling Pathways...............................40
   Yutaro Kumagai and Shizuo Akira
   Introduction 40
   Nucleic Acid-Sensing TLRs and Their Cofactors 41
   Adaptor Molecules and Their Signaling 43
   Intracellular Protein Trafficking as a Paradigm for Diversity
     in TLR Signaling.. 48
   Conclusion.. 50

4. Alternative Regulatory Mechanisms of TLR Signaling 58
   Claire E. McCoy
   Introduction 58
   Regulation by Alternative Splicing 60
   Regulation by RNA Binding Proteins 62
   Regulation by miRNA...63
   Discussion 64
   Conclusion...65

5. Intracellular Viral RNA Sensors: RIG-I Like Receptors...........................71
Seiji P. Yamamoto, Ryo Narita, Seigyoku Go, Kiyohiro Takahasi,
Hiroki Kato, and Takashi Fujita
    Introduction 71
    Specificity of RLRs in Recognition of Viral Infection 72
    RLR Ligands 73
    Positive and Negative Regulation of RLR-Mediated Signaling 75
    Structure.. 77
    Conclusions and Perspectives 79

6. Contribution of LGP2 to Viral Recognition Pathways 85
Osamu Takeuchi and Shizuo Akira
    Introduction 85
    LGP2—Characterization by In Vitro Studies 87
    LGP2 as a Positive Regulator of RNA Virus Recognition 88
    LGP2 Acts Upstream of MDA5 and RIG-I 89
    Role of LGP2 in Response to Transfection with Synthetic RNAs............ 89
    Structural Studies of LGP2... 89
    The Role of LGP2 ATPase Activity 90
    Potential Role of LGP2 in Cytoplasmic DNA Recognition 91
    Conclusion 92

7. The Mitochondrial Immune Signaling Complex 97
Yu Lei and Jenny P.-Y. Ting
    Introduction 97
    Molecules Important in the Recognition of Nucleic Acid Species............ 98
    The Significance of Mitochondrial-Localized Proteins in Host
        Innate Antiviral Responses 100
    The Roles of NLR Proteins in the Modulation
        of MAVS-RLR Signaling.. 101
    The Regulatory Components of the RLR Signaling Pathways.................. 103
    Connection of Autophagy, Innate Immunity
        and the Mitochondria 105
    Viruses Can Subvert MAVS-Dependent Type 1 IFN Production 106
    MAVS in Apoptotic Signaling... 107
    Conclusion 107

8. DNA Sensors and Anti-Viral Immune Responses 114
Susan Carpenter, Søren Beck Jensen and Katherine A. Fitzgerald
    Introduction 114
    DNA: A Key Activator of Innate Immune Signaling............................115
    PRRs: Essential Weapons in the Fight against Viral Infection 116
    DAI..116
    RNA Polymerase III 117
    HMGB1 118

Lrrfip1 118
DExD/H Box Helicases (DHX9 and DHX36)...................................118
IFI16..119
Small Molecule Ligands That Trigger TBK1-Dependent Type I
    IFN Gene Transcription 119
ci-di A/GMPs..120
PRRs Regulating Caspase-1 Dependent Maturation of IL-1β.................121
The NLRP3 Inflammasome 122
The AIM-2 Inflammasome 122
The IFI16 Inflammasome...122
Counterregulation of DNA Driven Immunity...................................124
Conclusion and Future Directions...125

9. Mechanisms of Interferon Antagonism by Poxviruses...........................131
    Xiangzhi Meng, Lloyd Rose and Yan Xiang
    Introduction 131
    Poxvirus Proteins That Inhibit the Induction of IFNs....................135
    Poxvirus Proteins That Inhibit Signaling of IFNs..........................137
    Poxvirus Proteins That Inhibit Effectors of IFN 138
    Conclusion..140

10. Innate Immune Evasion Strategies of HCV and HIV:
    Common Themes for Chronic Viral Infection 148
    Brian P. Doehle and Michael Gale Jr.
    Introduction 148
    HCV Structure and Infection..149
    Recognition of HCV Infection..151
    HCV Antagonism of Innate Immune Signaling Pathways..............151
    Human Immunodeficiency Virus 153
    HIV Structure and Infection 153
    Initial Stages of Infection: Exposure, Eclipse, and Acute 154
    Sensing of HIV by Cell Intrinsic Innate Immune Pathways 154
    Interferon and ISGs vs. HIV 157
    Viral Countermeasures: HIV Strikes Back...................................157
    The Innate Immune Activation: Paradox or Dysregulation?...........158
    Conclusions—Is Innate Immune Targeting a Path
        for Future Therapeutics and Vaccines? 159

11. Innate Immune Evasion Strategies of Influenza A Virus....................167
    Alesha Grant and Adolfo García-Sastre
    Introduction 167
    Recognition of IAV..168
    Induction and Propagation of Type I IFN 168
    IAV Type I IFN Antagonists..170
    Conclusion..172

12. **Autophagy in Antiviral Immunity**...178
   Brian Yordy and Akiko Iwasaki
   Introduction 178
   Autophagy Machinery as a "Delivery" Mechanism for Innate
      and Adaptive Antiviral Systems.. 182
   Autophagy and ATG Proteins Regulate Innate Signaling.................. 185
   Autophagy in Cell-Autonomous Antiviral Defense 185
   Viral Evasion Mechanisms 187
   Conclusion.. 190

13. **Synthetic and Natural Ligands of RLR** 197
   *Martin Schlee, Janos Ludwig, Christoph Coch, Jasper G. van den Boorn,
      Winfried Barchet and Gunther Hartmann*
   Introduction 197
   MDA5 198
   RIG-I 199
   Synthetic dsRNA Ligands.. 200
   Synthetic Triphosphorylated dsRNA Ligands.................................. 202
   Structural and Functional Insights into RNA Recognition
      by RIG-I Like Helicases... 206
   RNase Cleavage Products... 207
   In Vivo RNA Polymerase III Transcripts of Exogenous DNA 207
   Detection of Bacterial RNA 208
   Detection of Viral RNA by RIG-I 208
   Conclusion and Outlook... 210

14. **Antiviral Actions of Double-Stranded RNA** 218
   Saurabh Chattopadhyay, Michifumi Yamashita and Ganes C. Sen
   Introduction 218
   Sources of dsRNA 219
   Genes Regulated by dsRNA 219
   dsRNA Binding Proteins 220
   Functions of Specific dsRNA-Binding Proteins 221
   Conclusion... 233

15. **Ligands of Pathogen Sensors as Antiviral Agents** 240
   *Priya Ranjan, Victoria Jeisy-Scott, William G. Davis, Neetu Singh,
      J. Bradford Bowzard, Monika Chadwick, Shivaprakash Gangappa
      and Suryaprakash Sambhara*
   Introduction 240
   Cytosolic RNA Sensors 242
   Cytosolic DNA Sensors... 244
   Endosomal Nucleic Acid Sensors 245
   Non-Nucleic Acid Binding PRRs in Antiviral Immunity 246
   Conclusion... 246

   Index 257

EDITORS

Suryaprakash Sambhara
Influenza Division
National Center for Immunization and Respiratory Diseases
Centers for Disease Control and Prevention
Atlanta, Georgia, USA
Chapter 15

Takashi Fujita
Laboratory of Molecular Genetics
Institute for Virus Research
and
Laboratory of Molecular Cell Biology
Graduate School of Biostudies
Kyoto University
Kyoto, Japan
Chapter 5

CONTRIBUTORS

Shizuo Akira
Laboratory of Host Defense
World Premier International Immunology
  Frontier Research Center
and
Department of Host Defense
Research Institute for Microbial Diseases
Osaka University
Osaka, Japan
Chapters 3, 6

Winfried Barchet
Institute of Clinical Chemistry
  and Clinical Pharmacology
University Hospital Bonn
Bonn, Germany
Chapter 13

Bruce Beutler
Center for Genetics of Host Defense
University of Texas Southwestern
  Medical Center
Dallas, Texas, USA
Chapter 2

J. Bradford Bowzard
Influenza Division
National Center for Immunization
  and Respiratory Diseases
Centers for Disease Control
  and Prevention
Atlanta, Georgia, USA
Chapter 15

Susan Carpenter
Department of Medicine
Division of Infectious Diseases
  and Immunology
University of Massachusetts
  Medical School
Worcester, Massachusetts, USA
Chapter 8

Monika Chadwick
Influenza Division
National Center for Immunization
  and Respiratory Diseases
Centers for Disease Control
  and Prevention
Atlanta, Georgia, USA
Chapter 15

Saurabh Chattopadhyay
Department of Molecular Genetics
Lerner Research Institute
Cleveland Clinic
Cleveland, Ohio, USA
Chapter 14

Christoph Coch
Institute of Clinical Chemistry
   and Clinical Pharmacology
University Hospital Bonn
Bonn, Germany
Chapter 13

William G. Davis
Influenza Division
National Center for Immunization
   and Respiratory Diseases
Centers for Disease Control
   and Prevention
Atlanta, Georgia, USA
Chapter 15

Brian P. Doehle
Department of Immunology
University of Washington
Seattle, Washington, USA
Chapter 10

Katherine A. Fitzgerald
Department of Medicine
Division of Infectious Diseases
   and Immunology
University of Massachusetts
   Medical School
Worcester, Massachusetts, USA
Chapter 8

Michael Gale Jr.
Department of Immunology
University of Washington
Seattle, Washington, USA
Chapter 10

Shivaprakash Gangappa
Influenza Division
National Center for Immunization
   and Respiratory Diseases
Centers for Disease Control
   and Prevention
Atlanta, Georgia, USA
Chapter 15

Adolfo García-Sastre
Department of Microbiology
Department of Medicine
Global Health and Emerging
   Pathogens Institute
Mount Sinai School of Medicine
New York, New York, USA
Chapter 11

Seigyoku Go
Laboratory of Molecular Genetics
Institute for Virus Research
and
Laboratory of Molecular Cell Biology
Graduate School of Biostudies
Kyoto University
Kyoto, Japan
Chapter 5

Alesha Grant
Department of Microbiology
Department of Medicine
Global Health and Emerging
   Pathogens Institute
Mount Sinai School of Medicine
New York, New York, USA
Chapter 11

Gunther Hartmann
Institute of Clinical Chemistry
   and Clinical Pharmacology
University Hospital Bonn
Bonn, Germany
Chapter 13

Jules A. Hoffmann
CNRS-UPR9022
Institut de Biologie Moléculaire
  et Cellulaire
University of Strasbourg
Strasbourg, France
Chapter 1

Jean-Luc Imler
CNRS-UPR9022
Institut de Biologie Moléculaire
  et Cellulaire
University of Strasbourg
Strasbourg, France
Chapter 1

Akiko Iwasaki
Department of Immunobiology
Yale University School of Medicine
New Haven, Connecticut, USA
Chapter 12

Victoria Jeisy-Scott
Influenza Division
National Center for Immunization
  and Respiratory Diseases
Centers for Disease Control
  and Prevention
Atlanta, Georgia, USA
Chapter 15

Søren Beck Jensen
Department of Medicine
Division of Infectious Diseases
  and Immunology
University of Massachusetts
  Medical School
Worcester, Massachusetts, USA
and
Department of Medical Microbiology
  and Immunology
Aarhus University
Aarhus, Denmark
Chapter 8

Hiroki Kato
Laboratory of Molecular Genetics
Institute for Virus Research
and
Laboratory of Molecular Cell Biology
Graduate School of Biostudies
Kyoto University
Kyoto, Japan
Chapter 5

Yutaro Kumagai
Laboratory of Host Defense
World Premier International Immunology
  Frontier Research Center
and
Department of Host Defense
Research Institute for Microbial Diseases
Osaka University
Osaka, Japan
Chapter 3

Yu Lei
Lineberger Comprehensive Cancer Center
Chapel Hill, North Carolina, USA
Chapter 7

Janos Ludwig
Institute of Clinical Chemistry
  and Clinical Pharmacology
University Hospital Bonn
Bonn, Germany
Chapter 13

Claire E. McCoy
Monash Institute of Medical Research
Clayton, Victoria, Australia
Chapter 4

Xiangzhi Meng
Department of Microbiology
  and Immunology
The University of Texas Health Science
  Center at San Antonio
San Antonio, Texas, USA
Chapter 9

Ryo Narita
Laboratory of Molecular Genetics
Institute for Virus Research
Kyoto University
Kyoto, Japan
Chapter 5

Luke A.J. O'Neill
School of Biochemistry and Immunology
Trinity Biomedical Sciences Institute
Trinity College Dublin
Dublin, Ireland
Foreword

Priya Ranjan
Influenza Division
National Center for Immunization
    and Respiratory Diseases
Centers for Disease Control
    and Prevention
Atlanta, Georgia, USA
Chapter 15

Lloyd Rose
Department of Microbiology
    and Immunology
The University of Texas Health Science
    Center at San Antonio
San Antonio, Texas, USA
Chapter 9

Martin Schlee
Institute of Clinical Chemistry
    and Clinical Pharmacology
University Hospital Bonn
Bonn, Germany
Chapter 13

Ganes C. Sen
Department of Molecular Genetics
Lerner Research Institute
Cleveland Clinic
Cleveland, Ohio, USA
Chapter 14

Neetu Singh
Influenza Division
National Center for Immunization
    and Respiratory Diseases
Centers for Disease Control
    and Prevention
Atlanta, Georgia, USA
Chapter 15

Kiyohiro Takahasi
Laboratory of Molecular Genetics
Institute for Virus Research
and
Institute for Innovative NanoBio Drug
    Discovery and Development
Graduate School of Pharmaceutical
    Sciences
Kyoto University
Kyoto, Japan
Chapter 5

Osamu Takeuchi
Laboratory of Host Defense
World Premier International Immunology
    Frontier Research Center
and
Research Institute for Microbial Diseases
Osaka University
Osaka, Japan
Chapter 6

Jenny P.-Y. Ting
Lineberger Comprehensive Cancer Center
and
Institute for Inflammatory Diseases
and
Department of Microbiology
    and Immunology
School of Medicine
The University of North Carolina
    at Chapel Hill
Chapel Hill, North Carolina, USA
Chapter 7

Jasper G. van den Boorn
Institute of Clinical Chemistry
   and Clinical Pharmacology
University Hospital Bonn
Bonn, Germany
Chapter 13

Yan Xiang
Department of Microbiology
   and Immunology
The University of Texas Health Science
   Center at San Antonio
San Antonio, Texas, USA
Chapter 9

Seiji P. Yamamoto
Laboratory of Molecular Genetics
Institute for Virus Research
and
Laboratory of Biomass Conversion
Research Institute for Sustainable
   Humanosphere
Kyoto University
Kyoto, Japan
Chapter 5

Michifumi Yamashita
Department of Molecular Genetics
Lerner Research Institute
Cleveland Clinic
Cleveland, Ohio, USA
Chapter 14

Brian Yordy
Department of Immunobiology
Yale University School of Medicine
New Haven, Connecticut, USA
Chapter 12

FOREWORD

The discovery of Toll-like receptors (TLRs) in the late 1990s ushered in a new age of discovery for innate immunity. The importance of TLRs for immunology and biomedical research was recognized with the Nobel Prize for Medicine or Physiology in 2011. The prize was shared by three scientists: Ralph Steinman (for the discovery of dendritic cells, which express TLRs and whose activation by them provides a link between innate and adaptive immunity), Jules Hoffman (who made the pioneering observation of Toll in fruit fly anti-fungal immunity) and Bruce Beutler (who uncovered the role of TLR4 in the response to LPS). Work on TLRs inspired many researchers, and led to a search for other receptors in innate immunity. There are now several additional families of such receptors known, notably RIG-I-like receptors (RLRs), C-type lectin receptors (CLRs) and AIM2-like receptors (ALRs). A notable feature is the detection of nucleic acids from pathogens, but also from host cells in certain contexts, particularly in autoimmune diseases.

Nucleic Acid Sensors and Antiviral Immunity presents a timely and extensive account of the detection of nucleic acids in infection and inflammation. We have chapters by Beutler, Hoffman and Shizuo Akira, who is the most cited immunologist of the past ten years, for his work on innate immunity, which gives us an indication of the importance of the field. Several other pioneers in the field present comprehensive and highly lucid up-to-date accounts of their particular interests, revealing the large amount of activity in the past few years, as the literature continues to grow and become ever more complex. The fly yet again provides new insights, and anti-viral mechanisms in this key model organism are described. Other topics include the ability of viruses such as poxviruses, hepatitis C virus and HIV to interfere with detection and signalling; new insights into signalling including subcellular localization of signalling proteins, complex regulation of TLRs and RLRs by ubiquination and negative regulation by miRNAs; and the role of autophagy in antiviral defence. The importance of the RLRs in viral detection is widely reviewed. DNA sensing by ALRs and other receptors is extensively described, and the prospect of additional as yet unknown receptors for DNA debated, revealing a field that is still burgeoning. The prospect of therapeutic utility is covered in the context of using nucleic acids or other compounds as agents to promote anti-viral immunity.

This book therefore represents an unprecedented account of this important aspect of immunology, by a stellar cast of authors who have defined the field. We have a key resource which should act as a primary source of information. The chapters will inspire researchers to continue on their quest to provide mechanistic insights into anti-viral innate immunity. The discoveries provide us with new strategies in the never ending war between humanity and viral infection, and will help in the ultimate goal to provide treatments to use against viruses which continue to present a major threat to human health.

Luke A.J. O'Neill
School of Biochemistry and Immunology
Trinity Biomedical Sciences Institute
Trinity College Dublin
Dublin, Ireland
Email: laoneill@tcd.ie

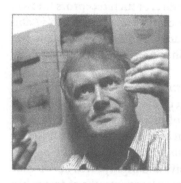 Professor Luke O'Neill holds the Chair of Biochemistry and is Director of the Trinity Biomedical Sciences Institute at Trinity College Dublin. His research aims to unravel the complex signaling pathways triggered during inflammation and innate immunity. He carried out pioneering work in the area of IL-1 signaling with Jeremy Saklatvala in Strangeways Research Laboratories, Cambridge UK. He has published extensively in the area of molecular immunology and inflammation. He has made several important findings in the area of toll-like receptors, providing the first evidence that TLRs might be anti-viral when he found Vaccinia proteins that inhibited TLR signaling. His laboratory subsequently found the TLR adapter protein Mal, and uncovered the complex regulation of TLR adaptors in signaling. More recently he has worked on regulation of TLRs by miRNAs, and the interplay between TLRs and inflammasomes in the production of IL-1β. He is a co-founder of Opsona Therapeutics which aims to develop anti-inflammatory agents that act on TLRs and inflammasomes. In 2009, he was awarded the Royal Dublin Society/ Irish Times Boyle Medal for Scientific Excellence.

PREFACE

Innate immunity is the front line of host defense and its importance was recognized over one hundred years ago by Metchnikoff with his landmark observation of phagocytosis. In his Nobel lecture, he stated

> The sum of the very numerous facts established in the archives of science leaves no room to doubt the major part played by the phagocytic system, as the organism's main defense against the danger from infectious agents of all kinds, as well as their poisons.
> ...when the microbes penetrate, the white corpuscles make use of the dilatation of the blood vessels and the nervous actions that control this, in order to reach the battle field in the shortest possible time. (http://www.nobelprize.org/nobel_prizes/medicine/laureates/1908/mechnikov-lecture.html)

thus setting the stage for the mechanisms of pathogen recognition by phagocytes and the receptors involved in this recognition. The advances in molecular biology, cell biology, immunology, biochemistry and other disciplines have unraveled the mysteries of innate immune recognition and effector functions. These would not have been possible without the innovative research of many investigators and it is rather impossible to acknowledge all for their contributions. Hence, we feel it appropriate to dedicate this volume to all those who contributed to the field of innate immunity. This book is intended to provide a comprehensive yet a thorough review of various aspects of innate immunity to enable the experts as well as junior investigators to appreciate the many unanswered questions of this exciting field. It is indeed a difficult task for the contributors as well as editors to bring the book as up to date as possible especially when research on innate immunity is progressing very rapidly.

The chapters are grouped with a theme for easy understanding. In the first two chapters, innate antiviral responses in invertebrates and an over view of Toll-like receptors in vertebrates are addressed at a great length respectively. Both these chapters touch on the phylogenetic relationship of pathogen sensing and the downstream adapter molecules, the functional consequences and provide a great introduction to the subsequent chapters.

Chapters 3-8 provide an in-depth coverage of and discussion of nucleic acid sensing pathways, alternative regulator mechanisms of TLR signaling, RIG-I-like receptors, contribution of LGP2 in antiviral immunity, mitochondrial immune signaling complex and DNA sensors. In these chapters, the readers will appreciate the complexities of downstream signaling, adapter molecules involved and the regulatory pathways.

The molecular mechanisms by which pathogens for example, pox viruses, HCV and HIV and influenza evade host innate immune mechanisms are discussed in Chapters 9-12. The viral virulence factors responsible and their interactions with the innate immune sensors will provide new targets for antiviral drug development. The important roles played by cellular mechanisms, autophagy in delivering pathogen ligands to the innate immune sensors and how viruses overcome autophagy are also discussed in detail.

In the final three chapters, the ligands of pathogen sensors, both natural and synthetic, their molecular interactions with one or more nucleic acid sensors and their potential application as antiviral agents are discussed. Ligands or small molecules that activate innate immune pathways have the potential pan-antiviral effects and perhaps can be used as molecular adjuvants for vaccines.

We hope the selection of chapters and topics satisfies the intellectual curiosity of both experts and novices in innate immunity and we sincerely thank all the contributors without whose cooperation and support we could not have bring this excellent collection of chapters to you. We thank Prof. Luke O'Neil for providing his insights and thoughts on innate immunity in the Foreword.

We also take this opportunity to thank the publishers, Landes Bioscience, Cynthia Conomos, Celeste Carlton and Erin O'Brien for their continued support throughout our journey to bring this book to you all.

Suryaprakash Sambhara, DVM, PhD
Influenza Division
National Center for Immunization and Respiratory Diseases
Centers for Disease Control and Prevention
Atlanta, Georgia, USA

Takashi Fujita, PhD
Laboratory of Molecular Genetics
Institute for Virus Research
and
Laboratory of Molecular Cell Biology
Graduate School of Biostudies
Kyoto University
Kyoto, Japan

CHAPTER 1

Antiviral Responses in Invertebrates

Jean-Luc Imler and Jules A. Hoffmann*

Abstract

Like all living organisms, invertebrates are constantly exposed to viruses and have evolved efficient antiviral defense mechanisms. We review here our current understanding on antiviral host-defense in invertebrates. Some invertebrate antiviral host-defense strategies such as apoptosis and inducible expression of antiviral molecules are shared with vertebrates, whereas others such as RNA interference are not. One common theme between antiviral innate immunity in vertebrates and invertebrates is the sensing of the presence of double-stranded RNA in infected cells, which involves molecules containing an evolutionarily conserved DExD/H box helicase domain.

Introduction

Viruses represent an important class of pathogens, causing serious concern for human health, as well as important economic losses in crops and animals. Because they replicate inside cells, and rely for the most part on host cell molecular machineries for their replication, viruses pose specific challenges to the immune system. It is therefore interesting to study antiviral immunity in a wide range of organisms, to get a grasp on the palette of different strategies evolved by different animals to fight-off viruses. More specifically, there are several reasons to work on virus-host interaction in invertebrate models. First, the study of antiviral defense mechanisms in genetically tractable invertebrate models such as the fruit fly *Drosophila melanogaster* and the nematode *Caenorhabditis elegans* can provide useful information on the genetic mechanisms operating, some of which may have been conserved through evolution. For example, antiviral apoptosis and viral suppressors of apoptosis were initially characterized while investigating resistance to baculovirus infection in Lepidopteran insects.[1] The use of viruses (e.g., baculoviruses) as biological control agents against insect pests is a second reason to investigate virus-host interactions in invertebrates.[2] A third motivation is that viral infection of invertebrates can cause important economic losses (e.g., contribution to colony-collapse disorder in honey-bees; infections with White Spot Syndrome virus (WSSV) in shrimp farming).[3,4] A fourth and final reason is of course that hematophagous invertebrates such as *Aedes* or *Culex* mosquitoes can transmit viral diseases (caused by so-called arthropod-borne viruses or arboviruses, e.g., dengue, yellow fever, West-Nile virus) to mammalian hosts.[5]

This chapter discusses our current understanding on antiviral defenses in invertebrates. Two efficient antiviral mechanisms, apoptosis and RNA interference have been identified. A poorly characterized inducible response also contributes to the control of viral infections in invertebrates. Whereas the degradation or inhibition of cellular inhibitors of apoptosis by an unknown mechanism plays a critical role in the detection of DNA virus infections, antiviral RNA interference and at least some inducible antiviral responses are triggered by double-stranded (ds)RNA. We discuss the involvement of Dicer- and RIG-I-like DExD/H box helicases in antiviral defenses in invertebrates.

*CNRS-UPR9022, Institut de Biologie Moléculaire et Cellulaire, University of Strasbourg, Strasbourg, France.
Corresponding Author: Jean-Luc Imler—Email: JL.Imler@unistra.fr

Nucleic Acid Sensors and Antiviral Immunity, edited by Suryaprakash Sambhara and Takashi Fujita.
©2013 Landes Bioscience.

Apoptosis and the Control of DNA Virus Infections

An efficient antiviral defense strategy for multicellular organisms relies on the induction of programmed cell death upon sensing viral infection. The rapid death of infected cells, before the virus achieves its replication cycle, provides an efficient mean to deal with viral infections, all the more so if the dying cell is rapidly and efficiently ingested by phagocytes. The role of programmed cell death in the control of viral infections is well illustrated by the interaction of a family of invertebrate DNA viruses, the baculoviruses, with their host.[6] These large double stranded DNA viruses (128kb genome for *Autographa californica M nucleopolyhedrovirus* (AcMNPV), the prototype species of *Baculoviridae*) are prolific pathogens that can be used for insect pest control. Viral particles are ingested by Lepidopteran larvae, and first enter midgut cells. The virus then spreads to tracheolar cells and hemocytes, thus initating systemic infection.[7] Baculovirus-induced apoptosis of midgut cells represents an efficient antiviral response in these insects.[8] Besides baculoviruses, experiments in insects and the nematode *C. elegans* showed that apoptosis is also an efficient antiviral defense against other types of DNA viruses, such as poxviruses.[9,10]

Apoptosis is regulated by a family of cysteine proteases that cut their substrates after an aspartic acid residue, the caspases (Fig. 1). They are synthesized as inactive precursors (the procaspases), which are activated through proteolytic cleavage. The so-called apical caspases contain in addition a large prodomain composed of a homotypic protein-protein interaction motif such as a dead box effector domain (DED) or a caspase recruitment domain (CARD). Recruitment and local concentration of apical procaspases through these domains trigger their activation. By contrast, effector caspases, which are activated upon cleavage by activated apical caspases, contain a short prodomain devoid of functional motifs.[11] Significantly, a tight association exists between programmed cell death and efficient mechanisms of phagocyte recruitment, leading to recognition

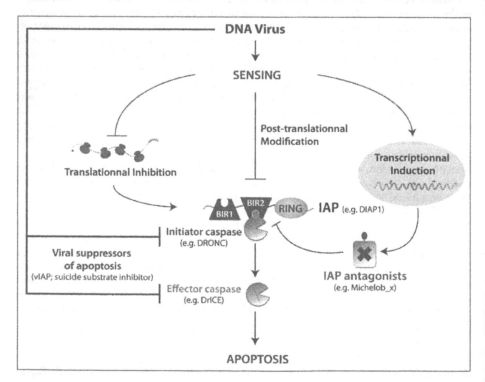

Figure 1. Induction of apoptosis in Lepidopteran cells infected by baculovirus. See the text for details.

and engulfment of apoptotic cells before any cellular material is released. This likely contributes to the efficient removal of virus infected cells.[12,13]

Caspase activity is controlled by inhibitors of apoptosis proteins (IAPs).[14] The existence of these proteins was first revealed by the identification of an apoptosis inhibitor in a baculovirus (see below), which led to the search of cellular orthologs. IAPs are characterized by the presence of one to three Baculovirus IAP Repeat (BIR) domains, coupled to a RING domain (Fig. 1). BIR domains (~80 amino-acids) function as protein-protein interaction domains and mediate interaction between IAPs and specific caspases. RING domains are 40–60 amino-acids domains present in proteins of the ubiquitination pathways. Importantly, many caspases only bind IAPs after they have been activated by proteolytic cleavage.[14] In these cases, the IAPs bind to a conserved IAP-binding motif (IBM) localized at the new N-terminus of the caspase uncovered by the proteolytic cleavage. The existence of this conserved motif provides a powerful way to regulate apoptosis in insect cells. IBM motif proteins (also known as IAP antagonists or RHG proteins, from the initials of the three first described members of this family in drosophila, Reaper, Hid and Grim) are expressed in cells destined to die.[15] These small proteins, induced at the transcriptional level by a range of signals such as UV irradiation, DNA damage or developmental cues, will bind to IAPs, thereby displacing the bound caspases and releasing them from the inhibitory effects of IAPs. In addition, in Drosophila, displacement of DIAP1 from caspases also promotes auto-ubiquitination of DIAP1, followed by its degradation.[11] Of note, IBM motif proteins acting as IAP antagonists also exist in mammals (e.g., Smac/DIABLO). In this case however, they are regulated by a post-translational mechanism rather than by transcriptional induction.[15]

The demonstration that apoptosis plays a critical role in the control of viral infections in insects came from the analysis of a viral mutant causing apoptosis in two cell lines permissive for replication of the wild-type virus.[1] The mutation affects the gene *p35*, which functions as a suppressor of apoptosis. Further experiments in vivo confirmed that apoptosis plays an important role in the control of AcMNPV infection, and that the lethal dose 50 for the p35 mutant was approximately 1000 fold higher than for the wild-type (wt) virus.[16] p35 is structurally distinct from any known protein. It functions as a potent substrate inhibitor for effector caspases, and remains associated with the caspase after cleavage.[17] The baculovirus *Spodoptera littoralis Nucleopolyhedrovirus* (SlNPV) and the entomopoxvirus *Amsacta moorei entomopoxvirus* (AmEPV) also express suicide substrates for caspases with weak sequence similarity to AnMNPV p35 (Fig. 1).[10,18,19] Interestingly, some mammalian viruses have independently co-opted similar solutions to counter host-cell death. In particular the cowpox virus gene *crmA* encodes a serpin inhibitor that forms a tight complex with and inhibits caspase-1, thus preventing apoptosis induced by viral infection.[20]

The identification of p35 in the genome of AcMNPV prompted the search for other viral suppressors of apoptosis. In an elegant set of experiments, L. Miller and colleagues identified a gene from the *Cydia pomenella granulovirus* (CpGV) which could complement a mutant p35-deleted AcMNPV.[21] The new suppressor of apoptosis, IAP, showed no sequence homology to p35, but its discovery led to the identification of a family of cellular homologs of this gene. Viral IAPs have been identified in multiple members of two families of insect DNA viruses, the *Baculoviridae* and the *Entomopoxviridae*.[22-24] Altogether, the studies on viral suppressors of apoptosis, either the caspase inhibitors or the vIAPs, reveal that virus production and spreading is severely reduced in the absence of these molecules, indicating that apoptosis is an efficient strategy to counter viral infections in insects,[8] and probably also in other invertebrates such as crustaceans.[4,25]

The importance of apoptosis in the control of infection by large DNA viruses, raises the question of the mechanisms used to detect infection and to trigger cell death. While the mechanisms for sensing viral infection remain poorly characterized, it is becoming apparent that three mechanisms can participate in the onset of apoptosis in virus-infected cells: (1) inhibition of the host cell translation machinery; (2) depletion of cellular IAP proteins; and (3) induction of IAP antagonist proteins (Fig. 1). Baculoviruses notoriously induce a dramatic shut-off of host protein synthesis.[26] This inhibition may reflect a viral strategy to recruit the translation machinery of the host for its benefit. Alternatively, it may help the host to counter viral infection by blocking viral gene expression, or by inducing programmed cell death. One consequence of the inhibition of host-cell protein synthesis is the arrest of the replenishment of short-lived proteins, such as the IAPs (half-life 30–45').[14] Thus, decreasing concentrations of IAPs in cells in which translation is diminished or abolished could provide a way to trigger apoptosis. Indeed, inhibition of IAPs is sufficient to trigger cell death, while their sustained expression can protect cells against apoptotic stimuli. For example, infection of drosophila Line-1 (DL-1) cells by the RNA virus FHV leads to a rapid decrease of host cell translation (within 4 to 8 hours), which trigger the rapid decline of the intracellular pool of DIAP1.[27] Significantly, apoptosis has little impact on FHV multiplication in DL-1 cells, indicating that cell death does not occur rapidly enough to affect viral growth in the case of this RNA virus.

Depletion of DIAP1 in DL-1 cells and of SfIAP in *Spodoptera frugiperda* cells is also observed upon infection with the baculovirus AcMNPV. In this case however, cellular IAP levels decrease 6h before host translation arrest becomes apparent, indicating that AcMNPV-induced IAP depletion cannot be entirely due to inhibition of host cell translation.[28] The rapid depletion of DIAP1/SfIAP in Drosophila/*Spodoptera* cells infected by AcMNPV depends on the activity of their RING domain, which functions as an E3 ubiquitin ligase, and is mediated in part by the proteasome. The fact that this inhibition is rapid and does not require protein synthesis points to the involvement of post-translational modifications triggered by viral infection. Indeed, both DIAP1 and SfIAP can be phosphorylated, and this phosphorylation affects the stability of the proteins.[29] Of note, one of the kinases phosphorylating DIAP1 in drosophila cells is DmIKKε[29], whose ortholog in mammals participates in the signaling pathway activated by viral RNAs and leading to interferon gene expression.[30] Altogether, these results indicate that IAPs can behave as sensors of viral infection in insect cells, their degradation in virus-infected cells unleashing the pro-apoptotic function of caspases.[28] It is tempting here to draw a parallel with the "guard" protection model in plants.[31]

Finally, a third, recently discovered, mechanism mediating the apoptosis response upon viral infection involves induction of IAP antagonists. The mosquito baculovirus *Culex nigripalpus nucleopolyhedrovirus* (CuniNPV) induces expression of *michelob_x* (*mx*), the ortholog of the Drosophila gene *reaper*, which encodes an IAP antagonist.[32] The induction is slow in the permissive species *C. quinquefasciatus* and fails to trigger timely apoptosis. As a result, infected cells support viral replication and ultimately die from necrosis with heavy loads of virus. By contrast, *mx* gene expression is rapidly induced in the midgut cells of the refractory mosquito *Aedes aegypti*, leading to apoptosis within 2 to 6 hours post-infection.[33] These data indicate that induction of the IBM-motif protein *mx* upon sensing viral infection can trigger apoptosis and result in containment of the viral infection. Interestingly, reoviruses inhibit cellular IAPs in mammalian cells by a similar mechanism, triggering the release of Smac/DIABLO from the outer mitochondrial membrane.[34] A key question raised by these observations now points to the nature of the receptors detecting the presence of viral infection and triggering translation shut-off, degradation of IAP proteins, or induction of IBM proteins.

In the course of viral DNA replication, short-lived stretches of single stranded DNA and double stranded DNA ends are generated, and can be recognized as damaged DNA.[35] Thus, as already shown in mammals, DNA virus replication in insects may trigger a DNA damage response, which shares many similarities between insects and mammals. Interestingly, two outcomes of this response, cell cycle arrest and apoptosis, are induced by baculovirus infections in insect cells. Furthermore, DNA damage in Drosophila and *Spodoptera* cells is sufficient to induce *reaper* expression. Further support for an involvement of the DNA damage response pathway in the sensing of DNA virus infection comes from a recent study demonstrating that infection of Sf9 cells by AcMNPV triggers induction of Sfp53 and phosphorylation of the histone variant protein H2AX.[36] Nevertheless, to date the exact role of the DNA damage response in the induction of apoptosis is still unclear, in part because the DNA damage response is required for optimal baculovirus replication.

RNA Interference Confers Sequence-Specific Antiviral Immunity

The mechanism of RNA interference relies on a family of molecules known as Argonautes (AGO). AGO molecules bind to small RNAs, and use them as guides to recognize complementary sequences in target RNA molecules. AGO molecules then inhibit translation of these RNAs, or trigger their degradation (slicer activity). Invertebrates contain several AGO molecules (five in drosophila: AGO1, -2, -3, Piwi and Aubergine), which interact with different types of small RNAs, thus defining three major pathways of RNA silencing, as detailed below for drosophila: (1) AGO1 interacts with 22–23nt long micro (mi)RNAs (miRNA pathway); (2) AGO2 interacts with 21nt long small interfering (si)RNAs (siRNA pathway); and (3) AGO3, Piwi and Aubergine (Aub) interact with Piwi-interacting (pi)RNAs (piRNA pathway). Both miRNAs and siRNAs are produced from double stranded (ds) RNA precursors, by RNaseIII enzymes of the Dicer family: Dicer-1 produces miRNAs from cellular short RNA precursors forming paired secondary structures, whereas Dicer-2 processes long dsRNAs into siRNAs. By contrast, biosynthesis of piRNAs does not involve a dsRNA precursor or an enzyme of the Dicer family, and remains poorly characterized.[37]

The origin of the dsRNAs processed by Dicer-2 can be cellular, when the two strands of a genomic region are transcribed simultaneously, or in the case of transcripts with complementary extremities folding back on themselves. Unlike the miRNAs, these endogenous siRNAs (endo-siRNAs) do not appear to play a crucial role in development, as *Dicer-2⁻/⁻* mutant flies are viable and fertile.[38] dsRNA in insect cells can also be of viral origin (e.g., replication intermediates in the case of most RNA viruses). The dsRNA binding protein R2D2 helps Dicer-2 to select long dsRNA substrates rather than pre-miRNAs, for example.[39] R2D2 forms a stable complex with Dicer-2, and also participates in the loading of the siRNA duplex onto AGO2. One strand of the duplex (passenger strand) is then cleaved by AGO2 and released, allowing the formation of the active siRISC (RNA induced silencing complex), containing the guide strand. Within this complex, AGO2 will cleave the target RNA between the positions 10 and 11 of the guide siRNA (slicer activity).[40]

The importance of the siRNA pathway for the control of viral infections is best illustrated by the strong susceptibility of *Dicer-2⁻/⁻*, *r2d2⁻/⁻* and *AGO2⁻/⁻* mutant flies to viral infections.[41-47] Mutant flies die more rapidly than wild-type controls, with higher viral loads, following infection by a number of RNA viruses, whether their genome is double- or single-stranded, of positive or negative polarity. It is therefore clearly established that the siRNA pathway plays a major role in the control of RNA virus infections. Deep sequencing of small RNAs produced in the course of a viral infection in flies and mosquitoes confirmed that the virus derived siRNAs (vsiRNAs) have a size of 21nt, as expected for the products of the enzyme Dicer-2 (Fig. 2).[43,48-55] In addition, the production of the vsiRNAs is strongly reduced or abolished in *Dicer-2⁻/⁻* mutant flies.[43] The vsiRNAs cover the whole length of the viral genome, and the ratio between the number of siRNAs matching the (+) strand and the (-) strand of the genome is close to one. These vsiRNAs therefore most likely derive from the cleavage of long dsRNA molecules produced in the course of viral replication (Fig. 2). The vsiRNAs are then loaded onto AGO2: indeed, they are protected from β-elimination following oxidation, which indicates that their 3′ end is methylated, a modification triggered by the methyl-transferase Hen1 on siRNAs loaded onto AGO2.[48] Altogether, the genetic and biochemical data support a model in which long dsRNA molecules generated in the course of viral replication are recognized by the Dicer-2/R2D2 complex, and processed into 21nt siRNAs. The vsiRNAs are then loaded onto AGO2 in the siRISC complex, to guide this molecule toward viral RNA molecules. AGO2 will then cleave the viral RNA through its slicer activity. This mechanism may also be used to protect cells that have not yet been infected. Indeed, insect cells in culture can take up exogenous dsRNA molecules, through scavenger receptor mediated endocytosis.[56,57] Thus, viral dsRNA molecules released following lysis of virus-infected cells can be taken up by non-infected cells and induce RNA interference, thereby protecting them against future challenges with the virus.[58]

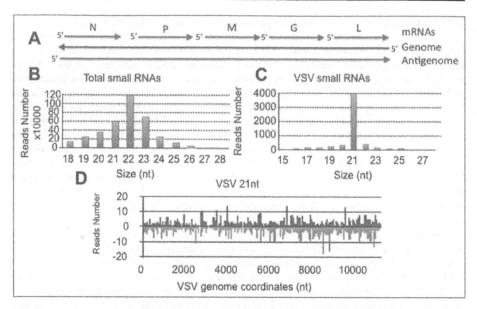

Figure 2. Virus-derived siRNAs in VSV infected flies. A) Representation of the viral RNAs present in virus infected cells. B) Size distribution of total small RNAs in VSV infected wt flies. C) Size distribution of small RNAs matching the VSV genome. D) Profile of 21nt siRNA reads along the VSV genome. Each siRNA is represented by the position of its first nucleotide. siRNAs matching the antigenome and genome are shown in dark gray (blue) and light gray (red), respectively. A color version is available online at www.landesbioscience.com/curie.

Interestingly, the piRNA pathway may also participate in the control of viral infections. Indeed, piRNAs corresponding to the sequence of two drosophila viruses, DCV and FHV, have been identified in cells of the line OSS, derived from the somatic sheet of the ovary and expressing Piwi.[55] Similar observations were made in the mosquito cell line C6/36, which appears to be defective in the siRNA pathway: when these cells are infected by the arboviruses dengue virus, La Crosse virus or Sindbis virus (SINV), virus-derived small RNAs of 26–27nt, rather than 21nt, are observed.[59,60] In addition, decreased resistance to infection by the RNA viruses DXV or WNV has been reported in *piwi*[-/-] mutant flies, suggesting that the piRNAs participate in the control of viral infections.[41,47]

As is often the case, viruses have adapted to the antiviral effects of RNAi, and can express viral suppressors of RNAi (VSR).[61] Originally identified in plant viruses, VSRs are also present in the genome of insect viruses, where three of them have so far been characterized in molecular detail. An efficient mechanism to counteract RNA interference is to prevent the interaction of Dicer-2 with dsRNA molecules, and prevent their dicing. The protein B2 from FHV functions in this way. In vitro, this 12kD protein binds dsRNA with nanomolar affinity, and prevents its cleavage by Dicer. B2 can also bind to siRNA duplexes, and thus pertubates their loading onto the RISC complex.[62] B2 interacts with the viral RNA polymerase, and is therefore tightly associated with the viral replication complex in infected cells.[48] The presence of B2 at the very site where dsRNAs are generated allows the suppressor to instantly bind to dsRNA, before it can be recognized by the Dicer-2/R2D2 complex. The protein 1A from DCV contains a canonical dsRNA binding domain and functions in a similar manner.[45] Thus, insect and mammalian viruses have evolved similar strategies based on the expression of dsRNA binding proteins to escape recognition by the innate immune system. As a result, some interferon antagonist viral proteins can function as VSRs when expressed in insect cells.[63] The third VSR characterized in insect viruses, CrPV-1A, behaves differently.[64] Although DCV and CrPV belong to the same family of viruses, and exhibit remarkable similarities in their sequence, the 5' end of the ORF1, where the sequences coding the VSR are located, are completely different. Unlike DCV-1A, CrPV-1A does not bind dsRNAs and does not interfere with the production of vsiRNAs. Rather, this suppressor blocks RNAi at a downstream step. CrPV-1A interacts with AGO2 and inhibits its function in the RISC complex.[64] Thus, the identification and characterization of the mode of action of new VSRs may provide useful tools to dissect molecularly the succesive steps of antiviral RNA interference.

VSRs represent an important determinant of pathogenicity in insect viruses. Indeed, a mutant FHV virus defective for B2 loses its virulence in drosophila.[42,51] Conversely, expression of B2 can strongly increase the pathogenicity of otherwise poorly pathogenic viruses, such as SINV.[52] The example of dicistroviruses is even more striking. In spite of the strong sequence homologies between the two viruses, CrPV is more pathogenic than DCV. This difference could be due to the strength of the CrPV VSR. Indeed, a recombinant SINV virus expressing CrPV-1A is more pathogenic than a similar recombinant virus expressing DCV-1A.[64]

The Antiviral Inducible Response

RNA interference and apoptosis are intrinsic systems of the host-defense in most invertebrate virus-infected cells. Importantly, viral infection in invertebrates also triggers an inducible antiviral response that contributes to the control of viral load and survival. Several studies monitoring gene expression in control and virus infected insects or crustaceans established that many genes are induced in response to viral infection.[4,65] For example, infection of drosophila by the picorna-related virus DCV triggers upregulation of at least one hundred genes,[66] whereas infection of *Aedes* mosquitoes with Flaviviruses (dengue, West-Nile virus or yellow fever virus) leads to induction of some two hundred genes.[67] The profile of induced genes during this response to virus infection differs from that of extracellular pathogens such as bacteria or fungi, pointing to a dedicated gene reprogramming pattern.

The analysis of the promoter of the DCV and FHV induced gene *vir-1* (virus-induced RNA1) revealed the importance of DNA motifs recognized by the transcription factor STAT92E, the sole STAT factor present in flies. In addition, *vir-1* as well as several other DCV-induced genes, are no longer induced following viral infection in flies mutant for the drosophila JAK kinase Hopscotch. In addition, *hopscotch*[-/-] mutant flies die more rapidly, with a higher viral load, than wild-type controls.[66] The JAK/STAT pathway also participates in the control of Dengue virus infections in *Aedes* mosquitoes.[68] In shrimps, infection by WSSV further activates the JAK/STAT pathway, but the virus subverts this response from the host, and uses the STAT transcription factor to express a subset of its own genes.[69] These data indicate that the JAK/STAT pathway plays an evolutionarily conserved role in antiviral immunity. As in mammals, the JAK/STAT pathway in drosophila is activated by cytokines. The drosophila receptor Domeless is an ortholog of the receptors for cytokines of the IL-6 family, and presents similarities with the gp130 subunit. Three cytokines, Unpaired-1, -2 and -3, activate the receptor Domeless and the JAK/STAT pathway in drosophila.[70] Expression of two of these cytokines, Upd2 and -3, is induced following DCV infection. Altogether, these data suggest that at least some viral infections trigger expression of Upd cytokines, which induce the JAK/STAT pathway and an antiviral state in non-infected cells.

Other genetic experiments in flies, but also in mosquitoes, suggest an involvement of the Toll and IMD pathways in antiviral immunity.[71-74] These pathways regulate the activity of transcription factors of the NF-κB family and play a well-characterized role in the induction of antimicrobial peptide gene expression, a hallmark of the inducible response of drosophila to bacterial and fungal infections.[75] However, we do not have a clear picture at this stage of the exact nature of the contribution of these pathways to the control of viral infections in insects, and this topic warrants clarification. In summary, the inducible antiviral defense in insects is complex, and may involve as many as three conserved signaling pathways, JAK/STAT, Toll and IMD. The existence of this inducible response raises two major questions concerning (1) the nature of the effector molecules induced by viral infections; and (2) the identity of the receptors sensing viral infection and triggering these responses.

One of the genes induced by DCV infection in drosophila, *Vago*, contributes to the control of viral infection. Indeed, the viral load increases by a factor 5 to 10 in the fat body (the tissue in which *Vago* is specifically expressed) of *Vago*[-/-] mutant flies compared with wild-type controls. The mode of action of Vago, a 16kDa protein containing 8 cysteines, however remains to be established.[76] In *Aedes* mosquitoes, two genes regulated by the JAK/STAT pathway in response to dengue virus infection encode factors restricting infection by this virus.[68] Here again, the modes of actions of these two molecules remain unknown. With regard to the Toll and IMD pathways, the informations available to date are too fragmentary and not sufficiently consistent to warrant a conclusion as to the putative involvement of the effector antimicrobial peptides regulated by these pathways in antiviral defenses. One induced effector mechanism involved in the control of viral infections in drosophila is autophagy. Indeed, VSV infection triggers autophagy in drosophila cells, and silencing of the autophagy genes *Atg7* and *Atg18* leads to decreased survival and increased virus titer in VSV infected flies. The sensitivity of these flies to DCV infection is not modified, indicating that autophagy does not represent a broad response to viral infections.[77] In other insects, activation of the hemolymph enzyme phenoloxidase, which catalyzes the oxidation of mono- and diphenol to orthoquinones and leads to melanization, can generate virucidal activities (reviewed in ref. 65). In the silk moth, phenoloxidase activity is regulated by hemolin,[78] a circulating immunoglobulin superfamily member, which is induced following baculovirus infection.[79] Other inducible antiviral proteins have been described in crustaceans, although their mode of action has not been characterized (e.g.,refs. 4,80,81).

The data available at this stage indicate that the inducible response can be triggered by sensing viral molecules (viral RNAs or proteins), or tissue degradation and cellular stress caused by the viruses. The detection of dsRNAs generated in the course of viral infections leads to the upregulation of *Vago* gene expression. Indeed, induction of this gene by DCV or SINV infection can be prevented in transgenic flies expressing the dsRNA binding VSR B2.[76] Induction of *Vago* is also impaired in *Dicer-2*[-/-] mutant flies, but not in *r2d2*[-/-] or *AGO2*[-/-] mutant flies. This result indicates that Dicer-2 acts both as a key component of the RNAi mechanism and as a receptor triggering an inducible response. Interestingly, the cytosolic receptors of the RIG-I-like receptor family contain a DExD/H box helicase domain phylogenetically related to that found at the N-terminal end of Dicer enzymes (Fig. 3).[76] This points to an evolutionarily common origin for these molecules (see below). The signaling pathway linking Dicer-2 to *Vago* gene expression remains unknown. dsRNA-triggered antiviral responses have been described in other invertebrates. For example, hemolin can be induced by dsRNA in Lepidoptera cells.[79] The receptor detecting dsRNA and mediating hemolin induction is currently unknown. Detection of dsRNA can also trigger some level of antiviral resistance in the marine shrimp *Litopenaus vannamei*,[82] although the resistance triggered appears limited compared with other mechanisms such as sequence specific RNA interference or apoptosis.[4,83]

In addition to nucleic acids, viral proteins can also trigger an antiviral response. Indeed, induction of autophagy in drosophila cells infected by VSV results from the recognition of the viral G glycoprotein. The receptor involved, which activates the PI3 kinase/AKT pathway to induce autophagy, is currently unknown.[77]

Induction of *vir-1*, or other genes regulated by the JAK/STAT pathway, is not affected by expression of B2, or the absence of Dicer-2, indicating that it is not the sensing of dsRNA that leads to the induction of the Upd cytokines.[76] As the JAK/STAT pathway can be activated by stress, this pathway may be induced by tissue-damage caused by viral infections.[70] This could also be the case for the induction of the Toll and Imd pathways. Indeed, accumulation of undigested DNA from apoptotic cells in flies mutant for DNaseII leads to induction of the genes *diptericin* and *attacin*, two markers of IMD pathway activation.[84] Furthermore, it has been shown that tissue damage in an epithelial tissue can lead to induction of the Toll pathway in the absence of infection, through activation of the Persephone circulating protease.[85] It will be interesting to elucidate the precise mechanism leading to activation of these pathways upon sensing the detrimental effects of viral infection on the tissues of the host.

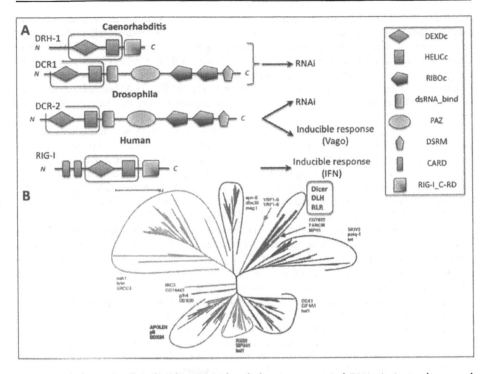

Figure 3. Phylogenetically related DExD/H box helicases sense viral RNAs in invertebrate and vertebrate cells. A) Domain architecture of DExD/H box helicases participating in antiviral immunity in nematodes, flies and mammals. The conserved DExD/H box helicase domain is boxed. B) Protein sequence-based dendrogram of the 389 DExD/H box helicase encoded by the genomes of *S. cerevisiae*, *C. elegans*, *D. melanogaster* and *H. sapiens*. The 11 sequences corresponding to the Dicers, the DLHs and the RLRs are boxed. Modified from reference 76, with permission.

In summary, the inducible antiviral response is complex and involves host- and virus-specific mechanisms. One viral molecular pattern sensed by the immune system in drosophila is dsRNA, which triggers in invertebrates both RNA interference and an inducible response. Interestingly, this viral molecular pattern is detected in invertebrates and vertebrates by molecules containing a conserved DExD/H box helicase domain (Fig. 3).

A Phylogenetic Perspective on RNA Sensing in Invertebrates

Vertebrates mainly rely on a subset of Toll-like receptors and on RIG-I like receptors to sense viral nucleic acids and trigger synthesis of interferons,[30] raising the question of the origin of these sensors in pre-vertebrate animals. Toll receptors also exist in invertebrates, including Cnidarians and Poriferans, indicating that Toll receptor related genes originated at the dawn of metazoan evolution, some 1 billion years ago. However, the sequences of these molecules have diverged to an extent that makes it delicate to assign orthology for members of this family between species, even for urochordates and cephalochordates.[86] Thus, it is not possible to trace back to pre-vertebrates the origin of the two groups of TLRs sensing viral nucleic acids (TLR3 and TLR7/9). Some other considerations suggest that the sensing of viral RNA or DNA by Toll receptors arose in vertebrates. For example, TLR7 and TLR9, the most important TLRs for the sensing of viral nucleic acids, are expressed in a mammalian specific cell-type, the plasmacytoid dendritic cells. This contrasts with the other important class of receptors sensing viral nucleic acids, the RIG-I like receptors, which are expressed in many cell types, including fibroblasts, epithelial cells, macrophages and conventional dendritic cells.[87] These data raise the question whether RLRs may represent the first line of sensors and activators of antiviral host-defense, and whether TLRs may alert dendritic cells to the presence of an infection when this initial response is inefficient, suppressed or overwhelmed.[88,89] Furthermore, experiments with influenza virus indicate that activation of TLR7 by viral RNA not only enforces the production of IFN, but also activates the adaptive immune response, a vertebrate-specific asset of antiviral immunity.[89] The structural similarities between the DExD/H box helicase domains of RLRs and Dicer enzymes (see below) also pleads for an evolutionarily ancient role of RLRs in sensing viral nucleic acids.

RNAi participates in the control of viral infections in plants, fungi and animals, indicating that it represents an ancestral host-defense system.[37] Indeed, Dicer and AGO proteins are also present in protists (e.g., the ciliate *Tetrahymena*), where dsRNA can trigger sequence-specific gene silencing.[90] All multicellular organisms have one *Dicer* gene for the production of miRNAs required for development and for fine-tuned responses to stress. Several of these organisms have additional *Dicer* genes, which may participate in endo- or exo-siRNA pathways. For example, the plant *Aribidopsis thaliana* has 4 *Dicer-like* (*DCL*) genes, one of which, *DCL-1*, is involved in the production of miRNAs. The others mediate host-response against RNA (*DCL2* and *-4*) or DNA viruses (*DCL3*).[91-93] Fungi have two *Dicer* genes, and studies in *Cryphonectria parasitica* showed that the product of one of these, DCR2, is required for the production of viral siRNAs and host-defense against a (+) strand RNA virus.[94] Most invertebrate animals also have several *Dicer* genes (Fig. 4): two are found in Cnidarians and insects, whereas up to five are observed in Porifera.[95] Based on the fungi, plant and insect paradigm it is tempting to postulate that these additional *Dicer* genes participate in antiviral defenses. One exception discussed below is *C. elegans* (a species which has notoriously lost many pathways over evolution), which contains a single *Dicer* gene. By contrast with protostomes, deuterostomes have a single *Dicer* gene, of the miRNA pathway *Dcr-1* type. However, these animals contain in addition RIG-I-like receptors (RLRs), which contain DExD/H box helicases phylogenetically related to the DExD/X box helicases found at the N-terminus of most Dicer molecules, but lack the RNaseIII domains. Mammals have three well-defined RLRs (RIG-I, MDA5 and LGP2). The number of RLRs is variable in deuterostome invertebrates: the urochordate *Ciona intestinalis* has two, whereas the cephalochordate *Branchiostoma floridae* (also known as amphioxus) and the sea urchin *Strongylocentrotus purpuratus* have respectively 13 and 16. The amplification of the RLR family in these species parallels that of other families of innate immunity receptors (e.g., TLRs).[96] Interestingly, RIG-I-like molecules are also found in protostomes: the nematode *C. elegans* has three, called Dicer-related helicase (DRH)-1, -2 and -3; the cnidarian *Nematostella vectensis* has two; the poriferan *Amphimedon queenslandica* has one. Insects do not have genes encoding such RLR-like molecules (Fig. 4). The function of RLRs outside of vertebrates remains unknown, with the exception of *C. elegans*. In nematodes, the DRH molecules function in the RNAi silencing pathway, and two of them have been molecularly characterized. DRH-3 is a core component of a cellular RNA-dependent RNA polymerase (RdRP) complex that produces secondary siRNAs.[97] It may be involved in the release of siRNA duplexes from Dicer.[98] DRH-1 also acts downstream of Dicer. Interestingly, although it is not directly involved in the sensing of viral RNAs, it is involved in antiviral RNAi in nematodes and helps control viral RNA replication in worms. Finally, the role of DRH-2 is less clearly defined molecularly, but this factor appears to play a negative regulatory role in antiviral defenses.[99] Thus, RLR-like molecules appear to be involved in two distinct types of antiviral defense in worms (i.e., RNAi) and in mammals (i.e., signaling to induce IFNs) (Fig. 3). In spite of their close sequence relationship (29% identity over 736 amino-acids for RIG-I and DRH-1), RLRs in mammals differ from DRHs in *C. elegans* by the presence at their N-terminus of CARD domains, which allows them to recruit the CARD domain signaling adaptor IPS-1 (also known as MAVS, VISA or CARDIF).[100] At least some of the RLR-like molecules found in urochordates, cephalochordates and echinoderms have N-terminal homotypic protein-protein interaction domain (CARD, DED or DD), in agreement with a putative signaling receptor function for these molecules. Interestingly, RLR-like

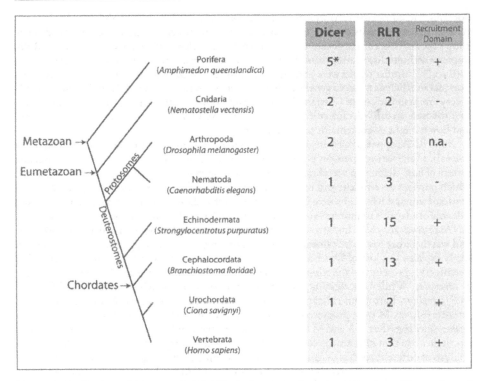

	Dicer	RLR	Recruitment Domain
Porifera (*Amphimedon queenslandica*)	5*	1	+
Cnidaria (*Nematostella vectensis*)	2	2	-
Arthropoda (*Drosophila melanogaster*)	2	0	n.a.
Nematoda (*Caenorhabditis elegans*)	1	3	-
Echinodermata (*Strongylocentrotus purpuratus*)	1	15	+
Cephalocordata (*Branchiostoma floridae*)	1	13	+
Urochordata (*Ciona savignyi*)	1	2	+
Vertebrata (*Homo sapiens*)	1	3	+

Figure 4. distribution of Dicer- and RIG-I like helicases in the animal kingdom. The number of genes in each species was estimated by blasting the protein sequence of Drosophila Dicer-2 or human RIG-I against the sequenced genomes of the indicated organisms. The presence of a DD or CARD recruitment domain in RLRs is indicated. *Data from reference 95; n.a.: not applicable.

molecules are also found in the *Nematostella* and *Amphimedon* genomes. Thus, it appears that insects represent an exception and that other invertebrate species, even if they have two or more Dicers, may contain RLRs. This raises the question whether these molecules function in RNAi (as in *C. elegans*) or in an inducible response (as in mammals) in these species. Whereas the two RLR molecules readily identified in the genome of the Cnidarian *Nematostella* are devoid of protein-protein interaction domain at their N-terminus, consistent with a role in RNAi, the single RLR identified in the Poriferan *Amphimedon* genome contains an N-terminal DD (Fig. 4). This indicates that RLR-dependent inducible antiviral responses may be very ancient and may co-exist with antiviral RNAi in some animals. Clearly, the family of RIG-I/Dicer-like helicases raises fascinating questions regarding the critical issue of sensing nucleic acids upon viral infection. Understanding their exact contribution to antiviral defenses in invertebrate models, in particular the genetically tractable *C. elegans* model, may shed light on currently poorly understood aspects of the biology of RLRs in mammals (e.g., the developmental roles of RIG-I and LGP2).[101,102]

The fact that the main sensors of viral RNAs in invertebrates and vertebrates share an evolutionarily conserved DExD/H box helicase domain raises the question of the function of this domain and of putative similarities in the sensing of RNA by Dicer and RIG-I like receptors. Recent data have shed light on these aspects. First, it is now clear that neither Dicer nor RLRs are real helicases. Rather, in vitro experiments conducted on DRH-3 and Dcr in *C. elegans*, Dicer-2 in *D. melanogaster* and RIG-I in mammals indicate that these molecules are dsRNA-stimulated ATPases.[39,98,103] In mammals, the cooperative tight binding of ATP and RNA to the helicase domain of RIG-I induces a major conformational change in the molecule, which liberates the CARD domains, and allows the recruitment of the signaling adaptor IPS-1.[104] However, the role of the ATPase activity remains unclear. In Dicer-2, in vitro experiments indicate that ATP hydrolysis allows the enzyme to translocate on long dsRNA molecules. Hence, Dicer-2 produces siRNA duplexes without dissociating from the dsRNA substrate, in a processive manner by moving along dsRNA.[39,103] Similar results were obtained in the case of the Dicer molecule from *C. elegans*. This provides an efficient mean to generate siRNAs, even when the amount of dsRNA present in cells is very low, as in the case of (-) strand RNA virus infections.[43] Interestingly, RIG-I was also shown to translocate on dsRNA molecules.[105] However, whether this movement contributes to signaling, and how it might do so, remains so far unknown.

Since RNAi appears to be an efficient antiviral pathway in protozoa, fungi, plants and many animals, a fascinating question pertains to the reason why it was supplanted by an inducible system of host-defense in vertebrates. One explanation may be the onset of adaptive immunity, which provides an efficient and highly specific way to deal with viral infections, and may have rendered antiviral RNAi obsolete. However, it seems that the common ancestor of deuterostomes –devoid of adaptive immunity- already had signaling RLRs. One hypothesis is that the antiviral RNAi pathway may have imparted a selective disadvantage under some particular circumstances, and was therefore lost in one lineage. Interestingly, a recent report suggests that such a scenario likely explains the loss of Dicer and AGO genes in some species of fungi. Indeed, the RNAi machinery is present and functional in *Saccharomyces castellii*, but was lost in the related species *S. cerevisiae*. While investigating the consequences of re-introducing Dicer and AGO genes in *S. cerevisiae*, Bartel and colleagues observed that the endogenous dsRNA virus L-A and its satellite dsRNA M were processed into siRNAs and eliminated.[106] This loss is detrimental to yeasts, since together L-A and M form the "killer" system, killing neighboring cells: M encodes a protein toxin that kills nearby cells while conferring immunity to producing cells. A thorough analysis of different species of fungi using whole genome sequencing confirmed that all species known to possess the killer dsRNA system have lost the RNAi machinery. Thus, one may propose that the advent of signaling RLRs in deuterostomes is connected to the acquisition of a novel viral element, which conferred to this lineage a net selective advantage (or, alternatively, which contained a potent suppressor of the antiviral RNAi pathway thus making it obsolete). An intringuing possibility is that the loss of antiviral RNAi is connected to the acquisition of the RAG1/2 genes encoding the components of the complex involved in V(D)J recombination in vertebrates.[107] Indeed, these genes appear to have originated from a Transib DNA transposon that infected the common ancestor of deuterostomes. Hence, the switch from an ancestral antiviral defense system based on RNAi to the interferon system may have been driven by the constant arms race between viruses and their hosts.

Conclusion

Compared with only a few years ago, remarkable progress was made recently on the characterization of the molecular and cellular mechanisms governing antiviral innate immunity in invertebrates. These mechanisms involve apoptosis, RNA interference and a poorly characterized inducible response. However, we are still far from understanding antiviral immunity in invertebrates. This applies in particular to the detection of viral infection, even though we now know that the sensing of viral nucleic acids plays an important role in some responses (e.g., RNAi).

Deciphering antiviral immunity is a complicated task because of the complex and intimate interactions between viruses and their host cells. The rapid evolution of viral genomes further triggers constant countermeasures from the host. Yet, some degree of conservation of sensing is apparent, as illustrated by the two families of molecules sharing an evolutionarily conserved DExD/H box helicase domain, the Dicers and the RLRs, which appear to be present in all invertebrate and vertebrate groups. These molecules represent a promising lead to further characterize the mechanisms involved in antiviral innate immunity in invertebrates.

Acknowledgments

We thank Carine Meignin for comments on the manuscript and assistance with the preparation of the figures.

About the Authors

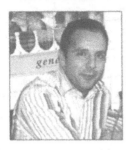

Jean-Luc Imler is Professor of Cell Biology in the Life Science Faculty of University of Strasbourg, and group leader in the Department of Insect Immunity and Development at the French National Research Agency CNRS. He obtained his Masters Degree in Life Science at Agro Paris Tech in Paris in 1985 and his PhD in Molecular and Cellular Biology at University Louis Pasteur in Strasbourg in 1988. After completing his PhD in the Department headed by Pierre Chambon, he performed his post-doctoral training at the DNAX Research Institute in Palo Alto (USA), working on cytokine-receptor interactions (1989-1991). He then briefly worked for the biotech company Transgene, before joining the University of Strasbourg and CNRS in 1994. He has been a close collaborator of Jules Hoffmann since, focusing on the immunobiology of Toll receptors in Drosophila, and more recently on antiviral immunity. Dr. Imler is a member of the Institut Universitaire de France.

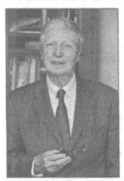

Jules A. Hoffmann is a Professor at the University of Strasbourg and has spent most of his career working with the French National Research Agency CNRS. The studies of the Hoffmann laboratory have been devoted over the last 30 years to unravelling the mechanisms of antimicrobial defenses in Diptera, namely in Drosophila. They have identified inducible antimicrobial peptides as primary immune response genes and have deciphered significant steps in the signaling cascade leading to gene reprogramming. They have further characterized the receptor proteins interacting with bacterial peptidoglycans and fungal β-glucans. Of major interest was the discovery of the involvement of the Toll receptor (initially identified by Ch. Nüsslein-Volhard for its role in embryonic development) in the response to fungal and Gram-positive bacterial infection. Altogether the studies of the Strasbourg laboratory have established Drosophila as an important model system for innate immunity and have contributed to a reevalution of this defense arm in the physiology of antimicrobial defense. Dr. Hoffmann is the recipient of many international awards, including the 2011 Nobel Prize in Medicine and Physiology.

References

1. Clem RJ, Fechheimer M, Miller LK. Prevention of apoptosis by a baculovirus gene during infection of insect cells. Science 1991; 254:1388-90; http://dx.doi.org/10.1126/science.1962198; PMID:1962198.
2. Moscardi F. Assessment of the application of baculoviruses for control of Lepidoptera. Annu Rev Entomol 1999; 44:257-89; http://dx.doi.org/10.1146/annurev.ento.44.1.257; PMID:15012374.
3. Cox-Foster DL, Conlan S, Holmes EC, Palacios G, Evans JD, Moran NA, et al. A metagenomic survey of microbes in honey bee colony collapse disorder. Science 2007; 318:283-7; http://dx.doi.org/10.1126/science.1146498; PMID:17823314.
4. Liu H, Soderhall K, Jiravanichpaisal P. Antiviral immunity in crustaceans. Fish Shellfish Immunol 2009; 27:79-88; http://dx.doi.org/10.1016/j.fsi.2009.02.009; PMID:19223016.
5. Mackenzie JS, Gubler DJ, Petersen LR. Emerging flaviviruses: the spread and resurgence of Japanese encephalitis, West Nile and dengue viruses. Nat Med 2004; 10:S98-109; http://dx.doi.org/10.1038/nm1144; PMID:15577938.
6. Clem RJ. The role of apoptosis in defense against baculovirus infection in insects. Curr Top Microbiol Immunol 2005; 289:113-29; http://dx.doi.org/10.1007/3-540-27320-4_5; PMID:15791953.

7. Friesen PD. Insect viruses. In: Fields Virology, Vol. 1. Knipe D, Howley P, eds. Philadelphia: Lippincott Williams & Wilkins, 2007: 707-736.

8. Chikhalya A, Luu DD, Carrera M, De La Cruz A, Torres M, Martinez EN, et al. Pathogenesis of Autographa californica multiple nucleopolyhedrovirus in fifth-instar Anticarsia gemmatalis larvae. J Gen Virol 2009; 90:2023-32; http://dx.doi.org/10.1099/vir.0.011718-0; PMID:19423548.

9. Liu WH, Lin YL, Wang JP, Liou W, Hou RF, Wu YC, et al. Restriction of vaccinia virus replication by a ced-3 and ced-4-dependent pathway in Caenorhabditis elegans. Proc Natl Acad Sci USA 2006; 103:4174-9; http://dx.doi.org/10.1073/pnas.0506442103; PMID:16537504.

10. Means JC, Penabaz T, Clem RJ. Identification and functional characterization of AMVp33, a novel homolog of the baculovirus caspase inhibitor p35 found in Amsacta moorei entomopoxvirus. Virology 2007; 358:436-47; http://dx.doi.org/10.1016/j.virol.2006.08.043; PMID:17010407.

11. Steller H. Regulation of apoptosis in Drosophila. Cell Death Differ 2008; 15:1132-8; http://dx.doi.org/10.1038/cdd.2008.50; PMID:18437164.

12. Cuttell L, Vaughan A, Silva E, Escaron CJ, Lavine M, Van Goethem E, et al. Undertaker, a Drosophila Junctophilin, links Draper-mediated phagocytosis and calcium homeostasis. Cell 2008; 135:524-34; http://dx.doi.org/10.1016/j.cell.2008.08.033; PMID:18984163.

13. Trudeau D, Washburn JO, Volkman LE. Central role of hemocytes in Autographa californica M nucleopolyhedrovirus pathogenesis in Heliothis virescens and Helicoverpa zea. J Virol 2001; 75:996-1003; http://dx.doi.org/10.1128/JVI.75.2.996-1003.2001; PMID:11134313.

14. Orme M, Meier P. Inhibitor of apoptosis proteins in Drosophila: gatekeepers of death. Apoptosis 2009; 14:950-60; http://dx.doi.org/10.1007/s10495-009-0358-2; PMID:19495985.

15. Shi Y. A conserved tetrapeptide motif: potentiating apoptosis through IAP-binding. Cell Death Differ 2002; 9:93-5; http://dx.doi.org/10.1038/sj.cdd.4400957; PMID:11840157.

16. Clem RJ, Miller LK. Apoptosis reduces both the in vitro replication and the in vivo infectivity of a baculovirus. J Virol 1993; 67:3730-8; PMID:8510202.

17. Xu G, et al. Covalent inhibition revealed by the crystal structure of the caspase-8/p35 complex. Nature 2001; 410:494-7; http://dx.doi.org/10.1038/35068604; PMID:11260720.

18. Pei Z, Cirilli M, Huang Y, Rich RL, Myszka DG, Wu H. Characterization of the apoptosis suppressor protein P49 from the Spodoptera littoralis nucleopolyhedrovirus. J Biol Chem 2002; 277:48677-84; http://dx.doi.org/10.1074/jbc.M208810200; PMID:12324475.

19. Zoog SJ, Schiller JJ, Wetter JA, Chejanovsky N, Friesen PD. Baculovirus apoptotic suppressor P49 is a substrate inhibitor of initiator caspases resistant to P35 in vivo. EMBO J 2002; 21:5130-40; http://dx.doi.org/10.1038/sj.emboj.7594736; PMID:12356729.

20. Tewari M, Dixit VM. Fas- and tumor necrosis factor-induced apoptosis is inhibited by the poxvirus crmA gene product. J Biol Chem 1995; 270:3255-60; http://dx.doi.org/10.1074/jbc.270.28.16526; PMID:7531702.

21. Crook NE, Clem RJ, Miller LK. An apoptosis-inhibiting baculovirus gene with a zinc finger-like motif. J Virol 1993; 67:2168-74; PMID:8445726.

22. Ikeda M, Yamada H, Ito H, Kobayashi M. Baculovirus IAP1 induces caspase-dependent apoptosis in insect cells. J Gen Virol 2011; 92:2654-63; http://dx.doi.org/10.1099/vir.0.033332-0; PMID:21795471.

23. Nogal ML, González de Buitrago G, Rodríguez C, Cubelos B, Carrascosa AL, Salas ML, et al. African swine fever virus IAP homologue inhibits caspase activation and promotes cell survival in mammalian cells. J Virol 2001; 75:2535-43; http://dx.doi.org/10.1128/JVI.75.6.2535-2543.2001; PMID:11222676.

24. Li Q, Liston P, Schokman N, Ho JM, Moyer RW. Amsacta moorei Entomopoxvirus inhibitor of apoptosis suppresses cell death by binding Grim and Hid. J Virol 2005; 79:3684-91; http://dx.doi.org/10.1128/JVI.79.6.3684-3691.2005; PMID:15731262.

25. Wang L, Zhi B, Wu W, Zhang X. Requirement for shrimp caspase in apoptosis against virus infection. Dev Comp Immunol 2008; 32:706-15; http://dx.doi.org/10.1016/j.dci.2007.10.010; PMID:18068223.

26. Schultz KL, Friesen PD. Baculovirus DNA replication-specific expression factors trigger apoptosis and shutoff of host protein synthesis during infection. J Virol 2009; 83:11123-32; http://dx.doi.org/10.1128/JVI.01199-09; PMID:19706708.

27. Settles EW, Friesen PD. Flock house virus induces apoptosis by depletion of Drosophila inhibitor-of-apoptosis protein DIAP1. J Virol 2008; 82:1378-88; http://dx.doi.org/10.1128/JVI.01941-07; PMID:17989181.

28. Vandergaast R, Schultz KL, Cerio RJ, Friesen PD. Active depletion of host cell inhibitor-of-apoptosis proteins triggers apoptosis upon baculovirus DNA replication. J Virol 2011; 85:8348-58; http://dx.doi.org/10.1128/JVI.00667-11; PMID:21653668.

29. Kuranaga E, et al. Drosophila IKK-related kinase regulates nonapoptotic function of caspases via degradation of IAPs. Cell 2006; 126:583-96; http://dx.doi.org/10.1016/j.cell.2006.05.048; PMID:16887178.

30. Beutler B, Eidenschenk C, Crozat K, Imler JL, Takeuchi O, Hoffmann JA, et al. Genetic analysis of resistance to viral infection. Nat Rev Immunol 2007; 7:753-66; http://dx.doi.org/10.1038/nri2174; PMID:17893693.

31. Jones JD, Dangl JL. The plant immune system. Nature 2006; 444:323-9; http://dx.doi.org/10.1038/nature05286; PMID:17108957.

32. Zhou L, Jiang G, Chan G, Santos CP, Severson DW, Xiao L. et al. Michelob_x is the missing inhibitor of apoptosis protein antagonist in mosquito genomes. EMBO Rep 2005; 6:769-74; http://dx.doi.org/10.1038/sj.embor.7400473; PMID:16041319.

33. Liu B, Becnel JJ, Zhang Y, Zhou L. Induction of reaper ortholog mx in mosquito midgut cells following baculovirus infection. Cell Death Differ 2011; 18:1337-45; http://dx.doi.org/10.1038/cdd.2011.8; PMID:21331076.

34. Kominsky DJ, Bickel RJ, Tyler KL. Reovirus-induced apoptosis requires mitochondrial release of Smac/DIABLO and involves reduction of cellular inhibitor of apoptosis protein levels. J Virol 2002; 76:11414-24; http://dx.doi.org/10.1128/JVI.76.22.11414-11424.2002; PMID:12388702.

35. Moody CA, Laimins LA. Human papillomaviruses activate the ATM DNA damage pathway for viral genome amplification upon differentiation. PLoS Pathog 2009; 5:e1000605; http://dx.doi.org/10.1371/journal.ppat.1000605; PMID:19798429.

36. Huang N, Wu W, Yang K, Passarelli AL, Rohrmann GF, Clem RJ. et al. Baculovirus infection induces a DNA damage response that is required for efficient viral replication. J Virol 2011; 85:12547-56; http://dx.doi.org/10.1128/JVI.05766-11; PMID:21917957.

37. Ding SW. RNA-based antiviral immunity. Nat Rev Immunol 2010; 10:632-44; http://dx.doi.org/10.1038/nri2824; PMID:20706278.

38. Lee YS, Nakahara K, Pham JW, Kim K, He Z, Sontheimer EJ, et al. Distinct roles for Drosophila Dicer-1 and Dicer-2 in the siRNA/miRNA silencing pathways. Cell 2004; 117:69-81; http://dx.doi.org/10.1016/S0092-8674(04)00261-2; PMID:15066283.

39. Cenik ES, Fukunaga R, Lu G, Dutcher R, Wang Y, Tanaka Hall TM, et al. Phosphate and R2D2 Restrict the Substrate Specificity of Dicer-2, an ATP-Driven Ribonuclease. Mol Cell 2011; 42:172-184; http://dx.doi.org/10.1016/j.molcel.2011.03.002; PMID:21419681.

40. Carthew RW, Sontheimer EJ. Origins and Mechanisms of miRNAs and siRNAs. Cell 2009; 136:642-55; http://dx.doi.org/10.1016/j.cell.2009.01.035; PMID:19239886.

41. Chotkowski HL, Ciota AT, Jia Y, Puig-Basagoiti F, Kramer LD, Shi PY, et al. West Nile virus infection of Drosophila melanogaster induces a protective RNAi response. Virology 2008; 377:197-206; http://dx.doi.org/10.1016/j.virol.2008.04.021; PMID:18501400.

42. Galiana-Arnoux D, Dostert C, Schneemann A, Hoffmann JA, Imler JL. Essential function in vivo for Dicer-2 in host defense against RNA viruses in drosophila. Nat Immunol 2006; 7:590-7; http://dx.doi.org/10.1038/ni1335; PMID:16554838.

43. Mueller S, Gausson V, Vodovar N, Deddouche S, Troxler L, Perot J, et al. RNAi-mediated immunity provides strong protection against the negative-strand RNA vesicular stomatitis virus in Drosophila. Proc Natl Acad Sci USA 2010; 107:19390-5; http://dx.doi.org/10.1073/pnas.1014378107; PMID:20978209.

44. Sabin LR, Zhou R, Gruber JJ, Lukinova N, Bambina S, Berman A, et al. Ars2 regulates both miRNA- and siRNA- dependent silencing and suppresses RNA virus infection in Drosophila. Cell 2009; 138:340-51; http://dx.doi.org/10.1016/j.cell.2009.04.045; PMID:19632183.

45. van Rij RP, Saleh MC, Berry B, Foo C, Houk A, Antoniewski C, et al. The RNA silencing endonuclease Argonaute 2 mediates specific antiviral immunity in Drosophila melanogaster. Genes Dev 2006; 20:2985-95; http://dx.doi.org/10.1101/gad.1482006; PMID:17079687.

46. Wang XH, Aliyari R, Li WX, Li HW, Kim K, Carthew R, et al. RNA interference directs innate immunity against viruses in adult Drosophila. Science 2006; 312:452-4; http://dx.doi.org/10.1126/science.1125694; PMID:16556799.

47. Zambon RA, Vakharia VN, Wu LP. RNAi is an antiviral immune response against a dsRNA virus in Drosophila melanogaster. Cell Microbiol 2006; 8:880-9; http://dx.doi.org/10.1111/j.1462-5822.2006.00688.x; PMID:16611236.

48. Aliyari R, Wu Q, Li HW, Wang XH, Li F, Green LD, et al. Mechanism of induction and suppression of antiviral immunity directed by virus-derived small RNAs in Drosophila. Cell Host Microbe 2008; 4:387-97; http://dx.doi.org/10.1016/j.chom.2008.09.001; PMID:18854242.

49. Brackney DE, Beane JE, Ebel GD. RNAi targeting of West Nile virus in mosquito midguts promotes virus diversification. PLoS Pathog 2009; 5:e1000502; http://dx.doi.org/10.1371/journal.ppat.1000502; PMID:19578437.

50. Flynt A, Liu N, Martin R, Lai EC. Dicing of viral replication intermediates during silencing of latent Drosophila viruses. Proc Natl Acad Sci USA 2009; 106:5270-5; http://dx.doi.org/10.1073/pnas.0813412106; PMID:19251644.

51. Han YH, Luo YJ, Wu Q, Jovel J, Wang XH, Aliyari R, et al. RNA-based immunity terminates viral infection in adult Drosophila in absence of viral suppression of RNAi: Characterization of viral siRNA populations in wildtype and mutant flies. J Virol 2011; 85:13153-63; http://dx.doi.org/10.1128/JVI.05518-11; PMID:21957285.

52. Myles KM, Wiley MR, Morazzani EM, Adelman ZN. Alphavirus-derived small RNAs modulate pathogenesis in disease vector mosquitoes. Proc Natl Acad Sci USA 2008; 105:19938-43; http://dx.doi.org/10.1073/pnas.0803408105; PMID:19047642.

53. Siu RW, Fragkoudis R, Simmonds P, Donald CL, Chase-Topping ME, Barry G, et al. Antiviral RNA interference responses induced by Semliki Forest virus infection of mosquito cells: characterization, origin, and frequency-dependent functions of virus-derived small interfering RNAs. J Virol 2011; 85:2907-17; http://dx.doi.org/10.1128/JVI.02052-10; PMID:21191029.

54. Vodovar N, Goic B, Blanc H, Saleh MC. In silico reconstruction of viral genomes from small RNAs improves virus-derived small interfering RNA profiling. J Virol 2011; 85:11016-21; http://dx.doi.org/10.1128/JVI.05647-11; PMID:21880776.

55. Wu Q, Luo Y, Lu R, Lau N, Lai EC, Li WX, et al. Virus discovery by deep sequencing and assembly of virus-derived small silencing RNAs. Proc Natl Acad Sci USA 2010; 107:1606-11; http://dx.doi.org/10.1073/pnas.0911353107; PMID:20080648.

56. Saleh MC, van Rij RP, Hekele A, Gillis A, Foley E, O'Farrell PH, et al. The endocytic pathway mediates cell entry of dsRNA to induce RNAi silencing. Nat Cell Biol 2006; 8:793-802; http://dx.doi.org/10.1038/ncb1439; PMID:16862146.

57. Ulvila J, Parikka M, Kleino A, Sormunen R, Ezekowitz RA, Kocks C, et al. Double-stranded RNA is internalized by scavenger receptor-mediated endocytosis in Drosophila S2 cells. J Biol Chem 2006; 281:14370-5; http://dx.doi.org/10.1074/jbc.M513868200; PMID:16531407.

58. Saleh MC, Tassetto M, van Rij RP, Goic B, Gausson V, Berry B, et al. Antiviral immunity in Drosophila requires systemic RNA interference spread. Nature 2009; 458:346-50; http://dx.doi.org/10.1038/nature07712; PMID:19204732.

59. Brackney DE, Scott JC, Sagawa F, Woodward JE, Miller NA, Schilkey FD, et al. C6/36 Aedes albopictus cells have a dysfunctional antiviral RNA interference response. PLoS Negl Trop Dis 2010; 4:e856; http://dx.doi.org/10.1371/journal.pntd.0000856; PMID:21049065.

60. Scott JC, Brackney DE, Campbell CL, Bondu-Hawkins V, Hjelle B, Ebel GD, et al. Comparison of dengue virus type 2-specific small RNAs from RNA interference-competent and -incompetent mosquito cells. PLoS Negl Trop Dis 2010; 4:e848; http://dx.doi.org/10.1371/journal.pntd.0000848; PMID:21049014.

61. Li H, Li WX, Ding SW. Induction and suppression of RNA silencing by an animal virus. Science 2002; 296:1319-21; http://dx.doi.org/10.1126/science.1070948; PMID:12016316.

62. Chao JA, Lee JH, Chapados BR, Debler EW, Schneemann A, Williamson JR. Dual modes of RNA-silencing suppression by Flock House virus protein B2. Nat Struct Mol Biol 2005; 12:952-7; PMID:16228003.

63. Li WX, Li H, Lu R, Li F, Dus M, Atkinson P, et al. Interferon antagonist proteins of influenza and vaccinia viruses are suppressors of RNA silencing. Proc Natl Acad Sci USA 2004; 101:1350-5; http://dx.doi.org/10.1073/pnas.0308308100; PMID:14745017.

64. Nayak A, Berry B, Tassetto M, Kunitomi M, Acevedo A, Deng C, et al. Cricket paralysis virus antagonizes Argonaute 2 to modulate antiviral defense in Drosophila. Nat Struct Mol Biol 2010; 17:547-54; http://dx.doi.org/10.1038/nsmb.1810; PMID:20400949.

65. Clem RJ, Popham HJ, Shelby KS. Antiviral responses in insects: apoptosis and humoral responses. In: Insect Virology. Asgari S, Johnson KD, eds. Norfolk: Caister Academic Press, 2010: 389-410.

66. Dostert C, Jouanguy E, Irving P, Troxler L, Galiana-Arnoux D, Hetru C, et al. The Jak-STAT signaling pathway is required but not sufficient for the antiviral response of drosophila. Nat Immunol 2005; 6:946-53; http://dx.doi.org/10.1038/ni1237; PMID:16086017.

67. Colpitts TM, Cox J, Vanlandingham DL, Feitosa FM, Cheng G, Kurscheid S, et al. Alterations in the Aedes aegypti transcriptome during infection with West Nile, dengue and yellow fever viruses. PLoS Pathog 2011; 7:e1002189; http://dx.doi.org/10.1371/journal.ppat.1002189; PMID:21909258.

68. Souza-Neto JA, Sim S, Dimopoulos G. An evolutionary conserved function of the JAK-STAT pathway in anti-dengue defense. Proc Natl Acad Sci USA 2009; 106:17841-6; http://dx.doi.org/10.1073/pnas.0905006106; PMID:19805194.

69. Liu WJ, Chang YS, Wang AH, Kou GH, Lo CF. White spot syndrome virus annexes a shrimp STAT to enhance expression of the immediate-early gene ie1. J Virol 2007; 81:1461-71; http://dx.doi.org/10.1128/JVI.01880-06; PMID:17079306.

70. Agaisse H, Perrimon N. The roles of JAK/STAT signaling in Drosophila immune responses. Immunol Rev 2004; 198:72-82; http://dx.doi.org/10.1111/j.0105-2896.2004.0133.x; PMID:15199955.

71. Avadhanula V, Weasner BP, Hardy GG, Kumar JP, Hardy RW. A novel system for the launch of alphavirus RNA synthesis reveals a role for the Imd pathway in arthropod antiviral response. PLoS Pathog 2009; 5:e1000582; http://dx.doi.org/10.1371/journal.ppat.1000582; PMID:19763182.

72. Costa A, Jan E, Sarnow P, Schneider D. The Imd pathway is involved in antiviral immune responses in Drosophila. PLoS ONE 2009; 4:e7436; http://dx.doi.org/10.1371/journal.pone.0007436; PMID:19829691.

73. Xi Z, Ramirez JL, Dimopoulos G. The Aedes aegypti toll pathway controls dengue virus infection. PLoS Pathog 2008; 4:e1000098; http://dx.doi.org/10.1371/journal.ppat.1000098; PMID:18604274.

74. Zambon RA, Nandakumar M, Vakharia VN, Wu LP. The Toll pathway is important for an antiviral response in Drosophila. Proc Natl Acad Sci USA 2005; 102:7257-62; http://dx.doi.org/10.1073/pnas.0409181102; PMID:15878994.

75. Ferrandon D, Imler JL, Hetru C, Hoffmann JA. The Drosophila systemic immune response: sensing and signalling during bacterial and fungal infections. Nat Rev Immunol 2007; 7:862-74; http://dx.doi.org/10.1038/nri2194; PMID:17948019.

76. Deddouche S, Matt N, Budd A, Mueller S, Kemp C, Galiana-Arnoux D, et al. The DExD/H-box helicase Dicer-2 mediates the induction of antiviral activity in drosophila. Nat Immunol 2008; 9:1425-32; http://dx.doi.org/10.1038/ni.1664; PMID:18953338.

77. Shelly S, Lukinova N, Bambina S, Berman A, Cherry S. Autophagy is an essential component of Drosophila immunity against vesicular stomatitis virus. Immunity 2009; 30:588-98; http://dx.doi.org/10.1016/j.immuni.2009.02.009; PMID:19362021.

78. Terenius O, Bettencourt R, Lee SY, Li W, Söderhäll K, Faye I. RNA interference of Hemolin causes depletion of phenoloxidase activity in Hyalophora cecropia. Dev Comp Immunol 2007; 31:571-5; http://dx.doi.org/10.1016/j.dci.2006.09.006; PMID:17129606.

79. Hirai M, Terenius O, Li W, Faye I. Baculovirus and dsRNA induce Hemolin, but no antibacterial activity, in Antheraea pernyi. Insect Mol Biol 2004; 13:399-405; http://dx.doi.org/10.1111/j.0962-1075.2004.00497.x; PMID:15271212.

80. Lei K, Li F, Zhang M, Yang H, Luo T, Xu X. et al. Difference between hemocyanin subunits from shrimp Penaeus japonicus in anti-WSSV defense. Dev Comp Immunol 2008; 32:808-13; http://dx.doi.org/10.1016/j.dci.2007.11.010; PMID:18234332.

81. Liu H, Jiravanichpaisal P, Soderhall I, Cerenius L, Soderhall K. Antilipopolysaccharide factor interferes with white spot syndrome virus replication in vitro and in vivo in the crayfish Pacifastacus leniusculus. J Virol 2006; 80:10365-71; http://dx.doi.org/10.1128/JVI.01101-06; PMID:17041217.

82. Robalino J, Browdy CL, Prior S, Metz A, Parnell P, Gross P, et al. Induction of antiviral immunity by double stranded RNA in a marine invertebrate. J Virol 2004; 78:10442-8; http://dx.doi.org/10.1128/JVI.78.19.10442-10448.2004; PMID:15367610.

83. Robalino J, Bartlett T, Shepard E, Prior S, Jaramillo G, Scura E, et al. Double-stranded RNA induces sequence-specific antiviral silencing in addition to nonspecific immunity in a marine shrimp: convergence of RNA interference and innate immunity in the invertebrate antiviral response? J Virol 2005; 79:13561-71; http://dx.doi.org/10.1128/JVI.79.21.13561-13571.2005; PMID:16227276.

84. Mukae N, Yokoyama H, Yokokura T, Sakoyama Y, Nagata S. Activation of the innate immunity in Drosophila by endogenous chromosomal DNA that escaped apoptotic degradation. Genes Dev 2002; 16:2662-71; http://dx.doi.org/10.1101/gad.1022802; PMID:12381665.

85. Tang H, Kambris Z, Lemaitre B, Hashimoto C. A serpin that regulates immune melanization in the respiratory system of Drosophila. Dev Cell 2008; 15:617-26; http://dx.doi.org/10.1016/j.devcel.2008.08.017; PMID:18854145.

86. Roach JC, Glusman G, Rowen L, Kaur A, Purcell MK, Smith KD, et al. The evolution of vertebrate Toll-like receptors. Proc Natl Acad Sci USA 2005; 102:9577-82; http://dx.doi.org/10.1073/pnas.0502272102; PMID:15976025.

87. Kawai T, Akira S. Toll-like receptors and their crosstalk with other innate receptors in infection and immunity. Immunity 2011; 34:637-50; http://dx.doi.org/10.1016/j.immuni.2011.05.006; PMID:21616434.

88. Kumagai Y, Takeuchi O, Kato H, Kumar H, Matsui K, Morii E, et al. Alveolar macrophages are the primary interferon-alpha producer in pulmonary infection with RNA viruses. Immunity 2007; 27:240-52; http://dx.doi.org/10.1016/j.immuni.2007.07.013; PMID:17723216.

89. Koyama S, Ishii KJ, Kumar H, Tanimoto T, Coban C, Uematsu S, et al. Differential role of TLR- and RLR-signaling in the immune responses to influenza A virus infection and vaccination. J Immunol 2007; 179:4711-20; PMID:17878370.

90. Batista TM, Marques JT. RNAi pathways in parasitic protists and worms. J Proteomics 2011; 74:1504-14; http://dx.doi.org/10.1016/j.jprot.2011.02.032; PMID:21385631.

91. Blevins T, Rajeswaran R, Shivaprasad PV, Beknazariants D, Si-Ammour A, Park HS, Vazquez F, et al. Four plant Dicers mediate viral small RNA biogenesis and DNA virus induced silencing. Nucleic Acids Res 2006; 34:6233-46; http://dx.doi.org/10.1093/nar/gkl886; PMID:17090584.
92. Deleris A, Gallego-Bartolome J, Bao J, Kasschau KD, Carrington JC, Voinnet O. et al. Hierarchical action and inhibition of plant Dicer-like proteins in antiviral defense. Science 2006; 313:68-71; http://dx.doi.org/10.1126/science.1128214; PMID:16741077.
93. Moissiard G, Voinnet O. RNA silencing of host transcripts by cauliflower mosaic virus requires coordinated action of the four Arabidopsis Dicer-like proteins. Proc Natl Acad Sci USA 2006; 103:19593-8; http://dx.doi.org/10.1073/pnas.0604627103; PMID:17164336.
94. Zhang X, Segers GC, Sun Q, Deng F, Nuss DL. Characterization of hypovirus-derived small RNAs generated in the chestnut blight fungus by an inducible DCL-2-dependent pathway. J Virol 2008; 82:2613-9; http://dx.doi.org/10.1128/JVI.02324-07; PMID:18199652.
95. de Jong D, Eitel M, Jakob W, Osigus HJ, Hadrys H, Desalle R, et al. Multiple dicer genes in the early-diverging metazoa. Mol Biol Evol 2009; 26:1333-40; http://dx.doi.org/10.1093/molbev/msp042; PMID:19276153.
96. Leulier F, Lemaitre B. Toll-like receptors—taking an evolutionary approach. Nat Rev Genet 2008; 9:165-78; http://dx.doi.org/10.1038/nrg2303; PMID:18227810.
97. Gu W, Shirayama M, Conte D Jr, Vasale J, Batista PJ, Claycomb JM, et al. Distinct argonaute-mediated 22G-RNA pathways direct genome surveillance in the C. elegans germline. Mol Cell 2009; 36:231-44; http://dx.doi.org/10.1016/j.molcel.2009.09.020; PMID:19800275.
98. Matranga C, Pyle AM. Double-stranded RNA-dependent ATPase DRH-3: insight into its role in RNAsilencing in Caenorhabditis elegans. J Biol Chem 2010; 285:25363-71; http://dx.doi.org/10.1074/jbc.M110.117010; PMID:20529861.
99. Lu R, Yigit E, Li WX, Ding SW. An RIG-I-Like RNA helicase mediates antiviral RNAi downstream of viral siRNA biogenesis in Caenorhabditis elegans. PLoS Pathog 2009; 5:e1000286; http://dx.doi.org/10.1371/journal.ppat.1000286; PMID:19197349.
100. Takeuchi O, Akira S. Pattern recognition receptors and inflammation. Cell 2010; 140:805-20; http://dx.doi.org/10.1016/j.cell.2010.01.022; PMID:20303872.
101. Kato H, Sato S, Yoneyama M, Yamamoto M, Uematsu S, Matsui K, et al. Cell Type-Specific Involvement of RIG-I in Antiviral Response. Immunity 2005; 23:19-28; http://dx.doi.org/10.1016/j.immuni.2005.04.010; PMID:16039576.
102. Satoh T, Kato H, Kumagai Y, Yoneyama M, Sato S, Matsushita K, et al. LGP2 is a positive regulator of RIG-I- and MDA5-mediated antiviral responses. Proc Natl Acad Sci USA 2010; 107:1512-7; http://dx.doi.org/10.1073/pnas.0912986107; PMID:20080593.
103. Welker NC, Maity TS, Ye X, Aruscavage PJ, Krauchuk AA, Liu Q, et al. Dicer's helicase domain discriminates dsRNA termini to promote an altered reaction mode. Mol Cell 2011; 41:589-99; http://dx.doi.org/10.1016/j.molcel.2011.02.005; PMID:21362554.
104. Kowalinski E, Lunardi T, McCarthy AA, Louber J, Brunel J, Grigorov B, et al. Structural Basis for the Activation of Innate Immune Pattern-Recognition Receptor RIG-I by Viral RNA. Cell 2011; 147:423-35; http://dx.doi.org/10.1016/j.cell.2011.09.039; PMID:22000019.
105. Myong S, Cui S, Cornish PV, Kirchhofer A, Gack MU, Jung JU, et al. Cytosolic viral sensor RIG-I is a 5'-triphosphate-dependent translocase on double-stranded RNA. Science 2009; 323:1070-4; http://dx.doi.org/10.1126/science.1168352; PMID:19119185.
106. Drinnenberg IA, Fink GR, Bartel DP. Compatibility with killer explains the rise of RNAi-deficient fungi. Science 2011; 333:1592; http://dx.doi.org/10.1126/science.1209575; PMID:21921191.
107. Fugmann SD, Messier C, Novack LA, Cameron RA, Rast JP. An ancient evolutionary origin of the Rag1/2 gene locus. Proc Natl Acad Sci USA 2006; 103:3728-33; http://dx.doi.org/10.1073/pnas.0509720103; PMID:16505374.

CHAPTER 2

Overview of TLRs

Bruce Beutler*

Abstract

Collectively, the mammalian Toll-like receptors (TLRs) sense host invasion by most microbes, including bacteria, fungi, protozoa, and viruses. They do so by recognizing signature molecules that herald infection: lipopeptides, lipopolysaccharides, flagellin, dsRNA, ssRNA and ssDNA. When such ligands engage TLRs, a conformational change is elicited leading to signaling via a chain of adaptor proteins, kinases, and ubiquitin ligases that ultimately cause the activation of transcription factors, including NF-κB, AP-1, and the IRFs. These transcription factors activate hundreds of genes, many of them encoding cytokines, and also change the entire cellular milieu. Other signaling events permit augmented translation of mRNAs encoding specific cytokines. Once released, the cytokines drive the inflammatory response that is usually witnessed in the setting of infection. It is remarkable that so few TLRs, and so few inciting molecules, are capable of initiating the inflammatory response to infection, with its myriad consequences. Moreover, the fact that similar signaling pathways are triggered by diverse microbes accounts for similarities in the mammalian response to many different kinds of infection. The role of TLRs in sterile inflammation, including certain autoimmune diseases, has begun to gain clarity with the recognition that endogenous nucleic acids can be detected by TLRs. In this sense, some kinds of autoimmunity may be viewed as a consequence of the limited resolving power of innate immune receptors.

Introduction

The story of the mammalian TLRs and their rise to prominence in immunology is one in which modern genetic methods were applied to a recalcitrant question. The question was: "How does the host recognize infection and begin to mount an immune response?"

The inherent ability of mammals to recognize microbes was known since microbes were shown to be the agents of infectious disease. "Innate" or "natural" immunity, as distinct from "adaptive" or "acquired" immunity, is a pre-programmed system for recognizing and killing microbes that breach physical defenses of the host. It is activated almost immediately upon contact with microbes. Its cellular executors include polymorphonuclear leukocytes and macrophages, to be sure; also dendritic cells (recognized as distinct from macrophages since the 1980s). But one might consider other cells as well. B cells, for example, were long known to undergo a mitogenic response to microbes and their products.[1] To some extent, almost all somatic cells might be included as executors of innate immunity, since they produce interferon in response to viral infection.[2] This has the effect of sounding an alarm to protect neighboring cells from infection, and may also slow the development of a viral infection within the cell itself, by way of an autocrine response to interferon.

In biological systems, molecular recognition usually implies the existence of specific receptors. While the receptors were mostly unknown until the end of the 20th century, the ligands recognized

*Center for Genetics of Host Defense, University of Texas Southwestern Medical Center, Dallas, Texas, USA.
Email: Bruce.Beutler@UTSouthwestern.edu

Nucleic Acid Sensors and Antiviral Immunity, edited by Suryaprakash Sambhara and Takashi Fujita.
©2013 Landes Bioscience.

by the innate immune system were not mysterious. Many of them were quite well known, and had been deduced through classical purification methods. Lipopolysaccharide (LPS; formerly "endotoxin") was the premiere example, capable of inducing such severe inflammation that it caused shock when administered systemically. Flagellin,[3] dsRNA analogs such as poly I:C,[4] and bacterial lipopeptides such as lipoprotein of *E. coli*[5] were all known to provoke inflammation or associated immune cellular responses as well.

The question as to which receptors mediated detection of these molecules defied the usual efforts at protein isolation, and remained relevant for many decades. Today we know of several types of microbe sensors: the Toll-like receptors (TLRs), RIG-I-like receptors (RLRs), C-type lectin receptors (CLRs), and NOD-like receptors (NLRs, which may not be authentic receptors at all). Among these, the TLRs are the most universal in coverage of the microbial universe, and the most potent in their capacity to generate inflammation. The TLRs were the first such sensors to be unequivocally identified.

They were found through a genetic approach, in which the question about recognition was narrowly addressed to the ligand LPS. The existence of an "endotoxin" was described by Pfeiffer in the 1890s.[6] The equivalence of endotoxin and LPS became evident in the 1940s through the work of Shear.[7]

The importance of LPS was 3-fold. First, it was widely believed to be a key inducer of shock and organ injury as observed in Gram-negative sepsis. Many thousands of investigators studied the effects of LPS over a period of nearly a century, each paying attention to one or more distal effects of LPS on different organ systems. Second, a discrete sensing system for LPS was known to exist in mammals, as certain mice, to be discussed in more detail shortly, were genetically refractory to LPS signaling. Third, LPS had effects that went beyond innate immune activation, extending to adaptive immune activation as well. By the 1950s, LPS had been clearly shown to be an adjuvant for antibody responses to co-injected proteins, indicating that it could help to drive the adaptive immune response to antigens.[8] By 1975, it had been shown that LPS could only function as an adjuvant in endotoxin-responsive mice.[9] LPS, itself a T-independent antigen, failed to elicit antibody against its own epitopes in LPS unresponsive mice.[10] And through a direct effect on B cells, it could elicit antibody responses against antigentic conjugates.[11] By identifying the LPS receptor, one could therefore hope to understand what ignites the inflammatory response to microbes, as well as the ability of microbes to help ignite an adaptive immune response.

C3H/HeJ and C57BL/10ScCr: Two Independent Lines of LPS-Refractory Mice

Heppner and Weiss[12] noted in 1965 that LPS toxicity was markedly attenuated in C3H mice of the HeJ substrain. Sultzer[13] subsequently observed that the peritoneal exudate response of mice injected with LPS was also attenuated in the C3H/HeJ strain. In years to come, the defect was seen to be global. The mitogenic response of B cells, cytokine production, and every other response of every cell type was found to be absent or severely depressed in the C3H/HeJ strain. Where responses persisted, we might, in retrospect, question the purity of the LPS preparation used to elicit them. The defect was also highly specific for LPS. Few problems, if any, were observed when cellular responses were induced using products of Gram-positive bacteria, dsRNA, or other agents.

Of critical importance, C3H/HeJ mice were hypersusceptible to infection by multiple Gram-negative bacteria.[14,15] Therefore, LPS sensing was linked to survival, mediated by the innate immune response.

The LPS-refractory state and survival following injection of normally lethal doses of LPS was dependent upon the host hematopoietic system. In reciprocal marrow transplantation experiments, the lethal effect of LPS was restored to C3H/HeJ mice by irradiation and reconstitution with C3H/HeN bone marrow. Conversely, C3H/HeN mice were rendered refractory to LPS by lethal irradiation and reconstitution with C3H/HeJ bone marrow.[16] However, this observation did not exclude the possibility that LPS might have direct effects on extrahematopoietic cells, and indeed, it is now quite clear that it does.

In 1977, Coutinho observed that mice of the strain C57BL/10ScCr had absent B-cell responses to LPS, much like mice of the C3H/HeJ strain.[17] Allelism testing showed that the mutation in C57BL/10ScCr mice affected the same locus as that which was defective in C3H/HeJ mice.[18]

By 1974, Watson and Riblet had demonstrated that in C3H/HeJ mice, a single locus mutation abolishes LPS responses,[19] taking B-cell mitogenesis and IgM production as the endpoints of interest. Moreover, they excluded linkage to the H-2 and Ig heavy chain loci. Later, using classical phenotypic markers and a total of 14 recombinant inbred strains of mice derived from C57BL/6 and C3H/HeJ parents, they established linkage between the so-called *Lps* locus and the *Major Urinary Protein* (*Mup1*) locus on chromosome 4.[20] Using a backcross strategy, the *Lps* locus was further confined to the interval between *Mup1* and *Polysyndactyly* (*Ps*) loci in 1978.[21] The interval spanning *Mup1* and *Ps* was immense, and no molecular markers lay between these loci at the time they were first used to map *Lps*. The *Ps* locus has not been identified to this day. Little progress followed for another 15 y, because the density of markers in the mouse genome remained exceedingly low. The extremely useful simple sequence length polymorphisms (SSLP, also referred to as "microsatellites") had yet to be identified.

CD14 and Its Crucial Role in LPS Sensing

In 1990, a key component of the LPS sensing apparatus was identified by Richard Ulevitch and his collaborators. Antibodies against the glycosylphosphoinositol-anchored cell surface protein CD14 were shown to prevent LPS sensing in myeloid cells.[22] Subsequently, transfection of 70Z3 pre-B cells with a CD14 expression construct was shown to greatly enhance LPS responsiveness.[23] CD14, a protein with leucine rich repeat (LRR) motifs, was at that time noted to be similar to Toll, Chaoptin, ribonuclease inhibitor, and several other proteins. But it had no obvious means of transducing a signal, nor was it encoded by a gene on mouse chromosome 4. The transducing subunit of the LPS receptor complex was therefore thought to depend upon another protein: possibly the protein encoded by the elusive *Lps* locus.

Positional Cloning of the *Lps* Locus, and the Discovery of TLR4

Between the years 1993 and 1998, the *Lps* locus was mapped on 2,093 meioses and confined to a 2.6 Mb interval on mouse chromosome 4. This level of confinement permitted the assembly of a contiguous array of 66 BAC (bacterial artificial chromosome) clones and two YAC (yeast artificial chromosome) clones. A minimum tiling pathway was established, the clones were shotgun sequenced, and the region thereby explored for genes. Approximately 90% of the contig had been sequenced in considerable depth, when within one of the BAC clones, a strong match with the orphan receptor encoding gene *Tlr4* was obtained using a BLAST search. In due course it was determined that the third exon of this gene differed between C3H/HeJ and C3H/HeN mice, in that a coding difference changed a highly conserved proline to a histidine (P712H). Moreover, in C57BL/10ScCr mice, the gene could not be detected on Southern blot (whereas it was readily detectible in the LPS-responsive C57BL/10ScSn strain).[24] Later, it was ascertained that the gene had been deleted in entirety from the C57BL/10ScCr genome.[25]

TLR4 was one of several mammalian homologs of Drosophila Toll known at the time its gene was discovered in the *Lps* critical region. Its ectodomain was mostly composed of LRR motifs and was approximately 650 residues in length. Its small cytoplasmic domain was similar in structure to the cytoplasmic domain of the IL-1 receptor, as noted for Toll in 1991 by Gay.[26] Later, the IL-18 receptor, and a number of other receptors of more obscure function, were noted to have similar domains as well. The same type of domain was observed in plant R (resistance) proteins; hence the domain was named a TIR domain (for Toll/IL-1R/Resistance motif).

The first mammalian TLR to be discovered, based on homology with Drosophila Toll, was denoted "TIL" (Toll/IL-1R like protein).[27] It is now known as TLR1. TLR1 was discovered prior to the understanding that Toll is involved in Drosophila immunity, at a time when the role of Toll was thought to be strictly developmental. TIL was therefore thought to be involved in mammalian development.[28]

Proceeding from the work of Hoffmann (discussed below), Medzhitov, Preston-Hurlburt, and Janeway[29] developed a modified TLR4 clone encoding a protein in which a CD4 ectodomain sequence was substituted for the native LRR ectodomain of TLR4. They showed that when expressed in mammalian cells, this construct would cause NF-κB activation. Moreover, when expressed in myeloid cells, it would cause upregulation of costimulatory proteins. They hypothesized that TLR4 might act as a "pattern recognition receptor"; that is, a receptor for evolutionarily conserved ligands of microbial origin. But they failed to demonstrate a receptor function for TLR4: whether for endogenous ligands (as in the case of Toll) or for microbial ligands of any kind.

The observation that two rare allelic variants of TLR4, one of them obviously deleterious, were associated with LPS unresponsiveness, allowed the unambiguous conclusion that TLR4, a putative cell surface protein, was part of the LPS sensing apparatus. It did not permit the conclusion that TLR4 acted as a receptor per se. Strong evidence of an actual interaction between TLR4 and LPS was adduced by genetic complementation studies. Advantage was taken of the fact that an LPS precursor known as Lipid IVa acts as an agonist for LPS responses in mouse cells, but an antagonist for LPS responses in human cells. Lipid IVa differs from Lipid A, the toxic center of LPS, by the absence of two acyl side chains. Could the structural difference between mouse and human TLR4 explain this? If so, one could infer that TLR4 from humans must "see" the difference between Lipid A and Lipid IVa: a relatively subtle difference indeed. This in turn would imply close contact between the ligands and the TLR4 protein.

A macrophage line derived from C3H/HeJ mice, LPS-unresponsive by virtue of the TLR4 mutation just mentioned, was transfected to express either human or mouse TLR4. Indeed, human TLR4 conferred responsiveness to Lipid A alone, while mouse TLR4 conferred responsiveness to both Lipid A and Lipid IVa.[30] A very similar result was reached independently using a different LPS-unresponsive host cell line.[31] Nearly nine years later, crystallographic studies confirmed that LPS does indeed have direct contact with TLR4: as well as another protein of the sensory complex known as MD-2, discussed below.

Discovery of MD-2

Miyake and colleagues had discovered MD-1 as a protein tightly associated with RP-105, an LRR protein similar to the TLRs, but differing in its lack of a cytoplasmic TIR motif that characterized all of the TLRs, the IL-1 receptor chains, and the IL-18 receptor chains. MD-2 was identified based on homology searches using MD-1 as a query sequence. It was found to be tightly associated with TLR4, and like TLR4, to be required for LPS sensing: a conclusion first reached using transfection studies[32] and later fully validated by gene targeting.[33] Today, MD-2 is known to be a subunit of a complex with TLR4, endowed with a deep, hydrophobic pocket, which engages most of the acyl chains of lipid A. While it might have been expected that CD14 would also be a part of the LPS receptor complex, close association with TLR4 and MD-2 has not been documented.

XA21 in Rice, and Toll in the Fly: the Importance of LRR Proteins

The discovery of the LPS receptor complex dovetailed beautifully behind two other stories, which remained unconnected with one another for some time, and which developed independently of one another. In 1995, Ronald and colleagues[34] used positional cloning to identify XA21, a cell surface LRR protein of domestic rice (*Oriza sativa*) with intrinsic tyrosine kinase activity, as a key mediator of resistance to *Xanthomonas oryzae*, a bacterial pathogen. Later, Ronald and colleagues identified the microbial ligand for XA21: a sulfated peptide produced by *X. oryzae*, called AX21.[35] While XA21 lacks a TIR domain, it had already been noted that the TIR motif (in cytoplasmic locations) could contribute to immunity in plants. Therefore, the ancient origins of the LRR/TIR recognition system were already evident when mediators of resistance in flies and mice began to emerge.

In 1996, Lemaitre et al.[36] showed that the classical mediator of dorsoventral polarity, Toll, a cell surface receptor activated by an endogenous ligand known as Spaetzle, had an equally important role in innate immunity: specifically, resistance to the fungal pathogen *Aspergillus fumigatus*. Mutations in Toll, Spaetzle, and downstream proteins needed for development would cripple the immune response of adult flies by preventing activation of the NF-κB homolog Dif, the Dorsal-related immunity factor, which promoted expression of hundreds of genes, including those encoding antimicrobial peptides.[37]

The Toll pathway was subsequently shown to mediate resistance to Gram-positive bacteria as well. But notably, no product of fungi or bacteria was ever shown to directly interact with Toll. On the contrary, upstream sensors of peptidoglycan, or proteases released from fungi, act to initiate a proteolytic cascade that ultimately cleaves Spaetzle to an active conformer, permitting its interaction with the Toll receptor. This in turn causes signaling quite similar to that observed in the TLR pathway of mammals.

Moreover, a single Drosophila Toll paralogue (of nine paralogues that exist in all) mediates immune responses. Toll itself has a dual function (in development and immunity), and all of the other Toll paralogues (Toll-2 through Toll-9) have only developmental functions where function is known. The mammalian TLRs, by contrast, are all devoted to immune perception, and have no clearly assigned roles in development.

How Many Mammalian TLRs Are There, and What Do They Each Detect?

In humans, we know of 10 TLRs (numbered 1 through 10). In the mouse, we know of 12 TLRs (numbered 1 through 13 with the exception of 10). Mouse *Tlr10* is a degenerate pseudogene that encodes no protein product; so too are human TLRs 11, 12, and 13. Mouse TLR8, once thought to be functionally inactive, has been shown to respond to a combination of polyT oligodeoxynucleotides and a synthetic imidazoquinoline agonist, similar to human TLR8.[38] The TLR genes are scattered widely in the genome, and TLRs 7, 8, and 13 are X-linked.

Table 1 indicates the ligand specificity of each of the TLRs. Notably, nucleic acids are sensed by TLRs 3, 7, 8, and 9. These TLRs are located principally or exclusively within endosomal compartments, and detect their ligands within a relatively narrow, acidic pH range. Hence alkalinization of the endosomal compartment abolishes detection, and excessive acidification does so as well.

Crystallographic studies demonstrated that the ectodomains of TLR4, TLR3, TLR2/1, and TLR2/6 fold into a horseshoe-like shape that is characteristic of LRR-containing proteins. TLRs are induced to dimerize by the simultaneous interaction of ligands with LRRs of distinct receptor chains. Most TLRs seem to operate as homodimers, but TLR2 engages either TLR1 or TLR6 to signal;[39] TLR4 has been reported to signal as a heterodimer with TLR6 as well.[40] In such cases, the ligand specificity is apparently altered, and it cannot be entirely excluded that other TLRs also act as heterodimers on some occasions. From the crystallographic studies performed to date, it is clear that TLRs engage their highly varied ligands in many different ways. In the case of TLR4, the interface between TLR4 and its required co-receptor MD-2 must form first, followed by LPS-induced dimerization of two TLR4:MD-2 dimers.[41] LPS simultaneously contacts a hydrophobic pocket within MD-2 (from one dimer) and the convex surface of TLR4 (from the other dimer). In contrast, two TLR3 molecules sandwich a 46-nucleotide dsRNA between them, with contacts by the N-terminus of each TLR3 with the ends of the dsRNA. The central portion of the dsRNA interacts with residues close to the C-terminus of each TLR3 chain.[42] Heterodimers of TLR2/TLR1 and TLR2/TLR6 interact with lipopeptides via a hydrophobic pocket formed by residues on the convex side of each ectodomain close to the center of the dimer.[43] Despite the variation in modes of ligand recognition, all known TLR dimer structures display the same arrangement, with the two C-terminal tails closely juxtaposed and the N termini at opposite ends of the dimer. This conformation is believed to bring the intracellular TIR domains into close proximity to recruit adapters and initiate signaling.

Table 1. The TLRs and their ligand specificity

TLR	Localization	Chromosomal Location		Subfamily; Dimer Association	Principal Ligand (Source)	Cofactor(s)	Adaptor(s)
		Mouse	Human				
TLR1	Plasma Membrane	Chr5: 65.316–65.324 Mb (-)	Chr4: 38.798–38.806 Mb (-)	TLR2 subfamily; Heterodimer with TLR2 or TLR6	Triacylated Lipopeptides with TLR2 (bacteria)	CD36; Gp96; PRAT4A	MyD88; TIRAP
TLR2	Plasma Membrane	Chr3: 83.640–83.646 Mb (-)	Chr4: 154.605–154.627 Mb (+)	TLR2 subfamily; Heterodimer with TLR1, TLR6 or TLR10	Lipopeptides with TLR1 and TLR6 (bacteria)	PRAT4A; Gp96; CD14; CD36	MyD88; TIRAP
TLR3	Endolysosome	Chr8: 46.481–46.496 Mb (-)	Chr4: 186.990–187.006 Mb (+)	TLR3 subfamily	Poly I:C (synthetic), dsRNA (viral)	CD14; Unc93b1; Gp96	TRIF
TLR4	Plasma Membrane	Chr4: 66.489–66.591 Mb (+)	Chr9: 120.466–120.480 Mb (+)	TLR4 subfamily; homodimer	LPS (Gram-negative bacteria)	MD-2; CD14; Gp96; PRAT4A; RP105/MD-1;	MyD88; TIRAP; TRAM; TRIF
TLR5	Plasma Membrane	Chr1: 184.885–184.906 Mb (+)	Chr1: 223.283–223.317 Mb (-)	TLR5 subfamily; homodimer	Flagellin (flagellated bacteria)	Gp96	MyD88
TLR7	Endolysosome	ChrX: 163.743–163.768 Mb (-)	ChrX: 12.885–12.908 Mb (-)	TLR9 subfamily; homodimer	ssRNA (virus); anti-viral drugs	CD14; Unc93b1; PRAT4A; Gp96	MyD88
TLR8	Endolysosome	ChrX: 163.681–163.702 Mb (-)	ChrX: 12.925–12.941 Mb (+)	TLR9 subfamily; homodimer	ssRNA	CD14	MyD88

continued on next page

Table 1. Continued

TLR	Localization	Chromosomal Location Mouse	Human	Subfamily; Dimer Association	Principal Ligand (Source)	Cofactor(s)	Adaptor(s)
TLR9	Endolysosome	Chr9: 106.125–106.129 Mb (+)	Chr3: 52.255–52.260 Mb (-)	TLR9 subfamily; homodimer	Unmethylated DNA, CpG-DNA (bacteria; protozoa, virus); Hemozoin (malaria parasites)	Granulin; CD14; HMGB1; LL37[*]; AP-3; BLOC-1; BLOC-2; Slc15a4; Unc93b1; PRAT4A; Gp96	MyD88
TLR10	Plasma Membrane	No mouse ortholog	Chr4: 38.774–38.785 Mb (-)	TLR2 subfamily; Heterodimer with TLR1 or TLR2; homodimer	Unknown	Unknown	MyD88
TLR11	Unknown	Chr14: 50.980–50.983 Mb (+)	No human ortholog	T-R11 subfamily	Protease-sensitive molecules (uropathogenic bacteria); profilin-like protein (T. gondii)	Unknown	MyD88
TLR12	Unknown	Chr4: 128.293–128.296 Mb (-)	Chr1: 33.932–33.934 Mb (+)	T-R11 subfamily	Unknown	Unknown	Unknown
TLR13	Unknown	ChrX: 103.338–103.356 Mb (+)	No human ortholog	T-R11 subfamily	Unknown	Unc93b1	Unknown

[*]LL37 (i.e., CAMP) is an antimicrobial peptide that stimulates TLR9 signaling to produce TNF-α.

The Need for Accessory Proteins in TLR Function

A number of accessory proteins are needed for TLRs to detect their ligands (Fig. 1). In some cases TLR ligands must initially or exclusively interact with transmembrane or membrane-bound proteins that associate with and regulate the conformation of TLRs to permit downstream signaling. As mentioned above, MD-2 is necessary for TLR4 to bind LPS, and makes direct contact with both LPS and TLR4. The GPI-anchored CD14 is required for TLR4 signaling in response to LPS, in particular for the O-glycosylated "smooth" LPS chemotype to stimulate either the MyD88-dependent or -independent pathways, and for "rough" LPS to stimulate the

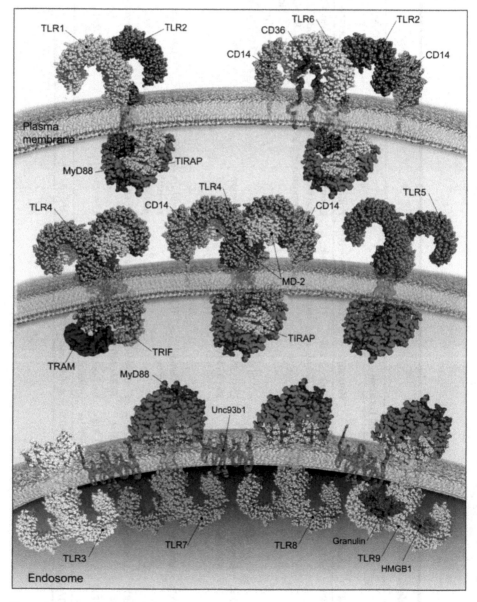

Figure 1. Please see figure legend on next page.

MyD88-independent pathway.[22,44] CD14 lacks intracellular signaling domains and is believed to function by binding to, and thereby concentrating, LPS at the cell membrane and then transferring it to the TLR4-MD-2 receptor complex.[45] Consistent with this idea, CD14 also exists in a soluble form that permits cells normally lacking CD14 to respond to LPS.[46,47] Both CD14 and CD36,[48] the latter a two transmembrane-spanning member of the class B scavenger receptor family, augment signaling from TLR2/6, although they are not absolutely required for it.

The nucleic acid-sensing TLRs (TLR3, TLR7, TLR8, and TLR9) detect their ligands and signal from the endosomal compartment, where they are trafficked with the aid of several accessory proteins from the endoplasmic reticulum (ER) via the secretory pathway. The general chaperones Gp96 and PRAT4A (also known as CNPY3) are necessary for TLR7 and TLR9 trafficking to endolysosomes, and for the plasma membrane localization of TLR1, TLR2, and TLR4.[49-52] Unc93b1, a 12 transmembrane spanning protein identified through genetic screening of ENU-mutagenized mice,[53] directly binds and transports TLR3, TLR7, and TLR9 from the ER to endolysosomes.[54,55] Once in endolysosomes, TLR9 is proteolytically cleaved within its ectodomain to generate a signaling-competent receptor capable of recruiting MyD88 and initiating downstream signaling.[56,57] Multiple proteases have been implicated in TLR9 cleavage,[56,57] an event that requires proper endolysosomal acidification.[58] A similar cleavage event has also been reported to occur in TLR7,[56,57] but not in TLR3.

Studies of TLR9 have provided evidence that granulin and HMGB proteins deliver CpG-DNA to TLR9 within endosomes, thus enabling TLR9 signaling to ensue.[59,60] Granulin and HMGB each simultaneously bind to both CpG-DNA and TLR9. However, whether they function in the same or distinct pathways to bring CpG-DNA to its receptor in endosomes remains unknown.

Finally, mention of the TLR signaling system in plasmacytoid dendritic cells (pDCs) is warranted here because its establishment requires a group of proteins not necessary in other cell types. pDCs exclusively express TLR7 and TLR9, which signal through the canonical MyD88-dependent pathway to produce proinflammatory cytokines. In addition, TLR7 and TLR9 activate a pathway absent from macrophages, conventional dendritic cells, and B cells to induce the IRF7-mediated production of abundant type I interferon (IFN) for which pDCs are known (see below). In addition to the chaperones Gp96, PRAT4A, and Unc93b1, lysosomal sorting proteins of the adaptor protein (AP)-3, biogenesis of lysosome-related organelle complex (BLOC)-1, and BLOC-2 complexes, and a transmembrane peptide/proton symporter channel called Slc15a4, are required for TLR9 signaling leading to both type I IFN and proinflammatory cytokine production by pDCs.[61,62] Future studies should shed light on the mechanism by which these proteins enable TLR signaling within pDCs.

Figure 1, viewed on previous page. The TLRs and their adaptor and accessory proteins. Shown are the TLR dimers in the plasma membrane (TLR1/2, TLR2/6, TLR4 and TLR5) or the endosomal membrane (TLR3, TLR7, TLR8 and TLR9). Upon ligand engagement (not shown, see Table 1), TLRs recruit adaptor proteins (MyD88, TRIF, TRAM, TIRAP) via homophilic TIR domain interactions. TLR4 signals from the plasma membrane through MyD88 and subsequently from the late endosome via TRIF. TLR3 signals exclusively through the TRIF-dependent pathway. Several accessory proteins associate with TLRs to permit downstream signaling (CD14, CD36, and MD-2) or aid in the trafficking of TLRs from the endoplasmic reticulum (ER) to the endosome (Unc93b1). The accessory proteins HMGB and Granulin assist in the delivery of CpG-DNA to TLR9 in the endosome. Note that only the death domain of MyD88 is shown. PDB IDs: TLR1/2 ectodomain (2Z7X); TLR2/6 ectodomain (3A79); TLR4 ectodomain + MD-2 (3FXI); TLR3 ectodomain (3CIY); 3FXI without MD-2 is shown for the ligand binding domain of all other TLRs; 1FYW is shown for the TIR domain of all TLRs. MyD88 (3MOP, death domain); TIRAP (2Y92); CD14 (1WWL); HMGB1 (2GZK, HMG box B domain only); Granulin (2JYE, human Granulin A, granulin/epithelin module). Structures for Unc93b1, TRAM and TRIF are unsolved and are, therefore, hypothetical. Docking interactions between proteins, except between TLR4 and MD-2, are hypothetical. 3D molecular models were generated at the same scale using the PyMOL Molecular Graphics System, Version 1.2r3pre, Schrödinger, LLC.

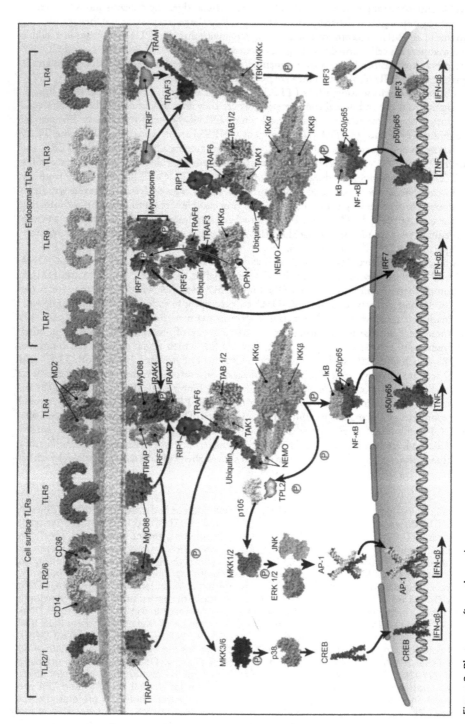

Figure 2. Please see figure legend on next page.

Signaling Pathways Activated by Mammalian TLRs

Much has been written of signaling pathways initiated by mammalian TLRs (Fig. 2). Initially, a putative adaptor protein termed MyD88, first identified in connection with signaling from the IL-1 receptor,[63,64] was implicated in TLR signaling. MyD88 has a well defined TIR domain, and also a death domain. The former is believed to engage the TIR domains of TLRs, while the latter propagates a signal by capturing downstream signaling intermediates.

MyD88 is the only adaptor required for signaling from some of the TLRs: the TLR2 complexes, TLR5, TLR7, TLR8, and TLR9. However, it soon became apparent that other adapters with a TIR domain structure also participated in TLR signaling. Tirap, also known as MAL, was the first to be identified because its structure was quite similar to that of MyD88. Tirap participates in signaling from the TLR2 and TLR4 complexes, but none of the other TLRs.

When MyD88 and/or Tirap are deleted by gene targeting, TLR signaling persists in a diminished form from TLR4, and persists normally from TLR3.[65-68] The so-called "MyD88-independent pathway" is responsible for this signaling, and the responsible adapters were identified in three ways. Rather sophisticated search algorithms were used to identify candidates, which were termed TRIF, or Ticam1,[69] and TRAM, or Ticam2.[70-72] These adapters were implicated in signaling through overexpression studies, and were also implicated as binding partners for the TIR domain of TLR3 and/or TLR4 by pull down and yeast 2-hybrid interaction studies.[71,73] Independently, ENU mutagenesis revealed the existence and essential functions of TRIF, which was mutated in the *Lps2* phenovariant strain.[74] *Lps2* mutants had diminished responses to LPS, and absent responses to poly I:C. BLAST searches with TRIF, in these studies, disclosed TRAM (which was implicated in LPS, but not poly I:C signaling).

The fact that an adaptor is shared between TLR4 (the LPS receptor) and TLR3 (the poly I:C receptor) raises interesting questions. LPS initiates strong responses in mammals, but not in most other vertebrate lineages. Conceivably, the ligand specificity has changed over several hundred million years of evolution, and in some species, the TLR4 ortholog may serve a nucleic acid (viral?) sensing role, as TLR3 is presumed to do.

In the MyD88-dependent pathway utilized by all TLRs except TLR3, MyD88 recruits several IRAK kinases (IRAK4, IRAK1, and IRAK2) through their death domains, which form a left-handed helical complex called the Myddosome.[75] The Myddosome is believed to represent the "active" conformation of the adaptor complex. IRAK4 phosphorylates and activates IRAK1

Figure 2, viewed on previous page. Overview of TLR signaling pathways. Shown are the signaling events downstream of TLR activation that lead to the induction of thousands of genes including those encoding the cytokines TNF and IFN-αβ. TLR1/2, TLR2/6, and TLR5 are located at the cell surface, while TLR3, TLR7, and TLR9 are localized in the endosome. TLR4 can signal from both the plasma membrane and the endosome. The MyD88-dependent pathway mediates signaling from all TLRs except TLR3; the TRIF-dependent pathway is utilized by TLR3 and TLR4. Note that TLR4 signals through the MyD88-dependent pathway from the cell membrane and is subsequently internalized into late endosomes to signal through the TRIF-dependent pathway. Small yellow circles labeled with a "P" represent phosphorylation events. PDB IDs: TLR1/2, TLR2/6, TLR3, TLR4, TLR5, TLR7, TLR9, MD-2, TIRAP, CD14, and MyD88 (see Figure 1); IRF5 (3DSH, transactivation domain); IRF3 (3QU6, DNA binding domain); IRF7 (3QU3, DNA binding domain); TAK1 (2EVA, kinase domain fused to TAB1 fragment); TAB1/2 (3A9J, TAB2 NZF domain complex with di-ubiquitin); NEMO (3BRV, IKK kinase association domain); IKKβ (3QA8); IκB (1IKN); NF-κB p65/p50 heterodimer (1VKX, Rel homology domains); CREB (1DH3, bZIP domain); MKK3/6 (3FME, kinase domain); MKK1/2 (2Y4I); ERK1/2 (3QYZ); JNK (3OY1); p105 (2DBF, death domain); ubiquitin chains (3DVN); Myddosome complex: MyD88, IRAK4, IRAK2 (3MOP, death domains); TRAF6 (1LB4, MATH domain); TRAF3 (1FLK, TRAF domain); p38 (3PG3); AP-1 (1FOS, bZIP domains). 3QA8 is shown for IKKα, IKKε, and TBK1. Structures for TRIF, TRAM, RIP1, TPL2, and OPN are unsolved and are, therefore, hypothetical. Docking interactions between proteins, except in the Myddosome, TLR4-MD-2, and NEMO-IKKβ complexes, are hypothetical. 3D molecular models were generated at the same scale using the PyMOL Molecular Graphics System, Version 1.2r3pre, Schrödinger, LLC.

and IRAK2, actions opposed by IRAKM, which is one of several inhibitory proteins in the TLR signaling pathway. TRAF6, an E3 ubiquitin ligase and ring finger domain protein, and IRF5 are also activated and recruited to this complex.

Ubiquitination plays a key role in signal transduction from the TLRs,[76] and signaling continues in this way: TRAF6, together with UBC13 and UEV1A, polyubiquitinates itself and NF-κB Essential Modulator (NEMO), a member of the IKK complex together with IKKα and IKKβ. The K63-linked polyubiquitin chains form a scaffold for the binding of the TAK1 complex, which binds through its ubiquitin-binding subunits TAB2/3.[77] TRAF6 activates TAK1, which phosphorylates IKKβ, activating the IKK complex to phosphorylate IκB, p105, and TPL2. As a consequence, IκBα and p105 are ubiquitinated and targeted for proteasome-mediated degradation, releasing NF-κB (to which IκBα was bound) and TPL2 (to which p105 was bound) as activated proteins. NF-κB enters the nucleus to regulate gene transcription, a function which also requires Akirin2, one of two mammalian orthologs of a Drosophila nuclear protein necessary for resistance to Gram-negative infections. Akirin2 is believed to function downstream of NF-κB in response to TLR and IL-1R signaling.[78] Activated TPL2 phosphorylates and activates MKK1 and MKK2. These MAP kinase kinases, together with MKK3 and MKK6 activated directly by TAK1, signal through p38, JNK, and ERK1/2 kinases to activate CREB and AP-1. NF-κB, CREB, and AP-1 induce transcription of numerous genes, including those for proinflammatory cytokines such as TNF, IL-6, and IL-1.

A study of mice with the hypomorphic mutation *panr2*, affecting *Ikbkg*, which encodes NEMO, provided evidence for a branchpoint in the MyD88-dependent pathway occurring at NEMO.[79] In macrophages from these mice, LPS-induced degradation of IκBα occurred normally, while p105 and ERK phosphorylation and NF-κB p65 nuclear translocation were impaired. An identical though less severe TLR2-dependent phenotype was observed in macrophages deficient in SHARPIN,[80] a component of the linear ubiquitin chain assembly complex (LUBAC) that acts on NEMO and promotes NF-κB activation.[81-83] SHARPIN appears to interact with NEMO to control p105 phosphorylation, and via Tpl2, ERK phosphorylation, leading to production of proinflammatory cytokines including IL-12, IL-1α, IL-1β, IL-18, and TNF. On the other hand, the branch of signaling involving IκBα degradation is independent of SHARPIN and NEMO. Thus, the function of NEMO extends beyond IκBα degradation and outside of this capacity, necessitates interaction with SHARPIN.

In the TRIF-dependent (MyD88-independent) signaling pathway stimulated by TLR3 or TLR4 activation, TRIF recruits polyubiquitinated RIP1, which interacts with the TRAF6/TAK1 complex, leading, as above, to NF-κB activation and proinflammatory cytokine induction.[84-87] TRIF signaling also induces type I IFN through phosphorylation and activation of IRF3 by a complex containing TRAF3, TBK1, and IKKε.[68,88,89]

In pDCs, activation of TLR7 and 9 in endosomes recruits MyD88 and IRAK4, which then interact with TRAF6, TRAF3, IRAK1, IKKα, osteopontin, and IRF7.[90,91] IRAK-1 and IKKα phosphorylate and activate IRF7, leading to transcription of interferon-inducible genes and production of large amounts of type I IFN.[92] pDCs also induce proinflammatory cytokine production downstream of TLR7 and TLR9 by signaling through the MyD88-dependent pathway resulting in NF-κB activation.

The Overall Importance of TLRs

When they were first discovered, an appealing view of TLRs held that they might be the proximal cause of everything that occurred during infection. "Everything" would embrace many complex phenomena, ranging from local inflammation and recruitment of other innate immune cells, the development of leukocytosis as a result of signals traveling from a nidus of infection to the bone marrow, the development of fever, shock, tissue injury, and other systemic problems; and of course, the development of an adaptive immune response (the well-known adjuvant effect of TLR signaling).

Subsequently, other means of detecting microbes were established: the RLRs, CLRs, and NLRs among them. Still more may await discovery. However, some aspects of TLR function are completely non-redundant. LPS has no other receptors of which we know, for example, nor do lipopeptides. And whatever redundancy may exist for nucleic acid perception, TLR mutations cause a dramatic enhancement of susceptibility to specific viral infections (notably infections by herpesviruses).[93] In the absence of all TLR signaling, a state observed in mice lacking both MyD88 and TRIF,[74] most animals fail to survive to weaning age, dying instead of opportunistic infections. Even adults succumb to large abscesses and systemic infection, but show a certain amount of resistance, perhaps mediated by adaptive immunity. In humans as well, mutations affecting MyD88 and IRAK4 are better tolerated as patients age and develop an adaptive response to compensate for their innate immune sensing defect.[94,95]

A particular point of controversy revolves around the oft-mentioned "requirement" of TLR signaling for the development of an adaptive immune response.[96-98] It has been suggested as well that B-cell responses are also TLR dependent.[99]

These studies appear to support, and may be based upon, the hypothesis that classical adjuvants such as Freund's adjuvant operate by activating TLR signaling, as postulated by Janeway.[100] However, a carefully controlled study by Gavin et al. revealed that TLR signaling is not necessary for strong adaptive responses to develop. On the contrary, responses of equal magnitude are observed when animals are immunized with antigens in Freund's complete adjuvant, Freund's incomplete adjuvant, Ribi adjuvant, or Alum, whether or not TLR signaling can occur.[101] A counter-argument was advanced, suggesting that only haptenated antigens behave in this way.[102] However, this argument is not tenable for two reasons. First, antibody responses to the protein antigen (in addition to the haptens attached to it) were unaffected by lack of TLR signaling (B. Beutler, unpublished observation). And second, lack of a requirement for TLR signaling has now been observed for antibody responses to numerous infectious agents, including recombinant Semliki Forest Virus,[103] enteric flora,[104] and mouse cytomegalovirus (C.N. Arnold and B. Beutler, unpublished observation).

Meanwhile, the C-type lectin mincle has been identified as a relevant receptor for trehalose dimycolate of mycobacteria[105,106] and it appears likely that mincle signaling, rather than TLR signaling, is responsible for at least part of the adjuvant effect of trehalose dimycolate and the mycobacterium Bacillus Calmette-Guerin.[107,108] Yet not all of the adjuvant effect of Freund's adjuvant likely proceeds via this pathway, since Freund's incomplete adjuvant is also quite effective at eliciting an immune response. In the end, it would appear that classical adjuvants operate through complex and redundant mechanisms. At the present time, no single mutation affecting the innate response can be said to be capable of abrogating adaptive immune responses.

The importance of TLR signaling to the maintenance of intestinal homeostasis has received much attention in light of the finding that inflammatory bowel disease (i.e., Crohn's disease and ulcerative colitis) arises from dysregulated innate immune responses to commensal intestinal bacteria. Patients with Crohn's disease benefit from blockade of TNF activity, supporting the contribution of TLR signaling to disease. Aberrant TLR signaling in hematopoietic cells is believed to drive chronic intestinal inflammation.[109] However, a large body of work also supports a protective role for TLR signaling in acute intestinal inflammation, where the function of TLRs is localized to intestinal epithelial cells (IECs). Mice deficient in MyD88, TLR2, or TLR4 displayed increased susceptibility to colitis induced by dextran sodium sulfate (DSS), a chemical that damages IECs and thereby permits luminal bacteria to access the lamina propria.[110-112] Using bone marrow chimeras generated from wild type and $Myd88^{-/-}Ticam1^{Lps2/Lps2}$ mice, it was demonstrated that TLR signaling in cells of the non-hematopoietic compartment, most probably IECs, is protective against DSS-induced colitis.[113] Within IECs, TLR signaling directs numerous cellular responses that promote epithelial barrier function and minimize inflammation, including proliferation induced by the EGF receptor ligands amphiregulin and epiregulin,[113] and possibly TGFα, HB-EGF, and β-cellulin. The function of the metalloprotease ADAM17 was also found to be necessary for resistance to DSS-induced colitis. In addition to promoting proliferation, the protective function of TLR signaling in IECs also includes induction of antimicrobial peptides and IgA2, and strengthening of tight junctions between IECs.[114]

Similarly to Crohn's disease, multiple disorders classified as autoimmune in nature, including rheumatoid arthritis, systemic lupus erythematosus (SLE), ankylosing spondylitis, and psoriasis, are improved by TNF blockade, raising the possibility that endogenous ligands may activate TLRs to initiate innate immune signaling. Indeed, a pathogenic role for intracellular TLR signaling is strongly supported in the case of SLE. Targeted deletion of *Tlr7* attenuated disease in the *Fas*[lpr] model of SLE,[115] as did MyD88[116] or Unc93b1 deficiency.[117] Consistent with these findings, mice with the Y-linked accelerator of autoimmunity (*Yaa*) mutation were demonstrated to harbor a duplication encompassing the *Tlr7* gene within the pseudoautosomal region of the Y chromosome;[118,119] the *Tlr7* duplication is believed to account for most aspects of the autoimmune phenotype associated with *Yaa*.[120-122] These findings support a role for TLR7 in the pathogenesis of SLE.

In contrast, TLR8 and TLR9 mediate a protective role distinct from that of TLR7. *Tlr8*[123] or *Tlr9* deletion in mice augmented disease[115,124-126] as a result of TLR7 overexpression via an unknown mechanism.[123,127] One possibility is that TLR7 competes with TLR8 and TLR9 for transport to endosomes, resulting in autoimmunity in TLR8- and TLR9-deficient mice. In support of this hypothesis, TLR7 and TLR9 have been shown to compete for association with Unc93b1.[128]

As mentioned above, the nucleic sensing TLRs (TLR3, TLR7, TLR8, and TLR9) are trafficked with the aid of multiple chaperones to endolysosomes, from which host DNA is usually excluded. It has been shown however, that B cells expressing antigen receptors specific for chromatin or small nuclear ribonucleoproteins (snRNPs) can internalize these autoantigens to endosomal compartments where they engage TLR7 or TLR9.[116,129,130] The combination of BCR and TLR engagement efficiently activates the B cell, leading to clonal expansion and thereby propagating an amplification loop that may explain the overrepresentation of antibodies directed against nuclear components observed in SLE.

So far, where it has been documented that endogenous molecules drive a TLR response leading to autoimmunity, these endogenous molecules are nucleic acids (or are tightly associated with nucleic acids). Nucleic acids appear to test the limits of self/non-self discrimination by the innate immune system. Although the nucleic acids of microbes have some molecular features that distinguish them from nucleic acids of the host (a 5'-triphosphate structure in some viruses, for example, and unmethylated CpG dinucleotides in all DNA from non-vertebrates), they cannot be distinguished with complete reliability. It remains to be seen whether endogenous activators of other TLRs exist, and whether they serve an important physiological function in vivo. It has been proposed, for example, that free fatty acids may sometimes activate TLR4, leading to an insulin-resistant state and "metabolic syndrome," which shares some characteristics with inflammation caused by microbes.[131-133] Oxidized phospholipids of endogenous origin have been proposed as activators of TLRs as well.[134]

Conclusion

The TLRs may be regarded as some of the keenest "eyes" of the innate immune system. They definitely protect against infection, but can also cause horrific injury or death: a dichotomy well known to clinicians concerned with inflammation. It is with the TLRs that the very first responses to an infection often begin, possibly within a few seconds, and certainly within a few minutes, after microbes find their way into the host. The future will tell us how we may best make use of this information. By using the TLRs for their adjuvant effects? By blocking TLR responses to quell inflammation? Or perhaps by harnessing TLRs for purposes they never evolved to fulfill? Already, certain drug responses, both intended[135-137] and unintended,[138] have been linked to TLRs. If highly specific drugs capable of blocking or activating TLRs can be designed, it may be possible to treat certain diseases with unprecedented specificity.

About the Author

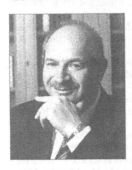

Dr. Bruce Beutler is a Professor and the Director of the Center for the Genetics of Host Defense at the University of Texas Southwestern Medical Center. He purified mouse tumor necrosis factor and identified it as a major mediator of the inflammatory response to lipopolysaccharide (LPS). Subsequently, the Beutler lab focused on uncovering the receptor that triggers the innate immune response to LPS, and determining the link between LPS sensing and host resistance. Their work with the C3H/HeJ and C57BL/10ScCr mice, two strains that are resistant to the toxic effects of LPS, identified Toll-like receptor 4 (TLR4) as the receptor for LPS and opened the way to discovery of the microbial ligands for each member of the TLR family. Approximately ten years ago, Dr. Beutler's lab began to utilize a classical forward genetic approach to study innate and adaptive immunity in mice. Since that time, more than 150,000 mutagenized mice have been screened for immune defects, leading to the identification of numerous genes required for TLR signaling, and for specific immunological phenomena including survival during infection with mouse cytomegalovirus, resistance to chemically-induced intestinal inflammation, and induction of antibody responses to an administered antigen. B. Beutler is the recipient of several prestigious international awards, including the 2011 Nobel Prize in Medicine and Physiology.

References

1. Andersson J, Sjöberg O, Möller G. Induction of immunoglobulin and antibody synthesis in vitro by lipopolysaccharides. Eur J Immunol 1972; 2:349-53; PMID:4563347; http://dx.doi.org/10.1002/eji.1830020410.
2. Bogdan C, Mattner J, Schleicher U. The role of type I interferons in non-viral infections. Immunol Rev 2004; 202:33-48; PMID:15546384; http://dx.doi.org/10.1111/j.0105-2896.2004.00207.x.
3. Ciacci-Woolwine F, Blomfield IC, Richardson SH, Mizel SB. Salmonella flagellin induces tumor necrosis factor alpha in a human promonocytic cell line. Infect Immun 1998; 66:1127-34; PMID:9488405.
4. Field AK, Tytell AA, Lampson GP, Hilleman MR. Inducers of interferon and host resistance. II. Multistranded synthetic polynucleotide complexes. Proc Natl Acad Sci U S A 1967; 58:1004 10; PMID:5233831; http://dx.doi.org/10.1073/pnas.58.3.1004.
5. Melchers F, Braun V, Galanos C. The lipoprotein of the outer membrane of Escherichia coli: a B-lymphocyte mitogen. J Exp Med 1975; 142:473-82; PMID:1095681; http://dx.doi.org/10.1084/jem.142.2.473.
6. Pfeiffer R. Untersuchungen über das Choleragift. Z Hyg 1892; 11:393-411; http://dx.doi.org/10.1007/BF02284303.
7. Shear MJ, Turner FC, Perrault A, et al. Chemical treatment of tumors. V. Isolation of the hemorrhage-producing fraction from Serratia marcescens (Baccillus prodigiosus) culture filtrate. J Natl Cancer Inst 1943; 4:81-97.
8. Johnson AG, Gaines S, Landy M. Studies on the O antigen of Salmonella typhosa. V. Enhancement of antibody response to protein antigens by the purified lipopolysaccharide. J Exp Med 1956; 103:225-46; PMID:13286429; http://dx.doi.org/10.1084/jem.103.2.225.
9. Skidmore BJ, Chiller JM, Morrison DC, Weigle WO. Immunologic properties of bacterial lipopolysaccharide (LPS): correlation between the mitogenic, adjuvant, and immunogenic activities. J Immunol 1975; 114:770-5; PMID:46249.
10. Coutinho A, Möller G. Thymus-independent B-cell induction and paralysis. Adv Immunol 1975; 21:113-236; PMID:1096578; http://dx.doi.org/10.1016/S0065-2776(08)60220-5.
11. Coutinho A, Gronowicz E, Bullock WW, Möller G. Mechanism of thymus-independent immunocyte triggering. Mitogenic activation of B cells results in specific immune responses. J Exp Med 1974; 139:74-92; PMID:4128449; http://dx.doi.org/10.1084/jem.139.1.74.
12. Heppner G, Weiss DW. High susceptibility of strain A mice to endotoxin and endotoxin-red blood cell mixtures. J Bacteriol 1965; 90:696-703; PMID:16562068.
13. Sultzer BM. Genetic control of leucocyte responses to endotoxin. Nature 1968; 219:1253-4; PMID:4877918; http://dx.doi.org/10.1038/2191253a0.

14. O'Brien AD, Rosenstreich DL, Scher I, Campbell GH, MacDermott RP, Formal SB. Genetic control of susceptibility to Salmonella typhimurium in mice: role of the LPS gene. J Immunol 1980; 124:20-4; PMID:6985638.
15. Hagberg L, Hull R, Hull S, McGhee JR, Michalek SM, Svanborg Edén C. Difference in susceptibility to gram-negative urinary tract infection between C3H/HeJ and C3H/HeN mice. Infect Immun 1984; 46:839-44; PMID:6389367.
16. Michalek SM, Moore RN, McGhee JR, Rosenstreich DL, Mergenhagen SE. The primary role of lymphoreticular cells in the mediation of host responses to bacterial endotoxim. J Infect Dis 1980; 141:55-63; PMID:6154108; http://dx.doi.org/10.1093/infdis/141.1.55.
17. Coutinho A, Forni L, Melchers F, Watanabe T. Genetic defect in responsiveness to the B cell mitogen lipopolysaccharide. Eur J Immunol 1977; 7:325-8; PMID:326565; http://dx.doi.org/10.1002/eji.1830070517.
18. Coutinho A, Meo T. Genetic basis for unresponsiveness to lipopolysaccharide in C57BL/10Cr mice. Immunogenetics 1978; 7:17-24; PMID:21302052; http://dx.doi.org/10.1007/BF01843983.
19. Watson J, Riblet R. Genetic control of responses to bacterial lipopolysaccharides in mice. I. Evidence for a single gene that influences mitogenic and immunogenic respones to lipopolysaccharides. J Exp Med 1974; 140:1147-61; PMID:4138849; http://dx.doi.org/10.1084/jem.140.5.1147.
20. Watson J, Riblet R, Taylor BA. The response of recombinant inbred strains of mice to bacterial lipopolysaccharides. J Immunol 1977; 118:2088-93; PMID:325138.
21. Watson J, Kelly K, Largen M, Taylor BA. The genetic mapping of a defective LPS response gene in C3H/HeJ mice. J Immunol 1978; 120:422-4; PMID:202651.
22. Wright SD, Ramos RA, Tobias PS, Ulevitch RJ, Mathison JC. CD14, a receptor for complexes of lipopolysaccharide (LPS) and LPS binding protein. Science 1990; 249:1431-3; PMID:1698311; http://dx.doi.org/10.1126/science.1698311.
23. Lee JD, Kato K, Tobias PS, Kirkland TN, Ulevitch RJ. Transfection of CD14 into 70Z/3 cells dramatically enhances the sensitivity to complexes of lipopolysaccharide (LPS) and LPS binding protein. J Exp Med 1992; 175:1697-705; PMID:1375269; http://dx.doi.org/10.1084/jem.175.6.1697.
24. Poltorak A, He X, Smirnova I, Liu MY, Van Huffel C, Du X, et al. Defective LPS signaling in C3H/HeJ and C57BL/10ScCr mice: mutations in Tlr4 gene. Science 1998; 282:2085-8; PMID:9851930; http://dx.doi.org/10.1126/science.282.5396.2085.
25. Poltorak A, Smirnova I, Clisch R, Beutler B. Limits of a deletion spanning Tlr4 in C57BL/10ScCr mice. J Endotoxin Res 2000; 6:51-6; PMID:11061032; http://dx.doi.org/10.1177/09680519000060010701.
26. Gay NJ, Keith FJ. Drosophila Toll and IL-1 receptor. Nature 1991; 351:355-6; PMID:1851964; http://dx.doi.org/10.1038/351355b0.
27. Nomura N, Miyajima N, Sazuka T, Tanaka A, Kawarabayasi Y, Sato S, et al. Prediction of the coding sequences of unidentified human genes. I. The coding sequences of 40 new genes (KIAA0001-KIAA0040) deduced by analysis of randomly sampled cDNA clones from human immature myeloid cell line KG-1. DNA Res 1994; 1:27-35; PMID:7584026; http://dx.doi.org/10.1093/dnares/1.1.27.
28. Taguchi T, Mitcham JL, Dower SK, Sims JE, Testa JR. Chromosomal localization of TIL, a gene encoding a protein related to the Drosophila transmembrane receptor Toll, to human chromosome 4p14. Genomics 1996; 32:486-8; PMID:8838819; http://dx.doi.org/10.1006/geno.1996.0150.
29. Medzhitov R, Preston-Hurlburt P, Janeway CA Jr. A human homologue of the Drosophila Toll protein signals activation of adaptive immunity. Nature 1997; 388:394-7; PMID:9237759; http://dx.doi.org/10.1038/41131.
30. Poltorak A, Ricciardi-Castagnoli P, Citterio S, Beutler B. Physical contact between lipopolysaccharide and toll-like receptor 4 revealed by genetic complementation. Proc Natl Acad Sci USA 2000; 97:2163-7; PMID:10681462; http://dx.doi.org/10.1073/pnas.040565397.
31. Lien E, Means TK, Heine H, Yoshimura A, Kusumoto S, Fukase K, et al. Toll-like receptor 4 imparts ligand-specific recognition of bacterial lipopolysaccharide. J Clin Invest 2000; 105:497-504; PMID:10683379; http://dx.doi.org/10.1172/JCI8541.
32. Shimazu R, Akashi S, Ogata H, Nagai Y, Fukudome K, Miyake K, et al. MD-2, a molecule that confers lipopolysaccharide responsiveness on Toll-like receptor 4. J Exp Med 1999; 189:1777-82; PMID:10359581; http://dx.doi.org/10.1084/jem.189.11.1777.
33. Nagai Y, Akashi S, Nagafuku M, Ogata M, Iwakura Y, Akira S, et al. Essential role of MD-2 in LPS responsiveness and TLR4 distribution. Nat Immunol 2002; 3:667-72; PMID:12055629.
34. Song WY, Wang GL, Chen LL, Kim HS, Pi LY, Holsten T, et al. A receptor kinase-like protein encoded by the rice disease resistance gene, Xa21. Science 1995; 270:1804-6; PMID:8525370; http://dx.doi.org/10.1126/science.270.5243.1804.
35. Lee SW, Han SW, Sririyanum M, Park CJ, Seo YS, Ronald PC. A type I-secreted, sulfated peptide triggers XA21-mediated innate immunity. Science 2009; 326:850-3; PMID:19892983; http://dx.doi.org/10.1126/science.1173438.

36. Lemaitre B, Nicolas E, Michaut L, Reichhart JM, Hoffmann JA. The dorsoventral regulatory gene cassette spätzle/Toll/cactus controls the potent antifungal response in Drosophila adults. Cell 1996; 86:973-83; PMID:8808632; http://dx.doi.org/10.1016/S0092-8674(00)80172-5.
37. Ferrandon D, Imler JL, Hetru C, Hoffmann JA. The Drosophila systemic immune response: sensing and signalling during bacterial and fungal infections. Nat Rev Immunol 2007; 7:862-74; PMID:17948019; http://dx.doi.org/10.1038/nri2194.
38. Gorden KK, Qiu XX, Binsfeld CC, Vasilakos JP, Alkan SS. Cutting edge: activation of murine TLR8 by a combination of imidazoquinoline immune response modifiers and polyT oligodeoxynucleotides. J Immunol 2006; 177:6584-7; PMID:17082568.
39. Ozinsky A, Underhill DM, Fontenot JD, Hajjar AM, Smith KD, Wilson CB, et al. The repertoire for pattern recognition of pathogens by the innate immune system is defined by cooperation between toll-like receptors. Proc Natl Acad Sci U S A 2000; 97:13766-71; PMID:11095740; http://dx.doi.org/10.1073/pnas.250476497.
40. Stewart CR, Stuart LM, Wilkinson K, van Gils JM, Deng J, Halle A, et al. CD36 ligands promote sterile inflammation through assembly of a Toll-like receptor 4 and 6 heterodimer. Nat Immunol 2010; 11:155-61; PMID:20037584; http://dx.doi.org/10.1038/ni.1836.
41. Park BS, Song DH, Kim HM, Choi BS, Lee H, Lee JO. The structural basis of lipopolysaccharide recognition by the TLR4-MD-2 complex. Nature 2009; 458:1191-5; PMID:19252480; http://dx.doi.org/10.1038/nature07830.
42. Liu L, Botos I, Wang Y, Leonard JN, Shiloach J, Segal DM, et al. Structural basis of toll-like receptor 3 signaling with double-stranded RNA. Science 2008; 320:379-81; PMID:18420935; http://dx.doi.org/10.1126/science.1155406.
43. Jin MS, Kim SE, Heo JY, Lee ME, Kim HM, Paik SG, et al. Crystal structure of the TLR1-TLR2 heterodimer induced by binding of a tri-acylated lipopeptide. Cell 2007; 130:1071-82; PMID:17889651; http://dx.doi.org/10.1016/j.cell.2007.09.008.
44. Jiang Z, Georgel P, Du X, Shamel L, Sovath S, Mudd S, et al. CD14 is required for MyD88-independent LPS signaling. Nat Immunol 2005; 6:565-70; PMID:15895089; http://dx.doi.org/10.1038/ni1207.
45. da Silva Correia J, Soldau K, Christen U, Tobias PS, Ulevitch RJ. Lipopolysaccharide is in close proximity to each of the proteins in its membrane receptor complex. transfer from CD14 to TLR4 and MD-2. J Biol Chem 2001; 276:21129-35; PMID:11274165; http://dx.doi.org/10.1074/jbc.M009164200.
46. Frey EA, Miller DS, Jahr TG, Sundan A, Bazil V, Espevik T, et al. Soluble CD14 participates in the response of cells to lipopolysaccharide. J Exp Med 1992; 176:1665-71; PMID:1281215; http://dx.doi.org/10.1084/jem.176.6.1665.
47. Haziot A, Rong GW, Silver J, Goyert SM. Recombinant soluble CD14 mediates the activation of endothelial cells by lipopolysaccharide. J Immunol 1993; 151:1500-7; PMID:7687634.
48. Hoebe K, Georgel P, Rutschmann S, Du X, Mudd S, Crozat K, et al. CD36 is a sensor of diacylglycerides. Nature 2005; 433:523-7; PMID:15690042; http://dx.doi.org/10.1038/nature03253.
49. Randow F, Seed B. Endoplasmic reticulum chaperone gp96 is required for innate immunity but not cell viability. Nat Cell Biol 2001; 3:891-6; PMID:11584270; http://dx.doi.org/10.1038/ncb1001-891.
50. Yang Y, Liu B, Dai J, Srivastava PK, Zammit DJ, Lefrançois L, et al. Heat shock protein gp96 is a master chaperone for toll-like receptors and is important in the innate function of macrophages. Immunity 2007; 26:215-26; PMID:17275357; http://dx.doi.org/10.1016/j.immuni.2006.12.005.
51. Takahashi K, Shibata T, Akashi-Takamura S, Kiyokawa T, Wakabayashi Y, Tanimura N, et al. A protein associated with Toll-like receptor (TLR) 4 (PRAT4A) is required for TLR-dependent immune responses. J Exp Med 2007; 204:2963-76; PMID:17998391; http://dx.doi.org/10.1084/jem.20071132.
52. Liu B, Yang Y, Qiu Z, Staron M, Hong F, Li Y, et al. Folding of Toll-like receptors by the HSP90 paralogue gp96 requires a substrate-specific cochaperone. Nat Commun 2010; 1:79; PMID:20865800; http://dx.doi.org/10.1038/ncomms1070.
53. Tabeta K, Hoebe K, Janssen EM, Du X, Georgel P, Crozat K, et al. The Unc93b1 mutation 3d disrupts exogenous antigen presentation and signaling via Toll-like receptors 3, 7 and 9. Nat Immunol 2006; 7:156-64; PMID:16415873; http://dx.doi.org/10.1038/ni1297.
54. Brinkmann MM, Spooner E, Hoebe K, Beutler B, Ploegh HL, Kim YM. The interaction between the ER membrane protein UNC93B and TLR3, 7, and 9 is crucial for TLR signaling. J Cell Biol 2007; 177:265-75; PMID:17452530; http://dx.doi.org/10.1083/jcb.200612056.
55. Kim YM, Brinkmann MM, Paquet ME, Ploegh HL. UNC93B1 delivers nucleotide-sensing toll-like receptors to endolysosomes. Nature 2008; 452:234-8; PMID:18305481; http://dx.doi.org/10.1038/nature06726.
56. Park B, Brinkmann MM, Spooner E, Lee CC, Kim YM, Ploegh HL. Proteolytic cleavage in an endolysosomal compartment is required for activation of Toll-like receptor 9. Nat Immunol 2008; 9:1407-14; PMID:18931679; http://dx.doi.org/10.1038/ni.1669.

57. Ewald SE, Lee BL, Lau L, Wickliffe KE, Shi GP, Chapman HA, et al. The ectodomain of Toll-like receptor 9 is cleaved to generate a functional receptor. Nature 2008; 456:658-62; PMID:18820679; http://dx.doi.org/10.1038/nature07405.

58. Häcker H, Mischak H, Miethke T, Liptay S, Schmid R, Sparwasser T, et al. CpG-DNA-specific activation of antigen-presenting cells requires stress kinase activity and is preceded by non-specific endocytosis and endosomal maturation. EMBO J 1998; 17:6230-40; PMID:9799232; http://dx.doi.org/10.1093/emboj/17.21.6230.

59. Park B, Buti L, Lee S, Matsuwaki T, Spooner E, Brinkmann MM, et al. Granulin is a soluble cofactor for toll-like receptor 9 signaling. Immunity 2011; 34:505-13; PMID:21497117; http://dx.doi.org/10.1016/j.immuni.2011.01.018.

60. Ivanov S, Dragoi AM, Wang X, Dallacosta C, Louten J, Musco G, et al. A novel role for HMGB1 in TLR9-mediated inflammatory responses to CpG-DNA. Blood 2007; 110:1970-81; PMID:17548579; http://dx.doi.org/10.1182/blood-2006-09-044776.

61. Blasius AL, Arnold CN, Georgel P, Rutschmann S, Xia Y, Lin P, et al. Slc15a4, AP-3, and Hermansky-Pudlak syndrome proteins are required for Toll-like receptor signaling in plasmacytoid dendritic cells. Proc Natl Acad Sci U S A 2010; 107:19973-8; PMID:21045126; http://dx.doi.org/10.1073/pnas.1014051107.

62. Sasai M, Linehan MM, Iwasaki A. Bifurcation of Toll-like receptor 9 signaling by adaptor protein 3. Science 2010; 329:1530-4; PMID:20847273; http://dx.doi.org/10.1126/science.1187029.

63. Wesche H, Henzel WJ, Shillinglaw W, Li S, Cao Z. MyD88: an adapter that recruits IRAK to the IL-1 receptor complex. Immunity 1997; 7:837-47; PMID:9430229; http://dx.doi.org/10.1016/S1074-7613(00)80402-1.

64. Muzio M, Ni J, Feng P, Dixit VM. IRAK (Pelle) family member IRAK-2 and MyD88 as proximal mediators of IL-1 signaling. Science 1997; 278:1612-5; PMID:9374458; http://dx.doi.org/10.1126/science.278.5343.1612.

65. Horng T, Barton GM, Flavell RA, Medzhitov R. The adaptor molecule TIRAP provides signalling specificity for Toll-like receptors. Nature 2002; 420:329-33; PMID:12447442; http://dx.doi.org/10.1038/nature01180.

66. Yamamoto M, Sato S, Hemmi H, Sanjo H, Uematsu S, Kaisho T, et al. Essential role for TIRAP in activation of the signalling cascade shared by TLR2 and TLR4. Nature 2002; 420:324-9; PMID:12447441; http://dx.doi.org/10.1038/nature01182.

67. Kawai T, Adachi O, Ogawa T, Takeda K, Akira S. Unresponsiveness of MyD88-deficient mice to endotoxin. Immunity 1999; 11:115-22; PMID:10435584; http://dx.doi.org/10.1016/S1074-7613(00)80086-2.

68. Kawai T, Takeuchi O, Fujita T, Inoue J, Mühlradt PF, Sato S, et al. Lipopolysaccharide stimulates the MyD88-independent pathway and results in activation of IFN-regulatory factor 3 and the expression of a subset of lipopolysaccharide-inducible genes. J Immunol 2001; 167:5887-94; PMID:11698465.

69. Yamamoto M, Sato S, Mori K, Hoshino K, Takeuchi O, Takeda K, et al. Cutting edge: a novel Toll/IL-1 receptor domain-containing adapter that preferentially activates the IFN-beta promoter in the Toll-like receptor signaling. J Immunol 2002; 169:6668-72; PMID:12471095.

70. Bin LH, Xu LG, Shu HB. TIRP, a novel Toll/interleukin-1 receptor (TIR) domain-containing adapter protein involved in TIR signaling. J Biol Chem 2003; 283:24526-32; PMID:12721283; http://dx.doi.org/10.1074/jbc.M303451200.

71. Fitzgerald KA, Rowe DC, Barnes BJ, Caffrey DR, Visintin A, Latz E, et al. LPS-TLR4 signaling to IRF-3/7 and NF-kappaB involves the toll adapters TRAM and TRIF. J Exp Med 2003; 198:1043-55; PMID:14517278; http://dx.doi.org/10.1084/jem.20031023.

72. Oshiumi H, Sasai M, Shida K, Fujita T, Matsumoto M, Seya T. TIR-containing adapter molecule (TICAM)-2, a bridging adapter recruiting to toll-like receptor 4 TICAM-1 that induces interferon-beta. J Biol Chem 2003; 278:49751-62; PMID:14519765; http://dx.doi.org/10.1074/jbc.M305820200.

73. Oshiumi H, Matsumoto M, Funami K, Akazawa T, Seya T. TICAM-1, an adaptor molecule that participates in Toll-like receptor 3-mediated interferon-beta induction. Nat Immunol 2003; 4:161-7; PMID:12539043; http://dx.doi.org/10.1038/ni886.

74. Hoebe K, Du X, Georgel P, Janssen E, Tabeta K, Kim SO, et al. Identification of Lps2 as a key transducer of MyD88-independent TIR signalling. Nature 2003; 424:743-8; PMID:12872135; http://dx.doi.org/10.1038/nature01889.

75. Lin SC, Lo YC, Wu H. Helical assembly in the MyD88-IRAK4-IRAK2 complex in TLR/IL-1R signalling. Nature 2010; 465:885-90; PMID:20485341; http://dx.doi.org/10.1038/nature09121.

76. Bhoj VG, Chen ZJ. Ubiquitylation in innate and adaptive immunity. Nature 2009; 458:430-7; PMID:19325622; http://dx.doi.org/10.1038/nature07959.

77. Kanayama A, Seth RB, Sun L, Ea CK, Hong M, Shaito A, et al. TAB2 and TAB3 activate the NF-kappaB pathway through binding to polyubiquitin chains. Mol Cell 2004; 15:535-48; PMID:15327770; http://dx.doi.org/10.1016/j.molcel.2004.08.008.

78. Goto A, Matsushita K, Gesellchen V, El Chamy L, Kuttenkeuler D, Takeuchi O, et al. Akirins are highly conserved nuclear proteins required for NF-kappaB-dependent gene expression in drosophila and mice. Nat Immunol 2008; 9:97-104; PMID:18066067; http://dx.doi.org/10.1038/ni1543.

79. Siggs OM, Berger M, Krebs P, Arnold CN, Eidenschenk C, Huber C, et al. A mutation of Ikbkg causes immune deficiency without impairing degradation of IkappaB alpha. Proc Natl Acad Sci U S A 2010; 107:3046-51; PMID:20133626; http://dx.doi.org/10.1073/pnas.0915098107.

80. Zak DE, Schmitz F, Gold ES, Diercks AH, Peschon JJ, Valvo JS, et al. Systems analysis identifies an essential role for SHANK-associated RH domain-interacting protein (SHARPIN) in macrophage Toll-like receptor 2 (TLR2) responses. Proc Natl Acad Sci U S A 2011; 108:11536-41; PMID:21709223; http://dx.doi.org/10.1073/pnas.1107577108.

81. Gerlach B, Cordier SM, Schmukle AC, Emmerich CH, Rieser E, Haas TL, et al. Linear ubiquitination prevents inflammation and regulates immune signalling. Nature 2011; 471:591-6; PMID:21455173; http://dx.doi.org/10.1038/nature09816.

82. Ikeda F, Deribe YL, Skånland SS, Stieglitz B, Grabbe C, Franz-Wachtel M, et al. SHARPIN forms a linear ubiquitin ligase complex regulating NF-κB activity and apoptosis. Nature 2011; 471:637-41; PMID:21455181; http://dx.doi.org/10.1038/nature09814.

83. Tokunaga F, Nakagawa T, Nakahara M, Saeki Y, Taniguchi M, Sakata S, et al. SHARPIN is a component of the NF-κB-activating linear ubiquitin chain assembly complex. Nature 2011; 471:633-6; PMID:21455180; http://dx.doi.org/10.1038/nature09815.

84. Sato S, Sugiyama M, Yamamoto M, Watanabe Y, Kawai T, Takeda K, et al. Toll/IL-1 receptor domain-containing adaptor inducing IFN-beta (TRIF) associates with TNF receptor-associated factor 6 and TANK-binding kinase 1, and activates two distinct transcription factors, NF-kappa B and IFN-regulatory factor-3, in the Toll-like receptor signaling. J Immunol 2003; 171:4304-10; PMID:14530355.

85. Jiang Z, Mak TW, Sen G, Li X. Toll-like receptor 3-mediated activation of NF-kappaB and IRF3 diverges at Toll-IL-1 receptor domain-containing adapter inducing IFN-beta. Proc Natl Acad Sci U S A 2004; 101:3533-8; PMID:14982987; http://dx.doi.org/10.1073/pnas.0308496101.

86. Meylan E, Burns K, Hofmann K, Blancheteau V, Martinon F, Kelliher M, et al. RIP1 is an essential mediator of Toll-like receptor 3-induced NF-kappa B activation. Nat Immunol 2004; 5:503-7; PMID:15064760; http://dx.doi.org/10.1038/ni1061.

87. Cusson-Hermance N, Khurana S, Lee TH, Fitzgerald KA, Kelliher MA. Rip1 mediates the Trif-dependent toll-like receptor 3- and 4-induced NF-kappaB activation but does not contribute to interferon regulatory factor 3 activation. J Biol Chem 2005; 280:36560-6; PMID:16115877; http://dx.doi.org/10.1074/jbc.M506831200.

88. Fitzgerald KA, McWhirter SM, Faia KL, Rowe DC, Latz E, Golenbock DT, et al. IKKepsilon and TBK1 are essential components of the IRF3 signaling pathway. Nat Immunol 2003; 4:491-6; PMID:12692549; http://dx.doi.org/10.1038/ni921.

89. Sharma S, tenOever BR, Grandvaux N, Zhou GP, Lin R, Hiscott J. Triggering the interferon antiviral response through an IKK-related pathway. Science 2003; 300:1148-51; PMID:12702806; http://dx.doi.org/10.1126/science.1081315.

90. Kawai T, Sato S, Ishii KJ, Coban C, Hemmi H, Yamamoto M, et al. Interferon-alpha induction through Toll-like receptors involves a direct interaction of IRF7 with MyD88 and TRAF6. Nat Immunol 2004; 5:1061-8; PMID:15361868; http://dx.doi.org/10.1038/ni1118.

91. Shinohara ML, Lu L, Bu J, Werneck MB, Kobayashi KS, Glimcher LH, et al. Osteopontin expression is essential for interferon-alpha production by plasmacytoid dendritic cells. Nat Immunol 2006; 7:498-506; PMID:16604075; http://dx.doi.org/10.1038/ni1327.

92. Honda K, Yanai H, Negishi H, Asagiri M, Sato M, Mizutani T, et al. IRF-7 is the master regulator of type-I interferon-dependent immune responses. Nature 2005; 434:772-7; PMID:15800576; http://dx.doi.org/10.1038/nature03464.

93. Tabeta K, Georgel P, Janssen E, Du X, Hoebe K, Crozat K, et al. Toll-like receptors 9 and 3 as essential components of innate immune defense against mouse cytomegalovirus infection. Proc Natl Acad Sci U S A 2004; 101:3516-21; PMID:14993594; http://dx.doi.org/10.1073/pnas.0400525101.

94. Ku CL, von Bernuth H, Picard C, Zhang SY, Chang HH, Yang K, et al. Selective predisposition to bacterial infections in IRAK-4-deficient children: IRAK-4-dependent TLRs are otherwise redundant in protective immunity. J Exp Med 2007; 204:2407-22; PMID:17893200; http://dx.doi.org/10.1084/jem.20070628.

95. von Bernuth H, Picard C, Jin Z, Pankla R, Xiao H, Ku CL, et al. Pyogenic bacterial infections in humans with MyD88 deficiency. Science 2008; 321:691-6; PMID:18669862; http://dx.doi.org/10.1126/science.1158298.

96. Schnare M, Barton GM, Holt AC, Takeda K, Akira S, Medzhitov R. Toll-like receptors control activation of adaptive immune responses. Nat Immunol 2001; 2:947-50; PMID:11547333; http://dx.doi.org/10.1038/ni712.

97. Pasare C, Medzhitov R. Toll pathway-dependent blockade of CD4+CD25+ T cell-mediated suppression by dendritic cells. Science 2003; 299:1033-6; PMID:12532024; http://dx.doi.org/10.1126/science.1078231.
98. Pasare C, Medzhitov R. Toll-like receptors: linking innate and adaptive immunity. Microbes Infect 2004; 6:1382-7; PMID:15596124; http://dx.doi.org/10.1016/j.micinf.2004.08.018.
99. Pasare C, Medzhitov R. Control of B-cell responses by Toll-like receptors. Nature 2005; 438:364-8; PMID:16292312; http://dx.doi.org/10.1038/nature04267.
100. Janeway CA Jr. Approaching the asymptote? Evolution and revolution in immunology. Cold Spring Harb Symp Quant Biol 1989; 54:1-13; PMID:2700931.
101. Gavin AL, Hoebe K, Duong B, Ota T, Martin C, Beutler B, et al. Adjuvant-enhanced antibody responses in the absence of toll-like receptor signaling. Science 2006; 314:1936-8; PMID:17185603; http://dx.doi.org/10.1126/science.1135299.
102. Palm NW, Medzhitov R. Immunostimulatory activity of haptenated proteins. Proc Natl Acad Sci U S A 2009; 106:4782-7; PMID:19255434; http://dx.doi.org/10.1073/pnas.0809403105.
103. Hidmark AS, McInerney GM, Nordström EK, Douagi I, Werner KM, Liljeström P, et al. Early alpha/ beta interferon production by myeloid dendritic cells in response to UV-inactivated virus requires viral entry and interferon regulatory factor 3 but not MyD88. J Virol 2005; 79:10376-85; PMID:16051830; http://dx.doi.org/10.1128/JVI.79.16.10376-10385.2005.
104. Slack E, Hapfelmeier S, Stecher B, Velykoredko Y, Stoel M, Lawson MA, et al. Innate and adaptive immunity cooperate flexibly to maintain host-microbiota mutualism. Science 2009; 325:617-20; PMID:19644121; http://dx.doi.org/10.1126/science.1172747.
105. Ishikawa E, Ishikawa T, Morita YS, Toyonaga K, Yamada H, Takeuchi O, et al. Direct recognition of the mycobacterial glycolipid, trehalose dimycolate, by C-type lectin Mincle. J Exp Med 2009; 206:2879-88; PMID:20008526; http://dx.doi.org/10.1084/jem.20091750.
106. Matsunaga I, Moody DB. Mincle is a long sought receptor for mycobacterial cord factor. J Exp Med 2009; 206:2865-8; PMID:20008525; http://dx.doi.org/10.1084/jem.20092533.
107. Marakalala MJ, Graham LM, Brown GD. The role of Syk/CARD9-coupled C-type lectin receptors in immunity to Mycobacterium tuberculosis infections. Clin Dev Immunol 2010; 2010: 567571.
108. Schoenen H, Bodendorfer B, Hitchens K, Manzanero S, Werninghaus K, Nimmerjahn F, et al. Cutting edge: Mincle is essential for recognition and adjuvanticity of the mycobacterial cord factor and its synthetic analog trehalose-dibehenate. J Immunol 2010; 184:2756-60; PMID:20164423; http://dx.doi.org/10.4049/jimmunol.0904013.
109. Asquith MJ, Boulard O, Powrie F, Maloy KJ. Pathogenic and protective roles of MyD88 in leukocytes and epithelial cells in mouse models of inflammatory bowel disease. Gastroenterology 2010; 139:519-29, 529, e1-2; PMID:20433840; http://dx.doi.org/10.1053/j.gastro.2010.04.045.
110. Fukata M, Michelsen KS, Eri R, Thomas LS, Hu B, Lukasek K, et al. Toll-like receptor-4 is required for intestinal response to epithelial injury and limiting bacterial translocation in a murine model of acute colitis. Am J Physiol Gastrointest Liver Physiol 2005; 288:G1055-65; PMID:15826931; http://dx.doi.org/10.1152/ajpgi.00328.2004.
111. Rakoff-Nahoum S, Paglino J, Eslami-Varzaneh F, Edberg S, Medzhitov R. Recognition of commensal microflora by toll-like receptors is required for intestinal homeostasis. Cell 2004; 118:229-41; PMID:15260992; http://dx.doi.org/10.1016/j.cell.2004.07.002.
112. Araki A, Kanai T, Ishikura T, Makita S, Uraushihara K, Iiyama R, et al. MyD88-deficient mice develop severe intestinal inflammation in dextran sodium sulfate colitis. J Gastroenterol 2005; 40:16-23; PMID:15692785; http://dx.doi.org/10.1007/s00535-004-1492-9.
113. Brandl K, Sun L, Neppl C, Siggs OM, Le Gall SM, Tomisato W, et al. MyD88 signaling in nonhematopoietic cells protects mice against induced colitis by regulating specific EGF receptor ligands. Proc Natl Acad Sci U S A 2010; 107:19967-72; PMID:21041656; http://dx.doi.org/10.1073/pnas.1014669107.
114. Abreu MT. Toll-like receptor signalling in the intestinal epithelium: how bacterial recognition shapes intestinal function. Nat Rev Immunol 2010; 10:131-44; PMID:20098461; http://dx.doi.org/10.1038/nri2707.
115. Christensen SR, Shupe J, Nickerson K, Kashgarian M, Flavell RA, Shlomchik MJ. Toll-like receptor 7 and TLR9 dictate autoantibody specificity and have opposing inflammatory and regulatory roles in a murine model of lupus. Immunity 2006; 25:417-28; PMID:16973389; http://dx.doi.org/10.1016/j.immuni.2006.07.013.
116. Lau CM, Broughton C, Tabor AS, Akira S, Flavell RA, Mamula MJ, et al. RNA-associated autoantigens activate B cells by combined B cell antigen receptor/Toll-like receptor 7 engagement. J Exp Med 2005; 202:1171-7; PMID:16260486; http://dx.doi.org/10.1084/jem.20050630.
117. Kono DH, Haraldsson MK, Lawson BR, Pollard KM, Koh YT, Du X, et al. Endosomal TLR signaling is required for anti-nucleic acid and rheumatoid factor autoantibodies in lupus. Proc Natl Acad Sci U S A 2009; 106:12061-6; PMID:19574451; http://dx.doi.org/10.1073/pnas.0905441106.

118. Pisitkun P, Deane JA, Difilippantonio MJ, Tarasenko T, Satterthwaite AB, Bolland S. Autoreactive B cell responses to RNA-related antigens due to TLR7 gene duplication. Science 2006; 312:1669-72; PMID:16709748; http://dx.doi.org/10.1126/science.1124978.

119. Subramanian S, Tus K, Li QZ, Wang A, Tian XH, Zhou J, et al. A Tlr7 translocation accelerates systemic autoimmunity in murine lupus. Proc Natl Acad Sci U S A 2006; 103:9970-5; PMID:16777955; http://dx.doi.org/10.1073/pnas.0603912103.

120. Deane JA, Pisitkun P, Barrett RS, Feigenbaum L, Town T, Ward JM, et al. Control of toll-like receptor 7 expression is essential to restrict autoimmunity and dendritic cell proliferation. Immunity 2007; 27:801-10; PMID:17997333; http://dx.doi.org/10.1016/j.immuni.2007.09.009.

121. Fairhurst AM, Hwang SH, Wang A, Tian XH, Boudreaux C, Zhou XJ, et al. Yaa autoimmune phenotypes are conferred by overexpression of TLR7. Eur J Immunol 2008; 38:1971-8; PMID:18521959; http://dx.doi.org/10.1002/eji.200838138.

122. Santiago-Raber ML, Kikuchi S, Borel P, Uematsu S, Akira S, Kotzin BL, et al. Evidence for genes in addition to Tlr7 in the Yaa translocation linked with acceleration of systemic lupus erythematosus. J Immunol 2008; 181:1556-62; PMID:18606711.

123. Demaria O, Pagni PP, Traub S, de Gassart A, Branzk N, Murphy AJ, et al. TLR8 deficiency leads to autoimmunity in mice. J Clin Invest 2010; 120:3651-62; PMID:20811154.

124. Christensen SR, Kashgarian M, Alexopoulou L, Flavell RA, Akira S, Shlomchik MJ. Toll-like receptor 9 controls anti-DNA autoantibody production in murine lupus. J Exp Med 2005; 202:321-31; PMID:16027240; http://dx.doi.org/10.1084/jem.20050338.

125. Wu X, Peng SL. Toll-like receptor 9 signaling protects against murine lupus. Arthritis Rheum 2006; 54:336-42; PMID:16385525; http://dx.doi.org/10.1002/art.21553.

126. Lartigue A, Courville P, Auquit I, François A, Arnoult C, Tron F, et al. Role of TLR9 in anti-nucleosome and anti-DNA antibody production in lpr mutation-induced murine lupus. J Immunol 2006; 177:1349-54; PMID:16818796.

127. Santiago-Raber ML, Dunand-Sauthier I, Wu T, Li QZ, Uematsu S, Akira S, et al. Critical role of TLR7 in the acceleration of systemic lupus erythematosus in TLR9-deficient mice. J Autoimmun 2010; 34:339-48; PMID:19944565; http://dx.doi.org/10.1016/j.jaut.2009.11.001.

128. Fukui R, Saitoh S, Matsumoto F, Kozuka-Hata H, Oyama M, Tabeta K, et al. Unc93B1 biases Toll-like receptor responses to nucleic acid in dendritic cells toward DNA- but against RNA-sensing. J Exp Med 2009; 206:1339-50; PMID:19451267; http://dx.doi.org/10.1084/jem.20082316.

129. Leadbetter EA, Rifkin IR, Hohlbaum AM, Beaudette BC, Shlomchik MJ, Marshak-Rothstein A. Chromatin-IgG complexes activate B cells by dual engagement of IgM and Toll-like receptors. Nature 2002; 416:603-7; PMID:11948342; http://dx.doi.org/10.1038/416603a.

130. Viglianti GA, Lau CM, Hanley TM, Miko BA, Shlomchik MJ, Marshak-Rothstein A. Activation of autoreactive B cells by CpG dsDNA. Immunity 2003; 19:837-47; PMID:14670301; http://dx.doi.org/10.1016/S1074-7613(03)00323-6.

131. Shi H, Kokoeva MV, Inouye K, Tzameli I, Yin H, Flier JS. TLR4 links innate immunity and fatty acid-induced insulin resistance. J Clin Invest 2006; 116:3015-25; PMID:17053832; http://dx.doi.org/10.1172/JCI28898.

132. Song MJ, Kim KH, Yoon JM, Kim JB. Activation of Toll-like receptor 4 is associated with insulin resistance in adipocytes. Biochem Biophys Res Commun 2006; 346:739-45; PMID:16781673; http://dx.doi.org/10.1016/j.bbrc.2006.05.170.

133. Poggi M, Bastelica D, Gual P, Iglesias MA, Gremeaux T, Knauf C, et al. C3H/HeJ mice carrying a toll-like receptor 4 mutation are protected against the development of insulin resistance in white adipose tissue in response to a high-fat diet. Diabetologia 2007; 50:1267-76; PMID:17426960; http://dx.doi.org/10.1007/s00125-007-0654-8.

134. Imai Y, Kuba K, Neely GG, Yaghubian-Malhami R, Perkmann T, van Loo G, et al. Identification of oxidative stress and Toll-like receptor 4 signaling as a key pathway of acute lung injury. Cell 2008; 133:235-49; PMID:18423196; http://dx.doi.org/10.1016/j.cell.2008.02.043.

135. Schaen L, Mercurio MG. Treatment of human papilloma virus in a 6-month-old infant with imiquimod 5% cream. Pediatr Dermatol 2001; 18:450-2; PMID:11737697; http://dx.doi.org/10.1046/j.1525-1470.2001.1980b.x.

136. Lacarrubba F, Potenza MC, Gurgone S, Micali G. Successful treatment and management of large superficial basal cell carcinomas with topical imiquimod 5% cream: a case series and review. J Dermatolog Treat 2011; 22:353-8; PMID:21781010; http://dx.doi.org/10.3109/09546634.2010.548503.

137. Lee SJ, Silverman E, Bargman JM. The role of antimalarial agents in the treatment of SLE and lupus nephritis. Nat Rev Nephrol 2011; 7:718-29; PMID:22009248; http://dx.doi.org/10.1038/nrneph.2011.150.

138. Sau K, Mambula SS, Latz E, Henneke P, Golenbock DT, Levitz SM. The antifungal drug amphotericin B promotes inflammatory cytokine release by a Toll-like receptor- and CD14-dependent mechanism. J Biol Chem 2003; 278:37561-8; PMID:12860979; http://dx.doi.org/10.1074/jbc.M306137200.

CHAPTER 3

Nucleic Acid-Sensing TLR Signaling Pathways

Yutaro Kumagai and Shizuo Akira*

Abstract

Our understanding of innate immunity has expanded rapidly since the discovery in 1996 of Toll as a cellular receptor in fruit flies that recognizes invading pathogens. Of the Toll-like receptors (TLRs) that have since been identified, mouse and human TLR3, TLR7, TLR8 and TLR9 recognize nucleic acids of pathogens. It has become apparent that the innate immune responses evoked by these nucleic acid-sensing TLRs are essential for inducing not only protective immunity but also vaccination against viruses. Current research is beginning to elucidate the intracellular signaling mechanisms downstream of these receptors on both molecular and cell biological levels, although the details of these intricate pathways remain incompletely defined. In this review, we describe the recent advances in nucleic acid-sensing TLR signaling research, with emphasis on the roles of these receptors in immune responses, their differential utilization of signaling pathways, and their intracellular trafficking.

Introduction

Mammals have two distinct immune systems; innate and acquired. One of the hallmarks of the acquired immune system is its almost infinite variety of receptors for antigen, which arise during genetic rearrangement and somatic hypermutation. Moreover, the acquired immune system has memory characteristics, which enable specific responses to secondary infection and form the principle underlying vaccination. In contrast, the innate immune system was previously thought of as primitive, unsophisticated, and only helpful up until the acquired immune system starts to work. However, the discovery of Toll as a receptor recognizing invading pathogens in the fruit fly *Drosophila melanogaster*,[1] followed by cloning of mammalian Toll-like receptor,[2] revealed that the innate immune system is able to recognize a variety of molecules derived from pathogens, and even to control acquired immunity. Ten and 13 Toll-like receptors (TLRs) have so far been identified in human and mouse, respectively.[3] These germ line-encoded receptors can sense a broad range of compounds called pathogen-associated molecular patterns (PAMPs), which include proteins, bacterial cell wall components such as sugars and lipids and nucleic acids. After recognition, TLRs induce intracellular signaling cascades that lead to pleiotropic responses, including the production of proinflammatory cytokines, and consequently contribute to the activation of the acquired immune response.

Mammalian TLR3, TLR7, TLR8 and TLR9 can recognize nucleic acids of pathogens and elicit pathogen-specific immune responses (Fig. 1).[3] These nucleic acid-sensing TLRs are essential for inducing protective vaccination against viruses. The intracellular signaling cascades downstream of these receptors have been recently described. In this review, we present the current understanding

*Laboratory of Host Defense, WPI Immunology Frontier Research Center, and Department of Host Defense, Research Institute for Microbial Diseases, Osaka University, Osaka, Japan. Corresponding Author: Yutaro Kumagai—Email: ykumagai@biken.osaka-u.ac.jp

Nucleic Acid Sensors and Antiviral Immunity, edited by Suryaprakash Sambhara and Takashi Fujita.

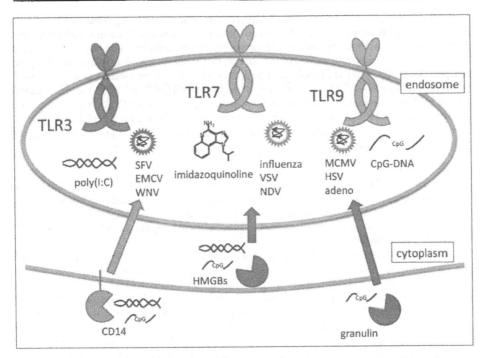

Figure 1. Nucleic acid-sensing TLRs. Human and mouse TLR3, 7, 8, and 9 recognize nucleic acid ligands. TLR3 recognizes poly(I:C), Semliki Forest virus (SFV), encephalomyocarditis virus (EMCV), and West Nile virus (WNV). TLR7 and TLR8 sense imidazoquinoline derivatives such as R-848 (resiquimod) and R-837 (imiquimod), and guanosine analogs such as loxoribine. Genomic ssRNA from viruses, such as influenza virus, vesicular stomatitis virus (VSV) and Newcastle disease virus (NDV), are also recognized by TLR7. TLR9 senses unmethylated CpG DNA. Viral DNA from mouse cytomegalovirus (MCMV), herpes simplex virus 1 (HSV 1), HSV-2, and adenovirus can also activate TLR9. These TLRs reside in intracellular membrane compartments, and their ligands are transported to these compartments by cofactors, including granulin, CD14, and HMGBs.

of nucleic acid-sensing TLRs, with emphasis on their roles in immune responses, their differential utilization of signaling pathways, and their intracellular trafficking.

Nucleic Acid-Sensing TLRs and Their Cofactors

TLR3

TLR3 was first identified as a receptor for a synthetic analog of double-stranded RNA (dsRNA) called poly(I:C).[4] TLR3 utilizes TRIF as its adaptor molecule, and both proinflammatory cytokines and IFN-inducible genes are induced upon stimulation of TLR3 by poly(I:C). A crystallographic study demonstrated that TLR3 forms a dimer when it binds to poly(I:C).[5]

poly(I:C) is a strong adjuvant, and loss of TLR3 or its adaptor TRIF impairs poly(I:C)-induced NK cell activation and antigen-specific T-cell responses.[6-8] Semliki Forest virus,[9] encephalomyocarditis virus (EMCV)[10] and West Nile virus (WNV)[11] are also recognized by TLR3. These single-stranded RNA (ssRNA) viruses produce dsRNA during their replication, which may serve as the ligand for TLR3. A pancreatic β-cell-trophic EMCV strain induces diabetes in TLR3-deficient mice but not in wild-type mice, suggesting a role of TLR3 in the protection against type I diabetes.[12]

TLR3 also confers resistance to DNA viruses such as mouse cytomegalovirus (MCMV),[13] although the TLR ligands produced by these viruses are unknown. An autosomal dominant mutation in *Tlr3* was found in patients with herpes simplex encephalitis caused by herpes simplex virus 1 (HSV-1).[14] An autosomal recessive mutation that results in complete loss of the *Tlr3* gene has been identified, and the fibroblasts of patients with this mutation were unable to respond to poly(I:C) and HSV-1.[15] However, the response against poly(I:C) and HSV-1 in the patients' peripheral blood mononuclear cells remained intact, suggesting that TLR3 is redundant for protection against HSV-1 outside the central nervous system. These patients exhibited no overt clinical manifestations other than herpes simplex encephalitis. Collectively, these results suggest that TLR3 is important in anti-HSV-1 immunity in central nervous system.

TLR7 and TLR8

The genes encoding TLR7 and TLR8 reside in proximity to one another on the X chromosome in both mouse and human. TLR7 was first identified as a receptor for imidazoquinoline derivatives such as R-848 (resiquimod) and R-837 (imiquimod).[16] It also recognizes guanosine analogs such as loxoribine.[17] MyD88-deficient cells do not respond to these compounds, indicating that TLR7 and TLR8 utilize MyD88 as an adaptor molecule.[16]

A cell type called plasmacytoid dendritic cells (pDC), which express high levels of B220 and intermediate levels of CD11c, is known to be an efficient producer of type I IFN, especially IFN-α, in response to viral infection.[18] A study using a reporter mouse strain in which IFN-α6 expression can be monitored with GFP showed that pDC are a major IFN-α producer in response to systemic viral infection.[19] TLR7-deficient pDC failed to respond to ssRNA viruses such as influenza virus[20] and vesicular stomatitis virus (VSV)[21] in vitro, and to Newcastle disease virus in vivo.[22] Deletion of TLR7 or its adaptor MyD88 impaired antigen-specific T-cell responses and immunoglobulin production upon secondary infection with influenza virus, indicating that vaccination with a live influenza virus vaccine strain requires TLR7-MyD88 signaling.[23] Recent studies have also indicated that TLR7 recognizes RNAs from specific bacteria and fungi, including *Streptococcus pneumoniae*[24] and *Candida albicans*.[25]

TLR9

TLR9 senses unmethylated CpG DNA.[26] The CpG motif is methylated in mammals but not in viruses and bacteria, and thus unmethylated CpG motifs can serve as a PAMP. TLR9 may also recognize hemozoin, which is generated by the malaria parasite *Plasmodium falciparum*.[27] In vitro binding assays have indicated that TLR9 directly binds to CpG DNA and hemozoin,[28] and surface plasmon resonance assays have revealed that base-free phosphodiester 2' deoxyribose binds directly to TLR9, consequently activating TLR9 signaling.[29] DNA bases achieve this effect even in the absence of CpG motifs. In contrast, phosphothioate modified 2' deoxyribose acts as an antagonist for both TLR9 and TLR7 if the CpG motif is absent.[29] Thus, the sugar backbone may determine the specificity of TLR9 ligands, although further molecular studies on the structures of TLR9 and its ligand are needed to elucidate how these specificities arise. TLR9 utilizes MyD88 as an adaptor molecule.[30]

pDC are also strong producers of IFN-α in response to TLR9 stimuli.[18] TLR9 recognizes MCMV,[31] HSV-1,[32] HSV-2[33] and adenovirus[34] in vivo, and is essential for antiviral responses against these viruses via pDC.

Cofactors for Nucleic Acid-Sensing TLRs

Several proteins act as cofactors for nucleic acid-sensing TLRs. Granulin and fragments derived from it by cleavage with elastase serve as soluble cofactors for TLR9. Granulin captures CpG oligodeoxynucleotide (CpG-ODN) and delivers it to the endosome. Loss of granulin impairs TLR9 signaling in response to CpG-ODN, while the addition of granulin protein restores this signaling.[35]

CD14 was originally characterized as a co-receptor for TLR4.[36] However, a recent study revealed that it also serves as a co-receptor for TLR3, TLR7 and TLR9. Deficiency in CD14 partially impairs CpG-ODN, imiquimod and poly(I:C)-induced responses such as proinflammatory cytokine production. CD14 is required for optimal uptake of CpG-ODN but is dispensable for uptake of the virus itself. However, it is required for virus-induced cytokine production.[37] In addition, HMGB proteins also bind to all immunogenic nucleic acids and facilitate TLR3, TLR7 and TLR9-dependent recognition of cognate nucleic acids.[38]

Adaptor Molecules and Their Signaling

Following the identification of TLRs in mammals, adaptor molecules which transmit information evoked by the engagement of a TLR with its ligands into intracellular signaling cascades began to be identified. At least five such adaptor molecules have been described in mammals; MyD88, TIRAP, TRIF, TRAM and SARM.[3] They all possess Toll-IL-1R homology (TIR) domains, which mediate the homotypic interaction between TIR domains in the cytosolic portion of TLR and those of adaptor proteins. Forward and reverse genetics, functional screening and bioinformatics approaches have revealed the roles of these molecules in TLR signaling.

MyD88 is the most frequently-used adaptor molecule, being used by all TLRs except TLR3 (Fig. 2). MyD88 also serves as an adaptor for IL-1R. TRIF and TIRAP are used by TLR3 and TLR4 and TLR2 and TLR4, respectively. TRAM appears to only transmit TLR4 signaling.

MyD88-Dependent Pathway for TLR4 Signaling

Injection of LPS into the blood stream of mice causes severe septic shock characterized by the production of pro-inflammatory cytokines and ultimately death. However, several inbred mouse strains exist that are resistant to LPS-induced septic shock. In the mid-1990s, it was revealed that some of these strains harbor mutations in the *Tlr4* locus, providing evidence that TLR4 is a receptor for LPS.[39,40] Analysis of TLR4-deficent mice also showed that the deletion of TLR4 impaired LPS-induced cytokine production from macrophages and septic shock in mice.[41] These results established the role of TLR4 as an LPS sensor.

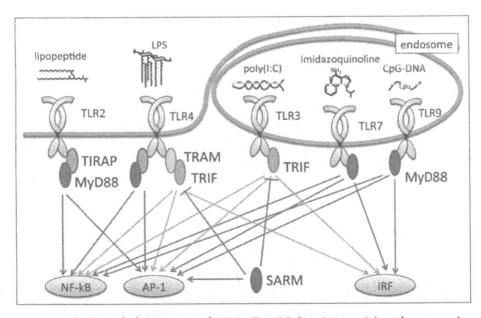

Figure 2. Utilization of adaptor proteins by TLRs. Five TIR domain-containing adaptor proteins have been identified. While MyD88 is involved in the signal transmission from all TLRs except TLR3, TRIF is specifically involved in TLR3 and TLR4, TIRAP transmits signaling of TLR2 which recognizes lipopeptide and TLR4 which recognizes LPS, and TRAM is used only by the TLR4 signaling pathway. SARM has been reported to suppress TRIF-dependent signaling and to control MAPK activation in neurons.

Another report showed that MyD88-deficient mice, in which IL-1 and IL-18 signaling is impaired,[42] also exhibit resistance to LPS-induced septic shock.[43] Furthermore, MyD88-deficient cells failed to produce cytokines in response to LPS, indicating that MyD88 serves as a downstream molecule of the LPS receptor TLR4. In this pathway, as also occurs in IL-1R signaling, MyD88 recruits IRAK via a death domain-mediated homotypic interaction between the two molecules. MyD88 deletion impairs activation of IRAK. These findings collectively defined the role of MyD88 as an adaptor molecule for TLR4, and subsequent analysis on MyD88-deficient mice showed that MyD88 is involved not only in TLR4 signaling but also in the TLR2, TLR7 and TLR9 signaling pathways.[3]

Discovery of the MyD88-Independent Pathway and Identification of TRIF

The identification of MyD88, however, led to new questions in the understanding of TLR signaling. Downstream signaling pathways, namely the MAP kinase, which activates transcription factor AP-1, and IKK-NF-κB pathways, were not abolished but only delayed in MyD88-deficient mice upon LPS stimulation, whereas TLR4-deficiency totally abolished activation of all of these pathways.[44] In contrast, the deletion of either MyD88 or TLR2 diminished activation of all the pathways following stimulation of TLR2 by its ligand MALP-2.[45,46] These data collectively suggested the existence of a TLR4-specific, MyD88-independent signaling mechanism which leads to the activation of NF-κB and MAPKs. Furthermore, the fact that LPS stimulation in the absence of MyD88 still induces maturation of dendritic cells (DC) also implied that other adaptor molecules are involved, not only in signaling but also in the physiological function of immune cells.[47]

Bioinformatics analysis had previously shown that a domain called the TIR domain is shared among insect Toll receptors, mammalian TLRs and IL-1Rs and MyD88.[48] Homology searches using this domain identified another adaptor candidate homologous to MyD88, which was named MyD88-adaptor-like (Mal)[49] or TIRAP.[50] In vitro studies suggested the involvement of TIRAP/Mal in the MyD88-independent pathway.[50] Reverse genetic studies, however, revealed that TIRAP is involved only in MyD88-dependent TLR2 and TLR4 signaling.[51,52]

Other groups used bioinformatics[53] and yeast two-hybrid screening[54] to identify another TIR domain-containing adaptor, called TRIF/TICAM-1. One of the hallmarks of the MyD88-indepdent TLR4 signaling pathway is the activation of the transcription factor IRF3 and subsequent induction of interferon-inducible genes. Overexpression of TRIF/TICAM-1 induced the activation of the IFN-β promoter. TRIF/TICAM-1 binds to the TIR domain of TLR3.[53,54] These results collectively indicated that TRIF/TICAM-1 is the adaptor molecule involved in MyD88-independent pathway for TLR4 signaling, and both forward and reverse genetic approaches established the role of TRIF in this pathway. Loss of TRIF results in the impaired induction of interferon-inducible genes upon LPS stimulation, and deletion of both MyD88 and TRIF totally abolishes NF-κB activation, MAPK activation, and maturation of DC upon LPS stimulation.[55] Cytokine production and interferon-inducible gene induction in response to poly (I:C), a TLR3 ligand, are also abrogated in TRIF-deficient cells.[55] Further evidence for this role for TRIF came from the identification of another LPS-unresponsive mutation, called *Lps2*, which was found to be localized in the *Trif* locus.[56] Taken together, these data indicate that TRIF is a genuine adaptor molecule for the MyD88-independent pathway. A microarray gene expression analysis study showed that gene induction in response to LPS stimulation is completely abolished in MyD88 and TRIF double deficient mice.[57] This suggests there is no additional pathway for TLR4 signaling other than the MyD88- and TRIF-dependent pathways.

Another adaptor molecule, TRAM, was found by both bioinformatics and yeast two-hybrid screening.[58-60] It is specifically involved in the MyD88-independent TRIF-dependent pathway of TLR4 signaling, but not during TLR3 signaling, as revealed by TRAM-deficient mice.[59]

SARM: Not a Genuine TLR Adaptor?

SARM also contains a TIR domain, and is thought to be an adaptor molecule for TLRs, having been described as a negative regulator of MyD88-independent TRIF-dependent signaling upon TLR3 or TLR4 stimulation. SARM associates with TRIF via its SAM and TIR domains. Knock-down of SARM led to increased expression of TRIF-dependent genes,[61] but SARM-deficient cells normally respond to TLR stimuli.[62] One study demonstrated that SARM interacts with JNK3 in neurons, and SARM-deficient neurons are defective in cell death after deprivation of oxygen and glucose.[62] Another report showed that SARM interacts with syndecan-2 and controls neuronal morphology.[63] These results suggest that SARM is also involved in physiological processes distinct from its role in innate immunity.

SARM provides the nematode *Caenorhabditis elegans* with innate immune responses via control of antimicrobial peptide gene expression,[64] although its binding partner is not the worm TLR TOL-1, but PMK-1, a worm p38 MAPK.[65] SARM has been shown to act as an inhibitor for TLR-mediated MAPK signaling in mammals.[66] SARM-deficient mice are susceptible for West Nile virus infection. Loss of SARM led to decreased activation of microglia and increased neuronal death in the brainstem.[67] Thus, it appears that SARM also acts as immune modulator, although the molecular mechanism by which SARM controls innate immune response and neuronal death and morphology remains to be clarified.

Signaling Cascades Downstream of MyD88 and TRIF

The MyD88 dependent signaling pathway has been extensively investigated (Fig. 3). Upon stimulation of MyD88, the downstream molecules IRAK1, 2, and 4 are recruited and activated.

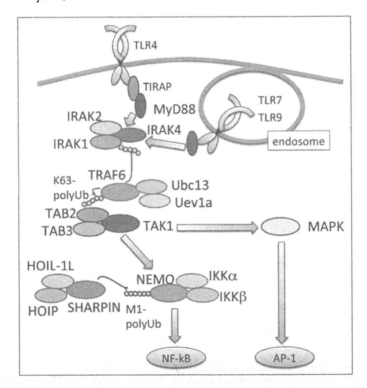

Figure 3. MyD88-dependent pathway. An overview of the MyD88-dependent pathway leading to NF-κB and MAPK activation is shown. MyD88 sequesters IRAK1, 2, and 4. The activation of IRAK kinases leads to an interaction with TRAF6, which catalyzes K63-type ubiquitination of target proteins such as TRAF6 itself, in conjunction with the E2 ubiquitin-conjugating enzymes Ubc13 and Uev1A. TAB2 and TAB3 in TAK1 complexes then bind to the polyubiquitin chain, resulting in a complex which activates the IKK complex and MAPK. LUBAC, consisted of HOIL-1L, HOIP, and SHARPIN, mediates linear M1 polyubiquitination of the IKK complex component NEMO and subsequently induces its activation leading to NF-κB activation.

Crystallography has recently revealed that MyD88 and IRAK proteins form a helical multimer.[68] Deletion of IRAK4 impaired cytokine production in response to various TLR stimuli, indicating a general role for IRAK4 in TLR signaling.[69] IRAK1 and IRAK2 have redundant but temporally differential roles in TLR2 and TLR4 signaling: IRAK1 is activated at earlier time points, upto 1 h after stimulation, and IRAK2 activation follows it to achieve robust signaling.[70] The activation of IRAK kinases leads to an interaction with TRAF6, which catalyzes K63-type ubiquitination of target proteins such as TRAF6 itself, in conjunction with the E2 ubiquitin-conjugating enzymes Ubc13 and Uev1A.[71] TAB2 and TAB3 in complexes with TAK1 then bind to the polyubiquitin chain, resulting in a complex which activates the IKK complex and MAPK.[72,73] Recent studies have indicated that both the K63 polyubiquitin chain and the linear M1 polyubiquitin chain are important for activation of NF-κB. The linear ubiquitin chain assembly complex (LUBAC) promotes the activation process. NEMO, one of the components in the IKK complex, is linearly polyubiquitinated and subsequently activated in a LUBAC-dependent manner.[74] Indeed, deficiency in SHARPIN, an essential component of LUBAC, has been shown to impair macrophage responses to TLR stimuli.[75]

NF-κB is also activated downstream of TRIF (Fig. 4). After recognition of LPS, TLR4 translocates from the cytoplasmic membrane to the endosome, where TLR4 associates with TRIF and TRAM.[76] TRIF binds to TRAF6 and activated IKK complexes.[77] TRIF-induced

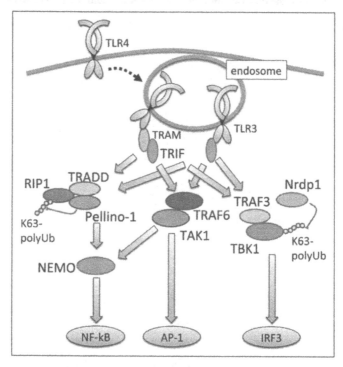

Figure 4. TRIF-dependent pathway. After recognition of LPS, TLR4 translocates from the cytoplasmic membrane to the endosome, where TLR4 associates with TRIF and TRAM. TRIF binds to TRAF6 and activated IKK complexes through TAK1, although TRIF-induced NF-κB activation is slower than that induced by the action of MyD88. TRIF also associates with RIP1 and RIP3 kinases and subsequently activates NF-κB via these kinases. TRADD serves as an adaptor protein by binding to RIP1. Pellino-1 has also been reported as a binding partner of RIP1, and it facilitates ubiquitination of RIP1. TRIF associates with TBK1 and in turn phosphorylates IRF3 molecules, which dimerize and translocate into the nucleus, where they serve to induce interferon-inducible genes. Nrdp1 K63-ubiquitinates TBK1 and activates the kinase. TRAF3 may also be a component of TRIF-dependent signaling.

NF-κB activation is slower than that of MyD88-induced activation, although the mechanism leading to this temporal difference is still unclear. TRIF can also associate with RIP1 and RIP3 kinases and subsequently activate NF-κB via these kinases.[78] TRADD serves as an adaptor protein and binds to RIP1, and TRADD-deficiency has been shown to impair NF-κB activation upon TLR3 stimulation.[79,80] Pellino-1 is another binding partner of RIP1 that facilitates K63-type ubiquitination of RIP1; Pellino-1-deficient cells show impaired TRIF-dependent gene expression upon TLR3 and TLR4 stimulation.[81]

TRIF also binds to TBK1, a kinase phosphorylating IRF3 upon stimulation.[77] The TRIF-dependent pathway in TLR3 and TLR4 signaling leads to TBK1-mediated IRF3 phosphorylation, and phosphorylated IRF3 molecules in turn dimerize and translocate into nucleus, where interferon-inducible genes are induced. A ubiquitin ligase called Nrdp1 associates with MyD88 and TBK1 upon TLR4 stimulation, catalyzing K48-type and K63-type polyubiquitination, respectively. The ubiquitination leads to degradation of MyD88 and activation of TBK1 and results in preferential activation of TRIF- and TBK1-dependent signaling.[82] TRAF3 is also involved in TRIF-dependent signaling. Interestingly, TRAF3 plays a similar role to Nrdp1: TRAF3 binds to both MyD88 and TRIF, but ubiquitinates only MyD88 to promote its degradation.[83] This preferential ubiquitination leads to suppression of MyD88-dependent signaling and promotion of TRIF-dependent signaling.

MyD88-Dependent Pathway in Nucleic Acid-Sensing TLR7 and TLR9

As mentioned above, TLR7 and TLR9 utilize MyD88 as an adaptor molecule and induce proinflammatory cytokines as well as IFN-inducible genes upon stimulation, similar to the effects seen following TLR3 and TLR4 stimulation. However, unlike TLR3 and TLR4, TLR7 and TLR9 do not utilize TRIF (Fig. 5).

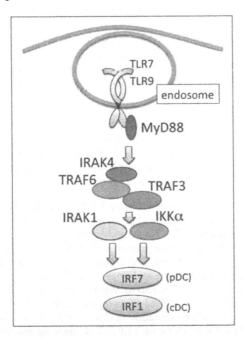

Figure 5. MyD88-dependent pathway under TLR7 and TLR9. When TLR7 or TLR9 on pDC are stimulated, IRF7 co-localizes with MyD88 and IRAK1, and IRAK1 phosphorylates IRF7. IKK-α may also serve as an IRF7 kinase, and IRAK4 may act upstream of IRAK1 and IKK-α. A precursor form of osteopontin is also recruited to the MyD88-IRF7 complex. In cDC, IRF1, instead of IRF7, associates with MyD88. Both IRAK1 and IKK-α are believed to be kinases for IRF1.

A yeast two-hybrid screen of proteins which bind to the death domain of MyD88 identified the transcription factor IRF7 as a binding partner of MyD88.[84] IFN-a4 and IFN-a6 promoters are synergistically activated by co-expression of MyD88 and IRF7, but not by MyD88 and IRF3. TRAF6 was also found to associate with and activate IRF7. These results indicate that IFN-α production from pDC is mediated by the MyD88-TRAF6-IRF7 axis. Interestingly, this IRF7 activation does not involve TBK1, since IFN-α production from TBK1-deficient Flt3L-induced bone marrow DC was comparable to wild-type DC. Subsequent studies using FRET analysis indicated that, following TLR7 or TLR9 stimulation, IRF7 co-localizes with MyD88 and IRAK1.[85,86] IRAK1-deficient pDC fail to produce IFN-α, but normally produce IL-12. IRAK1 phosphorylates IRF7, and may be an additional kinase for IRF7,[85,87] alongside IKK-α. In another study, IRAK4 kinase activity-deficient pDC failed to produce type I IFNs in response to either TLR7 or TLR9 stimulation, suggesting that IRAK4 acts upstream of IRAK1 and/or IKK-α in the signaling pathway.[88]

Additionally, a precursor form of osteopontin is induced upon TLR9 stimulation and is recruited to the MyD88-IRF7 complex in pDC.[89] Inhibition of PI3K, mTOR or p70S6K by specific inhibitors impairs the nuclear translocation of IRF7 and type I IFN production in response to TLR9 stimulation, suggesting that the PI3K-mTOR pathway plays a role in this signal transduction process, although the molecular mechanism for this remains to be elucidated.[90,91]

The signaling processes downstream of TLR7 or TLR9 are slightly different in CD11c high conventional DC (cDC). cDC produce IFN-β but not IFN-α in response to TLR9 stimulation,[92] and an analysis of IRF-1 deficient mice revealed that IRF1, rather than IRF3 and IRF7, is involved in this process,.[93-95] In cDC, IRF1 binds to MyD88, in contrast to the binding of IRF7 to MyD88 that occurs in pDC.[94,95] Again, both IRAK1 and IKK-α are suggested to be kinases for IRF1.[93,94]

Intracellular Protein Trafficking as a Paradigm for Diversity in TLR Signaling

During unstimulated conditions, nucleic acid-sensing TLRs are believed to be localized on intracellular membrane compartments such as the endoplasmic reticulum (ER). Upon activation, these TLRs translocate from the ER to the endosome, where they recognize their ligands.[96] This specialized location for ligand recognition may prevent accidental encounter of TLRs and host nucleic acids.[97]

However, the trigger for this translocation remains to be elucidated. TLR9 starts to translocate even in the absence of MyD88,[96] and DOCK2, which is essential for the activation of IKK-α in response to TLR9 stimulation in pDC, can be activated in a TLR-independent manner.[98] These data collectively suggest that pathways exist for TLR-independent sensing of TLR9 stimulation and subsequent translocation of proteins, and several molecules and mechanisms are already known to be involved in the translocation process (Fig. 6).

ER Proteins Conferring Translocation of TLR7 and TLR9

Cells from mice harboring the mutation known as *3d* are unresponsive to stimulation through all known nucleic acid-sensing TLRs.[99] A forward genetic study identified that the mutation responsible is in the *Unc93b* gene. The protein UNC93B resides in the ER in unstimulated cells, and it has been demonstrated that UNC93B is required for the translocation of nucleic acid-sensing TLRs from the ER to the endosome.[100] UNC93B directly binds to TLR7 and TLR9[101] and, upon stimulation, UNC93B as well as TLR7 and TLR9 relocate from the ER to the endolysosomal compartment.[100] TLR9 competes with TLR7 for UNC93B-dependent trafficking.[102] Interestingly, a D34A mutation in UNC93B has been found to skew the balance between TLR7 and TLR9 trafficking to TLR7. This skewing resulted into systemic lethal inflammation, suggesting that UNC93B plays a role in maintaining homeostasis in the innate immune system.[103] Patients harboring an autosomal recessive mutation in *UNC93B* suffer from herpes simplex encephalitis, underscoring the importance of UNC93B and the translocation process in antiviral responses.[104]

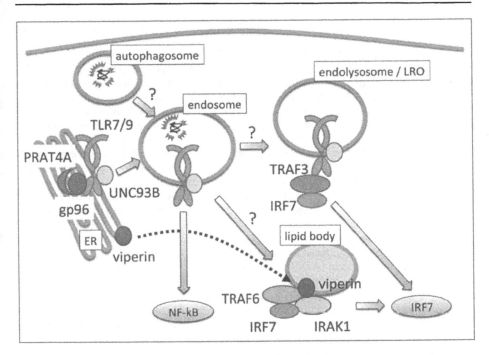

Figure 6. Trafficking of TLR7 and TLR9. During unstimulated conditions, nucleic acid-sensing TLRs are thought to be localized on intracellular membrane compartments such as the ER. Upon activation, the TLRs translocate from the ER to the endosome. On the ER, PRAT4A (also known as CNPY3) and the chaperon gp96 form complexes with TLRs, a process which is essential for translocation. UNC93B associates with TLRs and facilitates translocation from the ER to the endosome. After translocation, autophagy machinery serves as a platform for viral recognition by TLR7 and TLR9, as well as a bifurcation point leading to type I IFN production or to proinflammatory cytokine production. The endosomal protein AP3 is essential for translocation of TLR9 from VAMP3+ endosome to LAMP2+ lysosome-related organelle (LRO). The IFN-inducible protein viperin interacts with IRAK1 and TRAF6, and these molecules are localized at ADRP+ lipid bodies, where IRF7 is also recruited and activated.

Another ER protein, PRAT4A (also known as CNPY3), was identified as a binding partner of TLR4.[105] In knockout mice, PRAT4A-deficiency abrogates cytokine production in response to stimulation on a broad range of TLRs, including TLR7 and TLR9. TLR9 failed to relocate in PRAT4A-deficient cells, suggesting a role for PRAT4A in intracellular trafficking.[106] An ER Hsp90 homolog chaperon gp96 has been reported to associate with TLR9 and PRAT4A to form a multimolecular complex, and cells deficient in gp96 are defective in cytokine production in response to TLR1, 2, 4, 5, 7 and 9.[107] Thus, the chaperone gp96 and the "co-chaperone" PRAT4A are essential for proper translocation of TLR9 from the ER to the endosome.

Signaling at Intracellular Membrane Compartments

Cellular autophagy – the process by which intracellular proteins are degraded – is important for virus recognition by TLR7 in pDC.[108] The autophagy system captures replicating viruses in a specific membrane compartment called the autophagosome and then transfers them to the endosome, where TLR7 is located. Deficiency in Atg5, an essential component of the autophagy machinery, impairs type I IFN production but not IL-12p40 production in response to VSV. TLR9-dependent CpG-ODN- or HSV-1-induced type I IFN production is also impaired in Atg5-deficient pDC.[108] Thus, the autophagy machinery serves as a platform for viral recognition by TLR7 and TLR9, as well as a bifurcation point leading to type I IFN production or to proinflammatory cytokine production.

A recent study showed that AP3 is essential for proper trafficking of TLR9 in pDC. AP3-deficient pDC fail to translocate TLR9 from the VAMP3+ endosome to the LAMP2+ lysosome-related organelle (LRO) but not from the ER to the endosome, as is observed in UNC93B-deficient cells. At the LRO, TRAF3 and IRF7 are sequestered to the compartment and signaling leading to the induction of type I IFN is evoked. Similarly to the outcomes observed in Atg5-deficiency, AP3-deficiency impairs type I IFN production but not IL-12p40 production. Forced sequestration of TRAF3 onto the VAMP3+ endosome restores type I IFN production in the absence of AP3.[109] However, a forward genetic study demonstrated that a mutation in AP3 abrogated both type I IFN and IL-12p40 production in pDC upon TLR7 or TLR9 stimulation.[110] The precise role of AP3 in TLR9 signaling remains to be elucidated.

An IFN-inducible protein, viperin, is another protein that was recently reported to be involved in intracellular trafficking of TLR signaling components.[111] Viperin deficiency impairs type I IFN but not IL-12p40 production in response to TLR7 or TLR9 stimulation, as does either Atg5 or AP3 deficiency. Viperin interacts with IRAK1 and TRAF6, and these molecules are localized at lipid bodies. Lipid bodies are punctuate structures enriched with lipid and expressing adipocyte differentiation-related protein (ADRP). After stimulation, viperin translocates from the ER to ADRP+ lipid bodies and sequesters IRAK1, TRAF6, and IRF7.[111]

Taken together, these findings suggest that TLR7 and TLR9 signaling in pDC may require sequential translocation of receptors which induce different signaling cascades, which in turn are controlled by several molecules. However, the relationships and hierarchies between these molecules and cellular compartments remain to be clarified.

Cleavage of TLRs in Acidic Membrane Compartment

Acidification of the endosomal compartment is crucial for the recognition of nucleic acid by TLRs, and recent studies indicate that acidification is required for the activation of several endopeptidases which cleave TLRs.[112] Cathepsin K-deficiency impairs TLR9 activation,[113] and a forward genetic study using a mutant B-cell line indicates that cathepsin B is involved in TLR9 activation.[114] Subsequent studies demonstrated that cathepsin K and/or B cleave the N-terminus of TLRs.[115] In addition, AEP has also been shown to cleave TLR9, suggesting the involvement of multiple endopeptidases in the cleavage of TLR9. Deletion of asparagine endopeptidase (AEP) abrogated TLR7 and TLR9 responses.[116] Thus, the cleavage of TLRs may be critical for the recognition of their ligand, rendering acidification is essential for the activation of nucleic acid-sensing TLR signaling.

Conclusion

In the past 15 years since the identification of Drosophila Toll as an innate immune receptor, researchers have successfully identified many genes and pathways involved in innate immunity. Here, we have described the current knowledge of nucleic acid-sensing TLRs from the viewpoint of their role in antiviral responses, their signaling and their intracellular trafficking. One of the major focuses of ongoing research is the understanding of the complex networks in which these physiological layers are interconnected.[117] A major reason why an integrated approach to understanding these receptors is desirable is that these TLRs are directly involved in both innate and acquired immune responses. Thus, a better understanding of the mechanism by which these TLRs activate immune responses will help to establish effective therapeutics and vaccination for infectious diseases caused by viruses.

Acknowledgments

The authors are grateful for all the members in Shizuo Akira's lab for helpful discussions. The authors also thank E. Kamada and M. Kageyama for secretarial assistance.

About the Authors

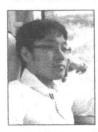

Yutaro Kumagai is an assistant professor in Laboratory of Host Defense, Immunology Frontier Research Center, and in Department of Host Defense, Research Institute for Microbial Diseases, Osaka University, Japan. He received his MS in 2004 from Tokyo Institute of Technology. He pursued his PhD in 2008 from Osaka University Graduate School of Medicine under the direction of Dr Shizuo Akira. From April to September 2008, he was a postdoc at Shizuo Akira's lab, where his research focused on identification of type I interferon producing cells in vivo, and its molecular mechanism. From October 2008, he is in the current position, aiming at systems analysis of innate immunity.

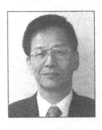

Shizuo Akira is Director of WPI Immunology Frontier Research Center at Osaka University, Japan since 2007, and a professor in Research Institute for Microbial Diseases at Osaka University since 1999. He was a professor in Department of Biochemistry, Hyogo College of Medicine from 1996 to 1999, where he became involved in Toll-like receptor research. He has shown by generating TLR family knockout mice that individual TLRs recognize different microbial components and established the role of TLR family as pathogen recognition receptors, and further clarified the whole picture of their signaling pathways. He is the top cited researcher in the immunological field since 2004. In 2006 and 2007 he was twice recognized the hottest scientist who had published the greatest number of Hot Papers over the preceding two years.

References

1. Lemaitre B, Nicolas E, Michaut L, Reichhart JM, Hoffmann JA, et al. The dorsoventral regulatory gene cassette spatzle/Toll/cactus controls the potent antifungal response in Drosophila adults. Cell 1996; 86:973-83; PMID:8808632; http://dx.doi.org/10.1016/S0092-8674(00)80172-5.
2. Medzhitov R, Preston-Hurlburt P, Janeway CA Jr. A human homologue of the Drosophila Toll protein signals activation of adaptive immunity. Nature 1997; 388:394-7; PMID:9237759; http://dx.doi.org/10.1038/41131.
3. Kawai T, Akira S. The role of pattern-recognition receptors in innate immunity: update on Toll-like receptors. Nat Immunol 2010; 11:373-84; PMID:20404851; http://dx.doi.org/10.1038/ni.1863.
4. Alexopoulou L, Holt AC, Medzhitov R, Flavell RA. Recognition of double-stranded RNA and activation of NF-kappaB by Toll-like receptor 3. Nature 2001; 413:732-8; PMID:11607032; http://dx.doi.org/10.1038/35099560.
5. Liu L, Botos I, Wang Y, Leonard JN, Shiloach J, Segal DM, et al. Structural basis of toll-like receptor 3 signaling with double-stranded RNA. Science 2008; 320:379-81; PMID:18420935; http://dx.doi.org/10.1126/science.1155406.
6. Miyake T, Kumagai Y, Kato H, Guo Z, Matsushita K, Satoh T, et al. Poly I:C-induced activation of NK cells by CD8 alpha+ dendritic cells via the IPS-1 and TRIF-dependent pathways. J Immunol 2009; 183:2522-8; PMID:19635904; http://dx.doi.org/10.4049/jimmunol.0901500.
7. Kumar H, Koyama S, Ishii KJ, Kawai T, Akira S. Cutting edge: cooperation of IPS-1- and TRIF-dependent pathways in poly IC-enhanced antibody production and cytotoxic T cell responses. J Immunol 2008; 180:683-7; PMID:18178804.
8. McCartney S, Vermi W, Gilfillan S, Cella M, Murphy TL, Schreiber RD, et al. Distinct and complementary functions of MDA5 and TLR3 in poly(I:C)-mediated activation of mouse NK cells. J Exp Med 2009; 206:2967-76; PMID:19995959; http://dx.doi.org/10.1084/jem.20091181.
9. Schulz O, Diebold SS, Chen M, Näslund TI, Nolte MA, Alexopoulou L, et al. Toll-like receptor 3 promotes cross-priming to virus-infected cells. Nature 2005; 433:887-92; PMID:15711573; http://dx.doi.org/10.1038/nature03326.
10. Hardarson HS, Baker JS, Yang Z, Purevjav E, Huang CH, Alexopoulou L, et al. Toll-like receptor 3 is an essential component of the innate stress response in virus-induced cardiac injury. Am J Physiol Heart Circ Physiol 2007; 292:H251-8; PMID:16936008; http://dx.doi.org/10.1152/ajpheart.00398.2006.

11. Daffis S, Samuel MA, Suthar MS, Gale M Jr, Diamond MS. Toll-like receptor 3 has a protective role against West Nile virus infection. J Virol 2008; 82:10349-58; PMID:18715906; http://dx.doi. org/10.1128/JVI.00935-08.

12. McCartney SA, Vermi W, Lonardi S, Rossini C, Otero K, Calderon B, et al. RNA sensor-induced type I IFN prevents diabetes caused by a beta cell-tropic virus in mice. J Clin Invest 2011; 121:1497-507; PMID:21403398; http://dx.doi.org/10.1172/JCI44005.

13. Tabeta K, Georgel P, Janssen E, Du X, Hoebe K, Crozat K, et al. Toll-like receptors 9 and 3 as essential components of innate immune defense against mouse cytomegalovirus infection. Proc Natl Acad Sci USA 2004; 101:3516-21; PMID:14993594; http://dx.doi.org/10.1073/pnas.0400525101.

14. Zhang SY, Jouanguy E, Ugolini S, Smahi A, Elain G, Romero P, et al. TLR3 deficiency in patients with herpes simplex encephalitis. Science 2007; 317:1522-7; PMID:17872438; http://dx.doi.org/10.1126/science.1139522.

15. Guo Y, Audry M, Ciancanelli M, Alsina L, Azevedo J, Herman M, et al. Herpes simplex virus encephalitis in a patient with complete TLR3 deficiency: TLR3 is otherwise redundant in protective immunity. J Exp Med 2011; 208:2083-98; PMID:21911422; http://dx.doi.org/10.1084/jem.20101568.

16. Hemmi H, Kaisho T, Takeuchi O, Sato S, Sanjo H, Hoshino K, et al. Small anti-viral compounds activate immune cells via the TLR7 MyD88-dependent signaling pathway. Nat Immunol 2002; 3:196-200; PMID:11812998; http://dx.doi.org/10.1038/ni758.

17. Heil F, Ahmad-Nejad P, Hemmi H, Hochrein H, Ampenberger F, Gellert T, et al. The Toll-like receptor 7 (TLR7)-specific stimulus loxoribine uncovers a strong relationship within the TLR7, 8 and 9 subfamily. Eur J Immunol 2003; 33:2987-97; PMID:14579267; http://dx.doi.org/10.1002/eji.200324238.

18. Reizis B, Bunin A, Ghosh HS, Lewis KL, Sisirak V. Plasmacytoid dendritic cells: recent progress and open questions. Annu Rev Immunol 2011; 29:163-83; PMID:21219184.

19. Kumagai Y, Takeuchi O, Kato H, Kumar H, Matsui K, Morii E, et al. Alveolar macrophages are the primary interferon-alpha producer in pulmonary infection with RNA viruses. Immunity 2007; 27:240-52; PMID:17723216; http://dx.doi.org/10.1016/j.immuni.2007.07.013.

20. Heil F, Hemmi H, Hochrein H, Ampenberger F, Kirschning C, Akira S, et al. Species-specific recognition of single-stranded RNA via toll-like receptor 7 and 8. Science 2004; 303:1526-9; PMID:14976262; http://dx.doi.org/10.1126/science.1093620.

21. Lund JM, Alexopoulou L, Sato A, Karow M, Adams NC, Gale NW, et al. Recognition of single-stranded RNA viruses by Toll-like receptor 7. Proc Natl Acad Sci USA 2004; 101:5598-603; PMID:15034168; http://dx.doi.org/10.1073/pnas.0400937101.

22. Kumagai Y, Kumar H, Koyama S, Kawai T, Takeuchi O, Akira S. Cutting Edge: TLR-Dependent viral recognition along with type I IFN positive feedback signaling masks the requirement of viral replication for IFN-{alpha} production in plasmacytoid dendritic cells. J Immunol 2009; 182:3960-4; PMID:19299691; http://dx.doi.org/10.4049/jimmunol.0804315.

23. Koyama S, Ishii KJ, Kumar H, Tanimoto T, Coban C, Uematsu S, et al. Differential role of TLR- and RLR-signaling in the immune responses to influenza A virus infection and vaccination. J Immunol 2007; 179:4711-20; PMID:17878370.

24. Mancuso G, Gambuzza M, Midiri A, Biondo C, Papasergi S, Akira S, et al. Bacterial recognition by TLR7 in the lysosomes of conventional dendritic cells. Nat Immunol 2009; 10:587-94; PMID:19430477; http://dx.doi.org/10.1038/ni.1733.

25. Bourgeois C, Majer O, Frohner IE, Lesiak-Markowicz I, Hildering KS, Glaser W, et al. Conventional dendritic cells mount a type I IFN response against Candida spp. requiring novel phagosomal TLR7-mediated IFN-beta signaling. J Immunol 2011; 186:3104-12; PMID:21282509; http://dx.doi. org/10.4049/jimmunol.1002599.

26. Hemmi H, Takeuchi O, Kawai T, Kaisho T, Sato S, Sanjo H, et al. A Toll-like receptor recognizes bacterial DNA. Nature 2000; 408:740-5; PMID:11130078; http://dx.doi.org/10.1038/35047123.

27. Coban C, Ishii KJ, Kawai T, Hemmi H, Sato S, Uematsu S, et al. Toll-like receptor 9 mediates innate immune activation by the malaria pigment hemozoin. J Exp Med 2005; 201:19-25; PMID:15630134; http://dx.doi.org/10.1084/jem.20041836.

28. Coban C, Igari Y, Yagi M, Reimer T, Koyama S, Aoshi T, et al. Immunogenicity of whole-parasite vaccines against Plasmodium falciparum involves malarial hemozoin and host TLR9. Cell Host Microbe 2010; 7:50-61; PMID:20114028; http://dx.doi.org/10.1016/j.chom.2009.12.003.

29. Haas T, Metzger J, Schmitz F, Heit A, Müller T, Latz E, et al. The DNA sugar backbone 2' deoxyribose determines toll-like receptor 9 activation. Immunity 2008; 28:315-23; PMID:18342006; http://dx.doi. org/10.1016/j.immuni.2008.01.013.

30. Häcker H, Vabulas RM, Takeuchi O, Hoshino K, Akira S, Wagner H. Immune cell activation by bacterial CpG-DNA through myeloid differentiation marker 88 and tumor necrosis factor receptor-associated factor (TRAF)6. J Exp Med 2000; 192:595-600; PMID:10952730; http://dx.doi.org/10.1084/jem.192.4.595.

31. Krug A, French AR, Barchet W, Fischer JA, Dzionek A, Pingel JT, et al. TLR9-dependent recognition of MCMV by IPC and DC generates coordinated cytokine responses that activate antiviral NK cell function. Immunity 2004; 21:107-19; PMID:15345224; http://dx.doi.org/10.1016/j.immuni.2004.06.007.

32. Hochrein H, Schlatter B, O'Keeffe M, Wagner C, Schmitz F, Schiemann M, et al. Herpes simplex virus type-1 induces IFN-alpha production via Toll-like receptor 9-dependent and -independent pathways. Proc Natl Acad Sci USA 2004; 101:11416-21; PMID:15272082; http://dx.doi.org/10.1073/pnas.0403555101.

33. Lund J, Sato A, Akira S, Medzhitov R, Iwasaki A. Toll-like receptor 9-mediated recognition of Herpes simplex virus-2 by plasmacytoid dendritic cells. J Exp Med 2003; 198:513-20; PMID:12900525; http://dx.doi.org/10.1084/jem.20030162.

34. Zhu J, Huang X, Yang Y. Innate immune response to adenoviral vectors is mediated by both Toll-like receptor-dependent and -independent pathways. J Virol 2007; 81:3170-80; PMID:17229689; http://dx.doi.org/10.1128/JVI.02192-06.

35. Park B, Buti L, Lee S,, et al. Matsuwaki T, Spooner E, Brinkmann MM, et al. Granulin is a soluble cofactor for toll-like receptor 9 signaling. Immunity 2011; 34:505-13; PMID:21497117; http://dx.doi.org/10.1016/j.immuni.2011.01.018.

36. Akira S, Uematsu S, Takeuchi O. Pathogen recognition and innate immunity. Cell 2006; 124:783-801; PMID:16497588; http://dx.doi.org/10.1016/j.cell.2006.02.015.

37. Baumann CL, Aspalter IM, Sharif O, Pichlmair A, Blüml S, Grebien F, et al. CD14 is a coreceptor of Toll-like receptors 7 and 9. J Exp Med 2010; 207:2689-701; PMID:21078886; http://dx.doi.org/10.1084/jem.20101111.

38. Yanai H, Ban T, Wang Z, Choi MK, Kawamura T, Negishi H, et al. HMGB proteins function as universal sentinels for nucleic-acid-mediated innate immune responses. Nature 2009; 462:99-103; PMID:19890330; http://dx.doi.org/10.1038/nature08512.

39. Poltorak A, He X, Smirnova I, Liu MY, Van Huffel C, Du X, et al. Defective LPS signaling in C3H/HeJ and C57BL/10ScCr mice: mutations in Tlr4 gene. Science 1998; 282:2085-8; PMID:9851930; http://dx.doi.org/10.1126/science.282.5396.2085.

40. Qureshi ST, Lariviere L, Leveque G, Clermont S, Moore KJ, Gros P, et al. Endotoxin-tolerant mice have mutations in Toll-like receptor 4 (Tlr4). J Exp Med 1999; 189:615-25; PMID:9989976; http://dx.doi.org/10.1084/jem.189.4.615.

41. Hoshino K, Takeuchi O, Kawai T, Sanjo H, Ogawa T, Takeda Y, et al. Cutting edge: Toll-like receptor 4 (TLR4)-deficient mice are hyporesponsive to lipopolysaccharide: evidence for TLR4 as the Lps gene product. J Immunol 1999; 162:3749-52; PMID:10201887.

42. Adachi O, Kawai T, Takeda K, Matsumoto M, Tsutsui H, Sakagami M, et al. Targeted disruption of the MyD88 gene results in loss of IL-1- and IL-18-mediated function. Immunity 1998; 9:143-50; PMID:9697843; http://dx.doi.org/10.1016/S1074-7613(00)80596-8.

43. Kawai T, Adachi O, Ogawa T, Takeda K, Akira S. Unresponsiveness of MyD88-deficient mice to endotoxin. Immunity 1999; 11:115-22; PMID:10435584; http://dx.doi.org/10.1016/S1074-7613(00)80086-2.

44. Kawai T, Takeuchi O, Fujita T, Inoue J, Mühlradt PF, Sato S, et al. Lipopolysaccharide stimulates the MyD88-independent pathway and results in activation of IFN-regulatory factor 3 and the expression of a subset of lipopolysaccharide-inducible genes. J Immunol 2001; 167:5887-94; PMID:11698465.

45. Takeuchi O, Hoshino K, Kawai T, Sanjo H, Takada H, Ogawa T, et al. Differential roles of TLR2 and TLR4 in recognition of gram-negative and gram-positive bacterial cell wall components. Immunity 1999; 11:443-51; PMID:10549626; http://dx.doi.org/10.1016/S1074-7613(00)80119-3.

46. Takeuchi O, Takeda K, Hoshino K, Adachi O, Ogawa T, Akira S. Cellular responses to bacterial cell wall components are mediated through MyD88-dependent signaling cascades. Int Immunol 2000; 12:113-7; PMID:10607756; http://dx.doi.org/10.1093/intimm/12.1.113.

47. Kaisho T, Takeuchi O, Kawai T, Hoshino K, Akira S. Endotoxin-induced maturation of MyD88-deficient dendritic cells. J Immunol 2001; 166:5688-94; PMID:11313410.

48. Rock FL, Hardiman G, Timans JC, Kastelein RA, Bazan JF. A family of human receptors structurally related to Drosophila Toll. Proc Natl Acad Sci USA 1998; 95:588-93; PMID:9435236; http://dx.doi.org/10.1073/pnas.95.2.588.

49. Fitzgerald KA, Palsson-McDermott EM, Bowie AG, Jefferies CA, Mansell AS, Brady G, et al. Mal (MyD88-adapter-like) is required for Toll-like receptor-4 signal transduction. Nature 2001; 413:78-83; PMID:11544529; http://dx.doi.org/10.1038/35092578.

50. Horng T, Barton GM, Medzhitov R. TIRAP: an adapter molecule in the Toll signaling pathway. Nat Immunol 2001; 2:835-41; PMID:11526399; http://dx.doi.org/10.1038/ni0901-835.

51. Horng T, Barton GM, Flavell RA, Medzhitov R. The adaptor molecule TIRAP provides signalling specificity for Toll-like receptors. Nature 2002; 420:329-33; PMID:12447442; http://dx.doi.org/10.1038/nature01180.

52. Yamamoto M, Sato S, Hemmi H, Sanjo H, Uematsu S, Kaisho T, et al. Essential role for TIRAP in activation of the signalling cascade shared by TLR2 and TLR4. Nature 2002; 420:324-9; PMID:12447441; http://dx.doi.org/10.1038/nature01182.

53. Yamamoto M, Sato S, Mori K, Hoshino K, Takeuchi O, Takeda K, et al. Cutting edge: a novel Toll/IL-1 receptor domain-containing adapter that preferentially activates the IFN-beta promoter in the Toll-like receptor signaling. J Immunol 2002; 169:6668-72; PMID:12471095.

54. Oshiumi H, Matsumoto M, Funami K, Akazawa T, Seya T. TICAM-1, an adaptor molecule that participates in Toll-like receptor 3-mediated interferon-beta induction. Nat Immunol 2003; 4:161-7; PMID:12539043; http://dx.doi.org/10.1038/ni886.

55. Yamamoto M, Sato S, Hemmi H, Hoshino K, Kaisho T, Sanjo H, et al. Role of adaptor TRIF in the MyD88-independent toll-like receptor signaling pathway. Science 2003; 301:640-3; PMID:12855817; http://dx.doi.org/10.1126/science.1087262.

56. Hoebe K, Du X, Georgel P, Janssen E, Tabeta K, Kim SO, et al. Identification of Lps2 as a key transducer of MyD88-independent TIR signalling. Nature 2003; 424:743-8; PMID:12872135; http://dx.doi.org/10.1038/nature01889.

57. Hirotani T, Yamamoto M, Kumagai Y, Uematsu S, Kawase I, Takeuchi O, et al. Regulation of lipopolysaccharide-inducible genes by MyD88 and Toll/IL-1 domain containing adaptor inducing IFN-beta. Biochem Biophys Res Commun 2005; 328:383-92; PMID:15694359; http://dx.doi.org/10.1016/j.bbrc.2004.12.184.

58. Fitzgerald KA, Rowe DC, Barnes BJ, Caffrey DR, Visintin A, Latz E, et al. LPS-TLR4 signaling to IRF-3/7 and NF-kappaB involves the toll adapters TRAM and TRIF. J Exp Med 2003; 198:1043-55; PMID:14517278; http://dx.doi.org/10.1084/jem.20031023.

59. Yamamoto M, Sato S, Hemmi H, Uematsu S, Hoshino K, Kaisho T, et al. TRAM is specifically involved in the Toll-like receptor 4-mediated MyD88-independent signaling pathway. Nat Immunol 2003; 4:1144-50; PMID:14556004; http://dx.doi.org/10.1038/ni986.

60. Oshiumi H, Sasai M, Shida K, Fujita T, Matsumoto M, Seya T. TIR-containing adapter molecule (TICAM)-2, a bridging adapter recruiting to toll-like receptor 4 TICAM-1 that induces interferon-beta. J Biol Chem 2003; 278:49751-62; PMID:14519765; http://dx.doi.org/10.1074/jbc.M305820200.

61. Carty M, Goodbody R, Schroder M, Stack J, Moynagh PN, Bowie AG. The human adaptor SARM negatively regulates adaptor protein TRIF-dependent Toll-like receptor signaling. Nat Immunol 2006; 7:1074-81; PMID:16964262; http://dx.doi.org/10.1038/ni1382.

62. Kim Y, Zhou P, Qian L, Chuang JZ, Lee J, Li C, et al. MyD88-5 links mitochondria, microtubules, and JNK3 in neurons and regulates neuronal survival. J Exp Med 2007; 204:2063-74; PMID:17724133; http://dx.doi.org/10.1084/jem.20070868.

63. Chen CY, Lin CW, Chang CY, Jiang ST, Hsueh YP. Sarm1, a negative regulator of innate immunity, interacts with syndecan-2 and regulates neuronal morphology. J Cell Biol 2011; 193:769-84; PMID:21555464; http://dx.doi.org/10.1083/jcb.201008050.

64. Couillault C, Pujol N, Reboul J, Sabatier L, Guichou JF, Kohara Y, et al. TLR-independent control of innate immunity in Caenorhabditis elegans by the TIR domain adaptor protein TIR-1, an ortholog of human SARM. Nat Immunol 2004; 5:488-94; PMID:15048112; http://dx.doi.org/10.1038/ni1060.

65. Liberati NT, Fitzgerald KA, Kim DH, Feinbaum R, Golenbock DT, Ausubel FM. Requirement for a conserved Toll/interleukin-1 resistance domain protein in the Caenorhabditis elegans immune response. Proc Natl Acad Sci USA 2004; 101:6593-8; PMID:15123841; http://dx.doi.org/10.1073/pnas.0308625101.

66. Peng J, Yuan Q, Lin B, Panneerselvam P, Wang X, Luan XL, et al. SARM inhibits both TRIF- and MyD88-mediated AP-1 activation. Eur J Immunol 2010; 40:1738-47; PMID:20306472; http://dx.doi.org/10.1002/eji.200940034.

67. Szretter KJ, Samuel MA, Gilfillan S, Fuchs A, Colonna M, Diamond MS. The immune adaptor molecule SARM modulates tumor necrosis factor alpha production and microglia activation in the brainstem and restricts West Nile Virus pathogenesis. J Virol 2009; 83:9329-38; PMID:19587044; http://dx.doi.org/10.1128/JVI.00836-09.

68. Lin SC, Lo YC, Wu H. Helical assembly in the MyD88-IRAK4-IRAK2 complex in TLR/IL-1R signalling. Nature 2010; 465:885-90; PMID:20485341; http://dx.doi.org/10.1038/nature09121.

69. Kawagoe T, Sato S, Jung A, Yamamoto M, Matsui K, Kato H, et al. Essential role of IRAK-4 protein and its kinase activity in Toll-like receptor-mediated immune responses but not in TCR signaling. J Exp Med 2007; 204:1013-24; PMID:17485511; http://dx.doi.org/10.1084/jem.20061523.

70. Kawagoe T, Sato S, Matsushita K, Kato H, Matsui K, Kumagai Y, et al. Sequential control of Toll-like receptor-dependent responses by IRAK1 and IRAK2. Nat Immunol 2008; 9:684-91; PMID:18438411; http://dx.doi.org/10.1038/ni.1606.

71. Deng L, Wang C, Spencer E, Yang L, Braun A, You J, et al. Activation of the IkappaB kinase complex by TRAF6 requires a dimeric ubiquitin-conjugating enzyme complex and a unique polyubiquitin chain. Cell 2000; 103:351-61; PMID:11057907; http://dx.doi.org/10.1016/S0092-8674(00)00126-4.

72. Kanayama A, Seth RB, Sun L, Ea CK, Hong M, Shaito A, et al. TAB2 and TAB3 activate the NF-kappaB pathway through binding to polyubiquitin chains. Mol Cell 2004; 15:535-48; PMID:15327770; http://dx.doi.org/10.1016/j.molcel.2004.08.008.

73. Wang C, Deng L, Hong M, Akkaraju GR, Inoue J, Chen ZJ. TAK1 is a ubiquitin-dependent kinase of MKK and IKK. Nature 2001; 412:346-51; PMID:11460167; http://dx.doi.org/10.1038/35085597.

74. Tokunaga F, Sakata S, Saeki Y, Satomi Y, Kirisako T, Kamei K, et al. Involvement of linear polyubiquitylation of NEMO in NF-kappaB activation. Nat Cell Biol 2009; 11:123-32; PMID:19136968; http://dx.doi.org/10.1038/ncb1821.

75. Zak DE, Schmitz F, Gold ES, Diercks AH, Peschon JJ, Valvo JS, et al. Systems analysis identifies an essential role for SHANK-associated RH domain-interacting protein (SHARPIN) in macrophage Toll-like receptor 2 (TLR2) responses. Proc Natl Acad Sci USA 2011; 108:11536-41; PMID:21709223; http://dx.doi.org/10.1073/pnas.1107577108.

76. Kagan JC, Su T, Horng T, Chow A, Akira S, Medzhitov R. TRAM couples endocytosis of Toll-like receptor 4 to the induction of interferon-beta. Nat Immunol 2008; 9:361-8; PMID:18297073; http://dx.doi.org/10.1038/ni1569.

77. Sato S, Sugiyama M, Yamamoto M, Watanabe Y, Kawai T, Takeda K, et al. Toll/IL-1 receptor domain-containing adaptor inducing IFN-beta (TRIF) associates with TNF receptor-associated factor 6 and TANK-binding kinase 1, and activates two distinct transcription factors, NF-kappa B and IFN-regulatory factor-3, in the Toll-like receptor signaling. J Immunol 2003; 171:4304-10; PMID:14530355.

78. Meylan E, Burns K, Hofmann K, Blancheteau V, Martinon F, Kelliher M, et al. RIP1 is an essential mediator of Toll-like receptor 3-induced NF-kappa B activation. Nat Immunol 2004; 5:503-7; PMID:15064760; http://dx.doi.org/10.1038/ni1061.

79. Ermolaeva MA, Michallet MC, Papadopoulou N, Utermöhlen O, Kranidioti K, Kollias G, et al. Function of TRADD in tumor necrosis factor receptor 1 signaling and in TRIF-dependent inflammatory responses. Nat Immunol 2008; 9:1037-46; PMID:18641654; http://dx.doi.org/10.1038/ni.1638.

80. Pobezinskaya YL, Kim YS, Choksi S, Morgan MJ, Li T, Liu C, et al. The function of TRADD in signaling through tumor necrosis factor receptor 1 and TRIF-dependent Toll-like receptors. Nat Immunol 2008; 9:1047-54; PMID:18641653; http://dx.doi.org/10.1038/ni.1639.

81. Chang M, Jin W, Sun SC. Peli1 facilitates TRIF-dependent Toll-like receptor signaling and proinflammatory cytokine production. Nat Immunol 2009; 10:1089-95; PMID:19734906; http://dx.doi.org/10.1038/ni.1777.

82. Wang C, Chen T, Zhang J, Yang M, Li N, Xu X, et al. The E3 ubiquitin ligase Nrdp1 'preferentially' promotes TLR-mediated production of type I interferon. Nat Immunol 2009; 10:744-52; PMID:19483718; http://dx.doi.org/10.1038/ni.1742.

83. Tseng PH, Matsuzawa A, Zhang W, Mino T, Vignali DA, Karin M, et al. Different modes of ubiquitination of the adaptor TRAF3 selectively activate the expression of type I interferons and proinflammatory cytokines. Nat Immunol 2010; 11:70-5; PMID:19898473; http://dx.doi.org/10.1038/ni.1819.

84. Kawai T, Sato S, Ishii KJ, Coban C, Hemmi H, Yamamoto M, et al. Interferon-alpha induction through Toll-like receptors involves a direct interaction of IRF7 with MyD88 and TRAF6. Nat Immunol 2004; 5:1061-8; PMID:15361868; http://dx.doi.org/10.1038/ni1118.

85. Uematsu S, Sato S, Yamamoto M, Hirotani T, Kato H, Takeshita F, et al. Interleukin-1 receptor-associated kinase-1 plays an essential role for Toll-like receptor (TLR)7- and TLR9-mediated interferon-{alpha} induction. J Exp Med 2005; 201:915-23; PMID:15767370; http://dx.doi.org/10.1084/jem.20042372.

86. Honda K, Yanai H, Mizutani T, Negishi H, Shimada N, Suzuki N, et al. Role of a transductional-transcriptional processor complex involving MyD88 and IRF-7 in Toll-like receptor signaling. Proc Natl Acad Sci USA 2004; 101:15416-21; PMID:15492225; http://dx.doi.org/10.1073/pnas.0406933101.

87. Hoshino K, Sugiyama T, Matsumoto M, Tanaka T, Saito M, Hemmi H, et al. IkappaB kinase-alpha is critical for interferon-alpha production induced by Toll-like receptors 7 and 9. Nature 2006; 440:949-53; PMID:16612387; http://dx.doi.org/10.1038/nature04641.

88. Kim TW, Staschke K, Bulek K, Yao J, Peters K, Oh KH, et al. A critical role for IRAK4 kinase activity in Toll-like receptor-mediated innate immunity. J Exp Med 2007; 204:1025-36; PMID:17470642; http://dx.doi.org/10.1084/jem.20061825.

89. Shinohara ML, Lu L, Bu J, Werneck MB, Kobayashi KS, Glimcher LH, et al. Osteopontin expression is essential for interferon-alpha production by plasmacytoid dendritic cells. Nat Immunol 2006; 7:498-506; PMID:16604075; http://dx.doi.org/10.1038/ni1327.

90. Guiducci C, Ghirelli C, Marloie-Provost MA, Matray T, Coffman RL, Liu YJ, et al. PI3K is critical for the nuclear translocation of IRF-7 and type I IFN production by human plasmacytoid predendritic cells in response to TLR activation. J Exp Med 2008; 205:315-22; PMID:18227218; http://dx.doi.org/10.1084/jem.20070763.

91. Cao W, Manicassamy S, Tang H, Kasturi SP, Pirani A, Murthy N, et al. Toll-like receptor-mediated induction of type I interferon in plasmacytoid dendritic cells requires the rapamycin-sensitive PI(3) K-mTOR-p70S6K pathway. Nat Immunol 2008; 9:1157-64; PMID:18758466; http://dx.doi.org/10.1038/ni.1645.

92. Hemmi H, Kaisho T, Takeda K, Akira S. The roles of Toll-like receptor 9, MyD88, and DNA-dependent protein kinase catalytic subunit in the effects of two distinct CpG DNAs on dendritic cell subsets. J Immunol 2003; 170:3059-64; PMID:12626561.

93. Hoshino K, Sasaki I, Sugiyama T, Yano T, Yamazaki C, Yasui T, et al. Critical role of IkappaB Kinase alpha in TLR7/9-induced type I IFN production by conventional dendritic cells. J Immunol 2010; 184:3341-5; PMID:20200270; http://dx.doi.org/10.4049/jimmunol.0901648.

94. Schmitz F, Heit A, Guggemoos S, Krug A, Mages J, Schiemann M, et al. Interferon-regulatory-factor 1 controls Toll-like receptor 9-mediated IFN-beta production in myeloid dendritic cells. Eur J Immunol 2007; 37:315-27; PMID:17273999; http://dx.doi.org/10.1002/eji.200636767.

95. Negishi H, Fujita Y, Yanai H, Sakaguchi S, Ouyang X, Shinohara M, et al. Evidence for licensing of IFN-gamma-induced IFN regulatory factor 1 transcription factor by MyD88 in Toll-like receptor-dependent gene induction program. Proc Natl Acad Sci USA 2006; 103:15136-41; PMID:17018642; http://dx.doi.org/10.1073/pnas.0607181103.

96. Latz E, Schoenemeyer A, Visintin A, Fitzgerald KA, Monks BG, Knetter CF, et al. TLR9 signals after translocating from the ER to CpG DNA in the lysosome. Nat Immunol 2004; 5:190-8; PMID:14716310; http://dx.doi.org/10.1038/ni1028.

97. Barton GM, Kagan JC, Medzhitov R. Intracellular localization of Toll-like receptor 9 prevents recognition of self DNA but facilitates access to viral DNA. Nat Immunol 2006; 7:49-56; PMID:16341217; http://dx.doi.org/10.1038/ni1280.

98. Gotoh K, Tanaka Y, Nishikimi A, Nakamura R, Yamada H, Maeda N, et al. Selective control of type I IFN induction by the Rac activator DOCK2 during TLR-mediated plasmacytoid dendritic cell activation. J Exp Med 2010; 207:721-30; PMID:20231379; http://dx.doi.org/10.1084/jem.20091776.

99. Tabeta K, Hoebe K, Janssen EM, Du X, Georgel P, Crozat K, et al. The Unc93b1 mutation 3d disrupts exogenous antigen presentation and signaling via Toll-like receptors 3, 7 and 9. Nat Immunol 2006; 7:156-64; PMID:16415873; http://dx.doi.org/10.1038/ni1297.

100. Kim YM, Brinkmann MM, Paquet ME, Ploegh HL. UNC93B1 delivers nucleotide-sensing toll-like receptors to endolysosomes. Nature 2008; 452:234-8; PMID:18305481; http://dx.doi.org/10.1038/nature06726.

101. Brinkmann MM, Spooner E, Hoebe K, Beutler B, Ploegh HL, Kim YM. The interaction between the ER membrane protein UNC93B and TLR3, 7, and 9 is crucial for TLR signaling. J Cell Biol 2007; 177:265-75; PMID:17452530; http://dx.doi.org/10.1083/jcb.200612056.

102. Fukui R, Saitoh S, Matsumoto F, Kozuka-Hata H, Oyama M, Tabeta K, et al. Unc93B1 biases Toll-like receptor responses to nucleic acid in dendritic cells toward DNA- but against RNA-sensing. J Exp Med 2009; 206:1339-50; PMID:19451267; http://dx.doi.org/10.1084/jem.20082316.

103. Fukui R, Saitoh S, Kanno A, Onji M, Shibata T, Ito A, et al. Unc93B1 restricts systemic lethal inflammation by orchestrating Toll-like receptor 7 and 9 trafficking. Immunity 2011; 35:69-81; PMID:21683627; http://dx.doi.org/10.1016/j.immuni.2011.05.010.

104. Casrouge A, Zhang SY, Eidenschenk C, Jouanguy E, Puel A, Yang K, et al. Herpes simplex virus encephalitis in human UNC-93B deficiency. Science 2006; 314:308-12; PMID:16973841; http://dx.doi.org/10.1126/science.1128346.

105. Wakabayashi Y, Kobayashi M, Akashi-Takamura S, Tanimura N, Konno K, Takahashi K, et al. A protein associated with toll-like receptor 4 (PRAT4A) regulates cell surface expression of TLR4. J Immunol 2006; 177:1772-9; PMID:16849487.

106. Takahashi K, Shibata T, Akashi-Takamura S, Kiyokawa T, Wakabayashi Y, Tanimura N, et al. A protein associated with Toll-like receptor (TLR) 4 (PRAT4A) is required for TLR-dependent immune responses. J Exp Med 2007; 204:2963-76; PMID:17998391; http://dx.doi.org/10.1084/jem.20071132.

107. Liu B, Yang Y, Qiu Z, Staron M, Hong F, Li Y, et al. Folding of Toll-like receptors by the HSP90 paralogue gp96 requires a substrate-specific cochaperone. Nat Commun 2010; 1:79; PMID:20865800.

108. Lee HK, Lund JM, Ramanathan B, Mizushima N, Iwasaki A. Autophagy-dependent viral recognition by plasmacytoid dendritic cells. Science 2007; 315:1398-401; PMID:17272685; http://dx.doi.org/10.1126/science.1136880.

109. Sasai M, Linehan MM, Iwasaki A. Bifurcation of Toll-like receptor 9 signaling by adaptor protein 3. Science 2010; 329:1530-4; PMID:20847273; http://dx.doi.org/10.1126/science.1187029.

110. Blasius AL, Arnold CN, Georgel P, Rutschmann S, Xia Y, Lin P, et al. Slc15a4, AP-3, and Hermansky-Pudlak syndrome proteins are required for Toll-like receptor signaling in plasmacytoid dendritic cells. Proc Natl Acad Sci USA 2010; 107:19973-8; PMID:21045126; http://dx.doi.org/10.1073/pnas.1014051107.

111. Saitoh T, Satoh T, Yamamoto N, Uematsu S, Takeuchi O, Kawai T, et al. Antiviral protein Viperin promotes Toll-like receptor 7- and Toll-like receptor 9-mediated type I interferon production in plasmacytoid dendritic cells. Immunity 2011; 34:352-63; PMID:21435586; http://dx.doi.org/10.1016/j.immuni.2011.03.010.

112. Ewald SE, Engel A, Lee J, Wang M, Bogyo M, Barton GM. Nucleic acid recognition by Toll-like receptors is coupled to stepwise processing by cathepsins and asparagine endopeptidase. J Exp Med 2011; 208:643-51; PMID:21402738; http://dx.doi.org/10.1084/jem.20100682.

113. Asagiri M, Hirai T, Kunigami T, Kamano S, Gober HJ, Okamoto K, et al. Cathepsin K-dependent toll-like receptor 9 signaling revealed in experimental arthritis. Science 2008; 319:624-7; PMID:18239127; http://dx.doi.org/10.1126/science.1150110.

114. Matsumoto F, Saitoh S, Fukui R, Kobayashi T, Tanimura N, Konno K, et al. Cathepsins are required for Toll-like receptor 9 responses. Biochem Biophys Res Commun 2008; 367:693-9; PMID:18166152; http://dx.doi.org/10.1016/j.bbrc.2007.12.130.

115. Ewald SE, Lee BL, Lau L, Wickliffe KE, Shi GP, Chapman HA, et al. The ectodomain of Toll-like receptor 9 is cleaved to generate a functional receptor. Nature 2008; 456:658-62; PMID:18820679; http://dx.doi.org/10.1038/nature07405.

116. Sepulveda FE, Maschalidi S, Colisson R, Heslop L, Ghirelli C, Sakka E, et al. Critical role for asparagine endopeptidase in endocytic Toll-like receptor signaling in dendritic cells. Immunity 2009; 31:737-48; PMID:19879164; http://dx.doi.org/10.1016/j.immuni.2009.09.013.

117. Germain RN, Meier-Schellersheim M, Nita-Lazar A, Fraser ID. Systems biology in immunology: a computational modeling perspective. Annu Rev Immunol 2011; 29:527-85; PMID:21219182.

CHAPTER 4

Alternative Regulatory Mechanisms of TLR Signaling

Claire E. McCoy*

Abstract

It is crucial that signaling pathways such as those induced by Toll-like receptors (TLR) are tightly regulated. This is to prevent over-production of pro-inflammatory mediators that would cause more harm than the good originally intended for the host. Classic mechanisms of regulation include post-translational modifications such as phosphorylation and ubiquitination, degradation of signaling components, transcriptional repressors and competition by inhibitory molecules. Alternative mechanisms of regulation, which will be the emphasis of this chapter, have focused our attention on the regulation of pathways post-transcriptionally. Regulation of TLR signaling pathways by mRNA splice variants, RNA binding proteins and microRNAs in particular will be discussed.

Introduction

Activation of TLR pathways results in a rapid and strong, dynamic and transient innate immune response, characterized by the transcription of a large range of genes, the products of which are required to fight infection. Post-transcriptional regulation plays a crucial role in controlling the expression of these gene transcripts and acts as an important regulatory step in modulating the TLR response. Post–transcriptional regulation is mediated by numerous events such as alternative splicing, processing, stability and ultimately translation of the mRNA transcript (Fig. 1).

Alternative splicing is a form of mRNA processing allowing individual genes to express multiple mRNAs to encode proteins with diverse and antagonistic functions as a method of regulation. Alternative splicing is a natural occurrence in eukaryotes and in humans up to 95% of genes are alternatively spliced.[1] There are many mechanisms of alternative splicing, the most common is exon skipping, where a particular exon may be included or omitted under particular conditions or in particular tissues. Other common mechanisms include alternative 5′ or 3′ splice junctions which change the boundaries of upstream and downstream exons. Splice variants may also be generated from multiple promoters that initiate transcription from different start points, or multiple polyadenylation sites which provide different 3′ end points for the transcript.[1,2]

The stability of mRNA transcripts is often mediated by sequence elements contained within their 5′ and 3′ untranslated regions (UTR). For example, many of the early gene products induced by TLR signaling, particularly cytokines, harbor adenylate-uridylate (AU)-rich elements (ARE) located within their 3′UTR. This sequence typically characterized by the presence of 'AUUUA' pentamers allows recruitment of specific RNA-binding proteins (RBP) to influence their stability.

*Monash Institute of Medical Research, Clayton, Victoria, Australia.
  Email: claire.mccoy@monash.edu

Nucleic Acid Sensors and Antiviral Immunity, edited by Suryaprakash Sambhara and Takashi Fujita.
©2013 Landes Bioscience.

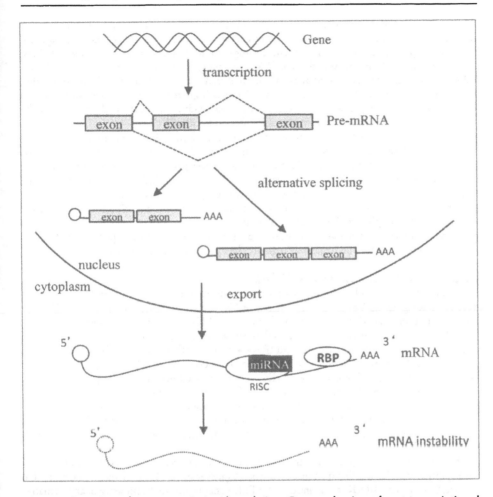

Figure 1. Overview of post-transcriptional regulation. One mechanism of post-transcriptional regulation involves alternative splicing which can generate multiple mRNA transcripts with diverse and antagonistic functions. Mature mRNA transcripts are exported to the cytoplasm after processing involving the addition of 5' cap and PolyA tail. In the cytoplasm they can undergo further regulation mediated by miRNA and RNA binding protein (RBP) which bind to sequence elements located in the 3' untranslated region (UTR). This results in mRNA instability, diminished translation and reduced protein output. TLRs can induce each of these mechanisms to feedback and negatively regulate the innate immune response.

Association with RBP initiates mechanisms of degradation that involve large multi-protein complexes such as exosomes and P-bodies.[3,4] Hundreds of RBPs exist, each of which has a unique RNA binding activity with specificity and affinity for different mRNA transcripts.

More recently, the 3'UTR of mRNA transcripts has been found to contain signature sequences for miRNAs, small RNA binding molecules. miRNAs are typically between 22–25 nucleotides in length containing what is known as a 'seed' sequence contained within nucleotides 2–8. This seed sequence is of importance as it acts in conjunction with the RNA-induced silencing complex (RISC) to guide the miRNA to complementary sequences located within the 3'UTR of target mRNA transcripts.[5] Pairing initiates Argonaute-catalyzed mRNA cleavage, ultimately leading to destabilization of mRNA transcripts and reduced protein output.[6-8]

The discovery of miRNAs has led to an increased interest in the study of post-transcriptional regulation. This is most likely brought about by the fact that the short length of the seed sequence increases the probability of the complement existing in multiple targets, thus one miRNA can have greater than 200 mRNA targets in the cell.[9,10] Software programs such as TargetScan, miRanda and miRTAR can predict targets based on the strength of seed complementarity, miRNA positioning within the 3′UTR and AU-rich composition.[11,12] Interestingly, there is evidence that miRNA may also regulate mRNA expression by binding to the open reading frame, the coding region or the 5′UTR of mRNA targets, an area worthy of further exploration.[9,13-15]

Even more staggering is the rate at which miRNAs are being identified. At their first emergence, it was thought that > 250 miRNA existed in mammalian cells. This has now expanded to > 500, cataloged in the miRBase database. With the popularity of deep sequencing and its ability to detect small non-coding RNA molecules, it suggests that many more are likely to exist. The sheer scale of potential miRNA-mRNA interactions means that complex networks must exist and heightens the requirement for sophisticated mechanisms of network analysis and bioinformatics to fully understand the complexity of miRNA regulation.

In all instances, TLR signaling has been shown to induce each of these post-transcriptional mechanisms to feedback and negatively regulate the innate immune response.

Regulation by Alternative Splicing

Each of the four members of the IL-1 receptor associated kinase (IRAK) family play a central role in TLR signaling. Upon TLR activation, IRAK1 and IRAK4 are recruited to MyD88 via their death domains (DD). IRAK4 phosphorylates IRAK1 within its kinase domain, resulting in IRAK1 hyper-autophosphorylation and their subsequent release from MyD88. In response to TLR2 and TLR4 stimulation, IRAK1 and IRAK4 interact with TRAF6 and the TAK1 complex that leads to NF-κB and MAPK activation, whereas in response to TLR7 and TLR9, they interact with IRF7.[16] Hyper-phoshorylation of IRAK1 is a signal for its degradation, an important response mediating negative regulation. In contrast, IRAK2 expression levels are sustained and required for maintaining late-phase NF-κB activation and the continuation of pro-inflammatory cytokine expression.[17-19] IRAKM is an inhibitory family member which is induced upon TLR signaling and acts to prevent IRAK1 and IRAK4 dissociation from MyD88, thereby blocking continuation of the signal.[20]

However additional regulation is mediated by the multiple splice variants that exist for IRAK family members. This was first demonstrated when 4 splice forms for IRAK2 were found present in mouse. One of these, IRAK2c, was induced by TLR signaling due to the presence of an alternative promoter. Overexpression of IRAK2c could inhibit NF-κB luciferase activation.[21] Furthermore, a 10 base pair deletion within the promoter region of IRAK2c, resulted in defective IRAK2c expression and higher expression levels of IL-6, TNF and IL-12 in response to TLR2 activation.[22] IRAK1c is a human splice variant which lacks the kinase domain found in IRAK1. This splice variant can still interact with MyD88, but fails to become phosphorylated by IRAK4. It therefore acts as a dominant negative variant remaining associated with MyD88 to block NF-κB activation and cytokine mediated induction.[23] Other IRAK1 variants exist, IRAK1b in mouse and human, and IRAK1s in mouse. Both these variants were shown to play a positive role in signaling rather than inhibitory.[24,25]

A splice variant of MyD88, termed MyD88s, lacks the intermediate domain located between the N-terminal DD and the C-terminal Toll/IL-1 receptor (TIR) homology domain found in MyD88.[26] Due to the expression of TIR and DD domains, MyD88s can still interact with both TLRs and IRAK1 but can no longer interact with IRAK4, the kinase responsible for IRAK1 phosphorylation and activation of MyD88 dependent signaling pathways.[26,27] Thus, overexpression of MyD88s was found to inhibit IRAK1 phosphorylation and block NF-κB activity.[26,27] It has still not been fully elucidated whether MyD88s is a predominant mechanism of TLR negative regulation. MyD88s appears to be solely expressed in the spleen with small amounts detected in the brain, whereas MyD88 is ubiquitously expressed in all tissues [Janssens 2002]. Furthermore, its expression is only just detected after prolonged exposure to LPS (~16hrs).[26] Nevertheless, it does suggest that under conditions of chronic inflammation, MyD88s may be playing an important role in tolerance and switching off TLR responses.

TAG, is a splice variant of the adaptor molecule TRAM. It differs from TRAM in that it is alternatively spliced to contain a Golgi dynamics (GOLD) homology domain within its N-terminus.[28] Both TLR3 and TLR4 use TRAM to recruit TRIF, activating the MyD88 independent pathway resulting in TRAF3 and TBK1 recruitment and activation of IRF3.[29,30] It appears that TAG plays a central role in switching this pathway off in response to TLR4 only. Upon LPS treatment, TAG co-localizes with TRAM in the late endosome, where it can bind to TRAM displacing TRIF, shutting down IRF3 activation and cytokine output as well as promoting TLR4 degradation.[28] TAG did not have this same effect on IRF3 signaling mediated downstream of TLR3, highlighting a specific effect on TLR4 only. Figure 2 summarizes the TLR signaling components that are regulated by the described splice variants.

The presence of single nucleotide polymorphisms (SNPs) located within the 5′UTR or promoter regions of genes may also contribute to the role of splice variants. For example, the TLR8 locus expresses two splice variants, where the presence of a SNP located in the upstream

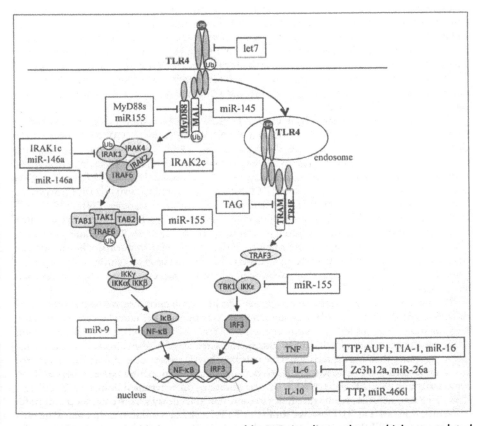

Figure 2. This diagram highlights components of the TLR signaling pathway which are regulated at the post-transcriptional level by splice variants, RBP and miRNAs. It is apparent that individual components such as IRAK1 and TNFα are targeted by multiple mechanisms that may work co-operatively and synergistically to mediate mRNA instability. Some components such as IRAK1, Mal and TLR4 are also regulated by post-translational degradation mediated by mechanisms such as ubiquitination.

open reading frame results in TLR8 splice variants with alternative translation start sites.[31] Although there appears to be no functional difference between these isoforms, the presence of the SNP interferes with ribosomal scanning of the start site and modulates the amount of TLR8 variants translated under particular conditions and in different cell types.[31] This could have direct impact on TLR8 sensing as presence of the SNP has been attributed to pulmonary tuberculosis and HIV susceptibility.[32,33] It is possible that other known SNPs associated with disease may post-transcriptionally regulate splice variants of TLR signaling components.[34]

Regulation by RNA Binding Proteins

TNFα is an important immediate early cytokine induced by the majority of TLRs. It is required for an acute immune reaction, acting as a potent chemoattractant for neutrophils, stimulating macrophage phagocytosis as well as inducing fever like symptoms. Its dysregulation has been implicated in a range of inflammatory diseases such as arthritis, inflammatory bowel disease as well as cancer.[35] It is therefore essential that this cytokine is appropriately regulated.

One such mechanism occurs via RNA binding proteins which was first demonstrated when the zinc-finger protein, tristetraprolin (TTP) was found to bind to the TNFα-ARE located in the 3'UTR, resulting in TNFα destabilization and degradation.[36,37] TTP deficient mice succumbed to a systemic inflammatory syndrome with severe arthritis and autoimmunity, characterized by a predominant increase in TNFα expression.[38,39] Furthermore, TNFα transgenic mice and mice lacking TNF-ARE elements, both created more stable TNFα transcripts and displayed similar disease phenotypes to TTP deficient mice.[40] TTP is induced in a similar time frame by the same ligands that stimulate TNFα production, including LPS and TNFα itself. Thus the induction of TTP is an important regulatory step by TLRs, as it feeds back to negatively regulate the mRNA expression of TNFα[40]. GM-CSF, IL-2, IL-1β and IL-10 transcripts are also destabilized upon association with TTP[39-43] (Fig. 2).

TNFα is not solely regulated by TTP, as other RBP have been shown to bind and regulate its expression. For example, AU-rich element RNA-binding protein 1 (AUF1) deficient mice display severe symptoms of endotoxic shock and display a 5-fold lower survival rate compared with wild-type controls. This was due to the selective overproduction of TNFα and IL-1β and the inability of AUF1 to mediate their rapid decay upon LPS exposure.[44] B-related factor 1 (BRF1) and KH-type splicing regulatory protein (KHSRP) have also been shown to play a role in mRNA instability, whereas Hu antigen R (HuR) RBP have been shown to stabilize TNFα mRNA.[45-47] RBP association with ARE-mRNAs not only promotes degradation of mRNA but can also induce translational arrest. For example, although cytotoxic granule associated RNA binding protein 1 (TIA-1) deficient macrophages produce more TNFα compared with normal cells, the half-life of TNFα transcripts remained unchanged. Instead, TIA-1 was found to significantly increase the proportion of TNFα transcripts associated with polysomes, suggesting that TIA-1 instead acts as a translational silencer.[48-50]

Recently, newly identified zinc-finger protein, Zc3h12a, has been shown to target the 3'UTR of IL-6 and IL-12, but not TNFα for degradation. Macrophages deficient in Zc3h12a produce larger amounts of IL-6 and IL-12 upon exposure to a range of TLR agonists.[51] Zc3h12a contains a RNA binding domain and a zinc finger domain characteristic of RBP involved in ARE-mediated decay, suggesting that IL-6 degradation is mediated via the AU repeats located in its 3'UTR. Instead it was discovered that degradation of IL-6 transcripts was due to an alternative conserved RNA region within its 3'UTR and RNase activity mediated by an N-terminal domain in Zc3h12a.[51] Thus TTP and Zc3h12a retain specificity to control mRNA decay via different mechanisms for different cytokines (Fig. 2). However similar to TTP, Zc3h12a is induced as an immediate early gene by a range of TLR agonists, suggesting that its induction is an important regulatory step for TLR induced immune responses. This is even more pertinent considering Zc3h12a deficient mice die within 12 weeks due to severe immune disorders.[51]

Co-operation between RBP and miRNAs may also exist to control mRNA stability (Fig. 2). This was first demonstrated when Dicer and Argonaute, key components of miRNA processing were shown to be required for the ARE mediated degradation of TNFα[52]. Furthermore, a binding site for miR-16 was identified in the TNFα-ARE, where binding could mediate TNF destabilization. This effect could no longer occur in the absence of TTP, suggesting that a TTP-miR-16 interaction was required.[52] TNF contains binding sites for other miRNAs and to date, two of these, miR-369-3 and miR-125b have also been shown to play a role in TNFα mRNA regulation.[53-55] miR-155 has also been suggested to play a role in the positive regulation of TNF in an as yet unknown mechanism.[55,56] miR-466l has the seed sequence 'AUAAAUA' which is complementary to typical ARE sequences 'AUUUA', it was postulated that miR-466l can bind to the 3'UTR of IL-10 and protect the ARE from TTP mediated degradation.[57] IL-6 has been shown to contain a binding for miR-26a, mediating IL-6 mRNA degradation.[58] However its association with Zc3h12a or other RBP remains unknown.

Regulation by miRNA

It has become increasingly clear that TLRs induce a range of miRNA required to mediate cellular function as well as feeding back to regulate the pathways in question. Although miRNA induction by TLRs is well reviewed elsewhere, see ref. 59, the induction of miRNA by nucleic acid sensing TLRs is much less characterized and will be discussed further (Table 1).

TLR3, TLR7/TLR8 and TLR9 family members mediate nucleic acid sensing, recognizing dsRNA, ssRNA and nonmethylated CpG DNA, respectively. Recognition of these viral components mediates an anti-viral response characterized by interferon (IFN) expression and induction of interferon-stimulated genes (ISG).[60] The first example of nucleic acid and interferon miRNA induction was demonstrated when miR-155 was identified as the only miRNA upregulated in PolyIC and IFNβ stimulated macrophages.[61] PolyIC induction of miR-155 was dependent on TRIF and occurred with earlier kinetics, whereas IFNβ induction was delayed and required TNF autocrine signaling. TLR9, TLR7, TLR2 and TLR4 have also been shown to induce miR-155, where TLR7 can also induce the antisense form miR-155[61,62]. Viruses such as Epstein-Barr virus (EBV) and Kaposi's sarcoma virus (KSV), which do not necessarily signal through TLRs, can also induce miR-155. In addition, viral homologs of miR-155 have been identified suggesting a mechanism that may be adapted by viruses to regulate the host immune response.[63]

miR-155 binding sites have been identified in TLR signaling components IKKε, TAK1-binding protein 2 (TAB2) and MyD88, suggesting that miR-155 may act to negatively regulate TLR responses[55,64,65] (Fig. 2). Indeed, suppression of miR-155 expression through the use of antisense oligonucleotides has increased the expression of cytokines and chemokines such as IL-1 and CXCL8 in a range of cells.[64-66] In contrast, other data suggests that miR-155 may act to promote the pro-inflammatory response as demonstrated in miR-155 deficient and transgenic mouse models that show a dependency for miR-155 and the expression of TNF, IL-6, IL-23 and type I IFNs.[56,67-69]

Table 1. Overview of miRNAs induced by nucleic acid sensing TLRs, other TLRs, viruses and cytokines

miRNA	Nucleic Acid Sensing TLR	Other TLR	Viral Induction	Cytokine Induction	Ref
miR-155	TLR3, TLR7, TLR9	TLR2, TLR4	EBV, KSV	IFNβ, TNF	61, 62
miR-146	-	TLR2, TLR4, TLR5	VSV, EBV	IL-1, TNF	74-77
miR-132	-	TLR4	KSHV, HSV-1, HCMV		74, 78
miR-9	TLR7/8	TLR2, TLR4			85
miR-147	TLR3	TLR2, TLR4			86

This is possibly due to its repressive effect on two negative regulators of cytokines, suppression of cytokine signaling (SOCS1) and Src homology-2 domain-containing inositol 5-phosphatase 1 (SHIP1).[69-71] However, a more recent study may help understand some of the discrepancies regarding miR-155 negative and positive regulation. For example, early induction of the antisense form, miR-155* by TLR7 can positively influence type I IFN expression mediated through its ability to suppress the negative regulator, IRAKM. On the other hand, suppression of type I IFN expression was mediated by the later induction of miR-155 and its ability to repress TAB2[62].

Overall, it would be informative to investigate the direct impact of TLR challenge in the range of miR-155 genetically modified mice that exist in order to fully understand the contribution of miR-155 to the innate immune response and whether it acts to positively or negatively it. There are indications that miR-155 will play an important role. For example, miR-155 deficient mice have defective dendritic cell function that could be playing a crucial role in the loss of adaptive capability well described in these mice.[56,68,72,73]

Two other miRNA, miR-146a and miR-132, were discovered in LPS-stimulated monocytes.[74] Although yet to be found induced by nucleic acid sensing TLRs, EBV-encoded latent membrane protein and vesicular stomatitis virus (VSV) that activates the RIG-I pathway, can induce miR-146a.[75-77] Similarly, miR-132 is induced in response to Kaposi's sarcoma-associated herpes virus (KSHV), herpes simplex virus-1 (HSV-1) and human cytomegalovirus (HCMV) suggesting that both these miRNA may play a role in the anti-viral response.[78]

miR-146a can bind to the 3′UTR of TRAF6 and IRAK1, two important signaling components for the majority of TLR pathways (Fig. 2). Induction of miR-146a therefore serves as a negative feedback loop, degrading TRAF6 and IRAK1 mRNA which acts to limit further signaling and TLR induced cytokine expression. This has been demonstrated in vitro where overexpression of miR-146a could reduce the expression of the pro-inflammatory cytokines IL-8 and RANTES in epithelial cells, IL-6 and IL-8 in fibroblasts and TNF in osteoarthritic tissue in response to IL-1; TNFα, IL-1β and IL-6 in ThP1 monocytes in response to LPS-tolerance and type I IFN in EBV and VSV infected cells.[75-77,79-83] The role for miR-146a in negatively regulating the inflammatory response has been confirmed in miR-146a deficient mice.[84] These mice have an exaggerated inflammatory response characterized by increased TNF, IL-6 and IL-1β and reduced survival when endotoxin challenged. Over time, these mice develop autoimmune diseases and display increased CD4 and CD8 positive T cells suggesting a role for miR-146a in shaping the adaptive response.

miR-9 and miR-147 are induced by TLR7/8 and TLR3 agonists respectively, as well as TLR2 and TLR4[85,86]. miR-9 and miR-147 were shown to negatively regulate TLR signaling when the p50 subunit of NFkB was shown to be targeted by the former, whereas miR-147 was shown to negatively regulate the expression of TNFα and IL-6 in response to both LPS and PolyIC through an unidentified mechansim[85,86]. Although not necessarily induced by TLRs, other miRNAs have been identified to regulate components of the TLR pathways (for detailed review see ref. 59). For example, TLR4 and TLR2 expression are regulated by members of the let7 family and miR-105 respectively.[70,87,88] Adaptor molecule, Mal is targeted by miR-145.[89] Together these studies highlight how miRNAs can fine-tune and time the inflammatory response, through their ability to target different components of the TLR signaling pathway.

Discussion

It is clear that mechanisms of mRNA processing and stability play a key role in regulating TLR pathways. One particular point of interest is that many of the TLR components regulated by these processes such as IRAK1, TAB2, TLR4 and Mal are also susceptible to protein instability suggesting that the two mechanisms may play a timed, synergistic role in negatively regulating TLR pathways (Fig. 2).

For example, shortly after its activation, IRAK1 is rapidly degraded with kinetics that varies depending on the TLR agonist.[90-92] The mechanism of degradation remains to be fully understood, but it is likely that K48-linked ubiquitination which targets proteins to the proteasome is required.[93,94] Interestingly, both mRNA and protein analysis of IRAK1 in response to LPS, CpG and IL-1 have demonstrated that although protein degradation is rapid (10 – 120 min), IRAK1 mRNA and protein can remain degraded for up to 24 h.[90,92] The later time points correlate with the induction of miR-146a and its ability to target IRAK1 mRNA for degradation. It is possible therefore that upon TLR activation and induction of signaling, IRAK1 is first degraded at the protein level and later targeted at the post-transcriptional level by miR-146a. Induction of regulatory isoforms such as IRAKM and splice variants further ensures that the levels of IRAK1 are carefully regulated.

Other examples include TAB2, post-translationally degraded by TRIM30a and post-transcriptionally regulated by miR-155.[64,95] Triad3A has been shown to target multiple components of the TLR pathway for K48-linked ubiquitination and proteasomal degradation.[96-98] To date, two of these, TLR4 and Mal are post-transcriptionally regulated by miRNAs.[70,87,89] It is plausible that both protein instability and miRNA regulation exist for other components of the TLR pathway and suggests that together they coordinate early and late mechanisms of regulation. It will be necessary that timed analysis of protein decay, miRNA induction and mRNA instability are appropriately studied to fully appreciate this point.

Conclusion

The discovery of miRNA has confirmed the importance of post-transcriptional regulation in the cell. However, one of the restrictive natures of miRNA study has been the temptation to focus on uni-directional miRNA-mRNA interactions through the use of overexpression and luciferase reporter assays. Although invaluable, it will be necessary to examine the impact of individual miRNA on pathways or systems as a whole, which can be achieved through the generation of genetically modified mice. It will be intriguing to understand the direct impact of TLR challenge in mice deficient for specific miRNAs, as examined in miR-146a deficient mice.[84]

Acknowledgments

The author would like to thank Michael Gantier for critical reading of the manuscript. The author is funded by the Health Research Board Ireland.

About the Author

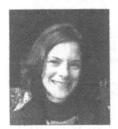Claire E. McCoy received her PhD in 2006 from the University of Dundee, where she investigated post-translational regulation of mitogen-activated protein kinase cascades. Her first post-doc with Prof Luke O'Neill in Trinity College Dublin investigated regulation of TLR signaling pathways, in particular the regulation mediated by microRNAs. During this time, she obtained a Health Research Board Ireland/Marie Curie mobility fellowship enabling further research with Prof Bryan Williams at Monash University, Melbourne. Her current area of interest investigates the role of microRNAs in TLR and cytokine signaling pathways.

References

1. Pan Q, Shai O, Lee LJ, Frey BJ, Blencowe BJ. Deep surveying of alternative splicing complexity in the human transcriptome by high-throughput sequencing. Nat Genet 2008; 40:1413-5; http://dx.doi.org/10.1038/ng.259; PMID:18978789.

2. Matlin AJ, Clark F, Smith CW. Understanding alternative splicing: towards a cellular code. Nat Rev Mol Cell Biol 2005; 6:386-98; http://dx.doi.org/10.1038/nrm1645; PMID:15956978.

3. Chen CY, Gherzi R, Ong SE, Chan EL, Raijmakers R, Pruijn GJ, et al. AU binding proteins recruit the exosome to degrade ARE-containing mRNAs. Cell 2001; 107:451-64; http://dx.doi.org/10.1016/S0092-8674(01)00578-5; PMID:11719186.

4. Barreau C. AU-rich elements and associated factors: are there unifying principles? Nucleic Acids Res 2005; 33:7138-50; http://dx.doi.org/10.1093/nar/gki1012; PMID:16391004.

5. Gregory RI, Chendrimada TP, Cooch N, Shiekhattar R. Human RISC couples microRNA biogenesis and posttranscriptional gene silencing. Cell 2005; 123:631-40; http://dx.doi.org/10.1016/j.cell.2005.10.022; PMID:16271387.

6. Hutvágner G, Zamore PD. A microRNA in a multiple-turnover RNAi enzyme complex. Science 2002; 297:2056-60; http://dx.doi.org/10.1126/science.1073827; PMID:12154197.

7. Liu J, Carmell MA, Rivas FV, Marsden CG, Thomson JM, Song JJ, et al. Argonaute2 is the catalytic engine of mammalian RNAi. Science 2004; 305:1437-41; http://dx.doi.org/10.1126/science.1102513; PMID:15284456.

8. Guo H, Ingolia NT, Weissman JS, Bartel DP. Mammalian microRNAs predominantly act to decrease target mRNA levels. Nature 2010; 466:835-40; http://dx.doi.org/10.1038/nature09267; PMID:20703300.

9. Lewis BP, Burge CB, Bartel DP. Conserved seed pairing, often flanked by adenosines, indicates that thousands of human genes are microRNA targets. Cell 2005; 120:15-20; http://dx.doi.org/10.1016/j.cell.2004.12.035; PMID:15652477.

10. Friedman RC, Farh KK, Burge CB, Bartel DP. Most mammalian mRNAs are conserved targets of microRNAs. Genome Res 2009; 19:92-105; http://dx.doi.org/10.1101/gr.082701.108; PMID:18955434.

11. Grimson A, Farh KK, Johnston WK, Garrett-Engele P, Lim LP, Bartel DP. MicroRNA targeting specificity in mammals: determinants beyond seed pairing. Mol Cell 2007; 27:91-105; http://dx.doi.org/10.1016/j.molcel.2007.06.017; PMID:17612493.

12. Hsu JB, Chiu CM, Hsu SD, Huang WY, Chien CH, Lee TY, Huang HD. miRTar: an integrated system for identifying miRNA-target interactions in Human. BMC Bioinformatics 2011; 12:300; http://dx.doi.org/10.1186/1471-2105-12-300; PMID:21791068.

13. Ørom UA, Nielsen FC, Lund AH. MicroRNA-10a binds the 5'UTR of ribosomal protein mRNAs and enhances their translation. Mol Cell 2008; 30:460-71; http://dx.doi.org/10.1016/j.molcel.2008.05.001; PMID:18498749.

14. Moretti F, Thermann R, Hentze MW. Mechanism of translational regulation by miR-2 from sites in the 5' untranslated region or the open reading frame. RNA 2010; 16:2493-502; http://dx.doi.org/10.1261/rna.2384610; PMID:20966199.

15. Lee EK, Gorospe M. Coding region: the neglected post-transcriptional code. RNA Biol 2011; 8:44-8; http://dx.doi.org/10.4161/rna.8.1.13863; PMID:21289484.

16. Gottipati S, Rao NL, Fung-Leung W-P. IRAK1: A critical signaling mediator of innate immunity. Cell Signal 2008; 20:269-76; http://dx.doi.org/10.1016/j.cellsig.2007.08.009; PMID:17890055.

17. Keating SE, Maloney GM, Moran EM, Bowie AG. IRAK-2 participates in multiple toll-like receptor signaling pathways to NFkappaB via activation of TRAF6 ubiquitination. J Biol Chem 2007; 282:33435-43; http://dx.doi.org/10.1074/jbc.M705266200; PMID:17878161.

18. Kawagoe T, Sato S, Matsushita K, Kato H, Matsui K, Kumagai Y, et al. Sequential control of Toll-like receptor-dependent responses by IRAK1 and IRAK2. Nat Immunol 2008; 9:684-91; http://dx.doi.org/10.1038/ni.1606; PMID:18438411.

19. Wan Y, Xiao H, Affolter J, Kim TW, Bulek K, Chaudhuri S, et al. Interleukin-1 receptor-associated kinase 2 is critical for lipopolysaccharide-mediated post-transcriptional control. J Biol Chem 2009; 284:10367-75; http://dx.doi.org/10.1074/jbc.M807822200; PMID:19224918.

20. Kobayashi K, Hernandez LD, Galán JE, Janeway CA, Medzhitov R, Flavell RA. IRAK-M is a negative regulator of Toll-like receptor signaling. Cell 2002; 110:191-202; http://dx.doi.org/10.1016/S0092-8674(02)00827-9; PMID:12150927.

21. Hardy MP, O'Neill LAJ. The murine IRAK2 gene encodes four alternatively spliced isoforms, two of which are inhibitory. J Biol Chem 2004; 279:27699-708; http://dx.doi.org/10.1074/jbc.M403068200; PMID:15082713.

22. Conner JR, Smirnova II, Poltorak A. A mutation in Irak2c identifies IRAK-2 as a central component of the TLR regulatory network of wild-derived mice. J Exp Med 2009; 206:1615-31; http://dx.doi.org/10.1084/jem.20090490; PMID:19564352.

23. Rao N, Nguyen S, Ngo K, Fung-Leung W-P. A novel splice variant of interleukin-1 receptor (IL-1R)-associated kinase 1 plays a negative regulatory role in Toll/IL-1R-induced inflammatory signaling. Mol Cell Biol 2005; 25:6521-32; http://dx.doi.org/10.1128/MCB.25.15.6521-6532.2005; PMID:16024789.

24. Jensen LE, Whitehead AS. IRAK1b, a novel alternative splice variant of interleukin-1 receptor-associated kinase (IRAK), mediates interleukin-1 signaling and has prolonged stability. J Biol Chem 2001; 276:29037-44; http://dx.doi.org/10.1074/jbc.M103815200; PMID:11397809.

25. Yanagisawa K, Tago K, Hayakawa M, Ohki M, Iwahana H, Tominaga S. A novel splice variant of mouse interleukin-1-receptor-associated kinase-1 (IRAK-1) activates nuclear factor-kappaB (NF-kappaB) and c-Jun N-terminal kinase (JNK). Biochem J 2003; 370:159-66; http://dx.doi.org/10.1042/BJ20021218; PMID:12418963.

26. Janssens S. MyD88S, a splice variant of MyD88, differentially modulates NF-κB- and AP-1-dependent gene expression. FEBS Lett 2003; 548:103-7; http://dx.doi.org/10.1016/S0014-5793(03)00747-6; PMID:12885415.

27. Burns K, Janssens S, Brissoni B, Olivos N, Beyaert R, Tschopp J. Inhibition of interleukin 1 receptor/ Toll-like receptor signaling through the alternatively spliced, short form of MyD88 is due to its failure to recruit IRAK-4. J Exp Med 2003; 197:263-8; http://dx.doi.org/10.1084/jem.20021790; PMID:12538665.

28. Palsson-McDermott EM, Doyle SL, McGettrick AF, Hardy M, Husebye H, Banahan K, et al. TAG, a splice variant of the adaptor TRAM, negatively regulates the adaptor MyD88–independent TLR4 pathway. Nat Immunol 2009; 10:579-86; http://dx.doi.org/10.1038/ni.1727; PMID:19412184.

29. Fitzgerald KA, Rowe DC, Barnes BJ, Caffrey DR, Visintin A, Latz E, et al. LPS-TLR4 signaling to IRF-3/7 and NF-kappaB involves the toll adapters TRAM and TRIF. J Exp Med 2003; 198:1043-55; http://dx.doi.org/10.1084/jem.20031023; PMID:14517278.

30. Yamamoto M, Sato S, Hemmi H, Uematsu S, Hoshino K, Kaisho T, et al. TRAM is specifically involved in the Toll-like receptor 4-mediated MyD88-independent signaling pathway. Nat Immunol 2003; 4:1144-50; http://dx.doi.org/10.1038/ni986; PMID:14556004.

31. Gantier MP, Irving AT, Kaparakis-Liaskos M, Xu D, Evans VA, Cameron PU, et al. Genetic modulation of TLR8 response following bacterial phagocytosis. Hum Mutat 2010; 31:1069-79; http://dx.doi.org/10.1002/humu.21321; PMID:20652908.

32. Dalgic N, Tekin D, Kayaalti Z, Cakir E, Soylemezoglu T, Sancar M. Relationship between toll-like receptor 8 gene polymorphisms and pediatric pulmonary tuberculosis. Dis Markers 2011; 31:33-8; PMID:21846947.

33. Davila S, Hibberd ML, Hari Dass R, Wong HE, Sahiratmadja E, Bonnard C, et al. Genetic association and expression studies indicate a role of toll-like receptor 8 in pulmonary tuberculosis. PLoS Genet 2008; 4:e1000218; http://dx.doi.org/10.1371/journal.pgen.1000218; PMID:18927625.

34. Corr SC. O rsquo Neill LA. Genetic Variation in Toll-Like Receptor Signalling and the Risk of Inflammatory and Immune Diseases. J Innate Immun 2009; 1:350-7; http://dx.doi.org/10.1159/000200774; PMID:20375592.

35. Locksley RM, Killeen N, Lenardo MJ. The TNF and TNF receptor superfamilies: integrating mammalian biology. Cell 2001; 104:487-501; http://dx.doi.org/10.1016/S0092-8674(01)00237-9; PMID:11239407.

36. Carballo E, Lai WS, Blackshear PJ. Feedback inhibition of macrophage tumor necrosis factor-alpha production by tristetraprolin. Science 1998; 281:1001-5; http://dx.doi.org/10.1126/science.281.5379.1001; PMID:9703499.

37. Lai WS, Carballo E, Strum JR, Kennington EA, Phillips RS, Blackshear PJ. Evidence that tristetraprolin binds to AU-rich elements and promotes the deadenylation and destabilization of tumor necrosis factor alpha mRNA. Mol Cell Biol 1999; 19:4311-23; PMID:10330172.

38. Taylor GA, Carballo E, Lee DM, Lai WS, Thompson MJ, Patel DD, et al. A pathogenetic role for TNF alpha in the syndrome of cachexia, arthritis, and autoimmunity resulting from tristetraprolin (TTP) deficiency. Immunity 1996; 4:445-54; http://dx.doi.org/10.1016/S1074-7613(00)80411-2; PMID:8630730.

39. Carrick DM, Lai WS, Blackshear PJ. The tandem CCCH zinc finger protein tristetraprolin and its relevance to cytokine mRNA turnover and arthritis. Arthritis Res Ther 2004; 6:248-64; http://dx.doi.org/10.1186/ar1441; PMID:15535838.

40. Carballo E, Blackshear PJ. Roles of tumor necrosis factor-alpha receptor subtypes in the pathogenesis of the tristetraprolin-deficiency syndrome. Blood 2001; 98:2389-95; http://dx.doi.org/10.1182/blood.V98.8.2389; PMID:11588035.

41. Ogilvie RL, Abelson M, Hau HH, Vlasova I, Blackshear PJ, Bohjanen PR. Tristetraprolin down-regulates IL-2 gene expression through AU-rich element-mediated mRNA decay. J Immunol 2005; 174:953-61; PMID:15634918.

42. Chen YL, Huang YL, Lin NY, Chen HC, Chiu WC, Chang CJ. Differential regulation of ARE-mediated TNFalpha and IL-1beta mRNA stability by lipopolysaccharide in RAW264.7 cells. Biochem Biophys Res Commun 2006; 346:160-8; http://dx.doi.org/10.1016/j.bbrc.2006.05.093; PMID:16759646.

43. Stoecklin G, Tenenbaum SA, Mayo T, Chittur SV, George AD, Baroni TE, et al. Genome-wide analysis identifies interleukin-10 mRNA as target of tristetraprolin. J Biol Chem 2008; 283:11689-99; http://dx.doi.org/10.1074/jbc.M709657200; PMID:18256032.

44. Lu JY, Sadri N, Schneider RJ. Endotoxic shock in AUF1 knockout mice mediated by failure to degrade proinflammatory cytokine mRNAs. Genes Dev 2006; 20:3174-84; PMID:17085481.

45. Schmidlin M, Lu M, Leuenberger SA, Stoecklin G, Mallaun M, Gross B, et al. The ARE-dependent mRNA-destabilizing activity of BRF1 is regulated by protein kinase B. EMBO J 2004; 23:4760-9; http://dx.doi.org/10.1038/sj.emboj.7600477; PMID:15538381.

46. Chou CF, Mulky A, Maitra S, Lin WJ, Gherzi R, Kappes J, Chen CY. Tethering KSRP, a decay-promoting AU-rich element-binding protein, to mRNAs elicits mRNA decay. Mol Cell Biol 2006; 26:3695-706; http://dx.doi.org/10.1128/MCB.26.10.3695-3706.2006; PMID:16648466.

47. Dean JL, Wait R, Mahtani KR, Sully G, Clark AR, Saklatvala J. The 3′ untranslated region of tumor necrosis factor alpha mRNA is a target of the mRNA-stabilizing factor HuR. Mol Cell Biol 2001; 21:721-30; http://dx.doi.org/10.1128/MCB.21.3.721-730.2001; PMID:11154260.

48. Piecyk M, Wax S, Beck AR, Kedersha N, Gupta M, Maritim B, et al. TIA-1 is a translational silencer that selectively regulates the expression of TNF-alpha. EMBO J 2000; 19:4154-63; http://dx.doi.org/10.1093/emboj/19.15.4154; PMID:10921895.

49. Saito K, Chen S, Piecyk M, Anderson P. TIA-1 regulates the production of tumor necrosis factor alpha in macrophages, but not in lymphocytes. Arthritis Rheum 2001; 44:2879-87; http://dx.doi.org/10.1002/1529-0131(200112)44:12<2879::AID-ART476>3.0.CO;2-4; PMID:11762949.

50. Anderson P. Post-transcriptional regulation of proinflammatory proteins. J Leukoc Biol 2004; 76:42-7; http://dx.doi.org/10.1189/jlb.1103536; PMID:15075353.

51. Matsushita K, Takeuchi O, Standley DM, Kumagai Y, Kawagoe T, Miyake T, et al. Zc3h12a is an RNase essential for controlling immune responses by regulating mRNA decay. Nature 2009; 458:1185-90; http://dx.doi.org/10.1038/nature07924; PMID:19322177.

52. Jing Q, Huang S, Guth S, Zarubin T, Motoyama A, Chen J, et al. Involvement of microRNA in AU-rich element-mediated mRNA instability. Cell 2005; 120:623-34; http://dx.doi.org/10.1016/j.cell.2004.12.038; PMID:15766526.

53. Vasudevan S, Tong Y, Steitz JA. Switching from repression to activation: microRNAs can up-regulate translation. Science 2007; 318:1931-4; http://dx.doi.org/10.1126/science.1149460; PMID:18048652.

54. El Gazzar M, McCall CE. MicroRNAs distinguish translational from transcriptional silencing during endotoxin tolerance. J Biol Chem 2010; 285:20940-51; http://dx.doi.org/10.1074/jbc.M110.115063; PMID:20435889.

55. Tili E, Michaille JJ, Cimino A, Costinean S, Dumitru CD, Adair B, et al. Modulation of miR-155 and miR-125b levels following lipopolysaccharide/TNF-alpha stimulation and their possible roles in regulating the response to endotoxin shock. J Immunol 2007; 179:5082-9; PMID:17911593.

56. Thai TH, Calado DP, Casola S, Ansel KM, Xiao C, Xue Y, et al. Regulation of the germinal center response by microRNA-155. Science 2007; 316:604-8; http://dx.doi.org/10.1126/science.1141229; PMID:17463289.

57. Ma F, Liu X, Li D, Wang P, Li N, Lu L, Cao X. MicroRNA-466l upregulates IL-10 expression in TLR-triggered macrophages by antagonizing RNA-binding protein tristetraprolin-mediated IL-10 mRNA degradation. J Immunol 2010; 184:6053-9; http://dx.doi.org/10.4049/jimmunol.0902308; PMID:20410487.

58. Jones MR, Quinton LJ, Blahna MT, Neilson JR, Fu S, Ivanov AR, et al. Zcchc11-dependent uridylation of microRNA directs cytokine expression. Nat Cell Biol 2009; 11:1157-63; http://dx.doi.org/10.1038/ncb1931; PMID:19701194.

59. O'Neill LA, Sheedy FJ, McCoy CE. MicroRNAs: the fine-tuners of Toll-like receptor signalling. Nat Rev Immunol 2011; 11:163-75; http://dx.doi.org/10.1038/nri2957; PMID:21331081.

60. Barton GM. Viral recognition by Toll-like receptors. Semin Immunol 2007; 19:33-40; http://dx.doi.org/10.1016/j.smim.2007.01.003; PMID:17336545.

61. O'Connell RM, Taganov KD, Boldin MP, Cheng G, Baltimore D. MicroRNA-155 is induced during the macrophage inflammatory response. Proc Natl Acad Sci USA 2007; 104:1604-9; http://dx.doi.org/10.1073/pnas.0610731104; PMID:17242365.

62. Zhou H, Huang X, Cui H, Luo X, Tang Y, Chen S, et al. miR-155 and its star-form partner miR-155* cooperatively regulate type I interferon production by human plasmacytoid dendritic cells. Blood 2010; 116: 5885-94 PMID:20852130.

63. Gottwein E, Mukherjee N, Sachse C, Frenzel C, Majoros WH, Chi JT, et al. A viral microRNA functions as an orthologue of cellular miR-155. Nature 2007; 450:1096-9; http://dx.doi.org/10.1038/nature05992; PMID:18075594.

64. Ceppi M, Pereira PM, Dunand-Sauthier I, Barras E, Reith W, Santos MA, Pierre P. MicroRNA-155 modulates the interleukin-1 signaling pathway in activated human monocyte-derived dendritic cells. Proc Natl Acad Sci USA 2009; 106:2735-40; http://dx.doi.org/10.1073/pnas.0811073106; PMID:19193853.

65. Tang B, Xiao B, Liu Z, Li N, Zhu ED, Li BS, et al. Identification of MyD88 as a novel target of miR-155, involved in negative regulation of Helicobacter pylori-induced inflammation. FEBS Lett 2010; 584:1481-6; http://dx.doi.org/10.1016/j.febslet.2010.02.063; PMID:20219467.

66. Stanczyk J, Pedrioli DM, Brentano F, Sanchez-Pernaute O, Kolling C, Gay RE, et al. Altered expression of MicroRNA in synovial fibroblasts and synovial tissue in rheumatoid arthritis. Arthritis Rheum 2008; 58:1001-9; http://dx.doi.org/10.1002/art.23386; PMID:18383392.

67. Costinean S, Sandhu SK, Pedersen IM, Tili E, Trotta R, Perrotti D, et al. Src homology 2 domain-containing inositol-5-phosphatase and CCAAT enhancer-binding protein beta are targeted by miR-155 in B cells of Emicro-MiR-155 transgenic mice. Blood 2009; 114:1374-82; http://dx.doi.org/10.1182/blood-2009-05-220814; PMID:19520806.

68. O'Connell RM, Kahn D, Gibson WS, Round JL, Scholz RL, Chaudhuri AA, et al. MicroRNA-155 promotes autoimmune inflammation by enhancing inflammatory T cell development. Immunity 2010; 33:607-19; http://dx.doi.org/10.1016/j.immuni.2010.09.009; PMID:20888269.

69. Wang P, Hou J, Lin L, Wang C, Liu X, Li D, et al. Inducible microRNA-155 Feedback Promotes Type I IFN Signaling in Antiviral Innate Immunity by Targeting Suppressor of Cytokine Signaling 1. J Immunol 2010; 185: 6226-33; PMID:20937844.

70. Androulidaki A, Iliopoulos D, Arranz A, Doxaki C, Schworer S, Zacharioudaki V, et al. The kinase Akt1 controls macrophage response to lipopolysaccharide by regulating microRNAs. Immunity 2009; 31:220-31; http://dx.doi.org/10.1016/j.immuni.2009.06.024; PMID:19699171.

71. O'Connell RM, Chaudhuri AA, Rao DS, Baltimore D. Inositol phosphatase SHIP1 is a primary target of miR-155. Proc Natl Acad Sci USA 2009; 106:7113-8; http://dx.doi.org/10.1073/pnas.0902636106; PMID:19359473.

72. Rodriguez A, Vigorito E, Clare S, Warren MV, Couttet P, Soond DR, et al. Requirement of bic/microRNA-155 for normal immune function. Science 2007; 316:608-11; http://dx.doi.org/10.1126/science.1139253; PMID:17463290.

73. Vigorito E, Perks KL, Abreu-Goodger C, Bunting S, Xiang Z, Kohlhaas S, et al. microRNA-155 regulates the generation of immunoglobulin class-switched plasma cells. Immunity 2007; 27:847-59; http://dx.doi.org/10.1016/j.immuni.2007.10.009; PMID:18055230.

74. Taganov KD, Boldin MP, Chang KJ, Baltimore D. NF-kappaB-dependent induction of microRNA miR-146, an inhibitor targeted to signaling proteins of innate immune responses. Proc Natl Acad Sci USA 2006; 103:12481-6; http://dx.doi.org/10.1073/pnas.0605298103; PMID:16885212.

75. Motsch N, Pfuhl T, Mrazek J, Barth S, Grasser FA. Epstein-Barr Virus-encoded latent membrane protein 1 (LMP1) induces the expression of the cellular microRNA miR-146a. RNA Biol 2007; 4:131-7; http://dx.doi.org/10.4161/rna.4.3.5206; PMID:18347435.

76. Cameron JE, Yin Q, Fewell C, Lacey M, McBride J, Wang X, et al. Epstein-Barr virus latent membrane protein 1 induces cellular MicroRNA miR-146a, a modulator of lymphocyte signaling pathways. J Virol 2008; 82:1946-58; http://dx.doi.org/10.1128/JVI.02136-07; PMID:18057241.

77. Hou J, Wang P, Lin L, Liu X, Ma F, An H, et al. MicroRNA-146a feedback inhibits RIG-I-dependent Type I IFN production in macrophages by targeting TRAF6, IRAK1, and IRAK2. J Immunol 2009; 183:2150-8; http://dx.doi.org/10.4049/jimmunol.0900707; PMID:19596990.

78. Lagos D, Pollara G, Henderson S, Gratrix F, Fabani M, Milne RS, et al. miR-132 regulates antiviral innate immunity through suppression of the p300 transcriptional co-activator. Nat Cell Biol 2010; 12:513-9; http://dx.doi.org/10.1038/ncb2054; PMID:20418869.

79. Perry MM, Moschos SA, Williams AE, Shepherd NJ, Larner-Svensson HM, Lindsay MA. Rapid changes in microRNA-146a expression negatively regulate the IL-1beta-induced inflammatory response in human lung alveolar epithelial cells. J Immunol 2008; 180:5689-98; PMID:18390754.

80. Bhaumik D, Scott GK, Schokrpur S, Patil CK, Orjalo AV, Rodier F, et al. MicroRNAs miR-146a/b negatively modulate the senescence-associated inflammatory mediators IL-6 and IL-8. Aging (Albany NY) 2009; 1:402-11; PMID:20148189.

81. Jones SW, Watkins G, Le Good N, Roberts S, Murphy CL, Brockbank SM, et al. The identification of differentially expressed microRNA in osteoarthritic tissue that modulate the production of TNF-alpha and MMP13. Osteoarthritis Cartilage 2009; 17:464-72; http://dx.doi.org/10.1016/j.joca.2008.09.012; PMID:19008124.

82. Nahid MA, Pauley KM, Satoh M, Chan EK. miR-146a is critical for endotoxin-induced tolerance: implication in innate immunity. J Biol Chem 2009; 284:34590-9; http://dx.doi.org/10.1074/jbc.M109.056317; PMID:19840932.

83. Tang Y, Luo X, Cui H, Ni X, Yuan M, Guo Y, et al. MicroRNA-146A contributes to abnormal activation of the type I interferon pathway in human lupus by targeting the key signaling proteins. Arthritis Rheum 2009; 60:1065-75; http://dx.doi.org/10.1002/art.24436; PMID:19333922.

84. Boldin MP, Taganov KD, Rao DS, Yang L, Zhao JL, Kalwani M, et al. miR-146a is a significant brake on autoimmunity, myeloproliferation, and cancer in mice. J Exp Med 2011; 208:1189-201; http://dx.doi.org/10.1084/jem.20101823; PMID:21555486.

85. Bazzoni F, Rossato M, Fabbri M, Gaudiosi D, Mirolo M, Mori L, et al. Induction and regulatory function of miR-9 in human monocytes and neutrophils exposed to proinflammatory signals. Proc Natl Acad Sci USA 2009; 106:5282-7; http://dx.doi.org/10.1073/pnas.0810909106; PMID:19289835.

86. Liu G, Friggeri A, Yang Y, Park YJ, Tsuruta Y, Abraham E. miR-147, a microRNA that is induced upon Toll-like receptor stimulation, regulates murine macrophage inflammatory responses. Proc Natl Acad Sci USA 2009; 106: 15819-24; PMID:19721002.

87. Chen XM, Splinter PL, O'Hara SP, LaRusso NF. A cellular micro-RNA, let-7i, regulates Toll-like receptor 4 expression and contributes to cholangiocyte immune responses against Cryptosporidium parvum infection. J Biol Chem 2007; 282:28929-38; http://dx.doi.org/10.1074/jbc.M702633200; PMID:17660297.

88. Benakanakere MR, Li Q, Eskan MA, Singh AV, Zhao J, Galicia JC, et al. Modulation of TLR2 protein expression by miR-105 in human oral keratinocytes. J Biol Chem 2009; 284:23107-15; http://dx.doi.org/10.1074/jbc.M109.013862; PMID:19509287.

89. Starczynowski DT, Kuchenbauer F, Argiropoulos B, Sung S, Morin R, Muranyi A, et al. Identification of miR-145 and miR-146a as mediators of the 5q- syndrome phenotype. Nat Med 2010; 16:49-58; http://dx.doi.org/10.1038/nm.2054; PMID:19898489.

90. Yamin TT, Miller DK. The interleukin-1 receptor-associated kinase is degraded by proteasomes following its phosphorylation. J Biol Chem 1997; 272:21540-7; http://dx.doi.org/10.1074/jbc.272.34.21540; PMID:9261174.

91. Jacinto R, Hartung T, McCall C, Li L. Lipopolysaccharide- and lipoteichoic acid-induced tolerance and cross-tolerance: distinct alterations in IL-1 receptor-associated kinase. J Immunol 2002;168(12):6136-6141.

92. Yeo SJ, Yoon JG, Hong SC, Yi AK. CpG DNA induces self and cross-hyporesponsiveness of RAW264.7 cells in response to CpG DNA and lipopolysaccharide: alterations in IL-1 receptor-associated kinase expression. J Immunol 2003;170(2):1052-1061.

93. Schauvliege R, Janssens S, Beyaert R. Pellino proteins are more than scaffold proteins in TLR/IL-1R signalling: A role as novel RING E3–ubiquitin-ligases. FEBS Lett 2006; 580:4697-702; http://dx.doi.org/10.1016/j.febslet.2006.07.046; PMID:16884718.

94. Ordureau A, Smith H, Windheim M, Peggie M, Carrick E, Morrice N, Cohen P. The IRAK-catalysed activation of the E3 ligase function of Pellino isoforms induces the Lys63-linked polyubiquitination of IRAK1. Biochem J 2008; 409:43-52; http://dx.doi.org/10.1042/BJ20071365; PMID:17997719.

95. Shi M, Deng W, Bi E, Mao K, Ji Y, Lin G, et al. TRIM30α negatively regulates TLR-mediated NF-κB activation by targeting TAB2 and TAB3 for degradation. Nat Immunol 2008; 9:369-77; http://dx.doi.org/10.1038/ni1577; PMID:18345001.

96. Chuang T-H, Ulevitch RJ. Triad3A, an E3 ubiquitin-protein ligase regulating Toll-like receptors. Nat Immunol 2004; 5:495-502; http://dx.doi.org/10.1038/ni1066; PMID:15107846.

97. Fearns C, Pan Q, Mathison JC, Chuang T-H. Triad3A regulates ubiquitination and proteasomal degradation of RIP1 following disruption of Hsp90 binding. J Biol Chem 2006; 281:34592-600; http://dx.doi.org/10.1074/jbc.M604019200; PMID:16968706.

98. Nakhaei P, Mesplede T, Solis M, Sun Q, Zhao T, Yang L, et al. The E3 ubiquitin ligase Triad3A negatively regulates the RIG-I/MAVS signaling pathway by targeting TRAF3 for degradation. PLoS Pathog 2009; 5:e1000650; http://dx.doi.org/10.1371/journal.ppat.1000650; PMID:19893624.

CHAPTER 5

Intracellular Viral RNA Sensors:
RIG-I Like Receptors

Seiji P. Yamamoto,[†,1,2] Ryo Narita,[†,1] Seigyoku Go,[†,1,3] Kiyohiro Takahasi,[1,4]
Hiroki Kato,[1,3] and Takashi Fujita[*,1,3]

Abstract

RIG-I-like receptors (RLRs) are DExD/H box RNA helicases that play an essential role in antiviral innate immunity. RLRs sense viral infection by recognizing the non-self structure of viral RNA in the cytoplasm and then trigger antiviral interferon (IFN) responses to eliminate invading viruses. Based on recent studies, here we describe how RLRs detect viruses and transduce antiviral signaling.

Introduction

RIG-I-like receptors (RLRs) are DExD/H box-containing RNA helicases that sense cytosolic pathogen-associated molecular patterns (PAMPs) within viral RNA.[1,2] Signals from RLRs activate transcription factors to induce type I interferon (IFN) and antiviral gene expression that give rise to rapid elimination of invading viruses.[3] So far, three family members have been identified: RIG-I (retinoic acid inducible gene I), melanoma differentiation associated gene 5 (MDA5) and laboratory of genetics and physiology 2 (LGP2).[4] These helicases are found only in higher vertebrates and are ubiquitously expressed in most tissues; therefore, it appears that RLRs provoke the first line of antiviral response by sensing peripheral infection.

All three RLR share structural similarities and contain a typical RNA helicase domain with RNA-dependent ATPase activity. RIG-I and MDA5 contain 3 domains: (1) the N-terminal domain (NTD) consisting of tandem caspase activation and recruitment domains (CARDs), (2) the central DExD/H box RNA helicase domain with ATPase activity, and (3) the C-terminal domain (CTD), which contributes to viral RNA recognition. Interestingly, LGP2 lacks CARDs and has been shown to positively regulate RIG-I- and MDA5-mediated signaling.[5]

When RIG-I and MDA5 recognize PAMPs, CARDs of RLR are implicated in the transmission of signals via interaction with a CARD-containing adaptor molecule on mitochondria, IFN-β promoter stimulator 1 (IPS-1) (also known as mitochondrial antiviral signaling (MAVS), virus-induced signaling adaptor (VISA), and CARD adaptor inducing IFN-β (Cardif)).[6-9] The RLR-IPS-1 complex serves as a scaffold for the assembly of a protein complex consisting of TRAF3/6, caspase-8/10, receptor interacting protein 1 (RIP1), and Fas-associated death domain (TRADD).[10] Formation of the complex of these molecules elicits the assembly of TRAF family

¹Laboratory of Molecular Genetics, Institute for Virus Research, Kyoto University, Kyoto, Japan; ²Laboratory of Biomass Conversion, Research Institute for Sustainable Humanosphere, Kyoto University, Kyoto, Japan; ³Laboratory of Molecular Cell Biology, Graduate School of Biostudies, Kyoto University, Kyoto, Japan; ⁴Institute for Innovative NanoBio Drug Discovery and Development, Graduate School of Pharmaceutical Sciences, Kyoto University, Kyoto, Japan.
†These authors contributed equally to this work.
*Corresponding Author: Takashi Fujita—Email: tfujita@virus.kyoto-u.ac.jp

Nucleic Acid Sensors and Antiviral Immunity, edited by Suryaprakash Sambhara and Takashi Fujita.
©2013 Landes Bioscience.

member-associated NF-κB activator (TANK) and NF-κB essential modulator (NEMO) to induce kinase activities of both IKKα/IKKβ/IKKγ and TBK1/IKKε complexes to activate NF-κB and IRF-3, respectively.[11] In addition, NAK-associated protein 1 (NAP1)[12] and similar to NAP1 and TBK1 adaptor (SINTBAD)[13] are reported to mediate the activation of IRFs through association with TBK1 and IKKε. Eventual activation of IRFs leads to the production of type I IFNs and proinflammatory cytokines.

Specificity of RLRs in Recognition of Viral Infection

Among RLRs, RIG-I and MDA5 exhibit a similar domain structure and share a common signaling pathway; however, their recognitions are virus-specific (Table 1). RIG-I detects a wide variety of viruses including Sendai virus (SeV), Newcastle disease virus (NDV), vesicular stomatitis virus (VSV), influenza A virus (IAV) and hepatitis C virus (HCV), which belong to subsets of ssRNA-genomed virus families.[4,14,15] Nonetheless, the viruses of *Picornavitidae* such as Encephalomyocarditis virus (EMCV), Theiler's virus and Mengo virus are not recognized by RIG-I, but are exclusively recognized by MDA5.[16,17] Vaccinia virus, a DNA virus which replicates in the cytoplasm, is specifically recognized by MDA5[18]; however, another poxvirus family, Myxoma virus, is recognized by RIG-I.[19] Moreover, it has been considered that both RIG-I and MDA5

Table 1. Viruses recognized by RIG-I and MDA5

RLRs	Viruses	References
RIG-I	*Paramyxoviridae*; ssRNA(-)/NS	
	Sendai virus	Yoneyama et al., Kato et al., 2005
	New Castle disease virus	Kato et al., 2005
	Respiratory syncytical virus	Loo et al., 2008
	Rhabdoviridae; ssRNA(-)/NS	
	Rabies virus	Hornung et al., 2006
	Vesicular stomatitis virus	Yoneyama et al., Kato et al., 2005
	Orthomyxoviridae; ssRNA(-)/S	
	Influenza A virus	Kato et al., 2006
	Influenza B virus	Loo et al., 2008
	Flaviviridae; ssRNA(+)/NS	
	Hepatitis C virus	Saito et al., 2007
	Japanese encephalitis virus	Kato et al., 2006
	Gammaherpesviridae; dsDNA	
	Epstein-Barr virus	Samanta et al., 2008
MDA5	*Picornaviridae*; ssRNA(+)/NS	
	Encephalomyocarditis virus	Kato et al., Gitlin et al., 2006
	Theiler's virus	Kato et al., 2006
	Mengo virus	Kato et al., 2006
	Poxviridae; dsDNA	
	Vaccinia virus	Pichlmair et al., 2009
RIG-I	*Flaviviridae*; ssRNA(+)/NS	
MDA5	West Nile virus	Loo et al., Fredericksen et al., 2008
	Dengue virus	Loo et al., 2008
	Reoviridae; dsRNA	
	Reovirus	Kato et al., Loo et al., 2008

RIG-I and MDA5 recognize distinct types of RNA viruses as indicated. Some types of viruses such as West Nile, Dengue and Reovirus are recognized by both RIG-I and MDA5.(-); negative-strand genome, (+); positive-strand genome, NS; non-segmented genome, S; segmented genome.

are required for a sufficient antiviral response against certain types of infections by viruses such as West Nile virus, dengue virus or reovirus.[20-22] It is quite possible that these differential roles in the recognition of viral infections are due to the distinct structures of viral RNA produced. Unlike RIG-I and MDA5, LGP2 lacks CARD. Because of this, this molecule was considered as a negative regulator in the IFN system; however, mice lacking LGP2 exhibit impaired IFN production upon NDV, VSV and EMCV infection, suggesting that LGP2 positively regulates the antiviral response against certain viruses. LGP2 may activate signaling by cooperation with either RIG-I or MDA5 through their CARD because double knockout of RIG-I and MDA5 barely produced IFN.[5]

RLR Ligands

dsRNAs as the Ligand of RIG-I and MDA5

Initially, RIG-I was identified as a cDNA clone, which augmented the poly(I:C)-induced activation of an IFN-responsive reporter construct.[1] Subsequent experiments revealed that the length of Poly(I:C) is one of the important determinants in ligand specificity of RIG-I and MDA5.[22] Long Poly(I:C) (> 4 kbp) was preferentially recognized by MDA5, whereas shorter Poly(I:C) (~300 bp) was an exclusive substrate of RIG-I (Table 2).

Also, the structure of RNA required for RIG-I activation was explored by using chemically-synthesized short (~25 bp) oligonucleotides; dsRNA. Synthetic blunt-ended and 5'-overhanged short dsRNA but not those with a 3'-overhang activate RIG-I.[23] This is consistent with another report,[24] which revealed that dsRNA with a 3' overhang is a good substrate for RIG-I helicase, but is a poor ligand for IFN production. Furthermore, it was shown that 5'-monophosphorylation at the ends of such dsRNA is required for RIG-I to elicit IFN induction.[24]

ssRNAs as the Ligand of RIG-I ?

Along with dsRNA, in vitro-transcribed ssRNA by phage polymerase (e.g., T7-Pol) was reported to be a good chemical inducer of IFN.[25] In theory, in vitro transcripts contain a 5' tri-phosphate and this appeared to be critical to induce IFN production in human primary monocytes in a RIG-I-dependent manner.[26] Also, genome RNA of influenza A virus, which contains 5' tri-phosphate, is sufficient to induce IFN by transfection.[27] These observations suggest that 5' tri-phosphate is the determinant for non-self RNA in the cytoplasm because 5'-triphosphate moiety of host RNA is removed or masked before being transported to the cytoplasm. Moreover, *Picornaviridae* is devoid of this structure by covalent attachment of viral protein, Vpg.[28]

However, later it was revealed that chemically-synthesized ssRNA with 5' tri-phosphate failed to activate RIG-I, suggesting that 5' tri-phosphate is not the sole determinant of non-self. Instead, it was revealed that in vitro transcription by phage polymerase results in partial double strands by the "copy-back" mechanism. Taken together, it is now accepted that short dsRNA (~25 bp) is a poor ligand for RIG-I but its activity is markedly enhanced by the presence of 5' tri-phosphate.[29,30] When dsRNA is relatively long (> 100 bp), the effect of 5' tri-phosphate is negligible, by an unknown mechanism.

Natural Viral RNA Ligands for RIG-I

The observations obtained by studies using artificially generated RNA provided the nature of ligands related to recognition by RIG-I. The next question is to identify natural viral RNA species produced during viral replication.

Of note, it was reported that not only dsRNA viruses but also positive strand ssRNA viruses (ssRNA(+)) produce substantial amounts of cytosolic dsRNA during the process of the viral lifecycle.[31] Consistent with the requirement of a double-stranded structure for recognition by RIG-I, some of these dsRNA-producing viruses are detected by RIG-I (Table 1). Negative strand RNA viruses (ssRNA(-)), on the other hand, do not produce a detectable amount of dsRNA during viral replication.[27,31] Nevertheless, most of these viruses are detected by RIG-I (Table 1). This conflict is explained by the characteristic structure of IAV genomic RNA. IAV contain a highly complementary sequence in their 5'- and 3'-non-coding regions, which causes the formation of a

Table 2. Structures of RIG-I and MDA5 ligands

RNAs	Structures	RLRs	References
Short Poly(I:C) dsRNA ~300bp		RIG-I	Kato et al., 2008
Long Poly(I:C) dsRNA >4kbp		MDA5	Kato et al., 2008
in vitro T7 transcript ssRNA (copy-back)		RIG-I	Schlee et al., 2009 Schmidt et al., 2009
IAV genomic RNA ssRNA (panhandle)		RIG-I	Rehwinkel et al., 2010
SeV genomic RNA ssRNA (DI, snap-back)		RIG-I	Strähle et al., 2007
HCV genomic RNA ssRNA (homopolymer)		RIG-I	Saito et al., 2008
EMCV genomic RNA ss/dsRNA (RNA web)		MDA5	Pichlmair et al., 2009

Summary of synthetic and viral RNA motifs recognized by RIG-I and MDA5. 5' triphosphate motif and short dsRNA are recognized by RIG-I. MDA5 recognizes long dsRNA and high-order structure by mixture of ss/dsRNA (RNA web).

short double-strand structure with a perfect blunt end (~15 bp), and this "panhandle" structure is supposed to be recognized by RIG-I (Table 2).[32] Likewise, SeV generates defective interfering (DI) viral genomes with a hairpin-like double-stranded structure (100–1,000 bp), and this "snap-back" structure likely represents a ligand of RIG-I.[33]

It was also demonstrated that the activation of RIG-I in response to HCV infection requires Poly(rU/rA) homomeric RNA composition in the HCV genome, implying the sequence dependency of RIG-I recognition in addition to specificity for the structures of the RNAs.[15] Furthermore, it was reported that synthetic dsDNA, poly(dA-dT) activates RIG-I indirectly by its RNA transcripts, which was produced by host RNA polymerase III.[34,35]

Concerning MDA5 activation, RNA extracted from cells infected with EMCV and Vaccinia virus was fractionated and assessed for IFN induction. It appeared that a large RNA complex, which was stuck at the top of agarose gel electrophoresis, activated the IFN gene in an MDA5-dependent manner.[36] Neither the precise structure of the complex nor its recognition mechanism by MDA5 has been elucidated.

Positive and Negative Regulation of RLR-Mediated Signaling

To date, numerous molecules have been reported as positive or negative regulators of RLR signaling, as indicated in Figure 1. Some regulators are mitochondrial proteins. NLRX1 (NOD9) belongs to the NOD-Like Receptor family and contains a highly conserved nucleotide-binding domain and leucine-rich-repeat, and uniquely localizes to the mitochondria and interacts with IPS-1.[37] NLRX1 knockdown augmented virus-induced IFN production and decreased viral replication, suggesting that NLRX1 is a negative modulator of RLR signaling by disrupting RLR

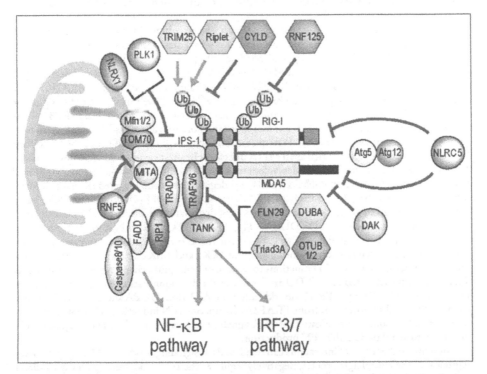

Figure 1. RIG-I and MDA5-mediated signaling and adaptor molecules. Various molecules are involved in RLR-mediated activation of NF-κB and IRF3/7 pathways via an adaptor molecule IPS-1. Positive and negative regulations are indicated by light gray (red) and dark gray (blue) lines, respectively. A color version of this figure is available online at www.landesbioscience.com/curie.

interaction with IPS-1. In contrast, other mitochondrion membrane-associated proteins have been reported as positive regulators of RLR signaling, including the Mediator of IRF-3 activation (MITA)(also known as the stimulator of interferon genes (STING)), translocases of outer membrane 70 (TOM70), and mitofusin 1 and 2. MITA, initially identified as a positive regulator of RLR signaling, directly interacts with both IPS-1 and IRF-3 and regulates the virus-dependent recruitment of TBK1 to the RIG-I/IPS-1 complex on mitochondria[38]; however, MITA is also an essential signaling adaptor protein that directs innate immune responses to DNA viruses, MITA may supply a platform important for both RLR signaling and the response to DNA virus infection.[39] TOM70 was identified as an interactor with IPS-1.[40] TOM70 also associates with Hsp90; thus, TBK1 and IRF3 assemble around IPS-1 together with HSP90, which enhances the activation of downstream signaling. Although there is controversy about the requirement of mitofusin 2 for signal transduction, mitofusin is thought to control mitochondrial fusion and affect IPS-1-dependent signal transduction during virus infection.[41-44] In contrast, NLRC5, another member of the NLR family, has been reported as a negative regulator of RLR signaling. Mechanistically, NLRC5 potently inhibits RLR-dependent IFN production by interacting with RLR but not IPS-1.[45] NLRC5 has further ability to bind to IKKα and IKKβ, prevents them from being phosphorylated, and impedes their NF-κB-activating activities. Interestingly, it has been reported that IPS-1-containing mitochondria huddle around the viral replication site in virus-infected cells.[43] This observation and the involvement of these mitochondrial proteins in RLR signaling imply that dynamic action of mitochondria is probably required for regulating proinflammatory cytokines and IFN production.

Other regulators are involved in the ubiquitination or deubiquitinaion of RLR signaling molecules. Three RING-type ubiquitin E3 ligases, Tripartite motif protein (TRIM) 25, Riplet (also termed RNF135 and REUL), and RNF125, have been reported to target RIG-I for ubiquitination. TRIM25 and Riplet conjugate Lys-63-linked ubiquitins to RIG-I independently from each other.[46-49] This ubiquitination promotes RIG-I-mediated IFN promoter activation. On the other hand, RNF125 catalyzes Lys-48-linked polyubiquitination.[50] This leads to proteasomal degradation of RIG-I. Moreover, since MDA5 and IPS-1 also undergo proteasomal degradation after conjugation of ubiquitination by RNF125, RNF125 suppresses RLR signaling. A20, RNF5 and Triad3A have also been reported as ubiquitin ligase, which negatively modulate RIG-I signaling but do not ubiquitinate RIG-I. A20 inhibits TBK1/IKKϵ kinases that activate IRF3.[51] A20 possesses a deubiquitination domain at its N terminus and ubiquitin ligase domain at its C terminus; however, deletion of the N-terminal deubiquitination domain does not influence the inhibitory function of A20. RNF5, identified as an MITA interactor by yeast two-hybrid screening, binds to MITA and IPS-1 in a virus-infection-dependent manner, and conjugates Lys-48-linked ubiquitin to MITA and IPS-1.[52,53] As a result of MITA and IPS-1 degradation, virus-triggered IRF3 activation is inhibited. Similarly, Triad3A, which has a TRAF-Interacting-Motif (TIM), binds to TRAF3 and mediates Lys-48 linked ubiquitination and subsequent degradation of TRAF3.[54] Deubiquitination enzymes, cylindromatosis (CYLD), DUBA, OTUB1 and OTUB2, were involved in the negative regulation of RIG-I-mediated signaling. CYLD, which is known as a tumor suppressor, has been shown to have a crucial role in preventing aberrant IKKϵ and TBK1 activation.[55] In addition, a recent report showed that CYLD functions to remove polyubiquitin chains from RIG-I as well as TBK1 to inhibit IRF3 signaling.[56] DUBA[57] is one of the deubiquitination enzymes for TRAF3, whereas OTUB1/2 [58] targets TRAF6 in addition to TRAF3. Both DUBA and OTUB1/2 remove the K63-linked ubiquitin chain from TRAF3/6, hampering IFN induction. These studies show that reversible ubiquitin modification of RLR signaling pathway molecules tightly regulates IFN induction to avoid undesirable IFN production.

Moreover, other types of interactors can regulate RLR signaling. Atg5-Atg12 conjugate, a key regulator of the autophagic process, negatively regulates the IFN production pathway by direct association with both RIG-I and IPS-1 through CARDs.[59,60] Polo-like kinase 1 (PLK1) was also characterized as an IPS-1 interactor and inhibited IFN production by disrupting IPS-1-TRAF3 interaction.[61] Similarly, FLN29, identified as an IFN-inducible gene, inhibits IPS-1-dependent activation of NF-κB and IRF3.[62] Since FLN29 associates with TRIF, IPS-1, TRAF3, and TRAF6, it is speculated that FLN29 negatively regulates the RLR signaling pathway at the level of IPS-1/ TRAF6 and IPS-1/TRAF3 complexes.[63] As an MDA5 interactor, dihydroaceotne kinase (DAK) was identified and shown to be a negative regulator of MDA5 signaling but not RIG-I, and inhibited polyI:C-induced IFN production.[64] Taken together, RLR signaling is regulated by functional interactors, suggesting the importance of precisely controlling IFN production.

Structure

CTD, an Essential RNA Binding Domain of RLRs

The C-terminal domain (CTD) of RIG-I was identified as a recognition domain for dsRNA and 5'pppRNA by two groups.[24,65] The structure of the CTD was determined by nuclear magnetic resonance (NMR) and X-ray crystal structure analyses. RIG-I CTD has a basic amino acid-rich cleft-like structure, whereas the opposite surface of CTD contains acidic patches. RLR CTD has about 30% amino acid similarity and both MDA5 and LGP2 CTDs have been identified as an RNA binding domain. The structure of each RLR CTD was demonstrated to have a similar overall structure and a similar basic surface. NMR titration and in vitro binding assay revealed that RIG-I CTD is sufficient to bind to dsRNA or 5'pppRNA. In addition, LGP2 CTD strongly binds to dsRNA or 5'pppRNA, whereas RNA binding activity of MDA5 CTD is much weaker because the basic surface of MDA5 CTD is extensively flat compared with that of RIG-I or LGP2.[66] The crystal structure of RIG-I CTD/RNA showed that RIG-I CTD recognizes the termini of RNA and RIG-I CTD has a pocket for 5'ppp moiety, which indicates that recognition mostly occurs at the end of RNA.[67,68] The crystal structure of LGP2 CTD/ dsRNA was also determined and LGP2 CTD was found to recognize the termini of dsRNA[69]; however, full-length RIG-I bound to dsRNA independent of the end structures,[24] suggesting that CTD per se does not represent RNA recognition by RIG-I.

Structural Biology of RIG-I and Model for Its Activation

Recently, the crystal structure of the helicase domain of RIG-I was reported by three groups. Luo et al.[70] and Jiang et al.[71] determined the structure of human RIG-I lacking CARDs complexed with dsRNA. Kowalinski et al.[72] determined the 3 different structures of duck RIG-I (dRIG-I): dRIG-I helicase domain alone; dRIG-I lacking CTD; dRIG-I lacking CARDs complexed with dsRNA. The domain structure of full-length RIG-I is shown in Figure 2A.

One of the interesting features of the RIG-I structure is its helicase domain. The helicase domain contains three parts, designated H-I–III from the N terminus. H-I and H-III are RecA-like helicase domains and H-II is a five-helix bundle domain that is inserted into the N-terminus of H-III. Importantly, in the structure of dRIG-I lacking CTD, H-II interacts with the second CARD (CII) and this interaction is speculated to repress the activation by CARDs (Fig. 2B). In the presence of dsRNA, all three parts of the helicase encircles dsRNA (H-I, H-III and H-II rotate clockwise, as described in Fig. 2C) and CTD captures the blunt end or 5' tri-phosphate of dsRNA, capping the edge. Notably, the surface of H-II interacting with CII in the basal state is involved in dsRNA binding. Thus, conformational change upon binding to viral RNA would release CARDs from restraint. The structure of RIG-I/RNA complex suggests that RIG-I binds at the end of dsRNA, not in the middle of dsRNA strands; however, these structures are inconsistent with the observation that RIG-I translocates along dsRNA.[73] Another interesting feature is linker 2 (L2), the structure between H-III and CTD, which consists of 62 aa, including an elbow-like structure, as shown in Figure 2B. This elbow interacts with both H-I and H-III in the basal state. The non-structured region of L2 allows flexible movement of CTD to catch the edge of dsRNA. Point mutations of the elbow confer constitutive activity, suggesting that the mutations release CARDs from H-II by conformational change.[74] Overexpression of L2 is sufficient to inhibit RIG-I-dependent activation of IFN signaling, although the mechanism is unknown.

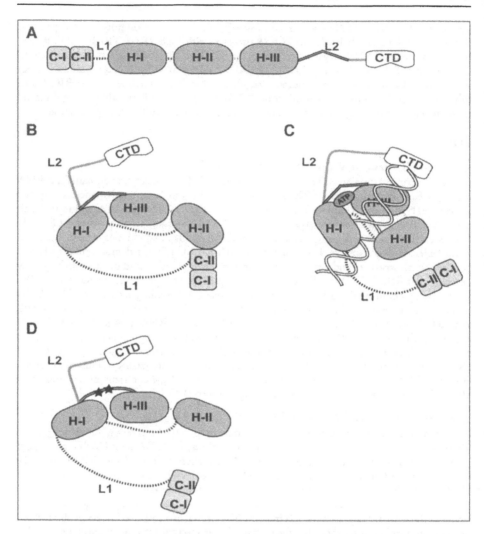

Figure 2. Model for RIG-I activation. A) Linear domain structure of full length RIG-I. CI and CII: CARD1 and CARD2. H-I, H-II, H-III: Helicase domain I II and III. CTD: C-terminal domain. L1: Linker 1. L2: Linker 2. B) Schematic representation of RIG-I in the basal state. Tandem CARDs are suppressed by the interaction with H-II. C) Schematic representation of RIG-I in complex with dsRNA. CTD binds the terminus of dsRNA and helicase domains (H-I to H-III) form ring like structure around dsRNA. Tandem CARDs are released. D) Proposed mechanism of constitutive active RIG-I, in which L2 structure is disrupted by point mutations (stars).

The possible model of RIG-I activation is:

1. Binding of RNA ligand to CTD, and ATP to H-I and H-III
2. Conformational change in the helicase region (encircling structure) and its binding to dsRNA
3. Conformational change (step 2) releases tandem CARDs

Further studies are still necessary to clarify the details of RLR activation.

Conclusions and Perspectives

Recently, much information about the mechanism by which RLR recognize viral RNA and induce IFN signaling has been accumulating. Also, we have noticed that viruses have many strategies to suppress RLR-mediated IFN responses.

As described here, it is clearly demonstrated that RLR are essential sensors of RNA viruses and that these RNA helicases discriminate self and non-self RNAs by precise recognition of RNA signatures specific to viruses; however, many interesting topics remain to be investigated further. The structure of RIG-I/RNA complex provides a clue to elucidate the mechanism of its activation; however, the details are still unclear. Also, the biological significance of helicase activity and translocation on dsRNA remain to be clarified. Even though the requirement for the dynamic action of mitochondria for IPS-1-dependent signaling has been demonstrated,[43] the reason why IPS-1 localizes to mitochondria should be determined. In addition, several phenotypes of RLR mutant mice suggest possible functions of RLR beyond the scope of viral RNA sensing, such as developmental defects in RIG-I-deficient mice.[14] For example, different from TBK1-deficient mice, liver degeneration of RIG-I-deficient mice is not rescued by a TNF-α-deficient background, which suggests that RIG-I-mediated IFN signaling is not involved in the defects of RIG-I-deficient mice. Some RNAs expressed in the embryonic liver during development might be regulated by RIG-I. Furthermore, the involvement of MDA5 in type I diabetes and possible tumor therapy by 5′ tri-phosphate siRNAs could be an interesting research target from a clinical aspect. It is important to explore and identify the physiological functions of RLR other than antiviral activities.

About the Authors

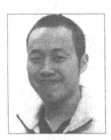

Seiji Yamamoto received his PhD at Kyoto University. He is currently a post-doctoral researcher in the Research Institute for Sustainable Humanosphere, and conducts experiments in Institute for Virus Research at Kyoto University.

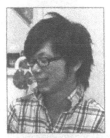

Seigyoku Go joined Dr. Takashi Fujita's laboratory as a doctoral student 4 years ago. He spent a happy time in the beautiful city of Kyoto, with his exciting research life. He is working hard to obtain PhD on his project concerning antiviral innate immunity.

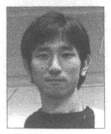

Ryo Narita is a research assistant in the Laboratory of Molecular Genetics, Institute for Virus Research. He is studying the mechanism of non-self RNA recognition by RLRs.

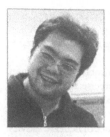

Kiyohiro Takahasi obtained his PhD from Hokkaido University in 2003 where he solved the crystal structure of Interferon regulatory factor 3 and revealed its activation mechanism. He joined the laboratory of Dr. Takashi Fujita at Kyoto University, Kyoto in 2009 where he is currently an Assistant Professor. His current research is focused on tertiary structure analysis of proteins in innate immunity using both NMR and X-ray crystallography.

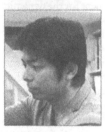

Hiroki Kato started his research in the field of innate immunity during a PhD course in Prof. Akira Shizuo's lab (Osaka University), generated knockout-mice of RIG-I like receptors (RLRs) and examined the functional role of RLRs in antiviral responses. After getting PhD, he worked with Prof. Craig Mello (University of Massachusetts Medical School) as a postdoctoral fellow and investigated a possible role of RLRs in RNA silencing pathway. Now he is an Associate Professor in Kyoto University. Currently his major interest is the involvement of RLRs in miRNA and RNA silencing pathways.

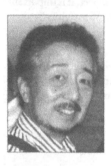

Takashi Fujita is Professor of Molecular Genetics in Institute for Virus Research, Kyoto University Japan. He obtained his PhD from Waseda University, Tokyo 1982 on studies on interferon priming. He joined Dr. T. Taniguchi's laboratory at Cancer Institute, then later at Osaka University as a postdoctoral fellow until 1990, where he worked on interferon-b gene and identified virus-inducible enhancer element and cloned IRF-1. He joined Prof. D. Baltimore's laboratory as a postdoctoral fellow at Whitehead Institute and Rockefeller University until 1993 and worked on transcriptional regulation by NF-κB. He started his own laboratory in Tokyo Metropolitan Institute for medical Sciences in 1993. His group discovered IRF-3 as a key regulator for interferon genes. In 2004, his group, including Dr. M. Yoneyama, discovered RIG-I and related sensors for viral RNA. In 2005, his group moved to Kyoto University.

References

1. Yoneyama M, Kikuchi M, Natsukawa T, Shinobu N, Imaizumi T, Miyagishi M, et al. The RNA helicase RIG-I has an essential function in double-stranded RNA-induced innate antiviral responses. Nat Immunol 2004; 5:730-7; http://dx.doi.org/10.1038/ni1087; PMID:15208624.
2. Schlee M, Hartmann G. The chase for the RIG-I ligand--recent advances. Mol Ther 2010; 18:1254-62; http://dx.doi.org/10.1038/mt.2010.90; PMID:20461060.
3. Takeuchi O, Akira S. Pattern recognition receptors and inflammation. Cell 2010; 140:805-20; http://dx.doi.org/10.1016/j.cell.2010.01.022; PMID:20303872.
4. Yoneyama M, Kikuchi M, Matsumoto K, Imaizumi T, Miyagishi M, Taira K, et al. Shared and unique functions of the DExD/H-box helicases RIG-I, MDA5, and LGP2 in antiviral innate immunity. J Immunol 2005; 175:2851-8; PMID:16116171.
5. Satoh T, Kato H, Kumagai Y, Yoneyama M, Sato S, Matsushita K, et al. LGP2 is a positive regulator of RIG-I- and MDA5-mediated antiviral responses. Proc Natl Acad Sci U S A 2010; 107:1512-7; http://dx.doi.org/10.1073/pnas.0912986107; PMID:20080593.
6. Kawai T, Takahashi K, Sato S, Coban C, Kumar H, Kato H, et al. IPS-1, an adaptor triggering RIG-I- and Mda5-mediated type I interferon induction. Nat Immunol 2005; 6:981-8; http://dx.doi.org/10.1038/ni1243; PMID:16127453.
7. Xu LG, Wang YY, Han KJ, Li LY, Zhai Z, Shu HB. VISA is an adapter protein required for virus-triggered IFN-beta signaling. Mol Cell 2005; 19:727-40; http://dx.doi.org/10.1016/j.molcel.2005.08.014; PMID:16153868.

8. Meylan E, Curran J, Hofmann K, Moradpour D, Binder M, Bartenschlager R, et al. Cardif is an adaptor protein in the RIG-I antiviral pathway and is targeted by hepatitis C virus. Nature 2005; 437:1167-72; http://dx.doi.org/10.1038/nature04193; PMID:16177806.

9. Seth RB, Sun L, Ea CK, Chen ZJ. Identification and characterization of MAVS, a mitochondrial antiviral signaling protein that activates NF-kappaB and IRF 3. Cell 2005; 122:669-82; http://dx.doi.org/10.1016/j.cell.2005.08.012; PMID:16125763.

10. Michallet MC, Meylan E, Ermolaeva MA, Vazquez J, Rebsamen M, Curran J, et al. TRADD protein is an essential component of the RIG-like helicase antiviral pathway. Immunity 2008; 28:651-61; http://dx.doi.org/10.1016/j.immuni.2008.03.013; PMID:18439848.

11. Kawai T, Akira S. The roles of TLRs, RLRs and NLRs in pathogen recognition. Int Immunol 2009; 21:317-37; http://dx.doi.org/10.1093/intimm/dxp017; PMID:19246554.

12. Sasai M, Shingai M, Funami K, Yoneyama M, Fujita T, Matsumoto M, et al. NAK-associated protein 1 participates in both the TLR3 and the cytoplasmic pathways in type I IFN induction. J Immunol 2006; 177:8676-83; PMID:17142768.

13. Ryzhakov G, Randow F. SINTBAD, a novel component of innate antiviral immunity, shares a TBK1-binding domain with NAP1 and TANK. EMBO J 2007; 26:3180-90; http://dx.doi.org/10.1038/sj.emboj.7601743; PMID:17568778.

14. Kato H, Sato S, Yoneyama M, Yamamoto M, Uematsu S, Matsui K, et al. Cell type-specific involvement of RIG-I in antiviral response. Immunity 2005; 23:19-28; http://dx.doi.org/10.1016/j.immuni.2005.04.010; PMID:16039576.

15. Saito T, Owen DM, Jiang F, Marcotrigiano J, Gale M Jr. Innate immunity induced by composition-dependent RIG-I recognition of hepatitis C virus RNA. Nature 2008; 454:523-7; http://dx.doi.org/10.1038/nature07106; PMID:18548002.

16. Kato H, Takeuchi O, Sato S, Yoneyama M, Yamamoto M, Matsui K, et al. Differential roles of MDA5 and RIG-I helicases in the recognition of RNA viruses. Nature 2006; 441:101-5; http://dx.doi.org/10.1038/nature04734; PMID:16625202.

17. Gitlin L, Barchet W, Gilfillan S, Cella M, Beutler B, Flavell RA, et al. Essential role of mda-5 in type I IFN responses to polyriboinosinic:polyribocytidylic acid and encephalomyocarditis picornavirus. Proc Natl Acad Sci U S A 2006; 103:8459-64; http://dx.doi.org/10.1073/pnas.0603082103; PMID:16714379.

18. Delaloye J, Roger T, Steiner-Tardivel QG, Le Roy D, Knaup Reymond M, Akira S, et al. Innate immune sensing of modified vaccinia virus Ankara (MVA) is mediated by TLR2-TLR6, MDA-5 and the NALP3 inflammasome. PLoS Pathog 2009; 5:e1000480; http://dx.doi.org/10.1371/journal.ppat.1000480; PMID:19543380.

19. Wang F, Gao X, Barrett JW, Shao Q, Bartee E, Mohamed MR, et al. RIG-I mediates the co-induction of tumor necrosis factor and type I interferon elicited by myxoma virus in primary human macrophages. PLoS Pathog 2008; 4:e1000099; http://dx.doi.org/10.1371/journal.ppat.1000099; PMID:18617992.

20. Loo YM, Fornek J, Crochet N, Bajwa G, Perwitasari O, Martinez-Sobrido L, et al. Distinct RIG-I and MDA5 signaling by RNA viruses in innate immunity. J Virol 2008; 82:335-45; http://dx.doi.org/10.1128/JVI.01080-07; PMID:17942531.

21. Fredericksen BL, Keller BC, Fornek J, Katze MG, Gale M Jr. Establishment and maintenance of the innate antiviral response to West Nile Virus involves both RIG-I and MDA5 signaling through IPS-1. J Virol 2008; 82:609-16; http://dx.doi.org/10.1128/JVI.01305-07; PMID:17977974.

22. Kato H, Takeuchi O, Mikamo-Satoh E, Hirai R, Kawai T, Matsushita K, et al. Length-dependent recognition of double-stranded ribonucleic acids by retinoic acid-inducible gene-I and melanoma differentiation-associated gene 5. J Exp Med 2008; 205:1601-10; http://dx.doi.org/10.1084/jem.20080091; PMID:18591409.

23. Marques JT, Devosse T, Wang D, Zamanian-Daryoush M, Serbinowski P, Hartmann R, et al. A structural basis for discriminating between self and nonself double-stranded RNAs in mammalian cells. Nat Biotechnol 2006; 24:559-65; http://dx.doi.org/10.1038/nbt1205; PMID:16648842.

24. Takahasi K, Yoneyama M, Nishihori T, Hirai R, Kumeta H, Narita R, et al. Nonself RNA-sensing mechanism of RIG-I helicase and activation of antiviral immune responses. Mol Cell 2008; 29:428-40; http://dx.doi.org/10.1016/j.molcel.2007.11.028; PMID:18242112.

25. Kim DH, Longo M, Han Y, Lundberg P, Cantin E, Rossi JJ. Interferon induction by siRNAs and ssRNAs synthesized by phage polymerase. Nat Biotechnol 2004; 22:321-5; http://dx.doi.org/10.1038/nbt940; PMID:14990954.

26. Hornung V, Ellegast J, Kim S, Brzózka K, Jung A, Kato H, et al. 5'-Triphosphate RNA is the ligand for RIG-I. Science 2006; 314:994-7; http://dx.doi.org/10.1126/science.1132505; PMID:17038590.

27. Pichlmair A, Schulz O, Tan CP, Näslund TI, Liljeström P, Weber F, et al. RIG-I-mediated antiviral responses to single-stranded RNA bearing 5'-phosphates. Science 2006; 314:997-1001; http://dx.doi.org/10.1126/science.1132998; PMID:17038589.

28. Paul AV. Possible unifying mechanism of picornavirus genome replication. In: Selmler B, Wiimmer E, eds. Molecular Biology of Picornaviruses. Washington DC: ASM Press, 2002:227-246.
29. Schlee M, Roth A, Hornung V, Hagmann CA, Wimmenauer V, Barchet W, et al. Recognition of 5' triphosphate by RIG-I helicase requires short blunt double-stranded RNA as contained in panhandle of negative-strand virus. Immunity 2009; 31:25-34; http://dx.doi.org/10.1016/j.immuni.2009.05.008; PMID:19576794.
30. Schmidt A, Schwerd T, Hamm W, Hellmuth JC, Cui S, Wenzel M, et al. 5'-triphosphate RNA requires base-paired structures to activate antiviral signaling via RIG-I. Proc Natl Acad Sci U S A 2009; 106:12067-72; http://dx.doi.org/10.1073/pnas.0900971106; PMID:19574455.
31. Weber F, Wagner V, Rasmussen SB, Hartmann R, Paludan SR. Double-stranded RNA is produced by positive-strand RNA viruses and DNA viruses but not in detectable amounts by negative-strand RNA viruses. J Virol 2006; 80:5059-64; http://dx.doi.org/10.1128/JVI.80.10.5059-5064.2006; PMID:16641297.
32. Rehwinkel J, Tan CP, Goubau D, Schulz O, Pichlmair A, Bier K, et al. RIG-I detects viral genomic RNA during negative-strand RNA virus infection. Cell 2010; 140:397-408; http://dx.doi.org/10.1016/j.cell.2010.01.020; PMID:20144762.
33. Strähle L, Marq JB, Brini A, Hausmann S, Kolakofsky D, Garcin D. Activation of the beta interferon promoter by unnatural Sendai virus infection requires RIG-I and is inhibited by viral C proteins. J Virol 2007; 81:12227-37; http://dx.doi.org/10.1128/JVI.01300-07; PMID:17804509.
34. Ablasser A, Bauernfeind F, Hartmann G, Latz E, Fitzgerald KA, Hornung V. RIG-I-dependent sensing of poly(dA:dT) through the induction of an RNA polymerase III-transcribed RNA intermediate. Nat Immunol 2009; 10:1065-72; http://dx.doi.org/10.1038/ni.1779; PMID:19609254.
35. Chiu YH, Macmillan JB, Chen ZJ. RNA polymerase III detects cytosolic DNA and induces type I interferons through the RIG-I pathway. Cell 2009; 138:576-91; http://dx.doi.org/10.1016/j.cell.2009.06.015; PMID:19631370.
36. Pichlmair A, Schulz O, Tan CP, Rehwinkel J, Kato H, Takeuchi O, et al. Activation of MDA5 requires higher-order RNA structures generated during virus infection. J Virol 2009; 83:10761-9; http://dx.doi.org/10.1128/JVI.00770-09; PMID:19656871.
37. Moore CB, Bergstralh DT, Duncan JA, Lei Y, Morrison TE, Zimmermann AG, et al. NLRX1 is a regulator of mitochondrial antiviral immunity. Nature 2008; 451:573-7; http://dx.doi.org/10.1038/nature06501; PMID:18200010.
38. Zhong B, Yang Y, Li S, Wang YY, Li Y, Diao F, et al. The adaptor protein MITA links virus-sensing receptors to IRF3 transcription factor activation. Immunity 2008; 29:538-50; http://dx.doi.org/10.1016/j.immuni.2008.09.003; PMID:18818105.
39. Ishikawa H, Barber GN. STING is an endoplasmic reticulum adaptor that facilitates innate immune signalling. Nature 2008; 455:674-8; http://dx.doi.org/10.1038/nature07317; PMID:18724357.
40. Liu XY, Wei B, Shi HX, Shan YF, Wang C. Tom70 mediates activation of interferon regulatory factor 3 on mitochondria. Cell Res 2010; 20:994-1011; http://dx.doi.org/10.1038/cr.2010.103; PMID:20628368.
41. Castanier C, Garcin D, Vazquez A, Arnoult D. Mitochondrial dynamics regulate the RIG-I-like receptor antiviral pathway. EMBO Rep 2010; 11:133-8; http://dx.doi.org/10.1038/embor.2009.258; PMID:20019757.
42. Koshiba T, Yasukawa K, Yanagi Y, Kawabata S. Mitochondrial membrane potential is required for MAVS-mediated antiviral signaling. Sci Signal 2011; 4:ra7; http://dx.doi.org/10.1126/scisignal.2001147; PMID:21285412.
43. Onoguchi K, Onomoto K, Takamatsu S, Jogi M, Takemura A, Morimoto S, et al. Virus-infection or 5'ppp-RNA activates antiviral signal through redistribution of IPS-1 mediated by MFN1. PLoS Pathog 2010; 6:e1001012; http://dx.doi.org/10.1371/journal.ppat.1001012; PMID:20661427.
44. Yasukawa K, Oshiumi H, Takeda M, Ishihara N, Yanagi Y, Seya T, et al. Mitofusin 2 inhibits mitochondrial antiviral signaling. Sci Signal 2009; 2:ra47; http://dx.doi.org/10.1126/scisignal.2000287; PMID:19690333.
45. Cui J, Zhu L, Xia X, Wang HY, Legras X, Hong J, et al. NLRC5 negatively regulates the NF-kappaB and type I interferon signaling pathways. Cell 2010; 141:483-96; http://dx.doi.org/10.1016/j.cell.2010.03.040; PMID:20434986.
46. Oshiumi H, Matsumoto M, Hatakeyama S, Seya T. Riplet/RNF135, a RING finger protein, ubiquitinates RIG-I to promote interferon-beta induction during the early phase of viral infection. J Biol Chem 2009; 284:807-17; http://dx.doi.org/10.1074/jbc.M804259200; PMID:19017631.
47. Oshiumi H, Miyashita M, Inoue N, Okabe M, Matsumoto M, Seya T. The ubiquitin ligase Riplet is essential for RIG-I-dependent innate immune responses to RNA virus infection. Cell Host Microbe 2010; 8:496-509; http://dx.doi.org/10.1016/j.chom.2010.11.008; PMID:21147464.

48. Gack MU, Shin YC, Joo CH, Urano T, Liang C, Sun L, et al. TRIM25 RING-finger E3 ubiquitin ligase is essential for RIG-I-mediated antiviral activity. Nature 2007; 446:916-20; http://dx.doi.org/10.1038/nature05732; PMID:17392790.

49. Gack MU, Kirchhofer A, Shin YC, Inn KS, Liang C, Cui S, et al. Roles of RIG-I N-terminal tandem CARD and splice variant in TRIM25-mediated antiviral signal transduction. Proc Natl Acad Sci U S A 2008; 105:16743-8; http://dx.doi.org/10.1073/pnas.0804947105; PMID:18948594.

50. Arimoto K, Takahashi H, Hishiki T, Konishi H, Fujita T, Shimotohno K. Negative regulation of the RIG-I signaling by the ubiquitin ligase RNF125. Proc Natl Acad Sci U S A 2007; 104:7500-5; http://dx.doi.org/10.1073/pnas.0611551104; PMID:17460044.

51. Lin R, Yang L, Nakhaei P, Sun Q, Sharif-Askari E, Julkunen I, et al. Negative regulation of the retinoic acid-inducible gene I-induced antiviral state by the ubiquitin-editing protein A20. J Biol Chem 2006; 281:2095-103; http://dx.doi.org/10.1074/jbc.M510326200; PMID:16306043.

52. Zhong B, Zhang L, Lei C, Li Y, Mao AP, Yang Y, et al. The ubiquitin ligase RNF5 regulates antiviral responses by mediating degradation of the adaptor protein MITA. Immunity 2009; 30:397-407; http://dx.doi.org/10.1016/j.immuni.2009.01.008; PMID:19285439.

53. Zhong B, Zhang Y, Tan B, Liu TT, Wang YY, Shu HB. The E3 ubiquitin ligase RNF5 targets virus-induced signaling adaptor for ubiquitination and degradation. J Immunol 2010; 184:6249-55; http://dx.doi.org/10.4049/jimmunol.0903748; PMID:20483786.

54. Nakhaei P, Mesplede T, Solis M, Sun Q, Zhao T, Yang L, et al. The E3 ubiquitin ligase Triad3A negatively regulates the RIG-I/MAVS signaling pathway by targeting TRAF3 for degradation. PLoS Pathog 2009; 5:e1000650; http://dx.doi.org/10.1371/journal.ppat.1000650; PMID:19893624.

55. Zhang M, Wu X, Lee AJ, Jin W, Chang M, Wright A, et al. Regulation of IkappaB kinase-related kinases and antiviral responses by tumor suppressor CYLD. J Biol Chem 2008; 283:18621-6; http://dx.doi.org/10.1074/jbc.M801451200; PMID:18467330.

56. Friedman CS, O'Donnell MA, Legarda-Addison D, Ng A, Cardenas WB, Yount JS, et al. The tumour suppressor CYLD is a negative regulator of RIG-I-mediated antiviral response. EMBO Rep 2008; 9:930-6; http://dx.doi.org/10.1038/embor.2008.136; PMID:18636086.

57. Kayagaki N, Phung Q, Chan S, Chaudhari R, Quan C, O'Rourke KM, et al. DUBA: a deubiquitinase that regulates type I interferon production. Science 2007; 318:1628-32; http://dx.doi.org/10.1126/science.1145918; PMID:17991829.

58. Li S, Zheng H, Mao AP, Zhong B, Li Y, Liu Y, et al. Regulation of virus-triggered signaling by OTUB1- and OTUB2-mediated deubiquitination of TRAF3 and TRAF6. J Biol Chem 2010; 285:4291-7; http://dx.doi.org/10.1074/jbc.M109.074971; PMID:19996094.

59. Jounai N, Takeshita F, Kobiyama K, Sawano A, Miyawaki A, Xin KQ, et al. The Atg5 Atg12 conjugate associates with innate antiviral immune responses. Proc Natl Acad Sci U S A 2007; 104:14050-5; http://dx.doi.org/10.1073/pnas.0704014104; PMID:17709747.

60. Takeshita F, Kobiyama K, Miyawaki A, Jounai N, Okuda K. The non-canonical role of Atg family members as suppressors of innate antiviral immune signaling. Autophagy 2008; 4:67-9; PMID:17921696.

61. Vitour D, Dabo S, Ahmadi Pour M, Vilasco M, Vidalain PO, Jacob Y, et al. Polo-like kinase 1 (PLK1) regulates interferon (IFN) induction by MAVS. J Biol Chem 2009; 284:21797-809; http://dx.doi.org/10.1074/jbc.M109.018275; PMID:19546225.

62. Mashima R, Saeki K, Aki D, Minoda Y, Takaki H, Sanada T, et al. FLN29, a novel interferon- and LPS-inducible gene acting as a negative regulator of toll-like receptor signaling. J Biol Chem 2005; 280:41289-97; http://dx.doi.org/10.1074/jbc.M508221200; PMID:16221674.

63. Sanada T, Takaesu G, Mashima R, Yoshida R, Kobayashi T, Yoshimura A. FLN29 deficiency reveals its negative regulatory role in the Toll-like receptor (TLR) and retinoic acid-inducible gene I (RIG-I)-like helicase signaling pathway. J Biol Chem 2008; 283:33858-64; http://dx.doi.org/10.1074/jbc.M806923200; PMID:18849341.

64. Diao F, Li S, Tian Y, Zhang M, Xu LG, Zhang Y, et al. Negative regulation of MDA5- but not RIG-I-mediated innate antiviral signaling by the dihydroxyacetone kinase. Proc Natl Acad Sci U S A 2007; 104:11706-11; http://dx.doi.org/10.1073/pnas.0700544104; PMID:17600090.

65. Cui S, Eisenächer K, Kirchhofer A, Brzózka K, Lammens A, Lammens K, et al. The C-terminal regulatory domain is the RNA 5'-triphosphate sensor of RIG-I. Mol Cell 2008; 29:169-79; http://dx.doi.org/10.1016/j.molcel.2007.10.032; PMID:18243112.

66. Takahasi K, Kumeta H, Tsuduki N, Narita R, Shigemoto T, Hirai R, et al. Solution structures of cytosolic RNA sensor MDA5 and LGP2 C-terminal domains: identification of the RNA recognition loop in RIG-I-like receptors. J Biol Chem 2009; 284:17465-74; http://dx.doi.org/10.1074/jbc.M109.007179; PMID:19380577.

67. Wang Y, Ludwig J, Schuberth C, Goldeck M, Schlee M, Li H, et al. Structural and functional insights into 5'-ppp RNA pattern recognition by the innate immune receptor RIG-I. Nat Struct Mol Biol 2010; 17:781-7; http://dx.doi.org/10.1038/nsmb.1863; PMID:20581823.

68. Lu C, Xu H, Ranjith-Kumar CT, Brooks MT, Hou TY, Hu F, et al. The structural basis of 5′ triphosphate double-stranded RNA recognition by RIG-I C-terminal domain. Structure 2010; 18:1032-43; http://dx.doi.org/10.1016/j.str.2010.05.007; PMID:20637642.
69. Li X, Ranjith-Kumar CT, Brooks MT, Dharmaiah S, Herr AB, Kao C, et al. The RIG-I-like receptor LGP2 recognizes the termini of double-stranded RNA. J Biol Chem 2009; 284:13881-91; http://dx.doi.org/10.1074/jbc.M900818200; PMID:19278996.
70. Luo D, Ding SC, Vela A, Kohlway A, Lindenbach BD, Pyle AM. Structural insights into RNA recognition by RIG-I. Cell 2011; 147:409-22; http://dx.doi.org/10.1016/j.cell.2011.09.023; PMID:22000018.
71. Jiang F, Ramanathan A, Miller MT, Tang GQ, Gale M Jr., Patel SS, et al. Structural basis of RNA recognition and activation by innate immune receptor RIG-I. Nature 2011; 479:423-7; http://dx.doi.org/10.1038/nature10537; PMID:21947008.
72. Kowalinski E, Lunardi T, McCarthy AA, Louber J, Brunel J, Grigorov B, et al. Structural basis for the activation of innate immune pattern-recognition receptor RIG-I by viral RNA. Cell 2011; 147:423-35; http://dx.doi.org/10.1016/j.cell.2011.09.039; PMID:22000019.
73. Myong S, Cui S, Cornish PV, Kirchhofer A, Gack MU, Jung JU, et al. Cytosolic viral sensor RIG-I is a 5′-triphosphate-dependent translocase on double-stranded RNA. Science 2009; 323:1070-4; http://dx.doi.org/10.1126/science.1168352; PMID:19119185.
74. Kageyama M, Takahasi K, Narita R, Hirai R, Yoneyama M, Kato H, et al. 55 Amino acid linker between helicase and carboxyl terminal domains of RIG-I functions as a critical repression domain and determines inter-domain conformation. Biochem Biophys Res Commun 2011; 415:75-81; http://dx.doi.org/10.1016/j.bbrc.2011.10.015; PMID:22020100.

CHAPTER 6

Contribution of LGP2 to Viral Recognition Pathways

Osamu Takeuchi and Shizuo Akira*

Abstract

RNA virus infection is recognized in the cell cytoplasm by retinoic acid-inducible gene (RIG)-I-like receptors (RLRs), comprised of RIG-I, melanoma differentiation-associated gene 5 (MDA5) and LGP2. RLRs are comprised of a DExD/H-box helicase domain and a C-terminal domain (CTD). Whereas RIG-I and MDA5 additionally harbor two caspase-recruitment domains (CARDs) for signaling, LGP2 lacks a CARD. Although LGP2 was hypothesized to function as the negative regulator in RLR-mediated virus recognition, a mouse study revealed that LGP2 is essential for positive regulation of MDA5-mediated viral recognition and is partially involved in the RIG-I-mediated responses. LGP2 induced Type I interferon production in an ATPase-dependent fashion. Although structural studies revealed that the CTD of LGP2 strongly binds dsRNA, transfected dsRNA activated cells independent of LGP2. Correctively, LGP2 functions upstream of MDA5 and RIG-I for sensing RNA virus infection; however, the precise mechanisms of its function are yet to be clarified.

Introduction

The innate immune system recognizes invasion of RNA viruses by utilizing specific pattern recognition receptors such as Toll-like receptors (TLRs) and Retinoic acid-inducible gene-I (RIG-I)-like receptors (RLRs).[1-5] Sensing of RNA viruses by these receptors leads to production of inflammatory mediators such as Type I interferons (IFNs), cytokines, chemokines and so on. The TLR system plays a critical role in the recognition of viruses in plasmacytoid dendritic cells (pDCs), a cell type known to produce vast amount of Type I IFNs in response to virus infection.[6] On the other hand, RLRs have been identified by Dr. Fujita and coworkers as cytoplasmic RNA virus sensors inducing Type I IFNs in virus-infected cells.[7,8] The RLRs are responsible for virus recognition in various cell types except pDCs.[9,10] The RLRs contain 3 family members, RIG-I (also known as DDX58), melanoma differentiation-associated gene 5 (MDA5) (also known as IFIH1) and LGP2 (Fig. 1). All 3 RLR family members harbor a DExD/H box RNA helicase domain and a C-terminal domain (CTD). In addition, RIG-I and MDA5, but not LGP2, have two caspase-recruitment domains (CARDs) at the N-terminus.

RIG-I and MDA5 are responsible for sensing different RNA viruses.[11] Analyses of RIG-I-deficient and MDA5-deficient mice revealed that RIG-I is essential for the production of Type I IFNs in response to various RNA viruses, including vesicular stomatitis virus (VSV), Sendai virus (SeV), Japanese encephalitis virus (JEV) and influenza virus, while MDA5 is critical for the detection of picornaviridae such as encephalomyocarditis virus (EMCV) and mengovirus.[9,11]

*Laboratory of Host Defense, WPI Immunology Frontier Research Center, and Research Institute for Microbial Diseases, Osaka University, Osaka, Japan.
Corresponding Author: Osamu Takeuchi—Email: otake@biken.osaka-u.ac.jp

Nucleic Acid Sensors and Antiviral Immunity, edited by Suryaprakash Sambhara and Takashi Fujita.
©2013 Landes Bioscience.

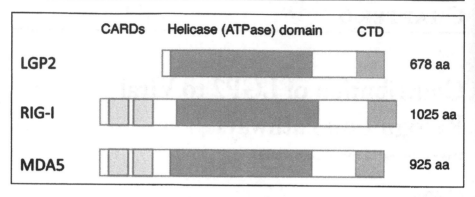

Figure 1. Domain structures of the RLR family. The RLR family members contain a DExD/H box helicase domain and a dsRNA binding C-terminal domain. Although LGP2 lacks a CARD, RIG-I and MDA5 also harbor two CARDs for triggering the intracellular signaling.

Hepatitis C virus is recognized by RIG-I in humans.[12,13] Some RNA viruses, such as West Nile virus and reovirus, are recognized by both RIG-I and MDA5.[14,15]

The RNA molecular structures sensed by RIG-1 and MDA5 have been extensively studied. RIG-I recognizes relatively short double-stranded (ds) RNAs (up to 1 kb) and the presence of a 5' triphosphate end greatly potentiates its Type I IFN-inducing activity (Fig. 2).[16-18] RIG-I has been shown to recognize influenza and Sendai virus viral genomic RNA bearing 5'-triphosphate, which form a panhandle conformation by pairing 5' and 3' ends.[19] On the other hand, MDA5 detects long dsRNAs (more than 2 kb), such as an dsRNA analog, polyinosinic polycytidylic acid (poly I:C). The CTDs of RIG-I and MDA5 are responsible for the binding with dsRNA.[20] The CARDs are responsible for activating downstream signaling pathways, by recruiting a cytoplasmic adaptor protein IFN-β promoter stimulator (IPS)-1 (also known as MAVS, VISA or CARDIF).[21-24] IPS-1 harbors a CARD on the N-terminus, and anchors on the mitochondrial outer membrane via a transmembrane domain at the C-terminus.[22] Mitochondrial fusion by mitofusin 1 is essential for downstream signaling,[25] and IPS-1 forms a prion-like aggregate on the mitochondrial membrane upon virus infection.[26] IPS-1 subsequently activates two IκB kinase (IKK)-related kinases, IKK-*i* (also known as IKKε) and TANK-binding kinase 1 (TBK1) via TNF receptor-associated factor 3 (TRAF3).[27,28] These kinases phosphorylate IFN-regulatory factor (IRF) 3 and IRF7, which activate the transcription of genes encoding Type I IFNs and IFN-inducible genes.[1,2]

Type I IFNs, including a large group of IFN-αs and the single IFN-β, share a common receptor, called the IFN-α/β receptor (IFN-α/βR).[2] Stimulation of IFN-α/βR leads to the phosphorylation of STAT proteins by members of the Janus kinase (JAK) family, inducing formation and nuclear translocation of a complex of STAT1, STAT2 and IFN-regulatory (IRF)-9. This results in the expression of a set of genes regulated by specific promoter sequences, the IFN-stimulated response elements (ISREs). Stimulation with Type I IFNs induces transcription of hundreds of genes, including IFN-regulatory factor (IRF)-7, protein kinase R (PKR), 2',5'-oligoadenylate synthetases (OASs), Mx proteins and several chemokines. PKR, a protein comprised of dsRNA-binding motifs and a kinase domain, is one of the dsRNA detectors in the cytoplasm. Binding of PKR with viral dsRNA results in the phosphorylation of the translation initiation factor, eIF2α, and translational inhibition. OASs catalyze the synthesis of 2',5'-oligoadenylates, which bind inactive RNase L, inducing its dimerization and activation. Activated RNase L cleaves both mRNA and rRNA in the cytoplasm of the cell, resulting in the suppression of protein expression. A report shows that the small self RNA cleaved by RNase L is further recognized by RIG-I to amplify the immune reaction.[29] IFN-inducible chemokines, such as CXCL10/IP-10 and CCL5/RANTES, are important for the regulation of chemotaxis mediated by IFNs.

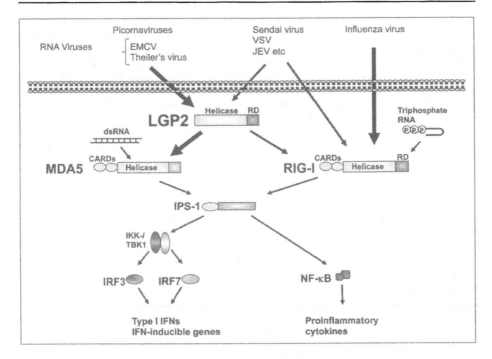

Figure 2. Role of LGP2 in the recognition of RNA viruses recognized by RIG-I and MDA5. LGP2 acts upstream of MDA5 and RIG-I for sensing RNA virus infection. Infection with Picornaviruses such as EMCV and Theiler's virus is first sensed by LGP2 followed by MDA5 to trigger signaling pathways, and some viruses such as Sendai virus, VSV and JEV partially require LGP2 before activating RIG-I. On the other hand, influenza virus does not require LGP2 and recognized by RIG-I. Synthetic dsRNAs activate MDA5 and RIG-I independent of LGP2 when transfected into the cells. RIG-I and MDA5 trigger intracellular signaling pathways via an adaptor, IPS-1, which induces production of Type I IFNs and proinflammatory cytokines via transcription factors, IRFs and NFκB.

The third RLR family member LGP2, also known as Dhx58, harbors a DExD/H-box helicase domain and a CTD, but lacks any CARDs.[7] In this chapter, we would like to focus on current knowledge of the role of LGP2 in antiviral responses.

LGP2—Characterization by In Vitro Studies

LGP2 was originally cloned as a functionally uncharacterized gene encoded on mouse chromosome 11 adjacent to STAT5 and STAT3.[30] Subsequently, the structural similarity between LGP2 and RIG-I was reported.[7,31] The helicase domain of human LGP2 showed 31% amino acid identity with RIG-I, and 41% identity with MDA5. The helicase domain of LGP2 and other RLR members are similar to that of Dicer, a nuclease responsible for the generation of microRNA and siRNA.[8] Drosophila, which lacks the IFN system, mounts antiviral responses via Dicer-2 in RNA interference-dependent and -independent mechanisms.[32,33] Therefore, this DExD/H box helicase family might function as the evolutionarily conserved sensors of viral infection. Further, the CTD of LGP2 exhibits 29% and 34% sequence identity with RIG-I and MDA5, respectively.

Like RIG-I and MDA5, the expression level of LGP2 is induced in response to virus infection or Type I IFN stimulation in human and mouse cells.[7,31,34] Human and mouse LGP2 genes encode proteins with 678 amino acid proteins with 79% overall identity. Since LGP2 itself does not have a CARD signaling domain, it was originally thought that LGP2 functions as a negative regulator of RNA virus infection.[7,31] Indeed, overexpression of LGP2 in cell lines suppressed virus-induced Type I IFN responses. Several models have been proposed for the mechanisms of this inhibition. The first model is that LGP2 binds to viral dsRNA and prevents RIG-I- and MDA5-mediated recognition.[31] However, LGP2 mutant proteins lacking dsRNA binding or ATPase activity still suppressed RIG-I signaling when overexpressed in HEK293 cells.[35] The second model is that LGP2 inhibits multimerization of RIG-I and its interaction with IPS-1 via the CTD of LGP2.[20] The third model is that LGP2 competes with IKK-*i* for recruitment to IPS-1, thereby suppressing RLR signaling.[36]

The RLRs are conserved among vertebrates,[37] and those in rainbow trout (*Oncorhynchus mykiss*) have been characterized.[38] The trout LGP2 has two variants; one contains a full-length CTD and the other has a shortened CTD with a deletion of 54 amino acids at the C-terminus. Overexpression of full length trout LGP2, but not its deletion mutant, induced expression of the IFN-inducible Mx gene similar to when MDA5 is overexpressed.[38] Furthermore, cells overexpressing LGP2 or MDA5 exhibited increased resistance to infection by RNA viruses. These results suggest that LGP2 functions as the positive regulator of RNA virus recognition in fish cells.

LGP2 as a Positive Regulator of RNA Virus Recognition

To investigate the role of LGP2, two different knockout mouse strains have been generated by homologous recombination of embryonic stem cells in two different laboratories.[34,39] The expression levels of RIG-I and MDA5 mRNA were not impaired in LGP2-deficient cells, indicating that LGP2 is not involved in the regulation of RIG-I and MDA5 expression.[34] The production of IFN-β in response to picornaviridae, EMCV and mengovirus were severely impaired in LGP2-deificient conventional dendritic cells (cDCs) compared with wild-type cells. IL-6 production induced by EMCV infection was also severely impaired in cells lacking LGP2. Consistently, upregulation of mRNA encoding CXCL10 and IL-6 in response to EMCV infection was severely impaired in LGP2-deficient macrophages.

RIG-I- and MDA5-deficient mice are susceptible to VSV and EMCV, respectively.[11] When LGP2-deficient mice were challenged with EMCV, production of IFN-β was abrogated in the sera. Furthermore, LGP2-deficient mice were highly susceptible to EMCV infection compared with their littermate controls. Consistent with the increased susceptibility to EMCV, the viral titer in the heart was remarkably higher in LGP2-deificient mice than in control mice. This phenotype is common to the two different LGP2 lacking mouse strains.[34,39] Thus, LGP2 is critical for cytokine and chemokine production in response to viruses recognized by MDA5. Furthermore, LGP2 is essential for host defense against infection with EMCV, a virus recognized by MDA5.

However, there is controversy regarding the responses against viruses recognized by RIG-I. One report showed that LGP2-deficient mice were more resistant to VSV infection together with increased IFN-β production in LGP2-deficient mice, implying that LGP2 negatively regulates RIG-I-mediated signaling.[39] In contrast, in the other report, the production of IFN-β in response to several RNA viruses recognized by RIG-I, such as VSV, SeV and JEV were impaired in LGP2-deficient cDCs.[34] IFN-β production in response to reovirus, a dsRNA virus, also required LGP2. On the other hand, the IFN-β production in response to infection with influenza virus was comparable between WT and LGP2-deficient cDCs. As mentioned below, the responses against RNA viruses recognized by RIG-I are also impaired in a mouse strain lacking LGP2 ATPase activity. These observations further suggest that LGP2 functions as the positive, rather than a negative, regulator of RNA virus recognition (Fig. 2).

Notably, the LGP2-deficient mice were partially embryonic lethal. In addition, adult female LGP2-deficient mice showed an enlarged uterus filled with fluid owing to vaginal atresia. Therefore, LGP2 is important for embryonic development, in addition to its role in antiviral responses.

LGP2 Acts Upstream of MDA5 and RIG-I

RIG-I and MDA5 are critical for initial recognition of invading RNA viruses in the cytoplasm and initiate intracellular signaling pathways. In the absence of LGP2, the activation of transcription factors NF-κB and IRFs in response to EMCV infection was severely impaired.[34] The activation of STAT1 also required LGP2, indicating that LGP2 is involved in the initial recognition of EMCV. Given that the expression of RIG-I and MDA5 is not impaired in LGP2-deficient cells, the expression of both LGP2 and MDA5 are required for recognizing EMCV.

The CARDs from RIG-I or MDA5 alone are sufficient to activate the IFN-b promoter by triggering intracellular signaling pathways. Indeed, overexpression of the RIG-I or MDA5 CARDs activated the IFN-β promoter in MEFs lacking LGP2, suggesting that LGP2 functions upstream of RIG-I and MDA5. These results suggest that LGP2 is required for the initial recognition of EMCV, leading to activation of transcription factors involved in the expression of Type I IFNs.

Consistent with the notion that LGP2 acts together with RIG-I and MDA5, LGP2 functions in a cell type-specific manner. Whereas LGP2 functions in recognizing virus infection in cell types such as MEFs and cDCs, LGP2 was dispensable for Type I IFN production in response to EMCV in plasmacytoid DCs derived from bone marrow cells.[34] These results indicate that LGP2 functions in cDCs, but not in pDCs, like other RLR family members.

Role of LGP2 in Response to Transfection with Synthetic RNAs

RIG-I recognizes short (less than 1 kb) dsRNA and the presence of 5' triphosphate greatly enhanced IFN-inducing activity. On the other hand, MDA5 recognizes long (more than 2 kb) dsRNA, although MDA5 is not involved in the sensing of dsRNAs detected by RIG-I. Again there disagreement between the two LGP2-deficient mouse strains with regard to the response to dsRNA stimulation. One study using a LGP2-deficient mouse strain revealed that LGP2-deficiency did not affect the IFN-β production in response to transfection with synthesized RNA, including triphosphate dsRNA and poly I:C.[34] These data suggest that LGP2 is dispensable for the recognition of transfected synthesized dsRNA and 5' triphosphate RNA. While one report showed that LGP2-deficient MEFs exhibit enhanced production of Type I IFNs in response to poly I:C transfection, suggesting that LGP2 negatively regulates poly I:C-mediated responses,[39] another study using the same mouse strain showed that LGP2 was not involved in poly I:C-induced IFN-β gene expression.[40] Thus, it is likely that LGP2 is dispensable for Type I IFN responses against transfection with synthetic dsRNAs activating RIG-I and MDA5, for unknown reasons.

Structural Studies of LGP2

Although LGP2 is dispensable for sensing transfected dsRNAs, all 3 RLR family members contain an RNA helicase domain and a CTD that binds dsRNA. The structure of an entire RLR protein has not been reported yet. However, there are several studies solving the structure of CTDs of RIG-I, MDA5 and LGP2 by nuclear magnetic resonance (NMR) and crystrography,[41-44] and a recent report revealed a crystal structure of the helicase domain and the CTD of RIG-I.[45]

Structural studies of the RIG-I CTD bound to a short dsRNA revealed that dsRNA forms a helical structure and recruits two RIG-I CTD molecules symmetrically. The RIG-I CTD preferentially binds 5' triphosphate dsRNA, and the 5' triphosphate of the dsRNA is recognized by a cluster of positively charged amino acid residues including Lys858, Lys861, Lys888 and His 847.[43,44] On the other hand, RIG-I was also reported to bind the blunt end of dsRNA in a different orientation such that it interacts with both strands of the dsRNA.[46] However, a recent structural study of the helicase domain and CTD of RIG-I bound to dsRNA showed that the way RIG-I binds with dsRNA is different from the binding of the CTD alone.[45] The RIG-I helicase and CTD associate with dsRNA with 1:1 stoichiometry. Although 5' triphosphate dsRNA binds RIG-I with higher affinity than blunt end dsRNA, the amino acid residues critical for binding of triphosphate with RIG-I CTD alone are no longer found to associate with the RNA. Rather, the CTD and the helicase appear to function synergistically in binding the dsRNA.

Structural analyses of the CTD of LGP2 have revealed that LGP2 can bind to the termini of dsRNAs more strongly than MDA5.[35,47,48] The LGP2 CTD contains a single Zn^{2+} binding Cys-X-X-Cys motif like other RLRs, and indeed contains a Zn^{2+} ion in solution.[47] The RNA binding activity of LGP2 CTD has been examined by several assays. A surface plasmon resonance (SPR) analysis showed that the LGP2 CTD was strongly bound to dsRNA and 5′ triphosphate RNA, and associates with ssRNA with low affinity. The affinity between dsRNA and LGP2 CTD looks stronger than those between dsRNA and RIG-I. An electrophoretic mobility shift assay (EMSA) also confirmed the interaction between the CTD and RNA. LGP2 was shown to bind blunt-ended dsRNA with 2:1 stoichiometry, suggesting that LGP2 homodimerizes on the termini of dsRNA. Upon binding with dsRNA, LGP2 can form a homodimer like RIG-I.[49] However, structural studies with full-length LGP2 are required to clarify the mechanisms of dsRNA recognition by LGP2, given the fact that the dsRNA-RIG-I structure is so different in the cases of CTD alone and CTD with the helicase domain.

A crystal structure study revealed that LGP2 CTD binds to the termini of dsRNA.[35] On the other hand, the affinity between dsRNA and MDA5 CTD was very low. When structures of RLR CTDs were compared, the LGP2 and RIG-I CTDs had a large basic surface, formed by the RNA-binding loop, and the LGP2 C-terminal domain bound to the termini of dsRNAs.[35,41,42,47,48] Although the MDA5 C-terminal domain also has a large basic surface, it is extensively flat because of the open conformation of the RNA-binding loop.[47] When basic lysine residues (KKK599/602/605) present in RNA binding loop in LGP2 CTD were substituted with alanines, dsRNA or 5′ triphosphate RNA no longer associated with LGP2. Furthermore, a phenialanine residue (F601) conserved between LGP2 and RIG-I was found to be essential for LGP2-dsRNA. The aromatic moiety of Phe stackes into the groove of the dsRNA via hydrophobic interactions with a ribose moiety in the dsRNA. The corresponding Phe residue is not conserved in MDA5, resulting in a flat RNA binding loop. Mutation of the corresponding Phe residue in RIG-I (F853), mimicking MDA5, reduced dsRNA binding activity, suggesting that the lack of this residue in the MDA5 CTD can explain the low dsRNA binding affinity of MDA5.

The analysis of LGP2-deficient mice revealed that LGP2 is more essential for the recognition of RNA viruses detected by MDA5 than for those detected by RIG-I.[34] MDA5 may require LGP2 for efficient recruitment of viral dsRNAs to facilitate the initiation of signaling, and LGP2 appears to be more important for MDA5 than for RIG-I, possibly because of differences in their affinities for dsRNAs.

The Role of LGP2 ATPase Activity

The helicase/ATPase domain of LGP2 is highly conserved among RLR family members. RIG-I and MDA5 have ATPase activity which is abrogated by introducing a point mutation in the Walker-type ATP-binding site.[7,8] Mutant RIG-I or MDA5 failed to induce IFN-responses in response to RNA virus infection, indicating that the ATPase activity is essential for their function. Although the RIG-I helicase domain has the ability to unwind dsRNA,[41,50] this activity is not correlated with the level of IFN production.[41] A recent report proposed that the RIG-I ATPase activity is required for translocation of RIG-I on dsRNA.[51] A recent RIG-I helicase-CTD structure supports a model wherein the RIG-I helicase domain acts as a translocase on dsRNA.[45,51] However, the meaning of this activity is not well understood. The helicase domain of LGP2 is reported to show structural similarity to that of the superfamily 2 DNA helicase Hef.[49] The Walker-type ATP-binding site is conserved in LGP2, and a point mutation of Lysine 30 to Alanine is reported to disrupt the ATPase activity. Indeed, reconstitution of LGP2-deficient MEFs with wild-type LGP2, but not the LGP2 K30A mutant, by retroviral transduction conferred IFN reporter activation in response to EMCV infection.

To investigate the role of LGP2 ATPase activity, a mouse strain harboring a K30A point mutation in LGP2 was been generated. Insertion of the point mutation did not affect the LGP2 expression levels in MEFs. The IFN-β productions in response to infections with EMCV, mengovirus, VSV, SeV and reovirus, but not with influenza virus, were severely impaired in cDCs lacking LGP2 ATPase activity. The defects observed in cells from LGP2 K30A mutant mice were as severe as those observed in LGP2-deficient cells, suggesting that the ATPase activity of LGP2 is essential for the recognition of viruses. The production of IFN-β in response to transfections of synthetic RNAs and poly I:C were comparable between WT and LGP2 K30A mutant cells. Taken together, these results indicate that the ATPase activity of LGP2 is essential for LGP2 to function as a positive regulator in MEFs. Similar to the results for LGP2-deficient mice, LGP2 K30A knock-in mice were highly susceptible to EMCV infection accompanied by highly increased viral titers in the heart. Furthermore, production of IFN-β in the sera was abrogated in mice lacking LGP2 ATPase activity.

These results demonstrate that the ATPase activity of LGP2 is a prerequisite for its function in recognizing RNA virus infection. However, the role of ATPase activity in sensing virus infection has not been clarified yet. The function of RIG-I ATPase activity has been hypothesized to induce a conformational change of RIG-I to facilitate CARD-mediated signaling. However, LGP2 does not have a CARD to trigger the signaling pathway. An alternative hypothesis of the role of the RIG-I ATPase domain is that it functions as a translocase on viral dsRNAs. Considering the similarity among RLR ATPase domains, it is possible that the LGP2 ATPase domain also functions as a translocase. However, it is still not clear how the translocation of LGP2 on dsRNA leads to the activation of RIG-I and MDA5. DExD/H-box helicase proteins are involved in all aspects of RNA and DNA metabolism including translation initiation, mRNA splicing and nuclear transport.[52] Hef, or its mammalian homolog FANCJ, encodes a LGP2-like helicase dissociating RNA:DNA hybrid generated in the course of transcription, probably to clear these hybrids. Although DExD/H-box proteins are known to exhibit ATP-dependent RNA helicase activity in vitro, many DExD/H-box proteins have a more general role in RNA conformational changes, rather than just duplex-unwinding activity. Therefore, LGP2 might function to modify viral RNA by removing proteins from viral ribonucleoprotein (RNP) complexes or unwinding complex RNA structures to facilitate MDA5- and RIG-I-mediated recognition of dsRNA. Picornaviruses replicate in association with the cytoplasmic membranes of infected cells.[53] It is therefore possible that LGP2 makes viral RNP complexes more accessible to MDA5 and RIG-I by changing their intracellular localization.

Whereas LGP2 K30A mutant mice and LGP2-deificient mice showed identical phenotype in terms of antiviral responses, there is a clear difference in embryonic development. Although some of the female LGP2-deificient mice showed a defect in the development of the vagina, LGP2 K30A mutant mice did not exhibit any developmental abnormalities. While the ATPase domain was essential for antiviral responses, the vaginal atresia was regulated by LGP2 independently of its ATPase activity. Not only LGP2, but also RIG-I is known to be involved in mouse embryonic development. However, further studies are required to determine the roles of the RLR family members in controlling mammalian development.

Potential Role of LGP2 in Cytoplasmic DNA Recognition

It has been reported that infection with intracellular bacteria such as Listeria monocytogenes leads to the production of IFN-β in a manner dependent of bacterial genomic DNA.[54] In addition, genomic RNAs of dsRNA viruses are reported to be recognized by potential cytoplasmic dsDNA receptor(s).[55] Currently, many potential cytoplasmic dsDNA receptors have been reported including DAI, IFI16, LRRFIP1, DDX41 and so on.[56-59] On the other hand, knockdown of RIG-I in human cells has been shown to impair IFN-β production in response to synthetic dsDNA, poly (dA:dT).[60] In the cell cytoplasm, transfected dsDNA is transcribed by polymerase III, and generated dsRNA stimulate RIG-I for producing Type I IFNs.[60,61] These molecules might function in a cell type-specific or stimulus specific- or species specific-fashion, although future studies are required for understanding the role of these molecules in cytoplasmic DNA recognition in vivo.

One study investigated the contribution of LGP2 in the responses against bacterial and DNA virus infection.[40] This report shows that LGP2-deficient MEFs and macrophages showed impaired production of IFN-β and inflammatory cytokines in response to poly (dA-dT) transfection and

Listeria monocytogenes infection. In addition, IFN responses to vaccinia virus infection was also impaired in LGP2-deficient MEFs. These results imply that LGP2 plays a role in the recognition of cytoplasmic dsDNA via dsRNA generated by polymerase III. However, LGP2 was shown to be dispensable for the recognition of transfected dsRNAs.[34] Furthermore, mouse cells recognize cytoplasmic dsRNA via a mechanism other than RIG-I. Therefore, further studies are required for clarifying the role of LGP2 in sensing bacteria and bacterial DNA-mediated responses.

Conclusion

In this chapter, we described current understanding of the role of LGP2, the third member of the RLR family. Although LGP2 lacks a CARD signaling domain, it functions as a positive regulator in RIG-I- and MDA5-mediated virus recognition. However, there remain many questions to be solved. For instance, the mechanism of how LGP2 is involved in the recognition of dsRNA has not been well understood, since transfected synthesized dsRNA induced Type I IFNs independent of LGP2. Furthermore, influenza virus infection does not require LGP2, although LGP2 is involved in the responses to various RNA viruses. Type I IFN production in response to influenza virus was dependent on RIG-I, but not on MDA5. It has been shown that removal of 5' triphosphate by phosphatase treatment of genomic RNA derived from influenza virus completely abolishes its Type I IFN-inducing activity via RIG-I,[16,62] indicating that a phosphate group at the 5' end of the influenza virus genome is responsible for RIG-I-mediated recognition. On the other hand, treatment of EMCV genomic RNA with phosphatase did not affect MDA5-mediated Type I IFN production. Therefore, the 5' triphosphate RNA present on viral genomes may be readily accessible to RIG-I without modification by LGP2.

Among RLR family members, RIG-I has been shown to undergo ubiquitination by E3 ubiquitin ligases such as TRIM25 and Riplet.[63-65] Furthermore, RIG-I was reported to interact with another helicase protein, DDX60, which facilitates RIG-I-mediated signaling.[66] It was reported that LGP2 also associates with DDX60, however, other modifications of LGP2 have not been studied yet.[66]

Future studies aimed at identifying the mechanisms by which LGP2 modifies viral RNP complexes will help us to understand the roles of the innate immune system in intracellular virus recognition, and will lead to the development of new strategies to manipulate antiviral responses.

Acknowledgments

We thank E. Kamada and M. Kageyama for secretarial assistance. This work was supported by the Special Coordination Funds of the Japanese Ministry of Education, Culture, Sports, Science and Technology, and grants from the Ministry of Health, Labour and Welfare in Japan, the Global Center of Excellence Program of Japan, and the NIH (P01 AI070167).

About the Author

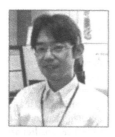Osamu Takeuchi is an associate professor in the Laboratory of Host Defense, Immunology Frontier Research Center, of Osaka University. He obtained his M.D. degree in 1995 at Osaka University, and finished PhD in Immunology in 2001 at Osaka University Osaka, Japan where he studied the differential roles of Toll-like receptors. During 2001, he worked as a postdoctoral fellow in Osaka University. During 2002–2004, he worked as a postdoctoral fellow in Dana Farber Cancer Institute and studied the role of Bcl2 family in immune cell activation in Dr. Standley Korsmeyer's laboratory. From 2004 to 2007 he was an assistant professor in the Department of Host Defense, Research Institute for Microbial Diseases, Osaka University. During the periods, he studied the role of the RIG-I family and its relation with TLR family in virus sensing. From 2007 to till date he is an associate professor in the Immunology Frontier Research Center, Osaka University.

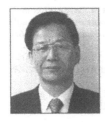

Shizuo Akira is Director of WPI Immunology Frontier Research Center at Osaka University, Japan since 2007, and a professor in Research Institute for Microbial Diseases at Osaka University since 1999. He was a professor in Department of Biochemistry, Hyogo College of Medicine from 1996 to 1999, where he became involved in Toll-like receptor research. He has shown by generating TLR family knockout mice that individual TLRs recognize different microbial components and established the role of TLR family as pathogen recognition receptors, and further clarified the whole picture of their signaling pathways. He is the top cited researcher in the immunological field since 2004. In 2006 and 2007 he was twice recognized the hottest scientist who had published the greatest number of Hot Papers over the preceding two years.

References

1. Akira S, Uematsu S, Takeuchi O. Pathogen recognition and innate immunity. Cell 2006; 124:783-801; PMID:16497588; http://dx.doi.org/10.1016/j.cell.2006.02.015.
2. Honda K, Takaoka A, Taniguchi T. Type I interferon [corrected] gene induction by the interferon regulatory factor family of transcription factors. Immunity 2006; 25:349-60; PMID:16979567; http://dx.doi.org/10.1016/j.immuni.2006.08.009.
3. Yoneyama M, Fujita T. Structural mechanism of RNA recognition by the RIG-I-like receptors. Immunity 2008; 29:178-81; PMID:18701081; http://dx.doi.org/10.1016/j.immuni.2008.07.009.
4. Takeuchi O, Akira S. Innate immunity to virus infection. Immunol Rev 2009; 227:75-86; PMID:19120477; http://dx.doi.org/10.1111/j.1600-065X.2008.00737.x.
5. Takeuchi O, Akira S. Pattern recognition receptors and inflammation. Cell 2010; 140:805-20; PMID:20303872; http://dx.doi.org/10.1016/j.cell.2010.01.022.
6. Gilliet M, Cao W, Liu YJ. Plasmacytoid dendritic cells: sensing nucleic acids in viral infection and autoimmune diseases. Nat Rev Immunol 2008; 8:594-606; PMID:18641647; http://dx.doi.org/10.1038/nri2358.
7. Yoneyama M, Kikuchi M, Matsumoto K, Imaizumi T, Miyagishi M, Taira K, et al. Shared and unique functions of the DExD/H-box helicases RIG-I, MDA5, and LGP2 in antiviral innate immunity. J Immunol 2005; 175:2851-8; PMID:16116171.
8. Yoneyama M, Kikuchi M, Natsukawa T, Shinobu N, Imaizumi T, Miyagishi M, et al. The RNA helicase RIG-I has an essential function in double-stranded RNA-induced innate antiviral responses. Nat Immunol 2004; 5:730-7; PMID:15208624, http://dx.doi.org/10.1038/ni1087
9. Kato H, Sato S, Yoneyama M, Yamamoto M, Uematsu S, Matsui K, et al. Cell type-specific involvement of RIG-I in antiviral response. Immunity 2005; 23:19-28; PMID:16039576; http://dx.doi.org/10.1016/j.immuni.2005.04.010.
10. Kumagai Y, Takeuchi O, Kato H, Kumar H, Matsui K, Morii E, et al. Alveolar macrophages are the primary interferon-alpha producer in pulmonary infection with RNA viruses. Immunity 2007; 27:240-52; PMID:17723216; http://dx.doi.org/10.1016/j.immuni.2007.07.013.
11. Kato H, Takeuchi O, Sato S, Yoneyama M, Yamamoto M, Matsui K, et al. Differential roles of MDA5 and RIG-I helicases in the recognition of RNA viruses. Nature 2006; 441:101-5; PMID:16625202; http://dx.doi.org/10.1038/nature04734.
12. Sumpter R Jr., Loo YM, Foy E, Li K, Yoneyama M, Fujita T, et al. Regulating intracellular antiviral defense and permissiveness to hepatitis C virus RNA replication through a cellular RNA helicase, RIG-I. J Virol 2005; 79:2689-99; PMID:15708988; http://dx.doi.org/10.1128/JVI.79.5.2689-2699.2005.
13. Saito T, Owen DM, Jiang F, Marcotrigiano J, Gale M Jr. Innate immunity induced by composition-dependent RIG-I recognition of hepatitis C virus RNA. Nature 2008; 454:523-7; PMID:18548002; http://dx.doi.org/10.1038/nature07106.
14. Fredericksen BL, Keller BC, Fornek J, Katze MG, Gale M Jr. Establishment and maintenance of the innate antiviral response to West Nile Virus involves both RIG-I and MDA5 signaling through IPS-1. J Virol 2008; 82:609-16; PMID:17977974; http://dx.doi.org/10.1128/JVI.01305-07.
15. Loo YM, Fornek J, Crochet N, Bajwa G, Perwitasari O, Martinez-Sobrido L, et al. Distinct RIG-I and MDA5 signaling by RNA viruses in innate immunity. J Virol 2008; 82:335-45; PMID:17942531; http://dx.doi.org/10.1128/JVI.01080-07.
16. Kato H, Takeuchi O, Mikamo-Satoh E, Hirai R, Kawai T, Matsushita K, et al. Length-dependent recognition of double-stranded ribonucleic acids by retinoic acid-inducible gene-I and melanoma differentiation-associated gene 5. J Exp Med 2008; 205:1601-10; PMID:18591409; http://dx.doi.org/10.1084/jem.20080091.

17. Schlee M, Roth A, Hornung V, Hagmann CA, Wimmenauer V, Barchet W, et al. Recognition of 5′ triphosphate by RIG-I helicase requires short blunt double-stranded RNA as contained in panhandle of negative-strand virus. Immunity 2009; 31:25-34; PMID:19576794; http://dx.doi.org/10.1016/j. immuni.2009.05.008.

18. Schmidt A, Schwerd T, Hamm W, Hellmuth JC, Cui S, Wenzel M, et al. 5′-triphosphate RNA requires base-paired structures to activate antiviral signaling via RIG-I. Proc Natl Acad Sci USA 2009; 106:12067-72; PMID:19574455; http://dx.doi.org/10.1073/pnas.0900971106.

19. Rehwinkel J, Tan CP, Goubau D, Schulz O, Pichlmair A, Bier K, et al. RIG-I detects viral genomic RNA during negative-strand RNA virus infection. Cell 2010; 140:397-408; PMID:20144762; http:// dx.doi.org/10.1016/j.cell.2010.01.020.

20. Saito T, Hirai R, Loo YM, Owen D, Johnson CL, Sinha SC, et al. Regulation of innate antiviral defenses through a shared repressor domain in RIG-I and LGP2. Proc Natl Acad Sci USA 2007; 104:582-7; PMID:17190814; http://dx.doi.org/10.1073/pnas.0606699104.

21. Kawai T, Takahashi K, Sato S, Coban C, Kumar H, Kato H, et al. IPS-1, an adaptor triggering RIG-I- and Mda5-mediated type I interferon induction. Nat Immunol 2005; 6:981-8; PMID:16127453; http:// dx.doi.org/10.1038/ni1243.

22. Seth RB, Sun L, Ea CK, Chen ZJ. Identification and characterization of MAVS, a mitochondrial antiviral signaling protein that activates NF-kappaB and IRF 3. Cell 2005; 122:669-82; PMID:16125763; http:// dx.doi.org/10.1016/j.cell.2005.08.012.

23. Meylan E, Curran J, Hofmann K, Moradpour D, Binder M, Bartenschlager R, et al. Cardif is an adaptor protein in the RIG-I antiviral pathway and is targeted by hepatitis C virus. Nature 2005; 437:1167-72; PMID:16177806; http://dx.doi.org/10.1038/nature04193.

24. Xu LG, Wang YY, Han KJ, Li LY, Zhai Z, Shu HB. VISA is an adapter protein required for virus-triggered IFN-beta signaling. Mol Cell 2005; 19:727-40; PMID:16153868; http://dx.doi. org/10.1016/j.molcel.2005.08.014.

25. Onoguchi K, Onomoto K, Takamatsu S, Jogi M, Takemura A, Morimoto S, et al. Virus-infection or 5¢ppp-RNA activates antiviral signal through redistribution of IPS-1 mediated by MFN1. PLoS Pathog 2010; 6:e1001012; PMID:20661427; http://dx.doi.org/10.1371/journal.ppat.1001012.

26. Hou F, Sun L, Zheng H, Skaug B, Jiang QX, Chen ZJ. MAVS forms functional prion-like aggregates to activate and propagate antiviral innate immune response. Cell 2011; 146:448-61; PMID:21782231; http://dx.doi.org/10.1016/j.cell.2011.06.041.

27. Oganesyan G, Saha SK, Guo B, He JQ, Shahangian A, Zarnegar B, et al. Critical role of TRAF3 in the Toll-like receptor-dependent and -independent antiviral response. Nature 2006; 439:208-11; PMID:16306936; http://dx.doi.org/10.1038/nature04374.

28. Häcker H, Redecke V, Blagoev B, Kratchmarova I, Hsu LC, Wang GG, et al. Specificity in Toll-like receptor signalling through distinct effector functions of TRAF3 and TRAF6. Nature 2006; 439:204-7; PMID:16306937; http://dx.doi.org/10.1038/nature04369.

29. Malathi K, Dong B, Gale M Jr., Silverman RH. Small self-RNA generated by RNase L amplifies antiviral innate immunity. Nature 2007; 448:816-9; PMID:17653195; http://dx.doi.org/10.1038/nature06042.

30. Cui Y, Li M, Walton KD, Sun K, Hanover JA, Furth PA, et al. The Stat3/5 locus encodes novel endoplasmic reticulum and helicase-like proteins that are preferentially expressed in normal and neoplastic mammary tissue. Genomics 2001; 78:129-34; PMID:11735219; http://dx.doi.org/10.1006/ geno.2001.6661.

31. Rothenfusser S, Goutagny N, DiPerna G, Gong M, Monks BG, Schoenemeyer A, et al. The RNA helicase Lgp2 inhibits TLR-independent sensing of viral replication by retinoic acid-inducible gene-I. J Immunol 2005; 175:5260-8; PMID:16210631.

32. Ding SW, Voinnet O. Antiviral immunity directed by small RNAs. Cell 2007; 130:413-26; PMID:17693253; http://dx.doi.org/10.1016/j.cell.2007.07.039.

33. Deddouche S, Matt N, Budd A, Mueller S, Kemp C, Galiana-Arnoux D, et al. The DExD/H-box helicase Dicer-2 mediates the induction of antiviral activity in drosophila. Nat Immunol 2008; 9:1425-32; PMID:18953338; http://dx.doi.org/10.1038/ni.1664.

34. Satoh T, Kato H, Kumagai Y, Yoneyama M, Sato S, Matsushita K, et al. LGP2 is a positive regulator of RIG-I- and MDA5-mediated antiviral responses. Proc Natl Acad Sci USA 2010; 107:1512-7; PMID:20080593; http://dx.doi.org/10.1073/pnas.0912986107.

35. Li X, Ranjith-Kumar CT, Brooks MT, Dharmaiah S, Herr AB, Kao C, et al. The RIG-I-like receptor LGP2 recognizes the termini of double-stranded RNA. J Biol Chem 2009; 284:13881-91; PMID:19278996; http://dx.doi.org/10.1074/jbc.M900818200.

36. Komuro A, Horvath CM. RNA- and virus-independent inhibition of antiviral signaling by RNA helicase LGP2. J Virol 2006; 80:12332-42; PMID:17020950; http://dx.doi.org/10.1128/JVI.01325-06.

37. Zou J, Chang M, Nie P, Secombes CJ. Origin and evolution of the RIG-I like RNA helicase gene family. BMC Evol Biol 2009; 9:85; PMID:19400936; http://dx.doi.org/10.1186/1471-2148-9-85.

38. Chang M, Collet B, Nie P, Lester K, Campbell S, Secombes CJ, et al. Expression and functional characterization of the RIG-I-like receptors MDA5 and LGP2 in Rainbow trout (Oncorhynchus mykiss). J Virol 2011; 85:8403-12; PMID:21680521; http://dx.doi.org/10.1128/JVI.00445-10.

39. Venkataraman T, Valdes M, Elsby R, Kakuta S, Caceres G, Saijo S, et al. Loss of DExD/H box RNA helicase LGP2 manifests disparate antiviral responses. J Immunol 2007; 178:6444-55; PMID:17475874.

40. Pollpeter D, Komuro A, Barber GN, Horvath CM. Impaired cellular responses to cytosolic DNA or infection with Listeria monocytogenes and vaccinia virus in the absence of the murine LGP2 protein. PLoS ONE 2011; 6:e18842; PMID:21533147; http://dx.doi.org/10.1371/journal.pone.0018842.

41. Takahasi K, Yoneyama M, Nishihori T, Hirai R, Kumeta H, Narita R, et al. Nonself RNA-sensing mechanism of RIG-I helicase and activation of antiviral immune responses. Mol Cell 2008; 29:428-40; PMID:18242112; http://dx.doi.org/10.1016/j.molcel.2007.11.028.

42. Cui S, Eisenacher K, Kirchhofer A, Brzózka K, Lammens A, Lammens K, et al. The C-terminal regulatory domain is the RNA 5'-triphosphate sensor of RIG-I. Mol Cell 2008; 29:169-79; PMID:18243112; http://dx.doi.org/10.1016/j.molcel.2007.10.032.

43. Lu C, Xu H, Ranjith-Kumar CT, Brooks MT, Hou TY, Hu F, et al. The structural basis of 5' triphosphate double-stranded RNA recognition by RIG-I C-terminal domain. Structure 2010; 18:1032-43; PMID:20637642; http://dx.doi.org/10.1016/j.str.2010.05.007.

44. Wang Y, Ludwig J, Schuberth C, Goldeck M, Schlee M, Li H, et al. Structural and functional insights into 5'-ppp RNA pattern recognition by the innate immune receptor RIG-I. Nat Struct Mol Biol 2010; 17:781-7; PMID:20581823; http://dx.doi.org/10.1038/nsmb.1863.

45. Jiang F, Ramanathan A, Miller MT, Tang GQ, Gale M, Patel SS, et al. Structural basis of RNA recognition and activation by innate immune receptor RIG-I. Nature 2011; 25:Epub ahead of print; PMID:21947008.

46. Lu C, Ranjith-Kumar CT, Hao L, Kao CC, Li P. Crystal structure of RIG-I C-terminal domain bound to blunt-ended double-strand RNA without 5' triphosphate. Nucleic Acids Res 2011; 39:1565-75; PMID:20961956; http://dx.doi.org/10.1093/nar/gkq974.

47. Takahasi K, Kumeta H, Tsuduki N, Narita R, Shigemoto T, Hirai R, et al. Solution structures of cytosolic RNA sensor MDA5 and LGP2 C-terminal domains: identification of the RNA recognition loop in RIG-I-like receptors. J Biol Chem 2009; 284:17465-74; PMID:19380577; http://dx.doi.org/10.1074/jbc.M109.007179.

48. Pippig DA, Hellmuth JC, Cui S, Kirchhofer A, Lammens K, Lammens A, et al. The regulatory domain of the RIG-I family ATPase LGP2 senses double-stranded RNA. Nucleic Acids Res 2009; 37:2014-25; PMID:19208642; http://dx.doi.org/10.1093/nar/gkp059.

49. Murali A, Li X, Ranjith-Kumar CT, Bhardwaj K, Holzenburg A, Li P, et al. Structure and function of LGP2, a DEX(D/H) helicase that regulates the innate immunity response. J Biol Chem 2008; 283:15825-33; PMID:18411269; http://dx.doi.org/10.1074/jbc.M800542200.

50. Marques JT, Devosse T, Wang D, Zamanian-Daryoush M, Serbinowski P, Hartmann R, et al. A structural basis for discriminating between self and nonself double-stranded RNAs in mammalian cells. Nat Biotechnol 2006; 24:559-65; PMID:16648842; http://dx.doi.org/10.1038/nbt1205.

51. Myong S, Cui S, Cornish PV, Kirchhofer A, Gack MU, Jung JU, et al. Cytosolic viral sensor RIG-I is a 5'-triphosphate-dependent translocase on double-stranded RNA. Science 2009; 323:1070-4; PMID:19119185; http://dx.doi.org/10.1126/science.1168352.

52. Linder P. Dead-box proteins: a family affair–active and passive players in RNP-remodeling. Nucleic Acids Res 2006; 34:4168-80; PMID:16936318; http://dx.doi.org/10.1093/nar/gkl468.

53. Salonen A, Ahola T, Kaariainen L. Viral RNA replication in association with cellular membranes. Curr Top Microbiol Immunol 2005; 285:139-73; PMID:15609503; http://dx.doi.org/10.1007/3-540-26764-6_5.

54. Stetson DB, Medzhitov R. Recognition of cytosolic DNA activates an IRF3-dependent innate immune response. Immunity 2006; 24:93-103; PMID:16413926; http://dx.doi.org/10.1016/j.immuni.2005.12.003.

55. Ishii KJ, Coban C, Kato H, Takahashi K, Torii Y, Takeshita F, et al. A Toll-like receptor-independent antiviral response induced by double-stranded B-form DNA. Nat Immunol 2006; 7:40-8; PMID:16286919; http://dx.doi.org/10.1038/ni1282.

56. Takaoka A, Wang Z, Choi MK, Yanai H, Negishi H, Ban T, et al. DAI (DLM-1/ZBP1) is a cytosolic DNA sensor and an activator of innate immune response. Nature 2007; 448:501-5; PMID:17618271; http://dx.doi.org/10.1038/nature06013.

57. Unterholzner L, Keating SE, Baran M, Horan KA, Jensen SB, Sharma S, et al. IFI16 is an innate immune sensor for intracellular DNA. Nat Immunol 2010; 11:997-1004; PMID:20890285; http://dx.doi.org/10.1038/ni.1932.

58. Yang P, An H, Liu X, Wen M, Zheng Y, Rui Y, et al. The cytosolic nucleic acid sensor LRRFIP1 mediates the production of type I interferon via a beta-catenin-dependent pathway. Nat Immunol 2010; 11:487-94; PMID:20453844; http://dx.doi.org/10.1038/ni.1876.

59. Zhang Z, Yuan B, Bao M, Lu N, Kim T, Liu YJ. The helicase DDX41 senses intracellular DNA mediated by the adaptor STING in dendritic cells. Nat Immunol 2011; 12:959-65; PMID:21892174.
60. Ablasser A, Bauernfeind F, Hartmann G, Latz E, Fitzgerald KA, Hornung V. RIG-I-dependent sensing of poly(dA:dT) through the induction of an RNA polymerase III-transcribed RNA intermediate. Nat Immunol 2009; 10:1065-72; PMID:19609254; http://dx.doi.org/10.1038/ni.1779.
61. Chiu YH, Macmillan JB, Chen ZJ. RNA polymerase III detects cytosolic DNA and induces type I interferons through the RIG-I pathway. Cell 2009; 138:576-91; PMID:19631370; http://dx.doi.org/10.1016/j.cell.2009.06.015.
62. Pichlmair A, Schulz O, Tan CP, Näslund TI, Liljeström P, Weber F, et al. RIG-I-mediated antiviral responses to single-stranded RNA bearing 5'-phosphates. Science 2006; 314:997-1001; PMID:17038589; http://dx.doi.org/10.1126/science.1132998.
63. Gack MU, Shin YC, Joo CH, Urano T, Liang C, Sun L, et al. TRIM25 RING-finger E3 ubiquitin ligase is essential for RIG-I-mediated antiviral activity. Nature 2007; 446:916-20; PMID:17392790; http://dx.doi.org/10.1038/nature05732.
64. Oshiumi H, Matsumoto M, Hatakeyama S, Seya T. Riplet/RNF135, a RING finger protein, ubiquitinates RIG-I to promote interferon-beta induction during the early phase of viral infection. J Biol Chem 2009; 284:807-17; PMID:19017631; http://dx.doi.org/10.1074/jbc.M804259200.
65. Oshiumi H, Miyashita M, Inoue N, Okabe M, Matsumoto M, Seya T. The ubiquitin ligase Riplet is essential for RIG-I-dependent innate immune responses to RNA virus infection. Cell Host Microbe 2010; 8:496-509; PMID:21147464; http://dx.doi.org/10.1016/j.chom.2010.11.008.
66. Miyashita M, Oshiumi H, Matsumoto M, Seya T. DDX60, a DEXD/H Box Helicase, Is a Novel Antiviral Factor Promoting RIG-I-Like Receptor-Mediated Signaling. Mol Cell Biol 2011; 31:3802-19; PMID:21791617; http://dx.doi.org/10.1128/MCB.01368-10.

CHAPTER 7

The Mitochondrial Immune Signaling Complex

Yu Lei[†,1] and Jenny P.-Y. Ting[*,1-3]

Abstract

The mitochondrion provides a coordinating platform to anchor and compartmentalize distinct and interactive protein complexes to sustain basic life functions. These include bioenergetics, reactive oxygen species regulation, autophagy, apoptosis and type 1 interferon innate immune response. A number of mitochondrial proteins that are actively shuttled between the mitochondria and other subcellular compartments have been shown to control key immune signaling pathways, such as NF-κB and IRFs, in response to PAMPs (Pathogen-Associated Molecular Patterns). We have previously proposed that these proteins form mitochondrial immune signaling complex(es) (MISC), which mediate(s) a host of immune functions, a primary one being the production of type 1 interferons and inflammatory cytokines. This chapter focuses on the composition and functions of MISC, its regulatory mechanisms, and its association with upstream and downstream signaling molecules.

Introduction

It was about a century ago when the serial endosymbiosis hypothesis was put forth to explain the origin of mitochondria.[1] This hypothesis postulates a prokaryotic origin of mitochondrion where this organelle serves as the cellular power plant. It is hypothesized that when an ancient species of alphaproteobacteria became an endosymbiont, this novel organelle in eukaryotes is subjected to constant interactions with host factors. Through co-evolution, the genetic material of bacterial ancestor of mitochondria has been transferred to the host nucleus; similarly mitochondria incorporated the protein import system to integrate nucleus-encoded proteins.[1] It is now evident that the mitochondria not only anchors a plethora of molecules engaged in bioenergetic functions, it also sustains a large number of crucial cellular functions such as metabolic balances, apoptotic signaling, organelle biogenesis and most relevant to this review, the innate immune response.[2-4] It has been increasingly appreciated that several key signaling molecules important for the detection of viral nucleic acids have a foundation in the mitochondrion. This review will focus on the role of the mitochondrion in this component of innate immunity.

¹Lineberger Comprehensive Cancer Center, Chapel Hill, North Carolina, USA; ²Department of Microbiology and Immunology, School of Medicine, The University of North Carolina at Chapel Hill, Chapel Hill, North Carolina, USA; ³Institute for Inflammatory Diseases, School of Medicine, The University of North Carolina at Chapel Hill, Chapel Hill, North Carolina, USA
†Present address: Department of Diagnostic Sciences, School of Dental Medicine, University of Pittsburgh Medical Center. Pittsburgh, Pennsylvania, USA.
*Corresponding Author: Jenny P.Y. Ting—Email: jpyting@gmail.com

Nucleic Acid Sensors and Antiviral Immunity, edited by Suryaprakash Sambhara and Takashi Fujita.
©2013 Landes Bioscience.

Molecules Important in the Recognition of Nucleic Acid Species

One of the primary functions of the innate defense system is to differentiate "self" from "non-self," which relies on several classes of extracellular and intracellular sensors to detect pathogen-associated molecular patterns (PAMPs) and/or other danger signals. Janeway first predicted the existence of pattern recognition receptors (PRRs) to engage their respective ligands and trigger immune activation.[5] Toll-like receptors (TLRs) represent the first identified class of PRRs[6] which are type I integral membrane glycoproteins that share an N-terminal extracellular leucine-rich-repeats (LRR) domain and a C-terminal cytoplasmic Toll/IL-1R (TIR) signaling domain.[7,8] TLRs detect both extracellular and endosomal/lysosomal microbial threats. Among the human and murine TLRs, many demonstrate specificity to distinct repertoires of microbial products of bacteria, viruses and fungi. TLR3, TLR7, TLR8 (human) and TLR9 recognize nucleic acids in the endolysosomal compartment. TLR3 binds to double-stranded RNA (dsRNA), TLR7 (or human TLR8) binds to single-stranded (ssRNA) and TLR9 recognizes CpG-DNA.[8] However, as early as 2004, López et al. found that the dendritic cells (DCs) matured normally in the absence of TLR3, TLR7, TLR8 or TLR9 signaling.[9] In addition, these TLR-deficient DCs could prime a normal Th1 response against Sendai virus (SeV) infection or influenza A virus infection.[9] Similarly, $Tlr3^{-/-}$ mice displayed uncompromised antiviral responses to lymphocytic choriomeningitis virus (LCMV), vesicular stomatitis virus (VSV), murine cytomegalovirus (MCMV) and reovirus infection.[10] Bacterial DNA causes septic shock,[11] and CpG DNA of *Listeria monocytogenes* can activate type 1 interferon (IFN) signaling, however, TLR signaling is dispensable for this response.[12] In addition, bacterial DNA activates B lymphocytes in a TLR9-independent fashion.[13] Finally, DNA viruses such as Herpes Simplex Virus type 1 induce type 1 IFN production in both TLR9-dependent and TLR9-independent pathways.[14] These cumulative data suggest the existence of other nucleotide-sensing pathways.

One of the early searches for novel nucleotides sensors was based on the screening of an expression cDNA library from IFN-β-treated human K562 cells, which responded poorly to viral infection unless the cells were treated with IFN-β.[15] One cDNA clone was identified to significantly augment poly (I:C)-induced IRF promoter activation and this clone encoded the N-terminal residues of the RNA helicase retinoic acid inducible gene I (RIG-I)[15] (Fig. 1). Together with the structurally similar proteins melanoma differentiation-associated gene 5 (MDA5) and laboratory of genetics and physiology 2 (LGP2), these proteins constitute the RIG-I-like receptors (RLRs) family. RIG-I contains two N-terminal caspase activation and recruitment domain (CARD), a central DExD/H box-containing helicase domain and a C-terminal regulatory domain (CTD). The helicase domain endows the protein with ATPase activity to drive the unwinding of dsRNA with 3′-terminal overhang (> 5nt).[16] Recent structure analysis reveals that the CTD domain forms a RNA-binding cleft.[16,17] Importantly, RIG-I and MDA5 exhibit distinct preferences for the molecular features of RNA ligands and RNA viruses.[18] RIG-I binds to short 5′-ppp dsRNA while MDA5 recognizes long dsRNA.[18-21] Although it was shown that in vitro transcribed 5′-ppp ssRNA could also induce type 1 IFN activation,[21] two recent reports showed that T7 RNA polymerase leads to the generation of dsRNA[22,23] while synthetic 5′-ppp ssRNA had no immune activation effect.[21] This suggests only dsRNA could be recognized by RLRs. The 5′-ppp moiety is the signature motif that activates RIG-I,[19,21] however, it has also been shown that 5′-p dsRNA and dsRNA bearing no 5′-triphosphate moiety could still potently induce type 1 IFN activation.[16,24] The source of dsRNA can be traced back to viral genomes, replication intermediates, viral transcripts or self-RNA generated by RNase L.[21,24,25] All these RNA species have been proposed to have immune stimulatory potential. However, a recent study showed that only viral genome RNA could potently induce type 1 IFN activation during influenza A virus and SeV infection while cleaved self-RNA does not induce type 1 IFN production during the infection.[26] Further studies are essential to evaluate the respective contributions of dsRNA from various sources in inducing type 1 IFN production upon viral challenges.

MDA5 recognizes higher-order structure of RNA complex involving dsRNA and ssRNA.[27] Due to the ligand binding properties of RIG-I and MDA5, they display specificity to different

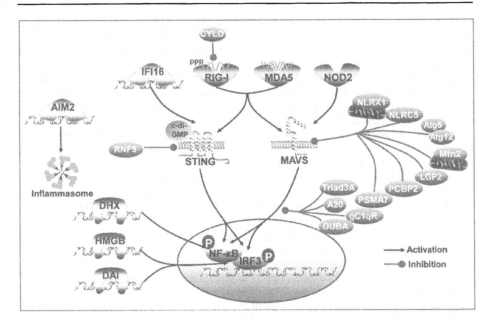

Figure 1. The mitochondrial immune signaling complex and its regulators. The MAVS and/ or STING-mediated RLR signaling activation is subjected to meticulous check mechanisms. Different regulatory factors employ molecular steric hindrance, autophagy-based strategies or protein proteasomal degradation pathway to modulate type 1 IFN activation. Black (green) arrows indicate enhancing functions, gray (red) lines indicates inhibitory functions. A color version of this image is available online at www.landesbioscience.com/curie.

viruses. RIG-I-deficient mouse fibroblasts and conventional dendritic cells (cDCs) fail to mount type 1 IFN activation in response to Newcastle disease virus (NDV), SeV, VSV, influenza A virus and Japanese encephalitis virus (JEV). However, MDA5-deficient cells respond normally to these viral challenges, yet fail to induce immune activation upon infection by picornaviruses such as encephalomyocarditis virus (EMCV), Mengo virus and the Theiler's virus.[28] Some flaviviruses such as Dengue virus and West Nile virus (WNV) can be recognized by both RIG-I and MDA5.[29,30]

RIG-I-mediated type 1 IFN signaling not only responds to certain RNA species but also to DNA. Two groups have independently identified DNA-dependent RNA polymerase III as the cytosolic DNA sensor that generates 5'-ppp RNA, which engages RIG-I and activates downstream signaling.[31,32] However, RIG-I-deficient cells still show competency in responding to cytoplasmic DNA, which raises the possibility that there are additional cytoplasmic DNA sensors. To qualify as an intracellular DNA sensor, it should contain a DNA-binding domain. The DNA-dependent activator of IFN-regulatory factors (DAI, also known as Z-DNA-binding protein) binds to dsDNA and associates with TBK1 as well as IRF3. DAI is an IFN-inducible protein, and could augment type 1 IFN induction by various DNA sources when overexpressed.[33] In addition, knockdown of DAI by RNA interference ablates immune activation by exogenous DNA.[33] The dimerization of DAI results in DNA-dependent type 1 IFN production.[34] DAI contains two receptor-interacting protein (RIP) homotypic interaction motifs (RHIMs) and binds to RIP1 and RIP3. Knockdown of RIP1 or RIP3 abrogated NF-κB activation induced by immunostimulatory DNA sequences.[35,36] However, DAI-deficient and wildtype control mice demonstrated no difference in DNA-dependent type 1 IFN activation in MEFs, and bone-marrow-derived dendritic cells differentiated by GM-CSF or by Flt3.[37] At this point, it was surmised that additional intracellular DNA sensors exist so that redundant mechanisms provide host cells another layer of safe-guard against DNA stimuli.

To identify novel DNA sensors, several high throughput biochemical screenings have been performed to seek DNA-interacting proteins (Fig. 1). One of the earliest identified members is the high-mobility group box (HMGB) protein family, which includes HMGB1, HMGB2 and HMGB3 which contribute to the initiation of type 1 IFN and proinflammatory cytokine responses to DNA stimuli.[38] Both HMGB1 and HMGB2 could be precipitated by immobilized B-DNA, and their deficiency resulted in impaired activation of NF-κB and IRF3. Furthermore, the absence of HMGBs also compromised the activation of TLR3, TLR7 and TLR9 by their cognate ligands nucleic acids.[38]

Another class of the intracellular DNA sensors is the PYHIN proteins, which contain two HIN DNA binding domains and one Pyrin domain. Two members in this family, including IFI16 and AIM2, have been shown to be engaged with DNA and activate innate immune system.[39-43] Interestingly, IFI16 and AIM2 trigger separate signaling pathways despite their structural similarity and affinity to DNA. IFI16 is essential for recruiting downstream adaptor proteins to mount type 1 IFN production in response to intracellular DNA. Targeted knockdown of IFI16 resulted in the ablation of DNA-induced but not RNA-induced activation of both NF-κB and IRF3.[39] In contrast, AIM2 has no effect in modulating host type 1 IFN responses to DNA; rather it forms a caspase-1 activating inflammasome necessary for IL-1β/IL-18 processing.[40-43]

The breadth of intracellular nucleic acid sensing system is additionally exemplified by the identification of two DExD/H-box helicases DHX36 and DHX9 in plasmacytoid dendritic cells.[44] Albeit these two proteins contain the DExD/H-box similar to RIG-I and MDA5, they exhibit different specificities. DHX36 primarily binds to CpG-A via the DEAH domain, while DHX9 binds to CpG-B via the DUF1605 domain. DHX36 is pivotal in activating IFN-α generation in response to CpG-A, while DHX9 preferentially activates NF-κB-dependent TNF-α and IL-6 production.[44]

Finally, the LRR (leucine-rich repeats) domain is postulated to function as ligands binding or protein-binding platforms.[8,45] A screening in mouse peritoneal macrophages with a siRNA library targeting LRR-containing and LRR-interacting proteins-encoding mRNA leads to the identification of LRRFIP1, which recognizes both exogenous RNA and DNA species to induce type 1 IFN production in a β-catenin-dependent fashion.[46]

The Significance of Mitochondrial-Localized Proteins in Host Innate Antiviral Responses

Two mitochondrial-localized adaptors have been identified in the type 1 IFN responses to intracellular RNA or DNA from microbes, these are MAVS[47-50] and Stimulator of Interferon Genes (STING, also known as MITA, MPYS and ERIS) (Fig. 1).[51-53] Both proteins are ubiquitously expressed and indispensable for transducing signals detected by upstream PRRs leading to type 1 IFNs production, albeit STING is less potent than MAVS in activating NF-κB or IRF3 when overexpressed.[52] Association between these two proteins has been also identified.[52] Importantly the integrity of this adaptor core is critical since deletion of either of these two proteins resulted in ablated type 1 IFNs even though the other remains intact. Some cell lines are exclusively dependent on MAVS for the cytosolic DNA-induced type 1 IFN response, yet MAVS-independent machinery has also been implicated in certain cell types such as MEF.[31] On the other hand, STING mediates cytosolic non-CpG DNA-induced type 1 IFN activation in MEF, BMDM (bone-marrow-derived macrophage), GM-DC and FL-DC.[54]

MAVS is located at the mitochondrial outer membrane, where it engages with upstream PRRs and recruits TBK1 and IKK complexes to activate NF-κB and IRF3. However, it becomes detergent-resistant when cells are infected with SeV, which indicates possible protein translocation.[47] Indeed, a recent study found MAVS is also located within peroxisomes, which are single-membrane-bound structures known to be involved in metabolic pathways.[55] The different locations of MAVS confer distinct antiviral signaling kinetics: the peroxisomal MAVS is unable to induce type 1 IFN production, however, it launches a quick interferon-independent transcription of ISG (Interferon-Stimulated Genes) to establish the early antiviral state of the cells; the mitochondrial-localized MAVS then assumes its function in type 1 IFN production and signaling, which in turn promotes the induction of ISGs. NDV (Newcastle disease virus) triggers RIG-I-mediated type 1 IFN production, a recent report found it also induced the redistribution of MAVS to form speckle-like aggregates.[56] Mfn1 (Mitofusin 1), which regulates mitochondrial fission and fusion, associates with MAVS and is responsible for its virus-induced redistribution. Indeed, disruption of mitochondrial fusion processes by knocking down Mfn1 abrogates both MAVS redistribution and type 1 IFN production in response to viral infections.[56] These findings support the notion that it is both the biochemical properties and localization of MAVS that determine its functional outcome.

A similar scenario seems to apply to the other adaptor, STING. The initial studies on STING showed discrepant findings regarding its subcellular localization: one group found this protein predominantly resides in the endoplasmic reticulum (ER) and interacts with a member of translocon-associated protein complex TRAPβ;[51] while another group demonstrated that STING is an exclusive mitochondrial outer membrane protein and associates with MAVS.[52] In two subsequent studies, STING was consistently identified in the microsomes fraction.[54,57] Microsomes are membrane structures comprised of ER, Golgi and vesicles that are generated during cell homogenization. However, the ER and mitochondria are not completely physically distinct organelles, but are connected by the mitochondria-associated ER membrane (MAM).[3] STING is also found in these structures, which may explain why it is also found in different cellular fractions. However, upon HSV-1 (Herpes Simplex Virus-1) infection, STING is only found in microsomes.[54] Furthermore STING could be degraded by an E3 ligase ring finger protein 5 (RNF5, also known as RMA1).[57] Such functional interaction and regulation occur predominantly in mitochondria. Although STING is barely detectable in the ER fraction at the resting state, it becomes more abundant when cells are infected with SeV (Sendai Virus) for 6h and diminishes from the ER again by 24h post-infection.[57] The function of STING in response to RNA virus infection was questioned by another report that showed STING-deficient BMDM were fully capable of producing IFN-β in response to SeV infection.[39] STING is consistently shown to mediate type 1 IFN signaling in response to intracellular DNA insults, which cover a wide spectrum of DNA species including DNA from virus, bacteria, plasmids and artificial DNA sequences such as poly(dA:dT), poly(dGC:dGC) and ISD (Interferon Stimulating DNA sequence).[39,51,54] Recent evidence suggests STING also directly binds to cyclic diguanylate monophosphate and serves as a sensor for intracellular cyclic dinucleotides, which are found in bacteria and thus possible PAMPs for innate immune activation.[58] *Sting* deficiency results in ablated type 1 IFNs production in response to these intracellular DNA challenges.[51,54,58] The significance of viral specific functions and subcellular compartmentalization of these adaptors in modulating host antiviral innate immunity require further investigations.

The Roles of NLR Proteins in the Modulation of MAVS-RLR Signaling

NLR (nucleotide-binding domain, leucine-rich repeats-containing) proteins (previously known as CATERPILLERs, NODs, NALPs or NACHT-LRRs) in mammals share sequence homology with the plants NBS-LRR proteins which are pivotal in delivering disease resistance.[59,60] Albeit there is scarce evidence showing the direct binding of NLRs to various cytosolic PAMPs and other DAMPs (damage-associated molecular patterns), these proteins are generally thought to be critically involved in the sensing, regulation and translation of hazardous stimuli to host pro-inflammatory responses including caspase-1-dependent IL-1β and IL-18 processing as well as NF-κB-dependent defensins and cytokines induction.[45,61] However, as evidence begins to accumulate, NLRs are also found pivotal in modulating cell death and interferon responses, both of which have links to the mitochondrion.

NLRs are characterized by a central NBD (nucleotide-binding domain), a C-terminal LRR domain and an N-terminal effector domain, which could be CARD, Pyrin, BIR (baculovirus inhibitor of apoptosis repeat), AD (transactivation domain) or an X domain that cannot be categorized as any known motifs.[61] NLRX1 is the first NLR shown to intersect the MAVS-RIG-I pathway. It is a unique NLR not only because of its mitochondrial localization but also its modes of functioning.[62,63] Instead of direct participation in response to microbial invasion, NLRX1 modulates the functions of a MAVS-dependent multimeric protein complex which could be > 600kDa in its quiescent state.[64] This complex is key in the induction of type 1 IFNs upon engagement with nucleic acids as described above, which then leads to the mitochondrial recruitment of TRAF3 and TRAF6 to induce subsequent signaling steps required for type 1 IFNs production. NLRX1 is a non-canonical NLR member in that its N-terminal effector domain does not share homology to any well-conserved motifs yet it contains a mitochondrial targeting sequence, and that its central nucleotide binding domain does not have a Walker A motif found in other NLRs. Overexpression of NLRX1 inhibits RIG-I- or MDA5-mediated activation of NF-κB-, IRF3-dependent and *IFNB1* promoter activity in a dose-dependent fashion. In addition, NLRX1 also inhibits *IFNB1* mRNA transcription upon RLR activation. Gene knockdown of NLRX1 by siRNA results in an enhanced type 1 IFN signaling which confers resistance to Sindbis virus infection.[62] NLRX1 is located on the outer membrane of mitochondria and interacts with the adaptor MAVS. Exogenous NLRX1 expression potently represses SeV-induced homotypic CARD:CARD interaction between RIG-I and MAVS.[62] Interestingly, the inhibitory function of NLRX1 is specific to mitochondrial MAVS rather than peroxisome-localized MAVS.[55] The role of NLRX1 in impeding MAVS-RIG-I interaction and the subsequent type 1 IFN induction has been further confirmed in gene deletion mice.[65] However, a recent study suggests that NLRX1 can be localized to the mitochondrial matrix and interacts with a matrix protein UQCRC2, although the physiological significance of such interaction is now known.[66] NLRX1 has been shown to be involved in the ROS production during *Shigella flexneri* and *Chlamydia trachomatis* infection.[67,68] The underlying reason for the discrepancy in localization is still not understood, but may be similar to the multiple localization of MAVS or STING. Thus the trafficking and localization of NLRX1 in the presence of virus needs further investigation.

NOD2 is the second NLR protein that intersects with the MAVS pathway. In a screening of NLR proteins, Sabbah et al. found that overexpression of NOD2 but not other NLRs endows HEK293 cells with the capability to activate IRF3 in response to ssRNA.[69] Interestingly, the endogenous level of NOD2 in A549 cells is inducible by viral infection. The authors also showed that depletion of NOD2 results in ablated IFN-β production upon viral challenge. Furthermore immunoprecipitation of overexpressed NOD2 leads to the recovery of RSV nucleocapsid protein specific RNA, which is substantiated in a cell-free system using HA-NOD2 bound-agarose beads as the bait. Although it's been shown NLRP3 is involved in the recognition of influenza A virus,[70,71] this finding represents the first piece of evidence that NLR can associate with viral ssRNA and activate the RLR signaling. However, it's still premature to define NOD2 as a bona fide PRR since it is not clear whether such association is direct or indirect. Immunoprecipitation of NOD2 would be very likely to pull down NOD2-interacting proteins. Since the adaptor MAVS associates with NOD2, and MAVS has been shown to interact with RIG-I, it is also possible that the recovery of RSV-specific RNA was the results of co-immunoprecipitation of RIG-I. In addition, the exact molecular features that activate NOD2 are still unknown. For example, is the 5'-triphosphate moiety a necessity in this recognition? Does dsRNA interact with NOD2? To demonstrate the direct binding of NOD2 to cytosolic RNA species, the use of highly purified recombinant NOD2 protein in a RNA-binding assay would be convincing. Evidence of direct binding would be compelling to establish the structural basis to group NOD2 into PRR.

The fact that certain NLR protein expression is inducible by viral infection also adds to the possibility that NLRs are actively involved in the antiviral signaling modulation. A novel NLR, NLRC5 has been recently characterized by several independent groups.[72-76] NLRC5 is highly expressed in hematopoietic cells and lowly expressed in epithelial cells. Two groups noticed NLRC5 expression was upregulated by poly (I:C) treatment, SeV or Cytomegalovirus (CMV) infection.[74,76] In fact, *NLRC5* contains the IFN-γ-responsive elements in its promoter region; and among a variety of treatments, only IFN-γ induces the expression of NLRC5.[77] Overexpression of NLRC5 leads to the activation of the IFN-responsive regulatory promoter elements and the upregulation of antiviral target genes, such as *IFN-α, OAS1 and PRKRIR*.[77] However, one group showed that overexpression of NLRC5 alone was not sufficient to activate type 1 IFN signaling, yet knockdown of NLRC5 reduced SeV- and poly (I:C)-mediated type 1 IFN induction in both THP-1 cells and human primary dermal fibroblasts.[76] In contrast to these reported immune-activation effects, two other groups found that NLRC5 is a negative regulator of NF-κB and type 1 IFN signaling pathways.[72,73] NLRC5 associates with RIG-I and MDA5 via the CARD domain to preclude their interaction with MAVS. Reduction of NLRC5 level by RNA interference significantly increased type 1 IFN production. In addition, NLRC5 also sequesters the IKKα/IKKβ complex to abolish their phosphorylation upon LPS challenges.[73] In congruent with the fact that NLRC5 overexpression inhibits NF-κB activity, reduction of NLRC5 leads to enhanced proinflammatory responses.[72,73] However all of these experiments relied on overexpression or RNA interference approaches. A gene-deletion approach has not been able to verify these findings.[78] Our own study in human cell lines and primary monocytes suggests that NLRC5 is important in in inflammasome activities;[79] while another paper suggests its role in the transcriptional activation of class I MHC genes.[75] Thus the role of NLRC5 is still debatable.

The Regulatory Components of the RLR Signaling Pathways

Given the great potential of MAVS and/or STING-mediated RLR signaling activation, this pathway is subjected to meticulous check mechanisms (Fig. 1). Thirteen host proteins have been identified up to date in the negative regulatory module of this complex including NLRX1, NLRC5, Atg5-Atg12 conjugate, gC1qR, Mfn2, RNF5, LGP2, CYLD, PCBP2, AIP4, A20, Triad3A and PSMA7 (Table 1).[57,62,64,73,80-88] RNAi-based reduction of these proteins levels results in enhanced type 1 IFN production in response to certain RNA viruses. The complexity of this regulatory module safeguards against overzealous immune activation. Although these proteins are functionally redundant, they primarily target RLR signaling via distinct mechanisms including molecular steric hindrance, autophagy as well as poly-ubiquitination (PUb)-mediated destabilization of adaptors and signaling modifications. It is worth noting that one regulatory protein could employ different mechanisms to function and structurally diverse proteins could fall into the same regulatory mechanism category.

The molecular steric hindrance hypothesis is based on the notion that some regulatory proteins could associate with the key molecules in the RLR signaling pathways, such as the PRRs, adaptors or downstream kinases; and such interaction competes them against their immune-activating engagement possibly by steric hindrance. This model has been supported by insights into the inhibitory mechanisms of NLRX1, NLRC5, LGP2, Atg5-Atg12 conjugate and Mfn2, all of which inhibit MAVS-mediated induction of type 1 IFN. In the case of NLRX1, it diminishes the interaction between RIG-I and MAVS in the resting state, and deficiency of NLRX1 results in higher resistance to Sindbis virus, which induces type 1 IFN production in a RIG-I-dependent manner.[62,65] Similarly, overexpressed NLRC5 preferentially binds to the CARD domain of RIG-I and strongly competes with MAVS for engagement. NLRC5 does not interact with MAVS, IKKi, TBK1, TRIF, TRAF3 or IRF3, which underlies the fact that NLRC5 potently inhibits RIG-I- and MDA5-induced *IFNB1* promoter activation yet only shows weak effect on MAVS- and TBK1-induced RLR signaling induction.[73]

A recent report also suggests that the Atg5-Atg12 conjugate, which is typically associated with autophagy, also intrudes between RIG-I and MAVS to abolish the homotypic CARD interactions and inhibits type 1 IFN production.[80] Another molecular break, Mfn2, targets the C-terminal region of MAVS instead of the N-terminal CARD for modulation; and reduction of Mfn2 by siRNA leads to a decrease in the MAVS apparent molecular mass.[64] In the current model, these regulatory proteins target different regions of MAVS for steric preclusion of its engagement with immune-activating molecules. Interestingly, the molecular steric hindrance mechanism can also be presented by the splice variants of the adaptor itself. A recent report identified two MAVS splice variants: MAVS1a lacking exon 2 and MAVS1b lacking exon 3.[89] During the excision of exons, a frame shift occurs. Both splice variants possess the CARD domain, which is essential to

Table 1. The modulators of RLR signaling

Regulatory Mechanisms		Regulators					
Molecular Steric Hindrance	Targeting MAVS CARD	NLRX1	NLRC5	Atg5-Atg12 conjugate	NOD2		
	Targeting MAVS C-terminus	Mfn2	LGP2				
Autophagy Disturbance	Deficiency in autophagy	Mfn2	Atg5	Atg5-Atg12 conjugate			
Ub-mediated modulation	Proteasomal degradation	A20	PCBP2	AIP4	PSMA7	RNF5	Triad3A
	Signaling modification	CYLD	DUBA	Unanchored PUb chain	TRIM23	TRIM25	
Unknown mechanism		gC1qR					

The regulators of RLR signaling could be classified into three categories based on their functioning mechanisms. The molecular steric hindrance hypothesis is based on the notion that some regulatory proteins could associate with the key molecules in RLR signaling to compete against their immune-activating engagement. Autophagy disturbance has been implicated in aberrant ROS production and damaged mitochondria accumulation, which cultivates in RLR signaling modification. PUb-mediated modulation is a set of delicate regulatory mechanisms composed of both PUb-mediated destabilization of the adaptors and PUb-mediated non-proteolytic signaling modification. Light gray background denotes negative RLR signaling regulators; dark gray background denotes positive regulators.

engage with upstream RLRs. However, MAVS1a does not have the essential signaling domains to transduce RLR interaction to downstream effector activation, while MAVS1b could interact with FADD and RIP1 to selectively induce type 1 IFN production.[89] Hence, MAVS1a functions as a steric blockade for full length MAVS to recruit downstream signaling complexes.

Connection of Autophagy, Innate Immunity and the Mitochondria

Autophagy represents another host strategy in keeping RLR signaling from over-reacting. Besides mitochondria, ER, MAM and peroxisomes, another membrane bound structure that has emerged to be a platform for antiviral signaling modulation is autophagosome. Autophagy is an evolutionarily conserved cellular function to recycle nutrients and maintain homeostasis. This process together with the proteosome-dependent mechanisms constitutes the major intracellular degradation system. It not only recycles damaged or aged organelles, misfolded proteins but it also sequesters invading microorganisms as a primary host defense strategy. Autophagy disturbance has been implicated in cellular components turnover, development, differentiation, tissue remodeling and numerous diseases such as cancer, muscular disorders, neurodegeneration and infectious diseases.[90,91]

Autophagy has been artificially categorized into four phases: (1) vesicle nucleation, in this phase the double-membrane structure begins to form and sequesters a part of the cytoplasm and damaged organelles; (2) vesicle elongation, in this phase, the membranes continue to grow until they reach the next phase; (3) docking and fusion, autophagosome formation is complete at this stage where the ends of isolated vesicles finally meet; (4) vesicle fusion and content breakdown, the autophagosome fuses with lysosome to deliver cargo into the newly formed autolysosome for content and inner membrane degradation.[91]

Inhibition of the TOR kinase is a major stimulus that activates autophagy,[92,93] which involves Atgs (Autophagy-related Genes encoded proteins). Among about 30 Atgs identified to date, there are two essential conjugation systems centering on Atg12 and Atg8 (also referred to as LC3 in mammals) for autophagosome formation. Similar to ubiquitin, Atg12 and Atg8 have conserved ubiquitin-fold regions despite their lack of amino acids sequence homology to ubiquitin.[94,95] Once activated, Atg12 will be transferred to Atg5 with the assistance of E1-like enzyme Atg7 and E2 enzyme Atg10. The Atg5-Atg12 conjugate also interacts with Atg16 to form a protein complex. Atg8 is conjugated to phosphatidylethanolamine (PE) (Atg8-PE or LC3-II) during autophagosome membrane expansion.[96] Hence biochemical detection of LC3-II is widely accepted as a measurement for autophagy.[97]

Besides being actively involved in autophagosome biogenesis, Atg5-Atg12 conjugate has been recently found to associate with RIG-I and MAVS via the CARD domain and inhibit downstream type 1 IFN signaling. Overexpression of Atg5-Atg12 results in dampened NF-κB and IRF3 activation; conversely, *Atg5−/−* MEFs are more resistant to VSV infection than controls due to enhanced type 1 IFN production.[80] The deficiency of autophagy also leads to the accumulation of damaged mitochondria, which results in the buildup of MAVS and enhanced levels of intracellular ROS. Either effect leads to the induction of type 1 IFN.[81]

The functions of autophagy in antiviral innate immune response are cell type specific. Plasmacytoid dendritic cells (pDCs) primarily rely on TLRs to recognize viral PAMPs in a MAVS-independent fashion. A recent study found that autophagy enhanced the transport of cytosolic viral replication intermediates into the endosomal/lysosomal compartment for TLR7 engagement.[98] In pDCs, absence of autophagy results in compromised antiviral innate immune response in contrast to the hyperactive type 1 IFN production in MEFs.

Mitochondria are closely associated with autophagosomes, and many proteins in both organelles have been functionally linked. For example, autophagic proteins Atg5 and Atg9 can be transiently localized onto the mitochondria;[99,100] similarly mitochondrial proteins Bif-1 and Sirt1 are essential for autophagy.[101,102] A recent study shows that both Atg5 and LC3 can be temporarily localized to punctae on mitochondria. Importantly, mitochondria provide membranes for the biogenesis of autophagosomes.[2] Mfn2 is responsible for tethering mitochondria to ER, and deficiency in Mfn2 leads to the disruption of the transfer of lipids from ER, which is necessary for proper mitochondrial functioning. Indeed *Mfn2*−/− cells have severely impaired autophagosome formation.[2] Given the fact that reduction of Mfn2 also leads to enhanced RLR signaling, it is plausible that Mfn2 not only contributes to the molecular steric hindrance in blocking MAVS association with downstream IKK complexes, but also inhibit this pathway via autophagy-mediated mechanism. However, further study is needed to understand how Mfn2 modulates autophagy in response to RLR signaling.

Viruses Can Subvert MAVS-Dependent Type 1 IFN Production

Given the broad consequences of type 1 IFN production in the viral life cycles, the mitochondrial-based MAVS pathway has been heavily targeted by different viruses to abrogate such response. Three simplified models have been proposed to explain how viruses subvert MAVS-mediated antiviral responses: (1) abrogating MAVS function by cleaving the protein off the mitochondria; (2) imposing steric hindrance by interfering with the association between MAVS and upstream RLRs; (3) destablizing MAVS by polyubiquitination-based mechanisms (Fig. 2).

Several viral proteins have been identified to cleave MAVS. HCV encodes a serine protease NS3/4A to cleave MAVS at the residue Cys508, dislodging MAVS from mitochondria.[50,103] Similarly a closely related virus GB virus B (GBV-B) employs NS3/4A to cleave MAVS.[104] A picornavirus HAV uses the 3ABC precursor of its 3C(pro) cysteine protease to cleave MAVS at the Gln428 site.[105]

In addition to cleaving MAVS, association with MAVS or upstream RLR to compete with their signaling-activating engagement is another widely used strategy by different classes of viruses. The non-structural protein NS1 encoded by influenza A virus inhibits host type 1 IFN response by not only binding to dsRNA to sequester activating RNA species from RLR but also by directly associating with RIG-I to prevent IRF3 nuclear translocation.[106-108] The PB2 subunit of influenza RNA polymerase can associate with MAVS and inhibits type 1 IFN production. Although the mitochondrial localization of PB2 is not essential for viral growth in vitro, non-mitochondrial PB2-encoding virus induces higher level of type 1 IFN.[109,110] The non-structural protein NS2 encoded by human Respiratory Syncytial Virus interacts with the CARD domain of RIG-I and blocks its association with MAVS to inhibit IFN promoter activation.[111] The Z proteins encoded

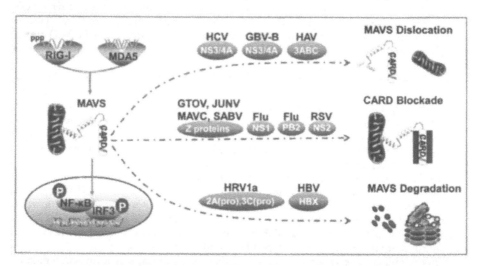

Figure 2. The subversion of RLR activation by viruses. Potent type 1 IFN production has profound effects in the viral life cycles. Hence, the mitochondrial-based MAVS pathway has been heavily targeted by different viruses to abrogate such response. Viral proteins employ diverse strategies including dislocating MAVS from mitochondria, interfering with the association between MAVS and upstream RLRs or targeting MAVS for degradation in both proteasome-dependent or independent mechanisms.

by four New World arenaviruses including Guanarito virus (GTOV), Junin virus (JUNV), Machupo virus (MAVC), and Sabia virus (SABV) have been found to interact with RIG-I and interfere with RIG-I:MAVS association.[112] The LCMV nucleoprotein interacts with both RIG-I and MDA5 to inhibit type 1 IFN signaling triggered by LCMV RNA or other RLR ligands.[113] V proteins encoded by paramyxoviruses associate with MDA5 and abrogate downstream type 1 IFN activation.[114] A recent report demonstrates that V proteins target a region within the MDA5 helicase domain to interrupt dsRNA binding and its homotypic dimerization.[115]

Destablizing MAVS is not only a host strategy to keep immune activation in-check, but also hijacked by viruses to evade immune surveillance. In a clinical samples analysis, MAVS was downregulated in hepatocellular carcinomas of Hepatitis B Virus (HBV) origin.[116] In fact the protein HBX encoded by HBV has been found to associate with MAVS and facilitate its proteasomal degradation through PUb at the Lys136 site. Consistently, HBX knock-in transgenic mice displayed enhanced susceptibility to VSV infection.[116] MAVS can also be disrupted by non-proteasomal pathway. For example, Human Rhinovirus 1a (HRV1a) infection can result in the degradation of MAVS. Ectopic expression of HRV1a and polioviral 2A(pro) and 3C(pro) resulted in the destabilization of MAVS.[117] Thus numerous viral proteins are known to target this critical pathway of mitochondrial-based immune signaling.

MAVS in Apoptotic Signaling

In addition to being a critical adaptor for type 1 IFN signaling induced by RLR engagement, we demonstrated that MAVS mediates virus-induced apoptosis in an IFN-independent fashion.[118] Two other groups reported similar results regarding the pro-apoptotic function of MAVS.[119,120] Overexpression of MAVS is similarly found to induce apoptosis in a caspase-3, -8, and -9 dependent manner. Anoikis is a type of apoptosis induced by the detachment of epithelial cells from the extracellular matrix. Not only can anoikis induce the upregulation of MAVS but also recruit caspase-8. Furthermore, MAVS binds to death-associated protein 3 (DAP3) and a reduction of MAVS protein level inhibits DAP3-mediated anoikis.[119] MAVS has been found to be involved in Sendai and Dengue virus-induced apoptosis while RNAi-based reduction of MAVS results in delayed caspases activation and attenuated cell death.[120] This process requires mitochondrial MAVS as dislocated MAVS not only loses its function in activating type 1 IFN, but become inert in activating the apoptotic pathway.[47,118]

The MAVS-mediated apoptotic signaling is also targeted by different classes of viruses. Truncating the transmembrane domain or cleavage of the protein by HCV NS3/4A completely abolished its apoptosis-inducing capacity. In addition, the NSP15 protein encoded by SARS-CoV can inhibit this pathway although the detailed molecular mechanism of its inhibitory function remains unclear.[118]

Conclusion

This review focuses on anti-viral signaling pathways that are centered on mitochondrial proteins. We propose that such mitochondrial immune signaling complex (MISC) plays pivotal roles in the host innate immune responses.[45] The adaptor MAVS or STING, both of which are reported in the mitochondria, associates with upstream PRRs when they are engaged in their respective ligands, and activates downstream signals such as NF-κB and IRF3 to mount type 1 IFN production.[47-50] Together with apoptosis, these constitute the first line of host defense against viruses. MAVS has dual roles in mounting type 1 IFN production and initiating virus-induced apoptosis. Both functions have been targeted by a variety of viral proteins for modulation. Additionally, an intricate regulatory network is employed to keep host immune responses in-check via distinct mechanisms including molecular steric hindrance, autophagy and poly-ubiquitination-based modulation. The network is also targeted by a variety of viruses which employ several common strategies such as cleavage of MAVS and the molecular steric hindrance to impede this pathway. Future identification of novel members and characterization of the relationship among the different regulators will be critical to better understand MISC and to design therapeutic target to modulate this pathway to its full potential.

About the Authors

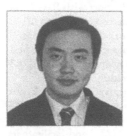

Yu Lei is currently completing a specialist residency in Oral and Maxillofacial Pathology at the University of Pittsburgh Medical Center. He received his DDS degree with an emphasis on prosthodontics in 2006 from the West China College of Stomatology, Sichuan University at Chengdu, China. He then joined Dr. Jenny Ting's laboratory at the University of North Carolina at Chapel Hill to investigate the regulation network of type 1 interferon production including the identification and characterization of novel partners of the mitochondrial immune signaling complex. He received his PhD degree in 2011 and completed a brief postdoctoral training with Dr. Jenny Ting. He is a recipient of the Freedland advanced dental education fellowship from the North Carolina Dental Foundation and the Turner Award from North Carolina-American Association of Dental Research. He is an editorial board member and peer-reviewer of many journals. His research interests include identification of novel innate immune genes in the oncogenesis of head and neck cancers.

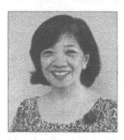

Jenny Ting is the co-Director of the Inflammatory Disease Institute and Director of the Center for Translational Immunology at the University of North Carolina at Chapel Hill, USA, since 2008. She is currently a William R. Kenan Professor of Microbiology and Immunology and the UNC Lineberger Comprehensive Cancer Center's Immunology program leader. She also serves as a council member of the National Institute of Allergy and Infectious Diseases. She has published extensively in the areas of molecular immunology, inflammation, infection and cancer. Her recent research concentrates on innate immunity, with a focus on the NLR and plexin gene families.

References

1. Gray MW, Burger G, Lang BF. Mitochondrial evolution. Science 1999; 283:1476-81; PMID:10066161.
2. Hailey DW, Rambold AS, Satpute-Krishnan P, Mitra K, Sougrat R, Kim PK, et al. Mitochondria supply membranes for autophagosome biogenesis during starvation. Cell 2010; 141:656-67; http://dx.doi.org/10.1016/j.cell.2010.04.009; PMID:20478256.
3. Hayashi T, Rizzuto R, Hajnoczky G, Su TP. MAM: more than just a housekeeper. Trends Cell Biol 2009; 19:81-8; http://dx.doi.org/10.1016/j.tcb.2008.12.002; PMID:19144519.
4. Hettema EH, Motley AM. How peroxisomes multiply. J Cell Sci 2009; 122:2331-6; http://dx.doi.org/10.1242/jcs.034363; PMID:19571112.
5. Janeway CA Jr. Approaching the asymptote? Evolution and revolution in immunology. Cold Spring Harb Symp Quant Biol 1989; 54:1-13; PMID:2700931.
6. Medzhitov R, Preston-Hurlburt P, Janeway CA Jr. A human homologue of the Drosophila Toll protein signals activation of adaptive immunity. Nature 1997; 388:394-7; http://dx.doi.org/10.1038/41131; PMID:9237759.
7. Medzhitov R, Janeway CA Jr. Innate immunity: the virtues of a nonclonal system of recognition. Cell 1997; 91:295-8; http://dx.doi.org/10.1016/S0092-8674(00)80412-2; PMID:9363937.
8. Akira S, Uematsu S, Takeuchi O. Pathogen recognition and innate immunity. Cell 2006; 124:783-801; http://dx.doi.org/10.1016/j.cell.2006.02.015; PMID:16497588.
9. López CB, Moltedo B, Alexopoulou L, Bonifaz L, Flavell RA, Moran TM. TLR-independent induction of dendritic cell maturation and adaptive immunity by negative-strand RNA viruses. J Immunol 2004; 173:6882-9; PMID:15557183.
10. Edelmann KH, Richardson-Burns S, Alexopoulou L, Tyler KL, Flavell RA, Oldstone MB. Does Toll-like receptor 3 play a biological role in virus infections? Virology 2004; 322:231-8; http://dx.doi.org/10.1016/j.virol.2004.01.033; PMID:15110521.
11. Sparwasser T, Miethke T, Lipford G, Borschert K, Häcker H, Heeg K, et al. Bacterial DNA causes septic shock. Nature 1997; 386:336-7; http://dx.doi.org/10.1038/386336a0; PMID:9121548.
12. Stockinger S, Reutterer B, Schaljo B, Schellack C, Brunner S, Materna T, et al. IFN regulatory factor 3-dependent induction of type I IFNs by intracellular bacteria is mediated by a TLR- and Nod2-independent mechanism. J Immunol 2004; 173:7416-25; PMID:15585867.

13. Cortez-Gonzalez X, Pellicciotta I, Gerloni M, Wheeler MC, Castiglioni P, Lenert P, et al. TLR9-independent activation of B lymphocytes by bacterial DNA. DNA Cell Biol 2006; 25:253-61; http://dx.doi.org/10.1089/dna.2006.25.253; PMID:16716115.

14. Hochrein H, Schlatter B, O'Keeffe M, Wagner C, Schmitz F, Schiemann M, et al. Herpes simplex virus type-1 induces IFN-alpha production via Toll-like receptor 9-dependent and -independent pathways. Proc Natl Acad Sci USA 2004; 101:11416-21; http://dx.doi.org/10.1073/pnas.0403555101; PMID:15272082.

15. Yoneyama M, Kikuchi M, Natsukawa T, Shinobu N, Imaizumi T, Miyagishi M, et al. The RNA helicase RIG-I has an essential function in double-stranded RNA-induced innate antiviral responses. Nat Immunol 2004; 5:730-7; http://dx.doi.org/10.1038/ni1087; PMID:15208624.

16. Takahasi K, Yoneyama M, Nishihori T, Hirai R, Kumeta H, Narita R, et al. Nonself RNA-sensing mechanism of RIG-I helicase and activation of antiviral immune responses. Mol Cell 2008; 29:428-40; http://dx.doi.org/10.1016/j.molcel.2007.11.028; PMID:18242112.

17. Cui S, Eisenacher K, Kirchhofer A, Brzózka K, Lammens A, Lammens K, et al. The C-terminal regulatory domain is the RNA 5¢-triphosphate sensor of RIG-I. Mol Cell 2008; 29:169-79; http://dx.doi.org/10.1016/j.molcel.2007.10.032; PMID:18243112.

18. Kato H, Takeuchi O, Sato S, Yoneyama M, Yamamoto M, Matsui K, et al. Differential roles of MDA5 and RIG-I helicases in the recognition of RNA viruses. Nature 2006; 441:101-5; http://dx.doi.org/10.1038/nature04734; PMID:16625202.

19. Myong S, Cui S, Cornish PV, Kirchhofer A, Gack MU, Jung JU, et al. Cytosolic viral sensor RIG-I is a 5¢-triphosphate-dependent translocase on double-stranded RNA. Science 2009; 323:1070-4; http://dx.doi.org/10.1126/science.1168352; PMID:19119185.

20. Nallagatla SR, Hwang J, Toroney R, Zheng X, Cameron CE, Bevilacqua PC. 5¢-triphosphate-dependent activation of PKR by RNAs with short stem-loops. Science 2007; 318:1455-8; http://dx.doi.org/10.1126/science.1147347; PMID:18048689.

21. Hornung V, Ellegast J, Kim S, Brzózka K, Jung A, Kato H, et al. 5¢-Triphosphate RNA is the ligand for RIG-I. Science 2006; 314:994-7; PMID:17038590.

22. Schlee M, Roth A, Hornung V, Hagmann CA, Wimmenauer V, Barchet W, et al. Recognition of 5¢ triphosphate by RIG-I helicase requires short blunt double-stranded RNA as contained in panhandle of negative-strand virus. Immunity 2009; 31:25-34; http://dx.doi.org/10.1016/j.immuni.2009.05.008; PMID:19576794.

23. Schmidt A, Schwerd T, Hamm W, Hellmuth JC, Cui S, Wenzel M, et al. 5¢-triphosphate RNA requires base-paired structures to activate antiviral signaling via RIG-I. Proc Natl Acad Sci USA 2009; 106:12067-72; http://dx.doi.org/10.1073/pnas.0900971106; PMID:19574455.

24. Kato H, Takeuchi O, Mikamo Satoh E, Hirai R, Kawai T, Matsushita K, et al. Length-dependent recognition of double-stranded ribonucleic acids by retinoic acid-inducible gene-I and melanoma differentiation-associated gene 5. J Exp Med 2008; 205:1601-10; http://dx.doi.org/10.1084/jem.20080091; PMID:18591409.

25. Malathi K, Dong B, Gale M Jr., Silverman RH. Small self-RNA generated by RNase L amplifies antiviral innate immunity. Nature 2007; 448:816-9; http://dx.doi.org/10.1038/nature06042; PMID:17653195.

26. Rehwinkel J, Tan CP, Goubau D, Schulz O, Pichlmair A, Bier K, et al. RIG-I detects viral genomic RNA during negative-strand RNA virus infection. Cell 2010; 140:397-408; http://dx.doi.org/10.1016/j.cell.2010.01.020; PMID:20144762.

27. Pichlmair A, Schulz O, Tan CP, Rehwinkel J, Kato H, Takeuchi O, et al. Activation of MDA5 requires higher-order RNA structures generated during virus infection. J Virol 2009; 83:10761-9; http://dx.doi.org/10.1128/JVI.00770-09; PMID:19656871.

28. Takeuchi O, Akira S. Pattern recognition receptors and inflammation. Cell 2010; 140:805-20; http://dx.doi.org/10.1016/j.cell.2010.01.022; PMID:20303872.

29. Loo YM, Fornek J, Crochet N, Bajwa G, Perwitasari O, Martinez-Sobrido L, et al. Distinct RIG-I and MDA5 signaling by RNA viruses in innate immunity. J Virol 2008; 82:335-45; http://dx.doi.org/10.1128/JVI.01080-07; PMID:17942531.

30. Fredericksen BL, Keller BC, Fornek J, Katze MG, Gale M Jr. Establishment and maintenance of the innate antiviral response to West Nile Virus involves both RIG-I and MDA5 signaling through IPS-1. J Virol 2008; 82:609-16; http://dx.doi.org/10.1128/JVI.01305-07; PMID:17977974.

31. Chiu YH, Macmillan JB, Chen ZJ. RNA polymerase III detects cytosolic DNA and induces type I interferons through the RIG-I pathway. Cell 2009; 138:576-91; http://dx.doi.org/10.1016/j.cell.2009.06.015; PMID:19631370.

32. Ablasser A, Bauernfeind F, Hartmann G, Latz E, Fitzgerald KA, Hornung V. RIG-I-dependent sensing of poly(dA:dT) through the induction of an RNA polymerase III-transcribed RNA intermediate. Nat Immunol 2009; 10:1065-72; http://dx.doi.org/10.1038/ni.1779; PMID:19609254.

33. Takaoka A, Wang Z, Choi MK, Yanai H, Negishi H, Ban T, et al. DAI (DLM-1/ZBP1) is a cytosolic DNA sensor and an activator of innate immune response. Nature 2007; 448:501-5; http://dx.doi.org/10.1038/nature06013; PMID:17618271.

34. Wang Z, Choi MK, Ban T, Yanai H, Negishi H, Lu Y, et al. Regulation of innate immune responses by DAI (DLM-1/ZBP1) and other DNA-sensing molecules. Proc Natl Acad Sci USA 2008; 105:5477-82; http://dx.doi.org/10.1073/pnas.0801295105; PMID:18375758.
35. Kaiser WJ, Upton JW, Mocarski ES. Receptor-interacting protein homotypic interaction motif-dependent control of NF-kappa B activation via the DNA-dependent activator of IFN regulatory factors. J Immunol 2008; 181:6427-34; PMID:18941233.
36. Rebsamen M, Heinz LX, Meylan E, Michallet MC, Schroder K, Hofmann K, et al. DAI/ZBP1 recruits RIP1 and RIP3 through RIP homotypic interaction motifs to activate NF-kappaB. EMBO Rep 2009; 10:916-22; http://dx.doi.org/10.1038/embor.2009.109; PMID:19590578.
37. Ishii KJ, Kawagoe T, Koyama S, Matsui K, Kumar H, Kawai T, et al. TANK-binding kinase-1 delineates innate and adaptive immune responses to DNA vaccines. Nature 2008; 451:725-9; http://dx.doi.org/10.1038/nature06537; PMID:18256672.
38. Yanai H, Ban T, Wang Z, Choi MK, Kawamura T, Negishi H, et al. HMGB proteins function as universal sentinels for nucleic-acid-mediated innate immune responses. Nature 2009; 462:99-103; http://dx.doi.org/10.1038/nature08512; PMID:19890330.
39. Unterholzner L, Keating SE, Baran M, Horan KA, Jensen SB, Sharma S, et al. IFI16 is an innate immune sensor for intracellular DNA. Nat Immunol 2010; 11:997-1004; http://dx.doi.org/10.1038/ni.1932; PMID:20890285.
40. Bürckstummer T, Baumann C, Bluml S, Dixit E, Dürnberger G, Jahn H, et al. An orthogonal proteomic-genomic screen identifies AIM2 as a cytoplasmic DNA sensor for the inflammasome. Nat Immunol 2009; 10:266-72; http://dx.doi.org/10.1038/ni.1702; PMID:19158679.
41. Fernandes-Alnemri T, Yu JW, Datta P, Wu J, Alnemri ES. AIM2 activates the inflammasome and cell death in response to cytoplasmic DNA. Nature 2009; 458:509-13; http://dx.doi.org/10.1038/nature07710; PMID:19158676.
42. Hornung V, Ablasser A, Charrel-Dennis M, Bauernfeind F, Horvath G, Caffrey DR, et al. AIM2 recognizes cytosolic dsDNA and forms a caspase-1-activating inflammasome with ASC. Nature 2009; 458:514-8; http://dx.doi.org/10.1038/nature07725; PMID:19158675.
43. Roberts TL, Idris A, Dunn JA, Kelly GM, Burnton CM, Hodgson S, et al. HIN-200 proteins regulate caspase activation in response to foreign cytoplasmic DNA. Science 2009; 323:1057-60; PMID:19131592.
44. Kim T, Pazhoor S, Bao M, Zhang Z, Hanabuchi S, Facchinetti V, et al. Aspartate-glutamate-alanine-histidine box motif (DEAH)/RNA helicase A helicases sense microbial DNA in human plasmacytoid dendritic cells. Proc Natl Acad Sci USA 2010; 107:15181-6; http://dx.doi.org/10.1073/pnas.1006539107; PMID:20696886.
45. Ting JP, Duncan JA, Lei Y. How the noninflammasome NLRs function in the innate immune system. Science 2010; 327:286-90; http://dx.doi.org/10.1126/science.1184004; PMID:20075243.
46. Yang P, An H, Liu X, Wen M, Zheng Y, Rui Y, et al. The cytosolic nucleic acid sensor LRRFIP1 mediates the production of type I interferon via a beta-catenin-dependent pathway. Nat Immunol 2010; 11:487-94; http://dx.doi.org/10.1038/ni.1876; PMID:20453844.
47. Seth RB, Sun L, Ea CK, Chen ZJ. Identification and characterization of MAVS, a mitochondrial antiviral signaling protein that activates NF-kappaB and IRF 3. Cell 2005; 122:669-82; http://dx.doi.org/10.1016/j.cell.2005.08.012; PMID:16125763.
48. Xu LG, Wang YY, Han KJ, Li LY, Zhai Z, Shu HB. VISA is an adapter protein required for virus-triggered IFN-beta signaling. Mol Cell 2005; 19:727-40; http://dx.doi.org/10.1016/j.molcel.2005.08.014; PMID:16153868.
49. Kawai T, Takahashi K, Sato S, Coban C, Kumar H, Kato H, et al. IPS-1, an adaptor triggering RIG-I- and Mda5-mediated type I interferon induction. Nat Immunol 2005; 6:981-8; http://dx.doi.org/10.1038/ni1243; PMID:16127453.
50. Meylan E, Curran J, Hofmann K, Moradpour D, Binder M, Bartenschlager R, et al. Cardif is an adaptor protein in the RIG-I antiviral pathway and is targeted by hepatitis C virus. Nature 2005; 437:1167-72; http://dx.doi.org/10.1038/nature04193; PMID:16177806.
51. Ishikawa H, Barber GN. STING is an endoplasmic reticulum adaptor that facilitates innate immune signalling. Nature 2008; 455:674-8; http://dx.doi.org/10.1038/nature07317; PMID:18724357.
52. Zhong B, Yang Y, Li S, Wang YY, Li Y, Diao F, et al. The adaptor protein MITA links virus-sensing receptors to IRF3 transcription factor activation. Immunity 2008; 29:538-50; http://dx.doi.org/10.1016/j.immuni.2008.09.003; PMID:18818105.
53. Sun W, Li Y, Chen L, Chen H, You F, Zhou X, et al. ERIS, an endoplasmic reticulum IFN stimulator, activates innate immune signaling through dimerization. Proc Natl Acad Sci USA 2009; 106:8653-8; http://dx.doi.org/10.1073/pnas.0900850106; PMID:19433799.
54. Ishikawa H, Ma Z, Barber GN. STING regulates intracellular DNA-mediated, type I interferon-dependent innate immunity. Nature 2009; 461:788-92; http://dx.doi.org/10.1038/nature08476; PMID:19776740.

55. Dixit E, Boulant S, Zhang Y, Lee AS, Odendall C, Shum B, et al. Peroxisomes are signaling platforms for antiviral innate immunity. Cell 2010; 141:668-81; http://dx.doi.org/10.1016/j.cell.2010.04.018; PMID:20451243.

56. Onoguchi K, Onomoto K, Takamatsu S, Jogi M, Takemura A, Morimoto S, et al. Virus-infection or 5¢ppp-RNA activates antiviral signal through redistribution of IPS-1 mediated by MFN1. PLoS Pathog 2010; 6:e1001012; http://dx.doi.org/10.1371/journal.ppat.1001012; PMID:20661427.

57. Zhong B, Zhang L, Lei C, Li Y, Mao AP, Yang Y, et al. The ubiquitin ligase RNF5 regulates antiviral responses by mediating degradation of the adaptor protein MITA. Immunity 2009; 30:397-407; http://dx.doi.org/10.1016/j.immuni.2009.01.008; PMID:19285439.

58. Burdette DL, Monroe KM, Sotelo-Troha K, Iwig JS, Eckert B, Hyodo M, et al. STING is a direct innate immune sensor of cyclic di-GMP. Nature 2011; 478(7370):515-8; PMID:21947006.

59. DeYoung BJ, Innes RW. Plant NBS-LRR proteins in pathogen sensing and host defense. Nat Immunol 2006; 7:1243-9; http://dx.doi.org/10.1038/ni1410; PMID:17110940.

60. Ting JP, Willingham SB, Bergstralh DT. NLRs at the intersection of cell death and immunity. Nat Rev Immunol 2008; 8:372-9; http://dx.doi.org/10.1038/nri2296; PMID:18362948.

61. Davis BK, Wen H, Ting JP. The Inflammasome NLRs in Immunity, Inflammation, and Associated Diseases. Annu Rev Immunol 2011; 29:707-35.; PMID:21219188.

62. Moore CB, Bergstralh DT, Duncan JA, Lei Y, Morrison TE, Zimmermann AG, et al. NLRX1 is a regulator of mitochondrial antiviral immunity. Nature 2008; 451:573-7; http://dx.doi.org/10.1038/nature06501; PMID:18200010.

63. Moore CB, Ting JP. Regulation of mitochondrial antiviral signaling pathways. Immunity 2008; 28:735-9; http://dx.doi.org/10.1016/j.immuni.2008.05.005; PMID:18549796.

64. Yasukawa K, Oshiumi H, Takeda M, Ishihara N, Yanagi Y, Seya T, et al. Mitofusin 2 inhibits mitochondrial antiviral signaling. Sci Signal 2009; 2:ra47; http://dx.doi.org/10.1126/scisignal.2000287; PMID:19690333.

65. Allen IC, Moore CB, Schneider M, Lei Y, Davis BK, Scull MA, et al. NLRX1 protein attenuates inflammatory responses to infection by interfering with the RIG-I-MAVS and TRAF6-NF-kappaB signaling pathways. Immunity 2011; 34:854-65; http://dx.doi.org/10.1016/j.immuni.2011.03.026; PMID:21703540.

66. Arnoult D, Soares F, Tattoli I, Castanier C, Philpott DJ, Girardin SE. An N-terminal addressing sequence targets NLRX1 to the mitochondrial matrix. J Cell Sci 2009; 122:3161-8; http://dx.doi.org/10.1242/jcs.051193; PMID:19692591.

67. Abdul-Sater AA, Said-Sadier N, Lam VM, Singh B, Pettengill MA, Soares F, et al. Enhancement of reactive oxygen species production and chlamydial infection by the mitochondrial Nod-like family member, NLRX1. J Biol Chem 2010; 285(53):41637-45; PMID:20959452.

68. Tattoli I, Carneiro LA, Jehanno M, Magalhaes JG, Shu Y, Philpott DJ, et al. NLRX1 is a mitochondrial NOD-like receptor that amplifies NF-kappaB and JNK pathways by inducing reactive oxygen species production. EMBO Rep 2008; 9:293-300; http://dx.doi.org/10.1038/sj.embor.7401161; PMID:18219313.

69. Sabbah A, Chang TH, Harnack R, Frohlich V, Tominaga K, Dube PH, et al. Activation of innate immune antiviral responses by Nod2. Nat Immunol 2009; 10:1073-80; http://dx.doi.org/10.1038/ni.1782; PMID:19701189.

70. Allen IC, Scull MA, Moore CB, Holl EK, McElvania-TeKippe E, Taxman DJ, et al. The NLRP3 inflammasome mediates in vivo innate immunity to influenza A virus through recognition of viral RNA. Immunity 2009; 30:556-65; http://dx.doi.org/10.1016/j.immuni.2009.02.005; PMID:19362020.

71. Ichinohe T, Lee HK, Ogura Y, Flavell R, Iwasaki A. Inflammasome recognition of influenza virus is essential for adaptive immune responses. J Exp Med 2009; 206:79-87; http://dx.doi.org/10.1084/jem.20081667; PMID:19139171.

72. Benko S, Magalhaes JG, Philpott DJ, Girardin SE. NLRC5 limits the activation of inflammatory pathways. J Immunol 2010; 185:1681-91; http://dx.doi.org/10.4049/jimmunol.0903900; PMID:20610642.

73. Cui J, Zhu L, Xia X, Wang HY, Legras X, Hong J, et al. NLRC5 negatively regulates the NF-kappaB and type I interferon signaling pathways. Cell 2010; 141:483-96; http://dx.doi.org/10.1016/j.cell.2010.03.040; PMID:20434986.

74. Kuenzel S, Till A, Winkler M, Häsler R, Lipinski S, Jung S, et al. The nucleotide-binding oligomerization domain-like receptor NLRC5 is involved in IFN-dependent antiviral immune responses. J Immunol 2010; 184:1990-2000; http://dx.doi.org/10.4049/jimmunol.0900557; PMID:20061403.

75. Meissner TB, Li A, Biswas A, Lee KH, Liu YJ, Bayir E, et al. NLR family member NLRC5 is a transcriptional regulator of MHC class I genes. Proc Natl Acad Sci USA 2010; 107:13794-9; http://dx.doi.org/10.1073/pnas.1008684107; PMID:20639463.

76. Neerincx A, Lautz K, Menning M, Kremmer E, Zigrino P, Hösel M, et al. A role for the human nucleotide-binding domain, leucine-rich repeat-containing family member NLRC5 in antiviral responses. J Biol Chem 2010; 285:26223-32; http://dx.doi.org/10.1074/jbc.M110.109736; PMID:20538593.

77. Kuenzel S, Till A, Winkler M, Häsler R, Lipinski S, Jung S, et al. The nucleotide-binding oligomerization domain-like receptor NLRC5 is involved in IFN-dependent antiviral immune responses. J Immunol 2010; 184:1990-2000; http://dx.doi.org/10.4049/jimmunol.0900557; PMID:20061403.

78. Kumar H, Pandey S, Zou J, Kumagai Y, Takahashi K, Akira S, et al. NLRC5 deficiency does not influence cytokine induction by virus and bacteria infections. J Immunol 2011; 186:994-1000; http://dx.doi.org/10.4049/jimmunol.1002094; PMID:21148033.

79. Davis BK, Roberts RA, Huang MT, Willingham SB, Conti BJ, Brickey WJ, et al. Cutting Edge: NLRC5-Dependent Activation of the Inflammasome. J Immunol 2011; 186(3):1333-7; PMID:21191067.

80. Jounai N, Takeshita F, Kobiyama K, Sawano A, Miyawaki A, Xin KQ, et al. The Atg5 Atg12 conjugate associates with innate antiviral immune responses. Proc Natl Acad Sci USA 2007; 104:14050-5; http://dx.doi.org/10.1073/pnas.0704014104; PMID:17709747.

81. Tal MC, Sasai M, Lee HK, Yordy B, Shadel GS, Iwasaki A. Absence of autophagy results in reactive oxygen species-dependent amplification of RLR signaling. Proc Natl Acad Sci USA 2009; 106:2770-5; http://dx.doi.org/10.1073/pnas.0807694106; PMID:19196953.

82. Xu L, Xiao N, Liu F, Ren H, Gu J. Inhibition of RIG-I and MDA5-dependent antiviral response by gC1qR at mitochondria. Proc Natl Acad Sci USA 2009; 106:1530-5; http://dx.doi.org/10.1073/pnas.0811029106; PMID:19164550.

83. Jia Y, Song T, Wei C, Ni C, Zheng Z, Xu Q, et al. Negative regulation of MAVS-mediated innate immune response by PSMA7. J Immunol 2009; 183:4241-8; http://dx.doi.org/10.4049/jimmunol.0901646; PMID:19734229.

84. Komuro A, Horvath CM. RNA- and virus-independent inhibition of antiviral signaling by RNA helicase LGP2. J Virol 2006; 80:12332-42; http://dx.doi.org/10.1128/JVI.01325-06; PMID:17020950.

85. Lin R, Yang L, Nakhaei P, Sun Q, Sharif-Askari E, Julkunen I, et al. Negative regulation of the retinoic acid-inducible gene I-induced antiviral state by the ubiquitin-editing protein A20. J Biol Chem 2006; 281:2095-103; http://dx.doi.org/10.1074/jbc.M510326200; PMID:16306043.

86. Friedman CS, O'Donnell MA, Legarda-Addison D, Ng A, Cárdenas WB, Yount JS, et al. The tumour suppressor CYLD is a negative regulator of RIG-I-mediated antiviral response. EMBO Rep 2008; 9:930-6; http://dx.doi.org/10.1038/embor.2008.136; PMID:18636086.

87. You F, Sun H, Zhou X, Sun W, Liang S, Zhai Z, et al. PCBP2 mediates degradation of the adaptor MAVS via the HECT ubiquitin ligase AIP4. Nat Immunol 2009; 10:1300-8; http://dx.doi.org/10.1038/ni.1815; PMID:19881509.

88. Nakhaei P, Mesplede T, Solis M, Sun Q, Zhao T, Yang L, et al. The E3 ubiquitin ligase Triad3A negatively regulates the RIG-I/MAVS signaling pathway by targeting TRAF3 for degradation. PLoS Pathog 2009; 5:e1000650; http://dx.doi.org/10.1371/journal.ppat.1000650; PMID:19893624.

89. Lad SP, Yang G, Scott DA, Chao TH, Correia Jda S, et al. Identification of MAVS splicing variants that interfere with RIGI/MAVS pathway signaling. Mol Immunol 2008; 45:2277-87; http://dx.doi.org/10.1016/j.molimm.2007.11.018; PMID:18207245.

90. Shintani T, Klionsky DJ. Autophagy in health and disease: a double-edged sword. Science 2004; 306:990-5; PMID:15528435.

91. Levine B, Kroemer G. Autophagy in the pathogenesis of disease. Cell 2008; 132:27-42; http://dx.doi.org/10.1016/j.cell.2007.12.018; PMID:18191218.

92. Kanazawa T, Taneike I, Akaishi R, Yoshizawa F, Furuya N, Fujimura S, et al. Amino acids and insulin control autophagic proteolysis through different signaling pathways in relation to mTOR in isolated rat hepatocytes. J Biol Chem 2004; 279:8452-9; http://dx.doi.org/10.1074/jbc.M306337200; PMID:14610086.

93. Ravikumar B, Vacher C, Berger Z, Davies JE, Luo S, Oroz LG, et al. Inhibition of mTOR induces autophagy and reduces toxicity of polyglutamine expansions in fly and mouse models of Huntington disease. Nat Genet 2004; 36:585-95; http://dx.doi.org/10.1038/ng1362; PMID:15146184.

94. Sugawara K, Suzuki NN, Fujioka Y, Mizushima N, Ohsumi Y, Inagaki F. The crystal structure of microtubule-associated protein light chain 3, a mammalian homologue of Saccharomyces cerevisiae Atg8. Genes Cells 2004; 9:611-8; http://dx.doi.org/10.1111/j.1356-9597.2004.00750.x; PMID:15265004.

95. Suzuki NN, Yoshimoto K, Fujioka Y, Ohsumi Y, Inagaki F. The crystal structure of plant ATG12 and its biological implication in autophagy. Autophagy 2005; 1:119-26; http://dx.doi.org/10.4161/auto.1.2.1859; PMID:16874047.

96. Geng J, Klionsky DJ. The Atg8 and Atg12 ubiquitin-like conjugation systems in macroautophagy. 'Protein modifications: beyond the usual suspects' review series. EMBO Rep 2008; 9:859-64; http://dx.doi.org/10.1038/embor.2008.163; PMID:18704115.

97. Klionsky DJ, Abeliovich H, Agostinis P, Agrawal DK, Aliev G, Askew DS, et al. Guidelines for the use and interpretation of assays for monitoring autophagy in higher eukaryotes. Autophagy 2008; 4:151-75; PMID:18188003.

98. Lee HK, Lund JM, Ramanathan B, Mizushima N, Iwasaki A. Autophagy-dependent viral recognition by plasmacytoid dendritic cells. Science 2007; 315:1398-401; PMID:17272685.

99. Yousefi S, Perozzo R, Schmid I, Ziemiecki A, Schaffner T, Scapozza L, et al. Calpain-mediated cleavage of Atg5 switches autophagy to apoptosis. Nat Cell Biol 2006; 8:1124-32; http://dx.doi.org/10.1038/ncb1482; PMID:16998475.

100. Reggiori F, Shintani T, Nair U, Klionsky DJ. Atg9 cycles between mitochondria and the pre-autophagosomal structure in yeasts. Autophagy 2005; 1:101-9; http://dx.doi.org/10.4161/auto.1.2.1840; PMID:16874040.

101. Takahashi Y, Coppola D, Matsushita N, Cualing HD, Sun M, Sato Y, et al. Bif-1 interacts with Beclin 1 through UVRAG and regulates autophagy and tumorigenesis. Nat Cell Biol 2007; 9:1142-51; http://dx.doi.org/10.1038/ncb1634; PMID:17891140.

102. Lee IH, Cao L, Mostoslavsky R, Lombard DB, Liu J, Bruns NE, et al. A role for the NAD-dependent deacetylase Sirt1 in the regulation of autophagy. Proc Natl Acad Sci USA 2008; 105:3374-9; http://dx.doi.org/10.1073/pnas.0712145105; PMID:18296641.

103. Li XD, Sun L, Seth RB, Pineda G, Chen ZJ. Hepatitis C virus protease NS3/4A cleaves mitochondrial antiviral signaling protein off the mitochondria to evade innate immunity. Proc Natl Acad Sci USA 2005; 102:17717-22; http://dx.doi.org/10.1073/pnas.0508531102; PMID:16301520.

104. Chen Z, Benureau Y, Rijnbrand R, Yi J, Wang T, Warter L, et al. GB virus B disrupts RIG-I signaling by NS3/4A-mediated cleavage of the adaptor protein MAVS. J Virol 2007; 81:964-76; http://dx.doi.org/10.1128/JVI.02076-06; PMID:17093192.

105. Yang Y, Liang Y, Qu L, Chen Z, Yi M, Li K, et al. Disruption of innate immunity due to mitochondrial targeting of a picornaviral protease precursor. Proc Natl Acad Sci USA 2007; 104:7253-8; http://dx.doi.org/10.1073/pnas.0611506104; PMID:17438296.

106. Mibayashi M, Martinez-Sobrido L, Loo YM, Cardenas WB, Gale M Jr., Garcia-Sastre A. Inhibition of retinoic acid-inducible gene I-mediated induction of beta interferon by the NS1 protein of influenza A virus. J Virol 2007; 81:514-24; http://dx.doi.org/10.1128/JVI.01265-06; PMID:17079289.

107. Opitz B, Rejaibi A, Dauber B, Eckhard J, Vinzing M, Schmeck B, et al. IFNbeta induction by influenza A virus is mediated by RIG-I which is regulated by the viral NS1 protein. Cell Microbiol 2007; 9:930-8; http://dx.doi.org/10.1111/j.1462-5822.2006.00841.x; PMID:17140406.

108. Guo Z, Chen LM, Zeng H, Gomez JA, Plowden J, Fujita T, et al. NS1 protein of influenza A virus inhibits the function of intracytoplasmic pathogen sensor, RIG-I. Am J Respir Cell Mol Biol 2007; 36:263-9; http://dx.doi.org/10.1165/rcmb.2006-0283RC; PMID:17053203.

109. Graef KM, Vreede FT, Lau YF, McCall AW, Carr SM, Subbarao K, et al. The PB2 subunit of the influenza virus RNA polymerase affects virulence by interacting with the mitochondrial antiviral signaling protein and inhibiting expression of beta interferon. J Virol 2010; 84:8433-45; http://dx.doi.org/10.1128/JVI.00879-10; PMID:20538852.

110. Iwai A, Shiozaki T, Kawai T, Akira S, Kawaoka Y, Takada A, et al. Influenza A virus polymerase inhibits type I interferon induction by binding to interferon beta promoter stimulator 1. J Biol Chem 2010; 285:32064-74; http://dx.doi.org/10.1074/jbc.M110.112458; PMID:20699220.

111. Ling Z, Tran KC, Teng MN. Human respiratory syncytial virus nonstructural protein NS2 antagonizes the activation of beta interferon transcription by interacting with RIG-I. J Virol 2009; 83:3734-42; http://dx.doi.org/10.1128/JVI.02434-08; PMID:19193793.

112. Fan L, Briese T, Lipkin WI. Z proteins of New World arenaviruses bind RIG-I and interfere with type I interferon induction. J Virol 2010; 84:1785-91; http://dx.doi.org/10.1128/JVI.01362-09; PMID:20007272.

113. Zhou S, Cerny AM, Zacharia A, Fitzgerald KA, Kurt-Jones EA, Finberg RW. Induction and inhibition of type I interferon responses by distinct components of lymphocytic choriomeningitis virus. J Virol 2010; 84:9452-62; http://dx.doi.org/10.1128/JVI.00155-10; PMID:20592086.

114. Andrejeva J, Childs KS, Young DF, Carlos TS, Stock N, Goodbourn S, et al. The V proteins of paramyxoviruses bind the IFN-inducible RNA helicase, mda-5, and inhibit its activation of the IFN-beta promoter. Proc Natl Acad Sci USA 2004; 101:17264-9; http://dx.doi.org/10.1073/pnas.0407639101; PMID:15563593.

115. Childs KS, Andrejeva J, Randall RE, Goodbourn S. Mechanism of mda-5 Inhibition by paramyxovirus V proteins. J Virol 2009; 83:1465-73; http://dx.doi.org/10.1128/JVI.01768-08; PMID:19019954.

116. Wei C, Ni C, Song T, Liu Y, Yang X, Zheng Z, et al. The hepatitis B virus X protein disrupts innate immunity by downregulating mitochondrial antiviral signaling protein. J Immunol 2010; 185:1158-68; http://dx.doi.org/10.4049/jimmunol.0903874; PMID:20554965.

117. Drahos J, Racaniello VR. Cleavage of IPS-1 in cells infected with human rhinovirus. J Virol 2009; 83:11581-7; http://dx.doi.org/10.1128/JVI.01490-09; PMID:19740998.

118. Lei Y, Moore CB, Liesman RM, O'Connor BP, Bergstralh DT, Chen ZJ, et al. MAVS-mediated apoptosis and its inhibition by viral proteins. PLoS ONE 2009; 4:e5466; http://dx.doi.org/10.1371/journal.pone.0005466; PMID:19404494.

119. Li HM, Fujikura D, Harada T, Uehara J, Kawai T, Akira S, et al. IPS-1 is crucial for DAP3-mediated anoikis induction by caspase-8 activation. Cell Death Differ 2009; 16:1615-21; http://dx.doi.org/10.1038/cdd.2009.97; PMID:19644511.

120. Yu CY, Chiang RL, Chang TH, Liao CL, Lin YL. The interferon stimulator mitochondrial antiviral signaling protein facilitates cell death by disrupting the mitochondrial membrane potential and by activating caspases. J Virol 2010; 84:2421-31; http://dx.doi.org/10.1128/JVI.02174-09; PMID:20032188.

CHAPTER 8

DNA Sensors and Anti-Viral Immune Responses

Susan Carpenter,[1] Søren Beck Jensen[1,2] and Katherine A. Fitzgerald*[1]

Abstract

The considerable potency of nucleic acids as triggers of the innate immune response has become clear over the last few years. It has been known for over a decade that DNA, the most recognizable unit of life elicits a robust inflammatory response in cells. The discovery of Toll-Like Receptor-9, a type I transmembrane receptor which drives inflammation in response to hypomethylated CpG-rich DNA partially explained these findings. A number of new DNA sensing molecules have since been uncovered which contribute to various aspects of DNA–driven immunity. Many of these molecules are present in the cytosolic compartment. Through recognition of microbial genomes or nucleic acids generated during replication, nucleic acid sensing from the cytosol has emerged as a central component of anti-viral and anti-bacterial defenses. Very recent developments have also revealed how in certain DNA virus infections, pathogen derived DNA can alert the innate immune system to the presence of infection. Inappropriate sensing of host-derived nucleic acids now appears to also be directly linked to immune-pathology and autoimmunity. The discovery of TLRs, cytosolic as well as nuclear DNA detection systems has therefore provided important new insights into a growing number of infectious diseases and contributed greatly to our understanding of the pathogenesis of autoimmune diseases.

Introduction

Successful elimination of invading pathogens is dependent on a tightly coordinated and interconnected innate and adaptive immune response. If successful, innate immunity can curb microbial growth until the adaptive response is activated to eliminate the pathogen. In recent years much work has focused on understanding how innate immunity, the body's first line of defense recognizes invading pathogens and orchestrate early inflammatory responses leading to transcriptional regulation of inflammatory cytokines, chemokines and Type I Interferons (IFNs). The microbial products recognized are often common to broad classes of microbes and are not normally present on or in cells of the host. The concept that pathogen associated molecular patterns (PAMPs) act as triggers of innate immunity therefore emerged leading to a decade or more of exciting discoveries that unveiled several classes of germline encoded pattern recognition receptors (PRRs) including the Toll-like receptors (TLRs), NOD-like receptors (NLRs) and the RIG-I like receptors (RLRs).[1] In many cases, microorganisms are recognized through unique PAMPs found in pathogens but absent from host cells. Additionally however, nucleic acids, the most recognizable units of life have emerged as potent triggers of innate responses during infection.[2]

[1]Division of Infectious Diseases and Immunology, Department of Medicine, University of Massachusetts Medical School, Worcester, Massachusetts, USA; [2]Department of Medical Microbiology and Immunology, Aarhus University, Aarhus, Denmark.
*Corresponding Author: Katherine A. Fitzgerald—Email: kate.fitzgerald@umassmed.edu

Nucleic Acid Sensors and Antiviral Immunity, edited by Suryaprakash Sambhara and Takashi Fujita.
©2013 Landes Bioscience.

Nucleic acids are not unique to pathogens therefore our immune system must exert tight and sophisticated control on nucleic acid sensing pathways to ensure that there is not inappropriate sensing of host nucleic acids. The ability to distinguish between pathogenic and self-nucleic acids is therefore central to human health.

It has been acknowledged for more than 50 years that nucleic acids are capable of triggering a strong Type I IFN response, the most important response needed for control of viral replication. It is only in recent years that we have begun to appreciate that a diverse range of infectious agents trigger immunity via nucleic acid detection systems.[3,4] In many cases, sensing of microbial pathogens appears to be exclusively through recognition of their nucleic acids. Considerable efforts from numerous laboratories have led to a much greater understanding of the molecular basis for this immune stimulatory activity. Several classes of PRR have evolved to recognize and respond to the presence of both RNA and DNA introduced to cells during infection or following tissue damage. Different cellular compartments where nucleic acids can be encountered are equipped with sensing receptors. The Toll-like receptors (TLRs) for example are a family of Type I transmembrane proteins capable of responding to a wide variety of PAMPs such as LPS, however RNA and DNA are also detected through these receptors. TLR3, 7/8 and TLR9 are Type I transmembrane proteins which recognize dsRNA, ssRNA and ssDNA respectively through leucine rich repeat domains located in the lumen of the endosomal compartment. Here in this acidic compartment these receptors detect nucleic acids following pathogen engulfment and phagocytosis. Additionally, viruses that traffic through the endosomal compartment expose their genomes to these sensors (reviewed in Chapters 1 and 2). The cytosol is also an environment rich in immune surveillance mechanisms. Cytosolic nucleic acid sensors have been discovered for RNA, such as the retinoic acid-inducible gene (RIG) like receptors (RLRs: RIG-I and MDA5, reviewed in Chapter 5), which recognize different RNA structures present on RNA viruses. These cytosolic RNA helicases provide the cytosol with a sensitive surveillance system analogous to that maintained by the TLRs in the endosome and if activated these sensors can turn on the expression of Type I Interferons and pro-inflammatory cytokines. In addition to RNA surveillance, exciting discoveries in recent years have uncovered a diversity of DNA sensing molecules, which act to preserve the sanctity of the cytosolic compartment. Finally, recent evidence indicates the existence of DNA sensors in the nucleus of cells to detect the genome of nuclear replicating herpesviruses. For the purposes of this chapter we will solely focus on sensing mechanisms in the cytosol and nucleus for DNA.

DNA: A Key Activator of Innate Immune Signaling

It has been known for sometime that microbial DNA can turn on inflammatory responses.[3,4] Before the discovery of TLR9, DNA derived from pathogens was known to activate fibroblasts to produce the anti-viral Type I IFNs, important in early control of virus infection.[5] The immune stimulatory property of microbial DNA was ascribed to the presence of unmethylated CG dinucleotides. These CpG motifs are present rarely in mammalian DNA, being more abundant in microbial DNA leading to the idea that innate immune sensing discriminates host from microbial DNA. The identification of TLR9 as a receptor for CpG rich DNA provided a framework to understand DNA driven immunity.[6] The ability of microbial DNA to drive immunity was re-evaluated in light of the findings that transfection of dsDNA derived from pathogens activated various immunological genes in TLR9 negative thyroid cells.[7] Subsequent studies showed that TLR9-deficient embryonic fibroblasts, which do not respond to CpG DNA, produce large amounts of IFN in response to transfection with genomic DNA isolated from bacteria, viruses or mammals.[7] Additional studies have since clearly established the ability of bacterial and viral DNA to trigger potent immune responses in a variety of cells including macrophages, dendritic cells and fibroblasts.[8,9] This cytosolic immune response to DNA has been the focus of investigation for several years now. The synthetic B-form dsDNA poly(dA-dT) and a ds 45 base pair oligonucleotide derived from the Listeria genome, termed IFN-stimulatory DNA (ISD) have been important tools that have aided in the dissection of the immune stimulatory activity of DNA. Critical early studies showed that the immune stimulatory activity of these DNA molecules did not utilize any known

TLRs prompting an active search for new molecules important in the recognition of DNA and signaling from the cytosolic compartment.

The primary response under scrutiny was the induction of the Type I IFNs, IFN-α and -β, Transcriptional regulation of the IFN-β gene requires the activation of IRF3, ATF-2/c-Jun and NF-κB. These transcription factors form a multiprotein complex, termed the enhanceosome on the IFN-β enhancer.[10] The determining factor in driving these events in particular is the transcription factor, Interferon regulatory factor (IRF3). In the resting state, IRF3 is localized to the cytoplasm. In response to a cytosolic dsDNA, IRF3 is phosphorylated on a cluster of C-terminal serine/threonine residues, which control its dimerization status. In this active dimeric form IRF3 translocates to the nucleus and associates with the coactivators CREB-binding protein (CBP)/p300 on the IFN-β enhancer where together with NF-κB as well as ATF-2/c-jun it drives IFNβ gene transcription. The IκB-related kinases, inhibitory protein κB kinase (IKK)ε (also called IKK*i*)[11] and TANK binding kinase (TBK1) (also called NAK[12] or T2K[13]), phosphorylate IRF3.[14,15] IKKε and TBK1 are structurally related to IKKα and IKKβ, but unlike IKKα or IKKβ, do not appear to be involved in NF-κB activation.[15,16] NF- κB and MAPK are also induced in dsDNA treated cells, however the precise mechanisms regulating their activation and their absolute requirement in driving IFNβ gene transcription are less clear.

In addition to TBK1 and IRF3, a further critical component of the response to intracellular DNA involves an ER resident protein, which is best known as STING (also called MITA, MPYS and ERIS).[17-20] STING was first identified as MPYS, a novel plasma membrane tetraspanner that was associated with MHC-II and found to mediate MHC-II-dependent death signaling.[21] STING-MPYS was found to be tyrosine phosphorylated upon MHC-II aggregation and associates with inositol lipid and tyrosine phosphatases. In the context of innate immunity, work from the Barber lab identified STING as a driver of Type I IFNβ induction in response to poly(dA-dT), ISD and live herpes simplex virus-1 (HSV-1).[18] STING-deficient animals are highly susceptible to HSV-1 in vivo owing to a severe defect in the Type I IFN response in these animals. Mechanistically, STING appears to act 'upstream' of TBK1, and in the presence of intracellular DNA, this molecule relocalizes from the endoplasmic recticulum to a cytoplasmic location where TBK1 is found.[18,22] A schematic representation of the TLR9 and TLR9-independent responses to DNA is shown in Figure 1.

PRRs: Essential Weapons in the Fight against Viral Infection

Although cytoplasmic IFNβ responses to intracellular DNA clearly involve STING, TBK1 and IRF3, the identity of the upstream DNA sensors that bind pathogen DNA and relay signals to converge on this STING-TBK1-IRF3 pathway are still incompletely characterized. Several key molecules have been identified which will be discussed in detail below.

DAI

DNA dependent activator of IRFs (DAI) (also known as DLM1 and ZBP1) was the first molecule to be identified as a possible cytosolic DNA sensor.[23] DAI was first shown through a series of in vitro studies to be an interferon inducible protein, which was capable of directly binding not only Z-DNA but also B-DNA.[23,24] DAI was discovered prior to the discovery of STING. The carboxyl terminus of DAI was shown to interact with TBK1, which subsequently leads to the activation of IRF3. Knocking down DAI using siRNA resulted in a decrease in Type I interferon production while overexpression of DAI had the opposite effect of enhancing the production of Type I IFNs in response to DNA. Whether DAI engages with the STING molecule as well as with TBK1 is still unclear and has not been examined to date. Surprisingly, DAI knockout mice showed essentially normal immune responses to in vivo challenge with DNA viruses (DNA). In vitro studies using DAI knockout cells also displayed normal Type I IFN and cytokine profiles in response to DNA.[24] These results suggest that either DAI is not involved in DNA driven Type I IFN responses or that DAI functions in a redundant manner with other sensors to detect dsDNA. This latter possibility might be the more relevant since several

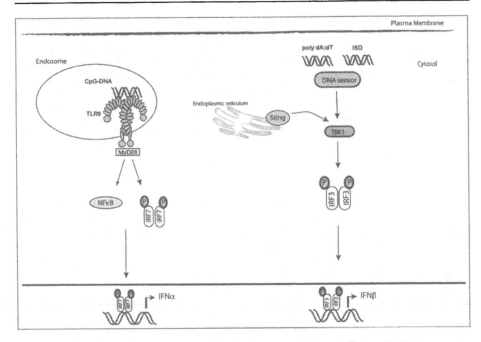

Figure 1. Intracelluar DNA recognition. Toll-Like Receptor-9 drives inflammation in response to hypomethylated CpG-rich DNA from the endosomal compartment resulting in the activation of the transcription factors NFκB and IRF7 leading to the production of IFN-α. Synthetic B-form dsDNA poly(dA-dT) and IFN-stimulatory DNA (ISD) derived from the listeria genome activate IFN-β production via the adaptor molecule Sting. Sting interacts with TBK1, which phosphorylates IRF3 resulting in the production of IFN-β.

additional DNA sensing molecules have since been implicated in driving STING-dependent DNA driven immune signaling.

Recently, two receptor-interacting protein (RIP) homotypic interaction motifs (RHIMs) were identified in the DAI protein sequence. These domains relay DAI-induced NF-κB signals through the recruitment of the RHIM-containing kinases RIP1 and RIP3. Knockdown of not only RIP1, but also RIP3 attenuated DAI-induced NF-κB activation.[25,26] Importantly, RIP recruitment to DAI is inhibited by a RHIM domain-containing murine cytomegalovirus (MCMV) protein M45. These latter findings delineate the DAI signaling pathway to NF-κB and suggest a possible new immune modulation strategy of MCMV.

RNA Polymerase III

One of the original studies that established the existence of the TLR-independent cytosolic DNA-recognition pathway to induce Type I IFNs suggested that MAVS (also called IPS1, VISA and CARDif), an adaptor molecule critical for RNA helicase signaling, was also an essential adaptor in DNA induced IFN production in HEK293 cells, a cell type widely used to study signaling from PRRs. What was surprising about these findings is that neither RIG-I nor MDA5, the only known molecules that could engage MAVS appeared to be involved in this DNA response. This was supported by earlier studies that had shown an inability of RIG-I or MDA-5 to bind to dsDNA.[27] This intriguing observation suggested that DNA and RNA sensing pathways converge on the MAVS adaptor molecule.[9] Later studies helped clarify this issue by revealing that cells from MAVS-deficient mice responded normally to dsDNA.[28,29] The molecular basis for this differential requirement for MAVS in DNA signaling in human vs. mouse cells was subsequently resolved with two studies identifying the DNA- dependent RNA polymerase III as a component of the DNA recognition machinery. RNA polymerase III could act in the cytosol to transcribe transfected poly-dAdT into short double stranded rArU intermediates containing 5'-triphosphate moieties that then signaled via RIG-I and MAVS to turn on Type I IFNs.[30-33] Interestingly this pathway appeared to be the sole mechanism involved in sensing B-form dsDNA in human HEK293 cells. This RNA polymerase III pathway was also active in mouse macrophages as indicated by the ability of DNA to generate an RNA intermediate that then signaled via RIG-I. However, it was not the only pathway involved in DNA recognition in mouse cells. An additional recognition-signaling pathway was therefore postulated to act in concert with this RNA polymerase III pathway to promote DNA driven responses. Exactly how DNA is sensed in mouse cells is still unclear. It is interesting to note that these findings provide some explanation as to why RNA Pol III might be present in the cytosolic compartment as well as the nucleus.[34]

HMGB1

Recently, the high mobility group (HMG) nuclear proteins HMGB1 and HMGB2 have been linked to nucleic acid sensing. HMG nuclear proteins are non-histone, chromatin- associated proteins involved in DNA organization and regulation of transcription. HMGB1 is released both passively as well as actively by immune cells during cellular necrosis. In this capacity, it serves to alert neighboring cells of ongoing damage and is as such considered an endogenous 'danger signal or alarmin'. HMGB1-DNA complexes are known to activate TLR9 signaling resulting in maturation of immune cells and cytokine secretion.[35] More recent studies have extended the role of HMGB1 and implicated it, as well as the related family members HMGB 2 and 3 as key mediators of all DNA and RNA driven immune responses. HMGBs bind to immune-stimulatory DNA and RNA, interactions that are important in driving not only TLR9 signaling but also cytosolic RNA and DNA sensing pathways. Hmgb1 and Hmgb2-deficient mouse cells are defective in Type-I interferon and inflammatory cytokine induction by DNA or RNA delivered to the cytosol,[36] suggesting that they function upstream of both the RLRs as well as all DNA sensing machineries identified to date.

Lrrfip1

Assembly of the IFN-β enhanceosome leads to transcriptional activation of the IFN-β promoter by recruiting the transcription machinery, including CBP/p300 and DNA dependent RNA polymerase II.[37] In the context of nucleic acid sensing the leucine-rich–repeat- containing protein Lrrfip1 has recently been described as a cytoplasmic RNA- and DNA- binding protein involved in transcriptional activation of the *IFN*-β gene.[38] Yang and colleagues showed that siRNA-mediated knock down of Lrrfip1 reduced IFN-β production in macrophages following transfection of nucleic acid ligands. Despite the impaired IFN-β induction in these cells, activation of NF-κB, IRF3 and ATF2-c-JUN was unaffected. This suggested that Lrrfip1 acts to regulate IFN-β via an alternative mechanism. In the search for an alternative mechanism for regulation of the IFN-β response, it was found that Lrrfip1 interacts with and activates β-catenin to mediate its nuclear translocation where it promotes p300 recruitment to the IFN-β enhancer. Furthermore it was shown that β-catenin is involved in both LPS- and nucleic acid-induced activation of the IFN-β promoter, whereas Lrrfip1 is only involved in the response to cytosolic nucleic acids. These results suggest that Lrrfip1 is a cytosolic sensor for nucleic acids that can enhance IFN-β transcription via a β-catenin dependent co-activator mechanism.

DExD/H Box Helicases (DHX9 and DHX36)

It is well established that plasmacytoid dendritic cells contribute greatly to systemic IFNα levels in response to extracellular DNA by signaling through a pathway that depends on TLR9. To drive IFNβ, TLR9 recruits the adaptor molecule MyD88 which signals via the IRAK kinases (IRAK1 and 4) to regulate activation of the IRF7 protein and drive IFNα gene expression (see Chapters 2 and 3). The primary mechanisms regulating IFN in pDCs is TLR-dependent, however, it has also been reported that pDCs can express IFNα and other cytokines in a

TLR9-independent but MyD88-dependent manner in response to the herpesvirus MCMV.[39] Using a biochemical approach with biotinylated CpG DNA coupled to streptavidin agarose beads, DHX9 and DHX36 were identified as cytoplasmic receptors for CpG-B and CpG-A, respectively.[40] DHX9 and DHX36 belong to the DExD/H family of helicases that also contain the Rig-I-like receptors. DHX36 binds to CpG-A via the DEAH-domain whereas DHX9 binds to CpG-B via a C-terminal DUF-domain. Furthermore it was found that the C-terminal HA2- and DUF-domains for DHX9 and DHX36 (helix domain may also be important in DHX9) are essential for interaction with the TIR domain of MyD88, which in turn relays signaling from both sensors. DHX9 drives activation of NFκB whereas DHX36 leads to IRF7 activation. Hence, DHX9 appears to induce an inflammatory cytokine response to CpG-B with a low level of IFNα induction, whereas DHX36 induces IRF7 activation in response to CpG-A leading to a cytokine response dominated by IFNα.

IFI16

In addition to the aforementioned DNA binding molecules, Interferon gamma induced protein-16 (IFI16) and its murine ortholog IFI204 (a member of the murine p200 or PYHIN (PYD and HIN200 domain) family of Type I IFN inducible genes were also recently linked to DNA-dependent Type I IFN responses. Using a vaccinia virus derived immune stimulatory DNA-motif with a strong capacity to induce IFN-β, IFI16 was identified in cytosolic extracts from DNA-precipitated THP1 cells.[41] Human IFI16 and its murine counterpart IFI204 have identical domain structures consisting of a pyrin domain followed by two HIN200 domains. The pyrin (PYD) domain (also known as a DAPIN or PAAD domain) is a member of the death domain (DD) superfamily of protein folds. The PYD domain forms homotypic interactions with other PYD-containing proteins to form higher complexes with known roles in apoptosis and the cell cycle. The HIN200 domains of IFI16 bound directly to DNA. Ligation of IFI16 by DNA leads to an interaction with STING and TBK1 resulting in IRF3 activation and transcriptional regulation of Type I IFNs. The importance of IFI16 and p204 in sensing HSV1 virus was also demonstrated using siRNA mediated knockdown of these proteins in human THP1 and mouse macrophages, respectively. Future studies will no doubt define the role of IFI16 in sensing other viruses and the relative contribution of IFI16 and other DNA sensors such as DAI or RNA polymerase III in driving DNA responses. A schematic highlighting the known cytosolic DNA sensing pathways is shown in Figure 2.

Small Molecule Ligands That Trigger TBK1-Dependent Type I IFN Gene Transcription

DMXAA

5,6-dimethylxanthenone-4-acetic acid (DMXAA) is a vasculature disrupting agent currently in phase II trials as an anti-cancer agent, however its exact mechanism of action is unknown. DMXAA has been shown to activate the TBK-1 and IRF3 signaling pathway in a TLR and MAVS independent manner.[42] DMXAA is a strong inducer of Type I IFNs but not MAPKs. It can also activate NFκB albeit with slower kinetics and reduced intensity in comparison to LPS stimulation. There is some evidence that this activation of NFκB is not dependent on the IKK kinase, IKKb but rather is dependent on TBK1. Exactly how TBK1 can control NFkB signaling in this system is still unclear. It was also shown that pretreatment of macrophages with either DMXAA or LPS induces a state of 'cross tolerance' in cells preventing further stimulation by either DMXAA or LPS. Further studies have examined the possible use of DMXAA as an antiviral agent.[43] DMXAA was shown to inhibit VSV cytotoxicity in vitro. In addition DMXAA exerted anti-viral activity against a number of strains of influenza. Both in vitro and in vivo DMXAA shows strong anti-viral responses to influenza and it even protects against the tamiflu® resistant strain A/Br in an IFNβ dependent manner. Together these data showcase the potential use of DMXAA as a treatment for drug resistant strains of influenza.

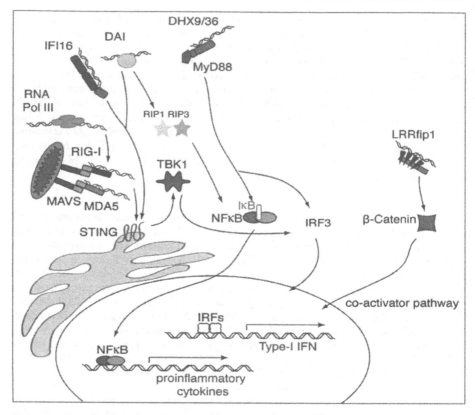

Figure 2. PRRs induce IFN production. A plethora of DNA receptors are present in the cytosolic compartment including, IFI16, RNA PolIII, DAI, LRRfip1 and DHX9/36. These receptors can activate proinflammatory cytokines through NFκB. In addition they share a common pathway consisting of Sting, TBK1 and the IRF proteins in order to activate Type I interferons.

ci-di A/GMPs

As mentioned previously our immune system is designed to respond to unique molecular signatures present in microbes. Cyclic di – adenosine monophosphate and cyclic di-guanosine monophosphate (ci-di-A/GMP) are second messengers, which play critical regulatory roles in many bacteria but are not present in eukaryotes. As such these molecules are classical PAMPs. Recent data has shown that these small molecules are capable of eliciting strong Type I IFN responses in macrophages.[44,45] Both ci-di-A and GMP trigger signaling independent of TLRs, RIG-I and MDA5. Like DMXAA, these small molecules require TBK1 and the transcription factors IRF3/7 and NFkB. DNA and ci-di-A/GMP activate similar cytosolic pathways however to date it has not been shown that they utilize similar receptors. Recently it has been shown that both DNA and ci-di-A/GMP require the adaptor protein STING in order to activate Type I IFN responses from the cytosol.[46] Sauer et al. showed that the mouse 'Goldenticket' (gt) harboring a point mutation within STING (T596A), which prevents the production of functional sting protein is unable to produce Type I IFNs in response to *Listeria monocytogenes*. Sauer et al. showed that Sting was required for Type I IFN responses to ci-di- A/GMP since Sting-deficient macrophages as well as macrophages from goldenticket mice failed to produce IFNβ in response to cytosolically delivered ci-di-A/GMP.These findings could indicate that *L. monocytogenes* utilizes ci-di-AMP in order to induce the production of IFN-β, however, since DNA from Listeria is also capable of driving

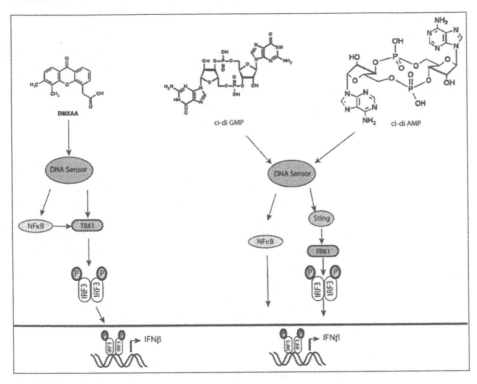

Figure 3. DMXAA and ci-di-A/GMP signaling. DMXAA and ci-di A/GMP activate unknown receptors present in the cytosol leading to the activation of Type I Interferons via the TBK1 and the transcription factors NFκB and IRF3.

IFNβ induction via STING, it is unclear at present whether DNA, ci-di-AMP or both ligands are central drivers of this response. A schematic representation of these pathways is shown in Figure 3.

PRRs Regulating Caspase-1 Dependent Maturation of IL-1β

The immune response to DNA in the cytosol is not limited to the activation of Type I interferon responses, but also stimulates the production of an important group of pro-inflammatory cytokines belonging to the Interleukin-1 family.[47] IL-1β and IL-18 play a central role in defending the host from a variety of bacterial and fungal pathogens.[48,49] Growing evidence also supports the importance of these cytokines in anti-viral host-defenses.[50] IL-1β stimulates innate and adaptive mechanisms of antimicrobial resistance through its action on neutrophils, macrophages, CD4 and CD8 T cells. Similarly, IL-18 is critical for IFN-γ production by NK cells and T cells.[51] Like other cytokines, IL-1β and IL-18 are regulated through transcription, however, in contrast to other proinflammatory cytokines, IL-1β and IL-18 are also regulated post-translationally. These cytokines are synthesized as inactive zymogen proteins following the stimulation of NFκB by PRRs such as the TLRs.[52] The conversion of proforms of IL-1β and IL-18 into their respective bioactive forms is achieved through the action of large multiprotein complexes in the cytosol referred to as inflammasomes.[48,53] In response to a distinct set of stimuli of microbial as well as endogenous origin, members of the NOD-like receptor family have been shown to be critical components of the pathways that control maturation of IL-1 and IL-18. The NLRs have a tripartite structure, consisting of a C-terminal leucine-rich repeat domain, a central nucleotide-binding oligomerization (NOD or NACHT) domain, and a variable N-terminal protein–protein interaction domain, which can be either a caspase recruitment and activation domain (CARD), a Pyrin domain (PYD) or a baculovirus inhibitor of apoptosis repeat domain (BIR).[54,55] The leucine-rich repeat domain has been implicated in ligand sensing, although no evidence exists to date revealing that any NLR binds directly to any ligand. The PYD, CARD or BIR domains facilitate downstream signaling through protein–protein interactions. Inflammasome complexes assemble upon activation by an appropriate stimulus (discussed in detail below), leading to the multimerization of the adaptor molecule ASC. Subsequently, procaspase-1 is recruited to ASC by means of interactions between the CARD domains of ASC and that of caspase-1. These events lead to the auto- cleavage of caspase-1. The two resulting subunits p10 and p20 assemble into the active caspase-1 that then cleaves IL-1β.

The NLRP3 Inflammasome

NLRP3 has been shown to recognize a wide range of microbial and endogenous danger signals. In the case of viruses, NLRP3 was the first NLR implicated in anti-viral defenses through recognition of adenovirus.[56] Muruve et al. implicated NLRP3 in the production of IL1β in vivo during adenovirus infection. There is however some conflicting evidence as to whether adenovirus induced inflammation is dependent on NLR inflammasomes, since the IL-1α pathway also appears to be tightly linked to adenovirus induced inflammation.[57] NLRP3 has also been shown to be involved in sensing modified vaccinia virus Ankara strain however this has not been examined in vivo.[58] More recent studies have revealed a more important role for NLRP3 in the recognition of RNA during viral infection. Purified dsRNA from rotavirus or brome mosaic virus and ssRNA from influenza A virus all activate NLRP3 (59–61). NLRP3 has also been implicated in sensing influenza virus in vivo. Additional evidence has recently shown that bacterial mRNA is also sensed via the NLRP3 inflammasome.[62] Exactly how NLRP3 is activated by viral or bacterial RNA or during virus infection is still unclear.

The AIM-2 Inflammasome

Recently absent in melanoma 2 (AIM2), a member of the PYHIN family of DNA binding proteins has been shown to regulate caspase-1 driven maturation of the pro-inflammatory cytokines, IL1β and IL18 in response to dsDNA.[63-66] AIM2 is an interferon inducible protein, which is characterized by HIN-200 DNA binding domains and pyrin domains. AIM2 does not appear to engage the signaling pathways which turn on Type I IFN gene transcription. Rather the AIM2 receptor binds double stranded DNA through the HIN-200 domain, which initiates a signaling cascade involving the recruitment of the inflammasome adaptor molecule ASC via its pyrin domain. ASC subsequently binds caspase-1 resulting in the formation of the inflammasome complex and the subsequent maturation of IL-1β and IL-18.

AIM2 appears to be important in sensing both cytosolic bacterial pathogens and DNA viruses.[51,67-71] AIM-2 has been shown to regulate IL-1 and IL-18 processing in response to both Vaccina virus and murine cytomegalovirus (mCMV).[51,63,70] Macrophages and dendritic cells from AIM2-deficient mice failed to activate caspase-1 and mature IL-1 in response to vaccina virus and mCMV infections.[51] AIM2 is also important in regulating the maturation of IL-18. IL-18 plays a key role in regulating NK cell-dependent production of IFNγ, events which are critical in the early control of mCMV infection in vivo. The inability of AIM2- deficient animals to regulate production of mature IL-18 results in a severe defect in the ability of NK cells to produce IFNγ and as such a reduced ability of AIM2-deficient animals to control viral loads. Interestingly, AIM2 does not sense all herpes viruses; for example, it has been shown that HSV-1-driven processing of IL-1β by macrophages does not require AIM2. This is somewhat surprising, since HSV-1 DNA has been shown to accumulate in the cytosol of infected cells where it activates IFI16.[72] It is of critical importance to determine the molecular basis for differential recognition of herpes viruses by AIM2.

The IFI16 Inflammasome

In addition to AIM2, recent evidence has suggested that IFI16 can sense viral DNA in the nucleus, leading to inflammasome activation.[73] In endothelial cells, IFI16 is required for Kaposi's sarcoma-associated herpesvirus (KSHV) mediated activation of the inflammasome. KSHV is a

DNA virus that establishes a latent infection, maintaining an episomal circular DNA genome in the nucleus of infected cells. IFI16 associates with ASC in the nucleus of endothelial cells and both proteins move out of the nucleus to the perinuclear region in KSHV- infected cells. IFI16 appears to have a dual function in the KSHV-induced production of proinflammatory cytokines in this system, as in addition to being required for inflammasome activation, pro-IL-1β and IL-6 transcription were also found to be regulated by IFI16. As pro-IL-1β and IL-6 are NFκB-dependent genes, this is consistent with the previously described function of IFI16 as an activator of this transcription factor during infection with the herpesvirus HSV-1.[72] It will be important to determine if the role of IFI16 as an inflammasome activator extends to viruses other than KSHV. The role of the NLRP3, AIM2 and IFI16 inflammasome in anti-viral defenses is shown in Figure 4.

The importance of inflammasome activation in anti-viral defenses is supported by the observations that viruses encode molecules to actively block inflammasome signaling. Poxviruses encode PYD domain containing molecules, e.g., M13L which block ASC activity.[49] A recent study has demonstrated that KSHV tegument protein ORF63 is an NLR homolog that can inhibit inflammasome activation by binding to NLRP1 and NLRP3.[74] This study also demonstrated that inflammasome activation suppresses KSHV reactivation from latency, suggesting that inflammasome activation and IL-1β mediated signaling facilitates KSHV latency. During primary KSHV infection and internalization, KSHV tegument ORF63 protein might be binding to NLRP3 and NLRP1 to prevent the detrimental effects of inflammasome activation. KSHV might therefore have evolved to hijack ORF63-mediated phenomenon to establish latency during

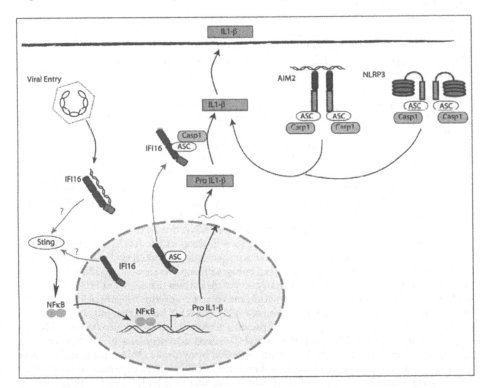

Figure 4. IFI16, NLRP3 and AIM-2 inflammasomes. Following viral infection IFI16 can interact with ASC in the nucleus prior to their trafficking out to the cytosol to form an inflammasome and activate IL-1β production. Both Aim-2 and NLRP3 form inflammasomes in the cyotoslic compartment where they interact with ASC and caspase-1 to activate IL-1β production.

primary infection. However, on the other hand, IFI16- mediated inflammasome activation after delivery of the viral genome to the nucleus could be aiding the virus to establish latency. Further studies are needed to understand the role of IFI16 in KSHV-induced inflammasome activation in other cell types including monocytes, KSHV and EBV transformed B-cell lymphoma cell lines.

Counterregulation of DNA Driven Immunity

A central question that arises from the identification of DNA receptors is what mechanisms govern self and non-self discrimination. This is particularly important in the nucleus where there are abundant levels of DNA. If IFI16 does indeed recognize the presence of viral DNA in the nucleus, understanding how IFI16 distinguishes viral genomic DNA from the abundance of cellular DNA in this location is of critical importance. Understanding how the host distinguishes between self and foreign DNA in the cytosol is also critical to understand how dysregulation of innate immune pathways might underlie the pathogenesis of diseases such as autoimmunity.

Many proteins interact with DNA and these interactions occur predominantly in the nucleus or the mitochondrion. Under normal circumstances, DNA is not found free within the cytosol. Deoxyribonuclease (DNase) enzymes serve the critical function of removal of DNA. Deoxyribonuclease I (DNase I) acts in the extracellular space where it digests endogenous DNA at sites of high cell turnover. Non-sense mutations in DNase I have been linked to Systemic Lupus Erythematosis where decreased DNase I activity correlates with disease severity.[75] Mice lacking one or both alleles of DNase I develop SLE-like disease. Both Toll- like receptor (TLR)-dependent and TLR-independent mechanisms likely become activated when extracellular DNA fails to be degraded.

The related enzyme, DNase II is confined to lysosomes where it degrades DNA from apoptotic or necrotic cells that have been phagocytosed or from nuclei expelled from erythroid precursors.[76,77] DNase II$^{-/-}$ mice accumulate undigested DNA in the lysosomes of macrophages, which activates the macrophages to produce IFNβ. The elevated level of IFNβ causes lethal anemia in mouse embryos).[76,77] DNase II$^{-/-}$ mice that also lack the Type I IFN receptor (IFN-IR$^{-/-}$) can live to adulthood, but develop chronic polyarthritis resembling rheumatoid arthritis.[78] The induction of IFNβ in DNase II-deficient mice is incompletely understood but is not mediated through TLR9. It does however depend on IRF3.[76] It is likely that one or more of the sensors outlined above contributes to the sensing of DNA in this context.

DNase III (also called TREX1) is the most abundant 3' to 5' exonuclease found on the endoplasmic reticulum. TREX1[79,80] digests single stranded DNA thereby preventing the accumulation of reverse- transcribed DNA from endogenous retroelements.[81] Mutations within TREX1 are associated with the autoimmune diseases Aicardi-Goutieres syndrome, Systemic Lupus Erythematosis (SLE) and Familial Chilbain Lupus (FCL).[82-84] Mice lacking TREX1 develop inflammatory myocarditis[81] that can be rescued by genetic ablation of IRF3 or of the Type I IFN receptor. TREX1 acts to metabolize reverse-transcribed DNA that accumulates from endogenous retroelements and as such acts as a negative regulator of the cytosolic DNA sensing pathway.

Recently, TREX1 has also been linked to innate immunity to human immunodeficiency virus Type I (HIV).[85] HIV enters T cells and macrophages through its envelope gp120 protein or by binding to lectins. Once the viral core gains entry to the cytosol the ssRNA of HIV is converted to DNA by HIV reverse transcriptase within the reverse transcription complex (RTC). The RTC matures into the preintegration complex (PIC).[86] TREX1 plays two roles in aiding HIV infection. It inhibits autointegration and prevents activation of Type I interferons.[85] TREX1 appears to inhibit Type I IFN production upon HIV infection by degrading HIV DNA generated during infection. This allows HIV to evade detection by cytosolic DNA sensors and prevents the induction of Type I IFNs which would curb viral replication. Recognition of HIV DNA, which accumulates in TREX1-deficient cells is dependent on STING and TBK1, however siRNA studies ruled out the involvement of TLR9, AIM2, RIG-I, Lrrfip1 and MAVS. The role of IFI16 in these recognition events remains to be determined. The role of DNase I, II and III (TREX1) is shown in Figure 5.

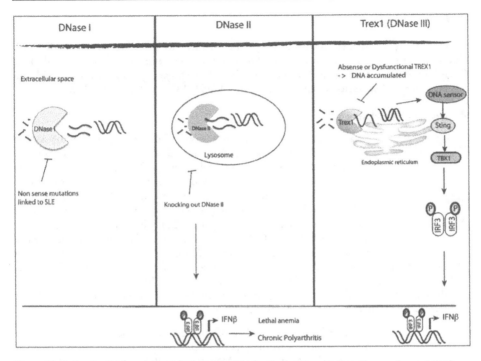

Figure 5. Roles for DNase I, II and Trex-1 in DNA recognition. Deoxyribonuclease I (DNase I) acts in the extracellular space where it digests exogenous DNA. Mutations in this gene as well as DNase I knockout mice links DNase I to SLE-like diseases. DNase II resides in lysosomes where it degrades DNA from apoptotic or necrotic cells or from nuclei expelled from erythroid precursors. DNase II knockout mice die at the embryo stage due to lethal anemia. Trex-1 is found in the endoplasmic reticulum where it degrades single stranded DNA. Trex-1 deficient mice develop inflammatory myocarditis due to single stranded DNA accumulating in the cytosol, leading to activation of cytosolic DNA sensors resulting in the production of IFN-β.

Conclusion and Future Directions

DNA sensors exist in the cytosol as essential surveyors of an environment that is normally DNA free. Significant progress has been made in understanding the mechanisms by which these sensors function in anti-viral immunity. Stimulation of these receptors by intracellular DNA results in transcriptional regulation of pro-inflammatory cytokines or Type I IFNs as well as caspase-1-dependent maturation of IL-1β and IL-18. Mutations within the pathway have been linked to a number of autoimmune diseases highlighting the need for a tightly regulated system to maintain homeostasis and prevent aberrant sensing of host DNA. There appears to be a considerable level of redundancy in the DNA receptors identified to date. In addition we believe that there are a number of DNA sensors still to be discovered. Another key question that emerges from recent findings is how nuclear DNA sensing by IFI16 is regulated and how IFI16 fails to be triggered by the abundance of DNA found free in the nuclear compartment. Overall it is important to gain a better understanding of the full repertoire of DNA sensors present in cells, how they all recognize DNA and their role in host-defenses and or disease. It will also be interesting to investigate mechanisms by which pathogens evade DNA driven immunity. This is a highly productive field of research and obtaining a better understanding of how cells respond to DNA should yield better therapeutic targets not only for viral and bacterial infections but also provide targets for therapeutic intervention in autoimmune disorders.

Acknowledgments

The authors would like to acknowledge Dr Cherilyn Sirois for providing graphics for Figure 2. This work is supported by a postdoctoral fellowship from the Health Research board and Marie Curie Post-doctoral Mobility Fellowship to S.C, by a PhD scholarship from the Faculty of Health Sciences, Aarhus University to S.B.J. and by grants AI083713 and AI067497 to K.A.F.

About the Authors

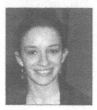

Susan Carpenter received her B.A Mod in Biochemistry and Immunology in 2004 from Trinity College Dublin, Ireland. She carried out her PhD in the laboratory of Professor Luke O'Neill in Trinity College Dublin, Ireland from 2004 to 2008. Her PhD work involved the characterization of a novel protein named TRIL, which was identified as a component of the TLR4 signaling pathway. Work carried out during her PhD was licensed to the Trinity based campus company Opsona Therapeutics Ltd, where she worked for part of 2008. From 2009 to 2010 she was a post-doctoral fellow in the Department of Biochemistry at Trinity College Dublin. She is currently working at the laboratory of Professor Katherine Fitzgerald at the Division of Infectious Disease at the University of Massachusetts Medical School. She is a recipient of a Health Research Board/ Marie Curie postdoctoral mobility fellowship enabling her to work at UMASS medical school from 2010 to 2012 and Trinity College Dublin from 2012 to 2013.

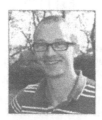

Søren Beck Jensen received his BSc in molecular biology in 2005 and spent six months in an exchange program with University of Victoria, British Columbia, Canada before he received his MSc degree in 2008, both degrees were received from the Faculty of Science, Aarhus University, Denmark. Currently, Søren is pursuing a PhD from the Laboratory of Professor Søren Riis Paludan at the Faculty of Health Sciences, Aarhus University, Denmark. Søren has worked the past two years in Kate Fitzgerald's laboratory as a visiting student.

His research interest is focused on innate immunity with emphasis on PAMP-PRR interaction and the intracellular signaling pathways. Induction of a Type I IFN response following virus infection is critical for control of the infection and protection of the host. Søren has recently contributed to our knowledge about how DNA and DNA-viruses are recognized by the innate immune system.

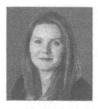

Katherine A. Fitzgerald received her BSc in Biochemistry in 1995 from University College Cork, Ireland, and her PhD in 1999 from the laboratory of Professor Luke O'Neill in Trinity College Dublin, Ireland. From 1999 to 2002, she was a post-doctoral fellow in the Department of Biochemistry at Trinity College Dublin, where her work was supported by a fellowship from the European Union. Dr. Fitzgerald joined the Division of Infectious Disease at the University of Massachusetts Medical School as a recipient of a Wellcome Trust International Award in 2001. In 2004 she joined the Faculty as an Assistant Professor and in 2007 became Associate Professor of Medicine where she received tenure in 2010. Her research interests focus on understanding the mechanisms responsible for recognition of microbial products and endogenous molecules released from damaged or dying cells and regulation of innate immunity. Optimal protection from infection requires complex immune responses involving both the innate and adaptive immune system. The innate immune system plays a key role in initiating and orchestrating host-defenses by regulating the production of pro-inflammatory cytokines, type I interferons and anti-microbial effectors. Her lab has been focused on uncovering innate sensors and associated signaling molecules regulating these events. Considerable progress has been made in her lab in understanding how pathogens or pathogen associated molecular patterns (PAMPs) are sensed by the innate immune system

References

1. Janeway CA Jr., Medzhitov R. Innate immune recognition. Annu Rev Immunol 2002; 20:197-216; PMID:11861602; http://dx.doi.org/10.1146/annurev.immunol.20.083001.084359.
2. Akira S, Uematsu S, Takeuchi O. Pathogen recognition and innate immunity. Cell 2006; 124:783-801; PMID:16497588; http://dx.doi.org/10.1016/j.cell.2006.02.015.
3. Isaacs A, Cox RA, Rotem Z. Foreign nucleic acids as the stimulus to make interferon. Lancet 1963; 2:113-6; PMID:13956740; http://dx.doi.org/10.1016/S0140-6736(63)92585-6.
4. Rotem Z, Cox RA, Isaacs A. Inhibition of virus multiplication by foreign nucleic acid. Nature 1963; 197:564-6; PMID:13975288; http://dx.doi.org/10.1038/197564a0.
5. Jensen KE, Neal AL, Owens RE, Warren J. Interferon Responses of Chick Embryo Fibroblasts to Nucleic Acids and Related Compounds. Nature 1963; 200:433-4; PMID:14076723; http://dx.doi.org/10.1038/200433a0.
6. Hemmi H, Takeuchi O, Kawai T, Kaisho T, Sato S, Sanjo H, et al. A Toll-like receptor recognizes bacterial DNA. Nature 2000; 408:740-5; PMID:11130078; http://dx.doi.org/10.1038/35047123.
7. Suzuki K, Mori A, Ishii KJ, Saito J, Singer DS, Klinman DM, et al. Activation of target-tissue immune-recognition molecules by double-stranded polynucleotides. Proc Natl Acad Sci USA 1999; 96:2285-90; PMID:10051633; http://dx.doi.org/10.1073/pnas.96.5.2285.
8. Stetson DB, Medzhitov R. Recognition of cytosolic DNA activates an IRF3-dependent innate immune response. Immunity 2006; 24:93-103; PMID:16413926; http://dx.doi.org/10.1016/j.immuni.2005.12.003.
9. Ishii KJ, Coban C, Kato H, Takahashi K, Torii Y, Takeshita F, et al. A Toll-like receptor-independent antiviral response induced by double-stranded B-form DNA. Nat Immunol 2006; 7:40-8; PMID:16286919; http://dx.doi.org/10.1038/ni1282.
10. Maniatis T. Mechanisms of human beta-interferon gene regulation. Harvey Lect 1986-1987; 82:71-104; PMID:3329166.
11. Shimada T, Kawai T, Takeda K, Matsumoto M, Inoue J, Tatsumi Y, et al. IKK-i, a novel lipopolysaccharide-inducible kinase that is related to IkappaB kinases. Int Immunol 1999; 11:1357-62; PMID:10421793; http://dx.doi.org/10.1093/intimm/11.8.1357.
12. Tojima Y, Fujimoto A, Delhase M, Chen Y, Hatakeyama S, Nakayama K, et al. NAK is an IkappaB kinase-activating kinase. Nature 2000; 404:778-82; PMID:10783893; http://dx.doi.org/10.1038/35008109.
13. Bonnard M, Mirtsos C, Suzuki S, Graham K, Huang J, Ng M, et al. Deficiency of T2K leads to apoptotic liver degeneration and impaired NF-kappaB-dependent gene transcription. EMBO J 2000; 19:4976-85; PMID:10990461; http://dx.doi.org/10.1093/emboj/19.18.4976.
14. Fitzgerald KA, McWhirter SM, Faia KL, Rowe DC, Latz E, Golenbock DT, et al. IKKepsilon and TBK1 are essential components of the IRF3 signaling pathway. Nat Immunol 2003; 4:491-6; PMID:12692549; http://dx.doi.org/10.1038/ni921.
15. Sharma S, tenOever BR, Grandvaux N, Zhou GP, Lin R, Hiscott J. Triggering the interferon antiviral response through an IKK-related pathway. Science 2003; 300:1148-51; PMID:12702806; http://dx.doi.org/10.1126/science.1081315.
16. McWhirter SM, Fitzgerald KA, Rosains J, Rowe DC, Golenbock DT, Maniatis T. IFN-regulatory factor 3-dependent gene expression is defective in Tbk1-deficient mouse embryonic fibroblasts. Proc Natl Acad Sci USA 2004; 101:233-8; PMID:14679297; http://dx.doi.org/10.1073/pnas.2237236100.
17. Ishikawa H, Barber GN. STING is an endoplasmic reticulum adaptor that facilitates innate immune signalling. Nature 2008; 455:674-8; PMID:18724357; http://dx.doi.org/10.1038/nature07317.
18. Ishikawa H, Ma Z, Barber GN. STING regulates intracellular DNA-mediated, type I interferon- dependent innate immunity. Nature 2009; 461:788-92; PMID:19776740; http://dx.doi.org/10.1038/nature08476.
19. Zhong B, Yang Y, Li S, Wang YY, Li Y, Diao F, et al. The adaptor protein MITA links virus-sensing receptors to IRF3 transcription factor activation. Immunity 2008; 29:538-50; PMID:18818105; http://dx.doi.org/10.1016/j.immuni.2008.09.003.
20. Sun W, Li Y, Chen L, Chen H, You F, Zhou X, et al. ERIS, an endoplasmic reticulum IFN stimulator, activates innate immune signaling through dimerization. Proc Natl Acad Sci USA 2009; 106:8653-8; PMID:19433799; http://dx.doi.org/10.1073/pnas.0900850106.
21. Jin L, Waterman PM, Jonscher KR, Short CM, Reisdorph NA, Cambier JC. MPYS, a novel membrane tetraspanner, is associated with major histocompatibility complex class II and mediates transduction of apoptotic signals. Mol Cell Biol 2008; 28:5014-26; PMID:18559423; http://dx.doi.org/10.1128/MCB.00640-08.
22. Saitoh T, Fujita N, Hayashi T, Takahara K, Satoh T, Lee H, et al. Atg9a controls dsDNA-driven dynamic translocation of STING and the innate immune response. Proc Natl Acad Sci USA 2009; 106:20842-6; PMID:19926846; http://dx.doi.org/10.1073/pnas.0911267106.
23. Takaoka A, Wang Z, Choi MK, Yanai H, Negishi H, Ban T, et al. DAI (DLM-1/ZBP1) is a cytosolic DNA sensor and an activator of innate immune response. Nature 2007; 448:501-5; PMID:17618271; http://dx.doi.org/10.1038/nature06013.

24. Wang Z, Choi MK, Ban T, Yanai H, Negishi H, Lu Y, et al. Regulation of innate immune responses by DAI (DLM-1/ZBP1) and other DNA-sensing molecules. Proc Natl Acad Sci USA 2008; 105:5477-82; PMID:18375758; http://dx.doi.org/10.1073/pnas.0801295105.
25. Kaiser WJ, Upton JW, Mocarski ES. Receptor-interacting protein homotypic interaction motif- dependent control of NF-kappa B activation via the DNA-dependent activator of IFN regulatory factors. J Immunol 2008; 181:6427-34; PMID:18941233.
26. Rebsamen M, Heinz LX, Meylan E, Michallet MC, Schroder K, Hofmann K, et al. DAI/ZBP1 recruits RIP1 and RIP3 through RIP homotypic interaction motifs to activate NF-kappaB. EMBO Rep 2009; 10:916-22; PMID:19590578; http://dx.doi.org/10.1038/embor.2009.109.
27. Yoneyama M, Kikuchi M, Natsukawa T, Shinobu N, Imaizumi T, Miyagishi M, et al. The RNA helicase RIG-I has an essential function in double-stranded RNA-induced innate antiviral responses. Nat Immunol 2004; 5:730-7; PMID:15208624; http://dx.doi.org/10.1038/ni1087.
28. Kawai T, Takahashi K, Sato S, Coban C, Kumar H, Kato H, et al. IPS-1, an adaptor triggering RIG-I- and Mda5-mediated type I interferon induction. Nat Immunol 2005; 6:981-8; PMID:16127453; http://dx.doi.org/10.1038/ni1243.
29. Sun Q, Sun L, Liu HH, Chen X, Seth RB, Forman J, et al. The specific and essential role of MAVS in antiviral innate immune responses. Immunity 2006; 24:633-42; PMID:16713980; http://dx.doi.org/10.1016/j.immuni.2006.04.004.
30. Chiu YH, Macmillan JB, Chen ZJ. RNA polymerase III detects cytosolic DNA and induces type I interferons through the RIG-I pathway. Cell 2009; 138:576-91; PMID:19631370; http://dx.doi.org/10.1016/j.cell.2009.06.015.
31. Ablasser A, Bauernfeind F, Hartmann G, Latz E, Fitzgerald KA, Hornung V. RIG-I-dependent sensing of poly(dA:dT) through the induction of an RNA polymerase III-transcribed RNA intermediate. Nat Immunol 2009; 10:1065-72; PMID:19609254; http://dx.doi.org/10.1038/ni.1779.
32. Hornung V, Ellegast J, Kim S, Brzozka K, Jung A, Kato H, et al. 5'-Triphosphate RNA Is the Ligand for RIG-I. Science 2006; 314:994-7; PMID:17038590; http://dx.doi.org/10.1126/science.1132505.
33. Pichlmair A, Schulz O, Tan CP, Naslund TI, Liljestrom P, Weber F, et al. RIG-I-mediated antiviral responses to single-stranded RNA bearing 5'-phosphates. Science 2006; 314:997-1001; PMID:17038589; http://dx.doi.org/10.1126/science.1132998.
34. Jaehning JA, Roeder RG. Transcription of specific adenovirus genes in isolated nuclei by exogenous RNA polymerases. J Biol Chem 1977; 252:8753-61; PMID:925020.
35. Tian J, Avalos AM, Mao SY, Chen B, Senthil K, Wu H, et al. Toll-like receptor 9-dependent activation by DNA-containing immune complexes is mediated by HMGB1 and RAGE. Nat Immunol 2007; 8:487-96; PMID:17417641; http://dx.doi.org/10.1038/ni1457.
36. Yanai H, Ban T, Wang Z, Choi MK, Kawamura T, Negishi H, et al. HMGB proteins function as universal sentinels for nucleic-acid-mediated innate immune responses. Nature 2009; 462:99-103; PMID:19890330; http://dx.doi.org/10.1038/nature08512.
37. Merika M, Williams AJ, Chen G, Collins T, Thanos D. Recruitment of CBP/p300 by the IFN beta enhanceosome is required for synergistic activation of transcription. Mol Cell 1998; 1:277-87; PMID:9659924; http://dx.doi.org/10.1016/S1097-2765(00)80028-3 .
38. Yang P, An H, Liu X, Wen M, Zheng Y, Rui Y, et al. The cytosolic nucleic acid sensor LRRFIP1 mediates the production of type I interferon via a beta-catenin-dependent pathway. Nat Immunol 2010; 11:487-94; PMID:20453844; http://dx.doi.org/10.1038/ni.1876.
39. Hokeness-Antonelli KL, Crane MJ, Dragoi AM, Chu WM, Salazar-Mather TP. IFN-alphabeta-mediated inflammatory responses and antiviral defense in liver is TLR9-independent but MyD88-dependent during murine cytomegalovirus infection. J Immunol 2007; 179:6176-83; PMID:17947693.
40. Kim T, Pazhoor S, Bao M, Zhang Z, Hanabuchi S, Facchinetti V, et al. Aspartate-glutamate-alanine-histidine box motif (DEAH)/RNA helicase A helicases sense microbial DNA in human plasmacytoid dendritic cells. Proc Natl Acad Sci USA 2010; 107:15181-6; PMID:20696886; http://dx.doi.org/10.1073/pnas.1006539107.
41. Unterholzner L, Keating SE, Baran M, Horan KA, Jensen SB, Sharma S, et al. IFI16 is an innate immune sensor for intracellular DNA. Nat Immunol 2010; 11:997-1004; PMID:20890285; http://dx.doi.org/10.1038/ni.1932.
42. Roberts ZJ, Goutagny N, Perera PY, Kato H, Kumar H, Kawai T, et al. The chemotherapeutic agent DMXAA potently and specifically activates the TBK1-IRF-3 signaling axis. J Exp Med 2007; 204:1559-69 PMID:17562815; http://dx.doi.org/10.1084/jem.20061845.
43. Shirey KA, Nhu QM, Yim KC, Roberts ZJ, Teijaro JR, Farber DL, et al. The anti-tumor agent, 5,6-dimethylxanthenone-4-acetic acid (DMXAA), induces IFN-beta-mediated antiviral activity in vitro and in vivo. J Leukoc Biol 2011; 89:351-7 PMID:21084628; http://dx.doi.org/10.1189/jlb.0410216.
44. McWhirter SM, Barbalat R, Monroe KM, Fontana MF, Hyodo M, Joncker NT, et al. A host type I interferon response is induced by cytosolic sensing of the bacterial second messenger cyclic-di-GMP. J Exp Med 2009; 206:1899-911 PMID:19652017; http://dx.doi.org/10.1084/jem.20082874.

45. Woodward JJ, Iavarone AT, Portnoy DA. c-di-AMP secreted by intracellular Listeria monocytogenes activates a host type I interferon response. Science 2010; 328:1703-5 PMID:20508090; http://dx.doi.org/10.1126/science.1189801.
46. Sauer JD, Sotelo-Troha K, von Moltke J, Monroe KM, Rae CS, Brubaker SW, et al. The N-ethyl-N-nitrosourea-induced Goldenticket mouse mutant reveals an essential function of Sting in the in vivo interferon response to Listeria monocytogenes and cyclic dinucleotides. Infect Immun 2011; 79:688-94 PMID:21098106; http://dx.doi.org/10.1128/IAI.00999-10.
47. Hornung V, Latz E. Intracellular DNA recognition. Nat Rev Immunol 2010; 10:123-30; PMID:20098460; http://dx.doi.org/10.1038/nri2690.
48. Martinon F, Mayor A, Tschopp J. The inflammasomes: guardians of the body. Annu Rev Immunol 2009; 27:229-65; PMID:19302040; http://dx.doi.org/10.1146/annurev.immunol.021908.132715.
49. Dinarello CA. The IL-1 family and inflammatory diseases. Clin Exp Rheumatol 2002; 20(Suppl 27):S1-13; PMID:14989423.
50. Kanneganti TD. Central roles of NLRs and inflammasomes in viral infection. Nat Rev Immunol 2010; 10:688-98; PMID:20847744; http://dx.doi.org/10.1038/nri2851.
51. Rathinam VA, Jiang Z, Waggoner SN, Sharma S, Cole LE, Waggoner L, et al. The AIM2 inflammasome is essential for host defense against cytosolic bacteria and DNA viruses. Nat Immunol 2010; 11:395-402; PMID:20351692; http://dx.doi.org/10.1038/ni.1864.
52. Dinarello CA. IL-1: discoveries, controversies and future directions. Eur J Immunol 2010; 40:599-606; PMID:20201008; http://dx.doi.org/10.1002/eji.201040319.
53. Martinon F, Burns K, Tschopp J. The inflammasome: a molecular platform triggering activation of inflammatory caspases and processing of proIL-beta. Mol Cell 2002; 10:417-26; PMID:12191486; http://dx.doi.org/10.1016/S1097-2765(02)00599-3.
54. Martinon F, Tschopp J. NLRs join TLRs as innate sensors of pathogens. Trends Immunol 2005; 26:447-54; PMID:15967716; http://dx.doi.org/10.1016/j.it.2005.06.004.
55. Franchi L, Warner N, Viani K, Nunez G. Function of Nod-like receptors in microbial recognition and host defense. Immunol Rev 2009; 227:106-28; PMID:19120480; http://dx.doi.org/10.1111/j.1600-065X.2008.00734.x.
56. Muruve DA, Petrilli V, Zaiss AK, White LR, Clark SA, Ross PJ, et al. The inflammasome recognizes cytosolic microbial and host DNA and triggers an innate immune response. Nature 2008; 452:103-7; PMID:18288107; http://dx.doi.org/10.1038/nature06664.
57. Di Paolo NC, Miao EA, Iwakura Y, Murali-Krishna K, Aderem A, Flavell RA, et al. Virus binding to a plasma membrane receptor triggers interleukin-1 alpha-mediated proinflammatory macrophage response in vivo. Immunity 2009; 31:110-21; PMID:19576795; http://dx.doi.org/10.1016/j.immuni.2009.04.015.
58. Delaloye J, Roger T, Steiner-Tardivel QG, Le Roy D, Knaup Reymond M, Akira S, et al. Innate immune sensing of modified vaccinia virus Ankara (MVA) is mediated by TLR2-TLR6, MDA-5 and the NALP3 inflammasome. PLoS Pathog 2009; 5:e1000480; PMID:19543380; http://dx.doi.org/10.1371/journal.ppat.1000480.
59. Allen IC, Scull MA, Moore CB, Holl EK, McElvania-Tekippe E, Taxman DJ, et al. The NLRP3 Inflammasome Mediates In Vivo Innate Immunity to Influenza A Virus through Recognition of Viral RNA. Immunity 2009; 30:556-65; PMID:19362020; http://dx.doi.org/10.1016/j.immuni.2009.02.005.
60. Ichinohe T, Lee HK, Ogura Y, Flavell R, Iwasaki A. Inflammasome recognition of influenza virus is essential for adaptive immune responses. J Exp Med 2009; 206:79-87; PMID:19139171; http://dx.doi.org/10.1084/jem.20081667.
61. Kanneganti TD, Body-Malapel M, Amer A, Park JH, Whitfield J, Franchi L, et al. Critical role for Cryopyrin/Nalp3 in activation of caspase-1 in response to viral infection and double-stranded RNA. J Biol Chem 2006; 281:36560-8; PMID:17008311; http://dx.doi.org/10.1074/jbc.M607594200.
62. Sander LE, Davis MJ, Boekschoten MV, Amsen D, Dascher CC, Ryffel B, et al. Detection of prokaryotic mRNA signifies microbial viability and promotes immunity. Nature 2011; 474:385-9; PMID:21602824; http://dx.doi.org/10.1038/nature10072.
63. Hornung V, Ablasser A, Charrel-Dennis M, Bauernfeind F, Horvath G, Caffrey DR, et al. AIM2 recognizes cytosolic dsDNA and forms a caspase-1-activating inflammasome with ASC. Nature 2009; 458:514-8; PMID:19158675; http://dx.doi.org/10.1038/nature07725.
64. Bürckstümmer T, Baumann C, Bluml S, Dixit E, Durnberger G, Jahn H, et al. An orthogonal proteomic-genomic screen identifies AIM2 as a cytoplasmic DNA sensor for the inflammasome. Nat Immunol 2009; 10:266-72; PMID:19158679; http://dx.doi.org/10.1038/ni.1702.
65. Fernandes-Alnemri T, Yu JW, Datta P, Wu J, Alnemri ES. AIM2 activates the inflammasome and cell death in response to cytoplasmic DNA. Nature 2009; 458:509-13; PMID:19158676; http://dx.doi.org/10.1038/nature07710.
66. Roberts TL, Idris A, Dunn JA, Kelly GM, Burnton CM, Hodgson S, et al. HIN-200 proteins regulate caspase activation in response to foreign cytoplasmic DNA. Science 2009; 323:1057-60; PMID:19131592; http://dx.doi.org/10.1126/science.1169841.

67. Warren SE, Armstrong A, Hamilton MK, Mao DP, Leaf IA, Miao EA, et al. Cutting edge: Cytosolic bacterial DNA activates the inflammasome via Aim2. J Immunol 2010; 185:818-21; PMID:20562263; http://dx.doi.org/10.4049/jimmunol.1000724.

68. Wu J, Fernandes-Alnemri T, Alnemri ES. Involvement of the AIM2, NLRC4, and NLRP3 inflammasomes in caspase-1 activation by Listeria monocytogenes. J Clin Immunol 2010; 30:693-702; PMID:20490635; http://dx.doi.org/10.1007/s10875-010-9425-2.

69. Sauer JD, Witte CE, Zemansky J, Hanson B, Lauer P, Portnoy DA. Listeria monocytogenes triggers AIM2-mediated pyroptosis upon infrequent bacteriolysis in the macrophage cytosol. Cell Host Microbe 2010; 7:412-9; PMID:20417169; http://dx.doi.org/10.1016/j.chom.2010.04.004.

70. Fernandes-Alnemri T, Yu JW, Juliana C, Solorzano L, Kang S, Wu J, et al. The AIM2 inflammasome is critical for innate immunity to Francisella tularensis. Nat Immunol 2010; 11:385-93; PMID:20351693; http://dx.doi.org/10.1038/ni.1859.

71. Kim S, Bauernfeind F, Ablasser A, Hartmann G, Fitzgerald KA, Latz E, et al. Listeria monocytogenes is sensed by the NLRP3 and AIM2 inflammasome. Eur J Immunol 2010; 40:1545-51; PMID:20333626; http://dx.doi.org/10.1002/eji.201040425.

72. Unterholzner L, Keating SE, Baran M, Horan KA, Jensen SB, Sharma S, et al. IFI16 is an innate immune sensor for intracellular DNA. Nat Immunol 2010; 11:997-1004; PMID:20890285; http://dx.doi.org/10.1038/ni.1932.

73. Kerur N, Veettil MV, Sharma-Walia N, Bottero V, Sadagopan S, Otageri P, et al. IFI16 Acts as a Nuclear Pathogen Sensor to Induce the Inflammasome in Response to Kaposi Sarcoma-Associated Herpesvirus Infection. Cell Host Microbe 2011; 9:363-75; PMID:21575908; http://dx.doi.org/10.1016/j.chom.2011.04.008.

74. Gregory SM, Davis BK, West JA, Taxman DJ, Matsuzawa S, Reed JC, et al. Discovery of a viral NLR homolog that inhibits the inflammasome. Science 2011; 331:330-4; PMID:21252346; http://dx.doi.org/10.1126/science.1199478.

75. Yasutomo K, Horiuchi T, Kagami S, Tsukamoto H, Hashimura C, Urushihara M, et al. Mutation of DNASE1 in people with systemic lupus erythematosus. Nat Genet 2001; 28:313-4; PMID:11479590; http://dx.doi.org/10.1038/91070.

76. Yoshida H, Okabe Y, Kawane K, Fukuyama H, Nagata S. Lethal anemia caused by interferon-beta produced in mouse embryos carrying undigested DNA. Nat Immunol 2005; 6:49-56; PMID:15568025; http://dx.doi.org/10.1038/ni1146.

77. Kawane K, Fukuyama H, Kondoh G, Takeda J, Ohsawa Y, Uchiyama Y, et al. Requirement of DNase II for definitive erythropoiesis in the mouse fetal liver. Science 2001; 292:1546-9; PMID:11375492; http://dx.doi.org/10.1126/science.292.5521.1546.

78. Kawane K, Tanaka H, Kitahara Y, Shimaoka S, Nagata S. Cytokine-dependent but acquired immunity-independent arthritis caused by DNA escaped from degradation. Proc Natl Acad Sci USA 2010; 107:19432-7; PMID:20974942; http://dx.doi.org/10.1073/pnas.1010603107.

79. Höss M, Robins P, Naven TJ, Pappin DJ, Sgouros J, Lindahl T. A human DNA editing enzyme homologous to the Escherichia coli DnaQ/MutD protein. EMBO J 1999; 18:3868-75; PMID:10393201; http://dx.doi.org/10.1093/emboj/18.13.3868.

80. Mazur DJ, Perrino FW. Identification and expression of the TREX1 and TREX2 cDNA sequences encoding mammalian 3'-5' exonucleases. J Biol Chem 1999; 274:19655-60; PMID:10391904; http://dx.doi.org/10.1074/jbc.274.28.19655.

81. Stetson DB, Ko JS, Heidmann T, Medzhitov R. Trex1 prevents cell-intrinsic initiation of autoimmunity. Cell 2008; 134:587-98; PMID:18724932; http://dx.doi.org/10.1016/j.cell.2008.06.032.

82. Crow YJ, Rehwinkel J. Aicardi-Goutieres syndrome and related phenotypes: linking nucleic acid metabolism with autoimmunity. Hum Mol Genet 2009; 18:R130-6; PMID:19808788; http://dx.doi.org/10.1093/hmg/ddp293.

83. Lee-Kirsch MA, Chowdhury D, Harvey S, Gong M, Senenko L, Engel K, et al. A mutation in TREX1 that impairs susceptibility to granzyme A-mediated cell death underlies familial chilblain lupus. J Mol Med 2007; 85:531-7; PMID:17440703; http://dx.doi.org/10.1007/s00109-007-0199-9.

84. Lee-Kirsch MA, Gong M, Chowdhury D, Senenko L, Engel K, Lee YA, et al. Mutations in the gene encoding the 3'-5' DNA exonuclease TREX1 are associated with systemic lupus erythematosus. Nat Genet 2007; 39:1065-7; PMID:17660818; http://dx.doi.org/10.1038/ng2091.

85. Yan N, Regalado-Magdos AD, Stiggelbout B, Lee-Kirsch MA, Lieberman J. The cytosolic exonuclease TREX1 inhibits the innate immune response to human immunodeficiency virus type 1. Nat Immunol 2010; 11:1005-13; PMID:20871604; http://dx.doi.org/10.1038/ni.1941.

86. Yan N, Lieberman J. Gaining a foothold: how HIV avoids innate immune recognition. Curr Opin Immunol 2011; 23:21-8; PMID:21123040; http://dx.doi.org/10.1016/j.coi.2010.11.004.

CHAPTER 9

Mechanisms of Interferon Antagonism by Poxviruses

Xiangzhi Meng, Lloyd Rose and Yan Xiang*

Abstract

The interferons (IFNs), a group of cytokines that induce the innate immune response and stimulate the adaptive immune response, pose a formidable barrier for viral replication in the host. In response, many viruses have evolved strategies to inhibit the induction and action of IFNs. Poxviruses, with a large genome and an entirely cytoplasmic life cycle, are particularly adept at evading IFNs. Almost every aspect of the IFN system is subject to modulation by specific poxvirus proteins. In recent years, great progress has been made in deciphering the molecular basis for IFN modulation by poxviruses. In particular, a number of poxvirus proteins have been identified to inhibit the signaling pathway that induces IFNs, and the structures of an increasing number of poxvirus IFN modulators have been determined. Here we review the multiple strategies used by poxviruses to modulate the induction, signaling and effectors of IFNs, with an emphasis on the molecular mechanisms of action of the poxvirus proteins.

Introduction

Interferons (IFNs) are a large family of cytokines that play an important role in the antiviral response.[1] They are classified into three types based on their receptor usage. Type I IFNs, consisting of multiple IFN-α subtypes, a single IFN-β, IFN-ε, IFN-κ and IFN-ω in humans, bind to a single cellular receptor composed of IFN-αR1 and IFN-αR2. Type I IFNs can be induced in many nucleated cells, and their receptor is expressed ubiquitously. Type II IFN, consisting of a single IFN-γ, binds to a distinct cellular IFN-γ receptor composed of IFN-γR1 and IFN-γR2. IFN-γ and its receptor are predominantly expressed in lymphocytes. Type III IFNs were discovered more recently and include IFN-λ1, IFN-λ2 and IFN-λ3.[2] They bind to an IFN-λ receptor complex composed of a unique IFN-λR1 chain and a shared IL-10R2 chain. Type III IFNs, like type I IFNs, can be induced in many cells but their receptor is largely restricted to cells of epithelial origin.[2]

The production of type I IFNs is induced after host pattern-recognition receptors (PRRs) are activated by pathogen-associated molecular patterns (PAMPs).[3] PRRs include Toll-like receptors (TLRs), retinoic acid-inducible gene I (RIG-I)-like receptors (RLRs), nucleotide-binding oligomerization domain (NOD)-like receptors (NLRs) and cytosolic DNA receptors. Viral nucleic acids, both RNA and DNA, are the most important PAMPs for the response to virus infection. The detection of PAMPs by PRRs leads to activation of transcription factors NF-κB and IFN regulatory factor (IRF) 3 or 7, which ultimately induce the production of type I IFNs.[4] Type II interferon is primarily produced in response to stimulation by pro-inflammatory cytokines, most notably IL-12 and IL-18.[5,6] Type III IFNs are induced by a mechanism that is similar to that of type I IFNs.[7]

*Department of Microbiology and Immunology, The University of Texas Health Science Center at San Antonio, San Antonio, Texas, USA.
Corresponding Author: Yan Xiang—Email: xiangy@uthscsa.edu

Nucleic Acid Sensors and Antiviral Immunity, edited by Suryaprakash Sambhara and Takashi Fujita.
©2013 Landes Bioscience.

Binding of IFNs to their corresponding cellular receptor complexes, despite their differences, induces similar signaling events in the JAK (Janus kinase) and STAT (signal transducer and activator of transcription) pathway.[1] The α and β chains of type I and type III IFN receptors associate respectively with Janus protein kinases Jak1 and Tyk2, while α and β chains of IFN-γR associate respectively with Jak1 and Jak2. IFNs binding to their respective receptors induce dimerization of the two receptor subunits. Receptor dimerization allows Janus kinases to phosphorylate the receptor, creating a binding site for STATs, which are present in the cytoplasm as latent transcription factors. Once bound to the receptor-JAK complex, STATs are phosphorylated and subsequently dissociate from the receptor and dimerize. Stimulation with type I and type III IFNs results in STAT1:STAT2 heterodimers, while IFN-γ stimulation results in STAT1 homodimers. STAT dimers translocate to the nucleus where they activate transcription. The STAT1:STAT2 heterodimer associates with IRF-9 to form active transcription factor ISGF3, which binds to a consensus binding motif referred to as the Interferon Stimulated Response Element (ISRE). The STAT1 homodimer binds to a consensus binding motif referred to as the Interferon-Gamma Activated Sequence (GAS). Activated STATs induce very similar sets of genes, including many genes that encode important mediators of the antiviral response. Consequently, all IFNs restrict viral replication via the induction of an antiviral state in cells bearing the appropriate receptor. They can also inhibit virus replication and spread via indirect immunoregulatory activities. In particular, IFN-γ activates natural killer (NK) and cytotoxic T cells that destroy infected cells.

The importance of IFN in defense against viruses is underscored by the discovery in many viruses of various strategies for circumventing IFN activities.[8] Poxviruses, in particular, have been found to encode a plethora of viral proteins that actively inhibit the induction, signaling and effectors of the IFNs, illustrating the fundamental importance of interferon blockage to poxviruses.[9] Poxviruses are large double-stranded DNA viruses that replicate entirely in the cytoplasm.[10] They typically contain a genome of around 200 kb and encode roughly 200 proteins. Among the vertebrate poxviruses, the orthopoxviruses include variola virus (VARV), monkeypox virus (MPXV), ectromelia virus (ECTV) and vaccinia virus (VACV). VARV is the most notorious poxvirus for being the causative agent of smallpox. MPXV is a zoonotic agent that causes a disease that is similar to smallpox. VACV is the vaccine for smallpox and the best studied poxvirus. Most immune evasion mechanisms of poxviruses were identified and studied in orthopoxviruses, particularly VACV.[11] Some immune evasion mechanisms have also been studied in the rabbit pathogen myxoma virus (MYXV) and the human pathogen molloscum contagiosum virus (MCV). Here we review the multiple strategies used by poxviruses to modulate IFN by using mostly VACV examples (Fig. 1 and Table 1), although similar proteins and mechanisms often exist in other poxviruses. VACV genes are historically named with a letter and a number

Figure 1, viewed on following page. Inhibition of the induction, signaling and effectors of interferons by vaccinia virus. Mechanisms of interferon induction are schematically shown on the left, while mechanisms of interferon signaling and antiviral effectors are shown on the right. Points of viral inhibition are shown along the pathways with the name of the viral protein underlined. Viral PAMPs are recognized by host PRRs that initiate signaling cascades to upregulate IRFs and NF-κB, leading to the production of type I interferons. VACV A46 blocks TLR signaling via interactions with TIR-containing adaptors including MyD88 and TRIF. VACV A52 blocks TLR signaling via inhibition of IRAK2. VACV E3 inhibits PKR and RLR signaling by binding to and preventing the recognition of viral dsRNA. VACV N1, C6 and K7 block activation of IRF3/7 and NF-κB via interactions with components of the TBK1 signaling complex. VACV M2 blocks ERK2-mediated activation of NF-κB. VACV B14 interacts with IKKβ to block IKK phosphorylation of IκBα. VACV K1 blocks degradation of phosphorylated IκBα. VACV C12 (IL-18BP) binds to IL-18 to prevent the binding to IL-18 receptor and the induction of IFN-γ. VACV B8 and B18 bind to IFN-γ and IFN-α/β respectively to prevent the binding to IFN receptors. VACV H1 dephosphorylates STAT1 and STAT2. VACV E3 inhibits dsRNA dependent activation of PKR. VACV K3 binds to PKR and prevents it from phosphorylating eIF2α. VACV K1 and C7 act on unidentified interferon effectors to prevent arrest of viral protein synthesis.

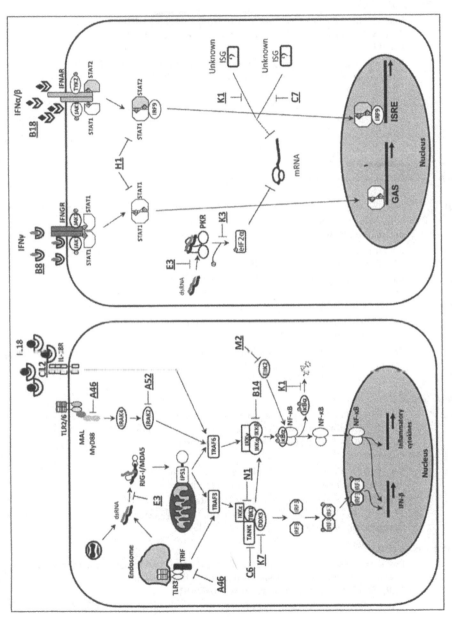

Figure 1. Please see figure legend on previous page.

Table 1. Vaccinia virus modulators of the interferon system

Protein	Function	Structure (PDB ID)
Inhibitors of IFN induction		
A46	Interacts directly with TIR domain-containing proteins MyD88, TRIF, MAL and TRAM to block activation of NF-κB and IRF3/7 via TLRs	Not known
A52	Interacts directly with IRAK2 to prevent NF-κB activation and interacts directly with TRAF6 to induce activation of p38 MAP kinase	2VVX[32]
B14	Interacts directly with the IKKβ, inhibiting the phosphorylation of its activation loop and the subsequent phosphorylation of IκBα	2VVY[32]
K1	Inhibits the degradation of phosphorylated IκBα by an unknown mechanism	3KEA[121]
M2	Blocks activation of NF-κB by inhibiting phosphorylation of ERK2 by an unknown mechanism	Not known
N1	Interacts directly with TBK1 to prevent NF-κB and IRF3/7 activation. Also interacts directly with BH3 domain-containing proteins to inhibit apoptosis	2UXE, 2I39[25,33]
C6	Interacts directly with TBK1 complex scaffold proteins TANK, NAP1 and SINTBAD to inhibit NF-κB and IRF3/7 activation	Not known
K7	Interacts directly with DDX3, a TBK1 complex protein, to prevent activation of IRF3/7	3JRV[30]
C12	Secreted protein that intercepts IL-18 by direct interaction, preventing its interaction with the IL-18 receptor and subsequent induction of IFN-γ	ECTV 3F62[46]
E3	Prevents activation of NF-κB and IRF3/7 by binding to dsRNA and preventing recognition of dsRNA by cellular pattern recognition receptors RLRs and PKR	N-terminus 1OYI[100]
Inhibitors of IFN signaling		
B18	Secreted protein that associates with glycosaminoglycans on the cell surface and intercepts type I interferons by direct interaction, preventing their interaction with the IFN-α/β receptor	ECTV 3BES
B8	Secreted protein that sequesters IFN-γ by direct interaction, preventing its interaction with the IFN-γ receptor	ECTV 3OQ3[63]
H1	Dual specificity phosphatase that dephosphorylates activated STAT1 and STAT2 following their activation, thereby preventing upregulation of interferon stimulated genes (ISGs)	3CM3[73]
Inhibitors of IFN effectors		
E3	Prevents activation of PKR and 2′-5′-oligoadenylate synthetase/RNaseL by sequestering dsRNA. Also interacts directly with PKR, ISG15, and adenosine deaminase 1 (ADAR1)	N-terminus 1OYI[100]
K3	A non-phosphorylable homolog of eIF2α that competitively binds to PKR, preventing it from interacting with its cellular substrate, eIF2α	1LUZ[112]
K1 and C7	Block activity of an unidentified ISG or ISGs, as loss of K1 and C7 result in IFN sensitivity down- stream of IFN signaling	K1: 3KEA,[121] C7: Not known

followed by the suffix 'L' or 'R', to indicate the direction of transcription. The suffix is omitted when referring to the corresponding protein. Some VACV proteins are secreted from infected cells and directly bind and inhibit IFNs or cytokines that induce IFNs, while other VACV proteins function intracellularly by inhibiting IFN signaling pathways and antiviral effectors of IFNs. VACV B18 and B8 are secreted binding proteins for IFNα/β and IFN-γ, respectively. VACV C12 is a secreted binding protein for IL-18, which induces the production of IFN-γ. In addition, a number of VACV proteins, including A46, A52, N1, K7, K1, M2, B14, and C6, block NF-κB and/or IRF activation. VACV H1 inhibits IFN signaling by dephosphorylating STATs. Both VACV E3 and K3 block the IFN-induced inhibition of protein synthesis by inhibiting the activation or action of the dsRNA-activated kinase PKR. VACV K1 and C7 block the action of a yet-unidentified IFN effector or effectors.

Poxvirus Proteins That Inhibit the Induction of IFNs

Viral replication in host cells produces a variety of PAMPs. These PAMPs are recognized by host PRRs, which signal to activate transcription factors NF-κB and IRFs, leading to the induction of type I IFNs. VACV E3 binds to double-stranded RNA (dsRNA), a major PAMP produced during viral replication. VACV A46 and A52 inhibit the signaling of TLRs. A variety of VACV proteins, including N1, K1, K7, B14, M2 and C6, inhibit NF-κB and/or IRFs activation at various steps along the signaling pathway. We will only briefly review here VACV proteins that inhibit NF-κB and IRFs, as they have been reviewed recently.[12,13] E3 and K1 will be discussed more extensively in a subsequent section. We will review in more detail the poxvirus binding protein for IL-18, a cytokine that induces IFN-γ production.

A46. TLRs signal through Toll/IL-1R (TIR) domain-containing adaptor proteins, which are recruited to TLRs via interaction with the TIR domain of the TLR.[14] With the exception of TLR3, which signals via TIR domain-containing adaptor inducing IFN-β ('TRIF), all other TLRs signals via MyD88. In addition, TLR2 and TLR4 signaling also require MyD88 adaptor-like (MAL), and TLR4 can signal through a MyD88-independent pathway that requires TRIF-related adaptor molecule (TRAM). A46 interacts with MyD88, TRIF, Mal and TRAM, inhibiting the signaling by all TLRs.[15]

A52. Recruitment of TIR domain-containing adaptor proteins leads to the recruitment of IL-1R-associated kinase (IRAK) family members, which subsequently activate TNFR-associated factor 6 ('TRAF6).[14] A52 functions downstream of A46 by interacting with IRAK2,[16] resulting in the inhibition of TLR-induced NF-κB activation. The N-terminal death domain of IRAK2 is essential for binding A52. A52 also interacts with TRAF6, but this interaction does not inhibit NF-κB activation but instead stimulates p38 MAP kinase activation.[17]

B14. The signaling pathways activated by many PRRs converge on the IκB kinase (IKK) complex, comprised of IKKα, IKKβ and IKKγ.[18] Once activated, IKK phosphorylates the inhibitor of NF-κB (IκBα) to initiate IκBα degradation. B14 interacts with IKKβ and prevents its activation by inhibiting the phosphorylation of its activation loop.[19]

K1. Once phosphorylated, IκBα is normally ubiquitinated and degraded by the 26S proteasome, releasing NF-κB and allowing its translocation into the nucleus.[20] K1 inhibits the degradation of phosphorylated IκBα by an unknown mechanism.[21] The function of K1 in NF-κB inhibition, however, is cell-type dependent and its molecular target is unknown.

M2. One alternative mechanism for activation of NF-κB is via ERK2, which is activated by Mitogen-activated ERK-regulating kinase (MEK). M2 inhibits the phorbol 12-myristate 13-acetate (PMA)-induced phosphorylation of ERK2 and subsequent activation of NF-κB, although the exact mechanism of this inhibition has not been identified.[22]

N1. Most of the PRR pathways, including TLR3, TLR4 and RLR, also converge at the level of the NF-κB activator (TANK)-binding kinase 1 (TBK1) and IκB kinase-ε (IKKε), leading to the phosphorylation and activation of IRF3 and 7.[23] N1 directly binds TBK1, inhibiting the activation of IRF3 and NF-κB.[24] In addition, N1 interacts with pro-apoptotic Bcl-2 proteins such as Bid, Bad, Bak and Bax, inhibiting apoptosis.[25]

C6. TBK1 and IKKε exist in complexes with the scaffold proteins TANK, NAP1 or SINTBAD.[26-28] C6 interacts with these scaffold proteins, without disrupting the formation of the signaling complexes containing the kinases TBK1 or IKKε.[29] This interaction inhibits TBK1/IKKε-induced IRF3 and IRF7 activation.

K7. K7 also inhibits TBK1/IKKε-mediated IRF activation. It forms a complex with the human DEAD-box RNA helicase DDX3, which was previously not known to be involved in IRF activation.[30,31] DDX3 binds to and is phosphorylated by IKKε and/or TBK1. The investigation of this K7-mediated viral evasion strategy revealed a novel function of DDX3 in innate immunity.

All the above-mentioned proteins except for K1 and M2 can be grouped into the same protein family based on their limited amino acid sequence homology.[12] Among them, the structures of A52,[32] N1,[25,33] B14[32] and K7[30] have been solved, revealing a similarity with the B-cell lymphoma 2 (Bcl-2) family of proteins, even though the poxvirus proteins share no significant sequence similarity with cellular Bcl-2–like proteins. The cellular Bcl-2 family members are small α-helical proteins containing a surface groove that binds BH3 motifs of pro-apoptotic family members and inhibits their cell death functions. The hydrophobic BH3-peptide binding grooves are occluded in A52, B14 and K7 but not in N1, thus explaining why only N1 inhibits apoptosis. The structure of K7 in complex with a peptide of DDX3 reveals that the DDX3 peptide binds to a negatively charged surface on K7 and buries two critical phenylalanine residues into a hydrophobic pocket on the surface of K7.[30] It is likely that an ancestral poxvirus acquired a Bcl-2 family gene from the host and that gene duplication events followed by extensive evolution gave rise to these structurally-related proteins with different functions.[12]

C12 (IL-18 Binding Protein)

IL-18, a proinflammatory cytokine of the IL-1 family, was formerly known as IFN-γ-inducing factor. Working synergistically with other cytokines such as IL-12, IL-18 activates natural killer (NK) cells, stimulates IFN-γ production from macrophages and T cells, and is required for an effective Th1 response.[6] The activities of IL-18 are regulated in vivo by a naturally-occurring soluble inhibitor of IL-18, the IL-18 binding protein (IL-18BP).[34] The binding of IL-18BP with IL-18 prevents IL-18 from activating the IL-18 receptor.[34] IFN-γ induces the expression of IL-18BP as part of a negative-feedback loop that regulates IL-18 activities.[35]

A poxvirus IL-18BP was first discovered in the human poxvirus molluscum contagiosum virus (MCV).[36] MCV encodes three secreted glycoproteins that share limited sequence homology to cellular IL-18BP, but only one of the three, MC54, binds IL-18 and inhibits IL-18 mediated IFN-γ production. Subsequently, a functional IL-18BP was also identified in orthopoxviruses and Yaba monkey tumor virus.[37-40] Studies with orthopoxviruses with deletion in IL-18BP showed that poxvirus IL-18BP contributes to virulence by down-modulating IL-18-mediated immune responses.[38,41]

Although poxvirus IL-18BPs share a very limited overall sequence homology (20-40% amino acid identities) with cellular IL-18BP, all IL-18BPs bind to IL-18 in a similar manner. A set of seven amino acids was identified in human IL-18BP to contribute to the binding to IL-18.[42] Among them, two aromatic residues, tyr-97 and phe-104, contribute most significantly. Corresponding residues in MCV and ECTV IL-18BPs were also found to be critical for the binding to IL-18.[43,44] The binding affinity of MCV IL-18BP to IL-18 is more than 10-fold weaker than that of human IL-18BP, largely due to a nonconservative phenylalanine to valine substitution at one of seven amino acids.[43] In human IL-18, three residues were identified to be part of the binding site for IL-18BP.[45] Among them, lys-53, contributes most significantly to the binding. These three residues are also part of the binding site for the α subunit of IL-18 receptor (IL-18Rα), suggesting that IL-18BP prevents IL-18 from binding to IL-18 receptor by competitive binding with IL-18Rα.[45] The binding interface identified through mutagenesis and binding studies was confirmed by the crystal structure of the complex between ECTV IL-18BP and human IL-18. IL-18BP adopts a canonical Ig fold, interacting via one edge of its β-sandwich with 3 cavities on the IL-18 surface involving the previously-identified seven residues on IL-18BP and lys-53 on IL-18.[46]

In addition to binding IL-18, MCV and several orthopoxvirus IL-18BPs also associate with cells or with extracellular matrix via interaction with glycosaminoglycans.[47,48] MCV IL-18BP has a long carboxyl tail of nearly 100 amino acids that are dispensable for IL-18 binding but mediate high-affinity binding with glycosaminoglycan.[47] The binding of poxvirus IL-18BPs with glycosaminoglycans may increase their IL-18 binding ability and concentrate them in the immediate vicinity of infected cells, where protection against IL-18 activity may be most needed.

Poxvirus Proteins That Inhibit Signaling of IFNs

Two secreted proteins of VACV bind IFNs and prevent their interactions with cellular receptors. In addition, a poxvirus phosphotase dephosphorylates STATs.

B18 (IFN-α/β Binding Protein)

VACV strain Western Reserve (WR) B18 was the first poxvirus protein that was found to bind and inhibit type I IFNs.[49,50] B18 binds to type III IFNs with a weaker affinity, but it does not block type III IFN-induced signaling.[51] B18 is a secreted glycoprotein with three Ig-like domains. There is only very limited sequence homology between B18 and the type I IFN receptor,[50] which has fibronectin type III domains. In contrast to the cellular receptors, B18 binds IFNs from a broad range of host species, including human, cow, rabbit, rat and mouse. Its affinity to mouse IFNs, however, is significantly lower than to other species.[49] VACV lacking the B18R gene is attenuated in intranasally infected mice.[49] The homologous IFN-α/β binding protein (IFN-α/βBP) in ECTV was found to be a more essential virulence factor in mice, as a 10^7-fold attenuation has been observed in its absence.[52] In addition, the ECTV IFN-α/βBP is an effective target for protective immunization.[52]

B18 binds to cells after secretion via an interaction with glycosaminoglycans (GAGs).[53] The binding is mediated by electrostatic interactions between positively charged amino acids in the first Ig domain of B18 and the sulfate GAG structure.[53] B18 mutants that lack GAG binding activity can still bind IFN with high affinity, but they are unable to block IFN signaling at the cell surface, a critical place for anti-IFN action. Homologous proteins from VARV, MPXV and the more distantly related yaba-like disease virus also bind to cells.[51,54,55]

B8 (IFN-γ Binding Protein)

MYXV M-T7, a major secreted protein from cells infected with MYXV, was the first poxvirus protein found to bind and inhibit IFN-γ.[36] Subsequently, IFN-γ binding proteins (IFN-γBP) were also identified in orthopoxviruses.[57,58] While M-T7 and cellular IFN-γR1 exhibit species-specific binding to their cognate ligand, orthopoxvirus IFN-γBPs show broad species specificity, binding and inhibiting the biological activity of human, bovine, and rat IFN-γ[57]. However, except for ECTV IFN-γBP, orthopoxviruses IFN-γBPs such as VACV B8 bind to murine IFN-γ with reduced affinity,[57,58] largely due to three amino acid difference between IFN-γBPs of ECTV and other orthopoxviruses.[59] The ECTV IFN-γBP is a critical virulence factor for ECTV in mice,[60] while there are conflicting reports as to whether B8 contributes to VACV virulence in mouse models.[61,62]

The N-terminal approximately 200 amino acids of orthopoxvirus IFN-γBP are homologous to the extracellular domain of the human cellular IFN-γR1 chain, while the C-terminal 60 amino acids share no identifiable sequence similarity with cellular proteins. A crystal structure of ECTV IFN-γBP complexed with IFN-γ confirmed that ECTV IFN-γBP residues 17–210 were structurally similar to the extracellular domain of the human cellular IFN-γR1,[63] composed of two fibronectin type III domains containing seven conserved β-strands. However, interactions between IFN-γBP and IFN-γ are more extensive than in the IFN-γR1/IFN-γ complex. In contrast to IFN-γR1, ECTV IFN-γBP forms extensive interactions with the C-terminal tail of IFN-γ,[63] which is highly conserved between IFN-γ from different species. In addition, some species-specific contacts between IFN-γR1 and α-helical regions of IFN-γ are absent in IFN-γBP/IFN-γ complex. These explain the broad species specificity of poxviral IFN-γBPs. The C-terminus of ECTV IFN-γBP adopts a helix-turn-helix structure that is similar to that of the transcription factor TFIIA.[63] It assembles four IFN-γBP chains into an "H"-shaped tetramer, sequestering two dimers of IFN-γ. This is another example of poxvirus acquisition of structural folds that have been adapted for additional functions. Both ECTV and VACV IFN-γBPs exist either as disulfide-linked homodimers or as larger oligomers in solution,[64,65] and the oligomerization is critical for antagonizing IFN-γ activity.[66]

H1

IFN-induced phosphorylation and nuclear transport of STAT1 and STAT2 is inhibited by VACV, and this inhibition is mediated by VACV H1, also known as VH1.[67,68] H1 is the first identified dual specificity phosphatase,[69] which dephosphorylates both phosphotyrosine and phosphoserine/threonine containing substrates. H1 dephosphorylates activated STAT1 and STAT2 but not STAT3 and STAT5.[67] It acts predominantly on the cytoplasmic pool of activated STAT1 prior to nuclear translocation, as it is inactive with respect to STAT1 bound to DNA. Two VACV virion membrane proteins, A17[70] and A14,[71] are also substrates of H1. Unlike other immune modulators, which are expressed early during infection, H1 is expressed late. However, it is packaged in the virion that enters into newly infected cells.[72]

The crystal structure of H1 reveals that H1 forms a stable dimer via an extensive domain swap of the N-terminal helix (residues 1–20).[73] The H1 dimerization domain is not conserved in other dual specificity phosphatases outside poxviruses. While there is no cross-talk between H1 active sites, dimerization appears essential for optimal catalytic activity of H1. Deletion of H1 residue 1–20 results in a monomeric phosphatase that is 120-fold less active than full-length H1.[74]

Poxvirus Proteins That Inhibit Effectors of IFN

The cellular factors that mediate antiviral effects of type I IFN are the products of interferon-stimulated genes (ISGs). Hundreds of ISGs have been identified, but only a few have been characterized with respect to antiviral activity.[75] One of the well-characterized ISGs is the dsRNA-dependent protein kinase R (PKR), consisting of an N-terminal dsRNA-binding domain and a C-terminal kinase domain.[76] PKR is activated by dsRNA produced during viral genome replication or gene transcription, and activated PKR binds and phosphorylates its substrate, the α subunit of translation initiation factor eIF2, on Ser-51.[77] The eIF2 is a GTP-binding protein that is responsible for binding the Met-tRNA to the small ribosomal subunit. Phosphorylation of eIF2α converts eIF2 from a substrate into an inhibitor of its guanine nucleotide exchange factor eIF2B and thereby arrests the exchange of GTP for GDP on eIF2 and consequently the synthesis of viral and host proteins.[78] VACV E3 and K3 inhibit PKR by two distinct mechanisms. In addition, VACV K1 and C7 inhibit a yet unidentified IFN effector or effectors.

E3

VACV E3 protein is comprised of two distinct functional domains.[79] The N-terminus of E3 is homologous to Z-DNA binding proteins,[80] while the C terminus contains a dsRNA binding domain.[81] The primary functions of E3 on IFN are related to its binding to dsRNA, and the C-terminus dsRNA binding domain is essential and sufficient for these functions.[82] E3 sequesters dsRNA produced during viral replication and prevents dsRNA from activating PKR and RLRs,[83-86] which in turn activate transcription factors IRF3, IRF7 and NF-κB, leading to the production of IFN-α/β and proinflammatory cytokines. E3 also blocks DNA-induced IFN-β production by inhibiting the RNA polymerase III-mediated dsDNA-sensing pathway.[87,88] In addition to blocking the induction of IFNs, E3 prevents dsRNA from activating IFN effectors PKR[89] and 2'-5'-oligoadenylate synthetase/RNase L,[90] activation of which results in a global inhibition of protein synthesis through the phosphorylation of eIF2α (for PKR) and degradation of RNA (for RNase L). A direct interaction between E3 and PKR may also contribute to the inhibition of PKR by E3.[91,92] PKR is the main host target of E3 in cultured cells, as deleting or knocking down the PKR gene from HeLa cells can compensate for the deletion of the E3L gene from VACV.[93] However, deleting both PKR and RNase L from the mouse host only partially compensates for the deletion of E3L,[94] suggesting that E3 does more than inhibit PKR and RNase L. Recently, E3 was reported to inhibit interferon-stimulated gene product 15 (ISG15),[95] a ubiquitin-like protein that can be reversibly conjugated to proteins and exerts antiviral effects.[96] E3 binds ISG15 through its C-terminal domain in a manner that is dependent on dsRNA but independent of PKR.[95]

Deletion of the E3L gene from the virus leads to sensitivity to type I IFN,[90] a restricted host range in cell culture[97] and profound attenuation in mice.[98] Although the N-terminal domain of E3 is not required for replication or IFN resistance in cultured cells,[82,99] it is required for full pathogenesis in mice.[98] The structures of the N-terminal domain of E3 and its homolog from Yaba-like disease virus have been determined,[100,101] revealing a helix-turn-helix with β-sheet fold that is very similar to the structure of the Z-DNA binding domain of adenosine deaminase 1 (ADAR1) and the DNA-dependent activator of IFN-regulatory factor (DAI). The N-terminal of E3 has very low affinity to Z-DNA in vitro,[102] but the Z-DNA-binding activity of E3 is required for viral pathogenicity in mice.[80] The N-terminal domain is also involved in the inhibition of ADAR1.[103]

K3

VACV K3 protein is a mimic of the N-terminal 88 amino acids of eIF2α, sharing 28% amino acid sequence identity.[104] K3 acts as a non-phosphorylable pseudosubstrate of PKR, interacting with active PKR to prevent PKR from phosphorylating and inactivating eIF2α.[105-108] Similar to the deletion of the E3L gene, the deletion of the K3L gene from the virus leads to sensitivity of the virus to type I IFN[104,109] and a restricted host range of the virus in cell culture.[110] The K3L deletion mutant is attenuated in mice of either WT or PKR knockout background, suggesting that PKR may not be the exclusive target of K3.[111]

The structure of K3 consists of a five-stranded β-barrel, strikingly similar to eIF2α structure.[112] Furthermore, the site for PKR recognition has been mapped to a surface that is highly conserved between K3 and eIF2α and is remote from the Ser-51 phosphorylation site in eIF2α.[113,114] However, K3 and eIF2α differ in a helix insert region,[112] which includes the Ser-51 phosphorylation site in eIF2α. The helix insert region of free eIF2α must undergo a conformational change in order to position the Ser-51 residue at the active cleft of PKR.[113] In contrast, the helix insert region of K3 directly contacts the active-site cleft of PKR to form a stable complex.[113]

Poxvirus K3 may have driven the rapid evolution of the PKR family. While eIF2α is essentially unchanged in simian primates, several residues of PKR that make direct contacts with eIF2α are among the fastest-evolving residues.[115,116] These residues affect recognition of K3 but not eIF2α, suggesting PKR has evolved to evade inhibition by K3 while maintaining recognition of the unchanging substrate eIF2α.[113,116]

K1 and C7

VACV K1 and C7 were recently shown to inhibit antiviral activities induced by type I IFNs. Deletion of both K1L and C7L render VACV sensitive to IFNs, which block the replication of the mutant virus at the step of translation of viral intermediate genes.[117] K1 and C7 function downstream of IFN signaling by antagonizing IFN effectors. However, the target of K1 or C7 is not among the well-characterized IFN effectors such as PKR and is yet to be identified.[117] Similar to E3 and K3, VACV K1 and C7 control the host-range of VACV.[118-120] VACV requires either K1 or C7 for productive replication in most mammalian cells.[120]

K1 and C7 function equivalently in most mammalian cells, despite having no sequence similarity. The crystal structure of K1 shows that it consists of nine ankyrin (ANK) repeats.[121] The ANK motif is quite common in eukaryotic proteins but is rarely encountered in viral proteins except the poxvirus proteins. ANK repeat adopts a helix-loop-helix-β-hairpin/loop fold, and multiple ANK repeats packs together forming an L shape structure. Different ANK proteins stack various numbers of the repeats with variable surface residues, performing diverse biological functions by interacting specifically with their targets.[122] The interaction usually occurs through a concave surface formed by the β turn and the first α helix of the ANK repeat.[122-125] However, residues that are critical for K1's function have been mapped to the surface opposite the consensus ANK interaction surface,[121] suggesting that K1 functions through ligand interaction with a novel ANK interaction surface. K1 binds to a cellular protein ACAP2,[126,127] a GTPase-activating protein for the small GTPase ARF6. However, this interaction is not essential for K1's functions in viral replication or antagonizing IFNs.[117,127]

Conclusion

Poxviruses have proved to be a gold mine for uncovering viral strategies of IFN modulation, providing insight into mechanisms of viral pathogenesis as well as the functions of IFN. Thirty years ago, soluble binding proteins for IFNs were discovered in poxviruses,[49,50,56] illustrating how viruses inhibit IFNs in the extracellular space. Around the same time, VACV E3 and K3 were found to inhibit IFN-induced antiviral effector PKR,[89,104,105] demonstrating how poxviruses use two different strategies to antagonize a critical intracellular effector of IFN. Over the years, additional cytokine binding proteins have been discovered in poxviruses, including the identification in many poxviruses of a binding protein for IL-18,[36] an IFN-γ-inducing factor. VACV phosphatase H1 was found to inhibit IFN signaling by dephosphorylating STATs.[68] A significant step forward in the last few years has been the identification of a number of poxvirus proteins that inhibit host innate immune signaling pathways such as the activation of transcription factors NF-κB and IRFs.[19,21,24,29,128] Among them is a family of Bcl-2-like proteins that, instead of modulating apoptosis like cellular Bcl-2 proteins, have evolved to inhibit various aspects of NF-κB and/or IRF signaling pathways.[12] Recent years have also witnessed significant progress in our understanding of the cellular innate immune system, particularly the RLR PRRs. Concomitantly, there has been an increased understanding on how E3 inhibits the dsRNA-mediated innate immune response pathways to prevent the induction of IFNs and inflammatory cytokines.[83-86] Most recently, VACV K1 and C7, long known to be critical host-range factors for VACV,[118-120] were found to confer IFN resistance to VACV by inhibiting IFN effector(s).[117]

There remain many unanswered questions with respect to how poxviruses evade IFN activities as well as how IFN exerts antiviral effects. Quite a number of poxvirus proteins have been shown to inhibit NF-κB and/or IRF activation when they are expressed individually in tissue culture cells.[19,21,24,29,128] However, it is less clear what role each of these poxvirus proteins plays in the context of viral infection. Many of these viral proteins target the same signaling pathway, but the deletion from the virus of any single one of the genes encoding these proteins often leads to reduction in virulence in animal models. The degree of virulence reduction also varies for different poxvirus genes. It is unclear whether these poxvirus proteins have redundant functions or whether they work synergistically in infected cells. It is also unclear whether their in vivo targets are the same as their targets in tissue culture cells. While IFN induction and signaling pathways have been well-characterized, comparatively little is known about the effector mechanisms of IFN. Only a few of the hundreds of ISGs have been shown to have antiviral effect. Conversely, very few viral inhibitors of IFN effectors have been discovered. It is thus interesting that K1 and C7 inhibit antiviral activities of IFNs but apparently do not target any well-characterized ISGs.[117] Studying the mechanism by which K1 and C7 antagonize IFN may lead to the identification of a novel IFN-inducible antiviral factor. Many poxvirus proteins that are involved in antagonizing IFNs appear to have been acquired from the host but have undergone extensive evolution in poxviruses. As a result, there is no or very limited primary sequence homology between the viral proteins and their host counterparts, and some viral proteins have acquired different or additional functions. Determination of 3D-structures of the poxvirus proteins often reveals similarity in structure that is not obvious in primary sequence. 3D-structure may also reveal critical differences between the viral proteins and their host counterparts that would explain the divergence of the poxvirus proteins from the traditional roles of their cellular homologs. Additional insights into the mechanisms of poxvirus IFN antagonism will likely be gained through continued studies of the structures of poxvirus proteins.

Acknowledgments

The work performed in Xiang laboratory is supported by NIH grant AI079217

About the Authors

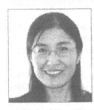

Xiangzhi Meng is a Research Scientist in the Department of Microbiology and Immunology at the University of Texas Health Science Center at San Antonio. Dr. Meng received an equivalent of MD degree from Jining Medical College in China and a PhD from the National Institute for Viral Disease Control and Prevention in China. From 1993 to 2004, she studied hantavirus pathogenesis in China. Since 2004, She has been a member of the Xiang laboratory in San Antonio working on immune evasion mechanisms of poxviruses.

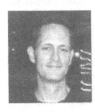

Lloyd Rose is a PhD candidate in the Department of Microbiology and Immunology at the University of Texas Health Science Center at San Antonio. He received his Bachelor of Science degree in Microbiology from the University of Texas at Austin in 2006 and began his graduate studies in San Antonio in the same year. He joined the Xiang laboratory in 2008 and is currently studying the interaction between vaccinia virus and the host cell environment.

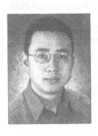

Yan Xiang is an Associate Professor in the Department of Microbiology and Immunology at the University of Texas Health Science Center at San Antonio. Dr. Xiang received his PhD in 1997 from Case Western Reserve University in Cleveland, Ohio studying retroviruses in the laboratory of Dr. Jonathan Leis. From 1998 to 2002, he was a postdoctoral fellow in the laboratory of Dr. Bernard Moss at National Institutes of Health studying the immune evasion mechanisms of poxviruses. In 2002, Dr. Xiang started as an Assistant Professor at the University of Texas Health Science Center at San Antonio, where his group has continued to study various aspects of poxvirus-host interactions.

References

1. Platanias LC. Mechanisms of type-I- and type-II-interferon-mediated signalling. Nat Rev Immunol 2005; 5:375-86; PMID:15864272; http://dx.doi.org/10.1038/nri1604.
2. Kotenko SV, Gallagher G, Baurin VV, Lewis-Antes A, Shen M, Shah NK, et al. IFN-lambdas mediate antiviral protection through a distinct class II cytokine receptor complex. Nat Immunol 2003; 4:69-77; PMID:12483210; http://dx.doi.org/10.1038/ni875.
3. Wilkins C, Gale M Jr. Recognition of viruses by cytoplasmic sensors. Curr Opin Immunol 2010; 22:41-7; PMID:20061127; http://dx.doi.org/10.1016/j.coi.2009.12.003.
4. Lee MS, Kim YJ. Signaling pathways downstream of pattern-recognition receptors and their cross talk. Annu Rev Biochem 2007; 76:447-80; PMID:17328678; http://dx.doi.org/10.1146/annurev. biochem.76.060605.122847.
5. Munder M, Mallo M, Eichmann K, Modolell M. Murine macrophages secrete interferon gamma upon combined stimulation with interleukin (IL)-12 and IL-18: A novel pathway of autocrine macrophage activation. J Exp Med 1998; 187:2103-8; PMID:9625771; http://dx.doi.org/10.1084/jem.187.12.2103.
6. Dinarello CA. Interleukin-18. Methods 1999; 19:121-32; PMID:10525448; http://dx.doi.org/10.1006/ meth.1999.0837.
7. Iversen MB, Paludan SR. Mechanisms of type III interferon expression. J Interferon Cytokine Res 2010; 30:573-8; PMID:20645874; http://dx.doi.org/10.1089/jir.2010.0063.
8. Randall RE, Goodbourn S. Interferons and viruses: an interplay between induction, signalling, antiviral responses and virus countermeasures. J Gen Virol 2008; 89:1-47; PMID:18089727; http://dx.doi. org/10.1099/vir.0.83391-0.
9. Perdiguero B, Esteban M. The interferon system and vaccinia virus evasion mechanisms. J Interferon Cytokine Res 2009; 29:581-98; PMID:19708815; http://dx.doi.org/10.1089/jir.2009.0073.
10. Moss B. Poxviridae: the viruses and their replication. In: Knipe DM, Howley PM, eds. Fields Virology, Vol 2. Philadelphia: Lippincott Williams & Wilkins, 2007:2905-2946.
11. Johnston JB, McFadden G. Poxvirus immunomodulatory strategies: current perspectives. J Virol 2003; 77:6093-100; PMID:12743266; http://dx.doi.org/10.1128/JVI.77.11.6093-6100.2003.

12. Bahar MW, Graham SC, Chen RA, Cooray S, Smith GL, Stuart DI, et al. How vaccinia virus has evolved to subvert the host immune response. J Struct Biol 2011; 175:127-34; PMID:21419849; http://dx.doi.org/10.1016/j.jsb.2011.03.010.

13. Rahman MM, McFadden G. Modulation of NF-kappaB signalling by microbial pathogens. Nat Rev Microbiol 2011; 9:291-306; PMID:21383764; http://dx.doi.org/10.1038/nrmicro2539.

14. Akira S, Takeda K. Toll-like receptor signalling. Nat Rev Immunol 2004; 4:499-511; PMID:15229469; http://dx.doi.org/10.1038/nri1391.

15. Stack J, Haga IR, Schroder M, Bartlett NW, Maloney G, Reading PC, et al. Vaccinia virus protein A46R targets multiple Toll-like-interleukin-1 receptor adaptors and contributes to virulence. J Exp Med 2005; 201:1007-18; PMID:15767367; http://dx.doi.org/10.1084/jem.20041442.

16. Harte MT, Haga IR, Maloney G, Gray P, Reading PC, Bartlett NW, et al. The poxvirus protein A52R targets Toll-like receptor signaling complexes to suppress host defense. J Exp Med 2003; 197:343-51; PMID:12566418; http://dx.doi.org/10.1084/jem.20021652.

17. Maloney G, Schroder M, Bowie AG. Vaccinia virus protein A52R activates p38 mitogen-activated protein kinase and potentiates lipopolysaccharide-induced interleukin-10. J Biol Chem 2005; 280:30838-44; PMID:15998638; http://dx.doi.org/10.1074/jbc.M501917200.

18. Israël A. The IKK complex, a central regulator of NF-kappaB activation. Cold Spring Harb Perspect Biol 2010; 2:a000158; PMID:20300203; http://dx.doi.org/10.1101/cshperspect.a000158.

19. Chen RA, Ryzhakov G, Cooray S, Randow F, Smith GL. Inhibition of IkappaB kinase by vaccinia virus virulence factor B14. PLoS Pathog 2008; 4:e22; PMID:18266467; http://dx.doi.org/10.1371/journal.ppat.0040022.

20. Oeckinghaus A, Hayden MS, Ghosh S. Crosstalk in NF-kappaB signaling pathways. Nat Immunol 2011; 12:695-708; PMID:21772278; http://dx.doi.org/10.1038/ni.2065.

21. Shisler JL, Jin XL. The vaccinia virus K1L gene product inhibits host NF-kappaB activation by preventing IkappaBalpha degradation. J Virol 2004; 78:3553-60; PMID:15016878; http://dx.doi.org/10.1128/JVI.78.7.3553-3560.2004.

22. Gedey R, Jin XL, Hinthong O, Shisler JL. Poxviral regulation of the host NF-kappaB response: the vaccinia virus M2L protein inhibits induction of NF-kappaB activation via an ERK2 pathway in virus-infected human embryonic kidney cells. J Virol 2006; 80:8676-85; PMID:16912315; http://dx.doi.org/10.1128/JVI.00935-06.

23. Chau TL, Gioia R, Gatot JS, Patrascu F, Carpentier I, Chapelle JP, et al. Are the IKKs and IKK-related kinases TBK1 and IKK-epsilon similarly activated? Trends Biochem Sci 2008; 33:171-80; PMID:18353649; http://dx.doi.org/10.1016/j.tibs.2008.01.002.

24. DiPerna G, Stack J, Bowie AG, Boyd A, Kotwal G, Zhang Z, et al. Poxvirus Protein N1L Targets the I-{kappa}B Kinase Complex, Inhibits Signaling to NF-{kappa}B by the Tumor Necrosis Factor Superfamily of Receptors, and Inhibits NF-{kappa}B and IRF3 Signaling by Toll-like Receptors. J Biol Chem 2004; 279:36570-8; PMID:15215253; http://dx.doi.org/10.1074/jbc.M400567200.

25. Cooray S, Bahar MW, Abrescia NG, McVey CE, Bartlett NW, Chen RA, et al. Functional and structural studies of the vaccinia virus virulence factor N1 reveal a Bcl-2-like anti-apoptotic protein. J Gen Virol 2007; 88:1656-66; PMID:17485524; http://dx.doi.org/10.1099/vir.0.82772-0.

26. Guo B, Cheng G. Modulation of the interferon antiviral response by the TBK1/IKKi adaptor protein TANK. J Biol Chem 2007; 282:11817-26; PMID:17327220; http://dx.doi.org/10.1074/jbc.M700017200.

27. Ryzhakov G, Randow F. SINTBAD, a novel component of innate antiviral immunity, shares a TBK1-binding domain with NAP1 and TANK. EMBO J 2007; 26:3180-90; PMID:17568778; http://dx.doi.org/10.1038/sj.emboj.7601743.

28. Sasai M, Shingai M, Funami K, Yoneyama M, Fujita T, Matsumoto M, et al. NAK-associated protein 1 participates in both the TLR3 and the cytoplasmic pathways in type I IFN induction. J Immunol 2006; 177:8676-83; PMID:17142768.

29. Unterholzner L, Sumner RP, Baran M, Ren H, Mansur DS, Bourke NM, et al. Vaccinia virus protein C6 is a virulence factor that binds TBK-1 adaptor proteins and inhibits activation of IRF3 and IRF7. PLoS Pathog 2011; 7:e1002247; PMID:21931555; http://dx.doi.org/10.1371/journal.ppat.1002247.

30. Kalverda AP, Thompson GS, Vogel A, Schröder M, Bowie AG, Khan AR, et al. Poxvirus K7 protein adopts a Bcl-2 fold: biochemical mapping of its interactions with human DEAD box RNA helicase DDX3. J Mol Biol 2009; 385:843-53; PMID:18845156; http://dx.doi.org/10.1016/j.jmb.2008.09.048.

31. Oda S, Schroder M, Khan AR. Structural basis for targeting of human RNA helicase DDX3 by poxvirus protein K7. Structure 2009; 17:1528-37; PMID:19913487; http://dx.doi.org/10.1016/j.str.2009.09.005.

32. Graham SC, Bahar MW, Cooray S, Chen RA, Whalen DM, Abrescia NG, et al. Vaccinia virus proteins A52 and B14 Share a Bcl-2-like fold but have evolved to inhibit NF-kappaB rather than apoptosis. PLoS Pathog 2008; 4:e1000128; PMID:18704168; http://dx.doi.org/10.1371/journal.ppat.1000128.

33. Aoyagi M, Zhai D, Jin C, Aleshin AE, Stec B, Reed JC, et al. Vaccinia virus N1L protein resembles a B cell lymphoma-2 (Bcl-2) family protein. Protein Sci 2007; 16:118-24; PMID:17123957; http://dx.doi.org/10.1110/ps.062454707.

34. Novick D, Kim SH, Fantuzzi G, Reznikov LL, Dinarello CA, Rubinstein M. Interleukin-18 binding protein: a novel modulator of the Th1 cytokine response. Immunity 1999; 10:127-36; PMID:10023777; http://dx.doi.org/10.1016/S1074-7613(00)80013-8.

35. Mühl H, Kampfer H, Bosmann M, Frank S, Radeke H, Pfeilschifter J. Interferon-gamma mediates gene expression of IL-18 binding protein in nonleukocytic cells. Biochem Biophys Res Commun 2000; 267:960-3; PMID:10673399; http://dx.doi.org/10.1006/bbrc.1999.2064.

36. Xiang Y, Moss B. IL-18 binding and inhibition of interferon gamma induction by human poxvirus-encoded proteins. Proc Natl Acad Sci USA 1999; 96:11537-42; PMID:10500212; http://dx.doi.org/10.1073/pnas.96.20.11537.

37. Calderara S, Xiang Y, Moss B. Orthopoxvirus IL-18 binding proteins: affinities and antagonist activities. Virology 2001; 279:22-6; PMID:11145885; http://dx.doi.org/10.1006/viro.2000.0689.

38. Born TL, Morrison LA, Esteban DJ, VandenBos T, Thebeau LG, Chen N, et al. A poxvirus protein that binds to and inactivates IL-18, and inhibits NK cell response. J Immunol 2000; 164:3246-54; PMID:10706717.

39. Smith VP, Bryant NA, Alcami A. Ectromelia, vaccinia and cowpox viruses encode secreted interleukin-18-binding proteins. J Gen Virol 2000; 81:1223-30; PMID:10769064.

40. Nazarian SH, Rahman MM, Werden SJ, Villeneuve D, Meng X, Brunetti C, et al. Yaba monkey tumor virus encodes a functional inhibitor of interleukin-18. J Virol 2008; 82:522-8; PMID:17959666; http://dx.doi.org/10.1128/JVI.00688-07.

41. Reading PC, Smith GL. Vaccinia Virus Interleukin-18-Binding Protein Promotes Virulence by Reducing Gamma Interferon Production and Natural Killer and T-Cell Activity. J Virol 2003; 77:9960-8; PMID:12941906; http://dx.doi.org/10.1128/JVI.77.18.9960-9968.2003.

42. Xiang Y, Moss B. Determination of the functional epitopes of human interleukin-18-binding protein by site-directed mutagenesis. J Biol Chem 2001; 276:17380-6; PMID:11278524; http://dx.doi.org/10.1074/jbc.M009581200.

43. Xiang Y, Moss B. Correspondence of the functional epitopes of poxvirus and human interleukin-18-binding proteins. J Virol 2001; 75:9947-54; PMID:11559827; http://dx.doi.org/10.1128/JVI.75.20.9947-9954.2001.

44. Esteban DJ, Buller RM. Identification of residues in an orthopoxvirus interleukin-18 binding protein involved in ligand binding and species specificity. Virology 2004; 323:197-207; PMID:15193916; http://dx.doi.org/10.1016/j.virol.2004.02.027.

45. Meng X, Leman M, Xiang Y. Variola virus IL-18 binding protein interacts with three human IL-18 residues that are part of a binding site for human IL-18 receptor alpha subunit. Virology 2007; 358:211-20; PMID:16979683; http://dx.doi.org/10.1016/j.virol.2006.08.019.

46. Krumm B, Meng X, Li Y, Xiang Y, Deng J. Structural basis for antagonism of human interleukin 18 by poxvirus interleukin 18-binding protein. Proc Natl Acad Sci USA 2008; 105:20711-5; PMID:19104048; http://dx.doi.org/10.1073/pnas.0809086106.

47. Xiang Y, Moss B. Molluscum contagiosum virus interleukin-18 (IL-18) binding protein is secreted as a full-length form that binds cell surface glycosaminoglycans through the C-terminal tail and a furin-cleaved form with only the IL-18 binding domain. J Virol 2003; 77:2623-30; PMID:12552001; http://dx.doi.org/10.1128/JVI.77.4.2623-2630.2003.

48. Esteban DJ, Nuara AA, Buller RM. Interleukin-18 and glycosaminoglycan binding by a protein encoded by Variola virus. J Gen Virol 2004; 85:1291-9; PMID:15105546; http://dx.doi.org/10.1099/vir.0.79902-0.

49. Symons JA, Alcami A, Smith GL. Vaccinia virus encodes a soluble type I interferon receptor of novel structure and broad species specificity. Cell 1995; 81:551-60; PMID:7758109; http://dx.doi.org/10.1016/0092-8674(95)90076-4.

50. Colamonici OR, Domanski P, Sweitzer SM, Larner A, Buller RM. Vaccinia virus B18R gene encodes a type I interferon-binding protein that blocks interferon alpha transmembrane signaling. J Biol Chem 1995; 270:15974-8; PMID:7608155; http://dx.doi.org/10.1074/jbc.270.27.15974.

51. Fernández de Marco Mdel M, Alejo A, Hudson P, Damon IK, Alcami A. The highly virulent variola and monkeypox viruses express secreted inhibitors of type I interferon. FASEB J 2010; 24:1479-88; PMID:20019241; http://dx.doi.org/10.1096/fj.09-144733.

52. Xu R-H, Cohen M, Tang Y, Lazear E, Whitbeck JC, Eisenberg RJ, et al. The orthopoxvirus type I IFN binding protein is essential for virulence and an effective target for vaccination. J Exp Med 2008; 205:981-92; PMID:18391063; http://dx.doi.org/10.1084/jem.20071854.

53. Alcamí A, Symons JA, Smith GL. The vaccinia virus soluble alpha/beta interferon (IFN) receptor binds to the cell surface and protects cells from the antiviral effects of IFN. J Virol 2000; 74:11230-9; PMID:11070021; http://dx.doi.org/10.1128/JVI.74.23.11230-11239.2000.
54. Montanuy I, Alejo A, Alcami A. Glycosaminoglycans mediate retention of the poxvirus type I interferon binding protein at the cell surface to locally block interferon antiviral responses. FASEB J 2011; 25:1960-71; PMID:21372110; http://dx.doi.org/10.1096/fj.10-177188.
55. Huang J, Smirnov SV, Lewis-Antes A, Li W, Tang S, Silke GV, et al. Inhibition of type I and type III interferons by a secreted glycoprotein from Yaba-like disease virus. Proc Natl Acad Sci USA 2007; 104:9822-7; PMID:17517620; http://dx.doi.org/10.1073/pnas.0610352104.
56. Upton C, Mossman K, McFadden G. Encoding of a homolog of the IFN-gamma receptor by myxoma virus. Science 1992; 258:1369-72; PMID:1455233; http://dx.doi.org/10.1126/science.1455233.
57. Alcami A, Smith GL. Vaccinia, cowpox, and camelpox viruses encode soluble gamma interferon receptors with novel broad species specificity. J Virol 1995; 69:4633-9; PMID:7609027.
58. Mossman K, Upton C, Buller RM, McFadden G. Species specificity of ectromelia virus and vaccinia virus interferon-gamma binding proteins. Virology 1995; 208:762-9; PMID:7747448; http://dx.doi.org/10.1006/viro.1995.1208.
59. Nuara AA, Buller RM, Bai H. Identification of residues in the ectromelia virus gamma interferon-binding protein involved in expanded species specificity. J Gen Virol 2007; 88:51-60; PMID:17170436; http://dx.doi.org/10.1099/vir.0.82324-0.
60. Sakala IG, Chaudhri G, Buller RM, Nuara AA, Bai H, Chen N, et al. Poxvirus-encoded gamma interferon binding protein dampens the host immune response to infection. J Virol 2007; 81:3346-53; PMID:17229697; http://dx.doi.org/10.1128/JVI.01927-06.
61. Symons JA, Tscharke DC, Price N, Smith GL. A study of the vaccinia virus interferon-gamma receptor and its contribution to virus virulence. J Gen Virol 2002; 83:1953-64; PMID:12124459.
62. Verardi PH, Jones LA, Aziz FH, Ahmad S, Yilma TD. Vaccinia virus vectors with an inactivated gamma interferon receptor homolog gene (B8R) are attenuated In vivo without a concomitant reduction in immunogenicity. J Virol 2001; 75:11-8; PMID:11119568; http://dx.doi.org/10.1128/JVI.75.1.11-18.2001.
63. Nuara AA, Walter LJ, Logsdon NJ, Yoon SI, Jones BC, Schriewer JM, et al. Structure and mechanism of IFN-gamma antagonism by an orthopoxvirus IFN-gamma-binding protein. Proc Natl Acad Sci USA 2008; 105:1861-6; PMID:18252829; http://dx.doi.org/10.1073/pnas.0705753105.
64. Alcamí A, Smith GL. The vaccinia virus soluble interferon-gamma receptor is a homodimer. J Gen Virol 2002; 83:545-9; PMID:11842249.
65. Bai H, Buller RM, Chen N, Green M, Nuara AA. Biosynthesis of the IFN-gamma binding protein of ectromelia virus, the causative agent of mousepox. Virology 2005; 334:41-50; PMID:15749121; http://dx.doi.org/10.1016/j.virol.2005.01.015.
66. Nuara AA, Bai H, Chen N, Buller RM, Walter MR. The unique C termini of orthopoxvirus gamma interferon binding proteins are essential for ligand binding. J Virol 2006; 80:10675-82; PMID:16928759; http://dx.doi.org/10.1128/JVI.01015-06.
67. Mann BA, Huang JH, Li P, Chang HC, Slee RB, O'Sullivan A, et al. Vaccinia virus blocks Stat1-dependent and Stat1-independent gene expression induced by type I and type II interferons. J Interferon Cytokine Res 2008; 28:367-80; PMID:18593332; http://dx.doi.org/10.1089/jir.2007.0113.
68. Najarro P, Traktman P, Lewis JA. Vaccinia virus blocks gamma interferon signal transduction: viral VH1 phosphatase reverses Stat1 activation. J Virol 2001; 75:3185-96; PMID:11238845; http://dx.doi.org/10.1128/JVI.75.7.3185-3196.2001.
69. Guan KL, Broyles SS, Dixon JEA. Tyr/Ser protein phosphatase encoded by vaccinia virus. Nature 1991; 350:359-62; PMID:1848923; http://dx.doi.org/10.1038/350359a0.
70. Derrien M, Punjabi A, Khanna M, Grubisha O, Traktman P. Tyrosine phosphorylation of A17 during vaccinia virus infection: involvement of the H1 phosphatase and the F10 kinase. J Virol 1999; 73:7287-96; PMID:10438817.
71. Traktman P, Liu K, DeMasi J, Rollins R, Jesty S, Unger B. Elucidating the essential role of the A14 phosphoprotein in vaccinia virus morphogenesis: construction and characterization of a tetracycline-inducible recombinant. J Virol 2000; 74:3682-95; PMID:10729144; http://dx.doi.org/10.1128/JVI.74.8.3682-3695.2000.
72. Chung CS, Chen CH, Ho MY, Huang CY, Liao CL, Chang W. Vaccinia virus proteome: identification of proteins in vaccinia virus intracellular mature virion particles. J Virol 2006; 80:2127-40; PMID:16474121; http://dx.doi.org/10.1128/JVI.80.5.2127-2140.2006.
73. Koksal AC, Nardozzi JD, Cingolani G. Dimeric quaternary structure of the prototypical dual specificity phosphatase VH1. J Biol Chem 2009; 284:10129-37; PMID:19211553; http://dx.doi.org/10.1074/jbc.M808362200.

74. Koksal AC, Cingolani G. Dimerization of Vaccinia Virus VH1 Is Essential for Dephosphorylation of STAT1 at Tyrosine 701. J Biol Chem 2011; 286:14373-82; PMID:21362620; http://dx.doi.org/10.1074/jbc.M111.226357.

75. de Veer MJ, Holko M, Frevel M, Walker E, Der S, Paranjape JM, et al. Functional classification of interferon-stimulated genes identified using microarrays. J Leukoc Biol 2001; 69:912-20; PMID:11404376.

76. Pindel A, Sadler A. The role of protein kinase R in the interferon response. J Interferon Cytokine Res 2011; 31:59-70; PMID:21166592; http://dx.doi.org/10.1089/jir.2010.0099.

77. Dey M, Cao C, Dar AC, Tamura T, Ozato K, Sicheri F, et al. Mechanistic link between PKR dimerization, autophosphorylation, and eIF2alpha substrate recognition. Cell 2005; 122:901-13; PMID:16179259; http://dx.doi.org/10.1016/j.cell.2005.06.041.

78. Sonenberg N, Dever TE. Eukaryotic translation initiation factors and regulators. Curr Opin Struct Biol 2003; 13:56-63; PMID:12581660; http://dx.doi.org/10.1016/S0959-440X(03)00009-5.

79. Ho CK, Shuman S. Physical and functional characterization of the double-stranded RNA binding protein encoded by the vaccinia virus E3 gene. Virology 1996; 217:272-84; PMID:8599212; http://dx.doi.org/10.1006/viro.1996.0114.

80. Kim YG, Muralinath M, Brandt T, Pearcy M, Hauns K, Lowenhaupt K, et al. A role for Z-DNA binding in vaccinia virus pathogenesis. Proc Natl Acad Sci USA 2003; 100:6974-9; PMID:12777633; http://dx.doi.org/10.1073/pnas.0431131100.

81. Chang HW, Jacobs BL. Identification of a conserved motif that is necessary for binding of the vaccinia virus E3L gene products to double-stranded RNA. Virology 1993; 194:537-47; PMID:8099244; http://dx.doi.org/10.1006/viro.1993.1292.

82. Shors T, Kibler KV, Perkins KB, Seidler-Wulff R, Banaszak MP, Jacobs BL. Complementation of vaccinia virus deleted of the E3L gene by mutants of E3L. Virology 1997; 239:269-76; PMID:9434718; http://dx.doi.org/10.1006/viro.1997.8881.

83. Langland JO, Kash JC, Carter V, Thomas MJ, Katze MG, Jacobs BL. Suppression of Proinflammatory Signal Transduction and Gene Expression by the Dual Nucleic Acid Binding Domains of the Vaccinia Virus E3L Proteins. J Virol 2006; 80:10083-95; PMID:17005686; http://dx.doi.org/10.1128/JVI.00607-06.

84. Myskiw C, Arsenio J, van Bruggen R, Deschambault Y, Cao J. Vaccinia virus E3 suppresses expression of diverse cytokines through inhibition of the PKR, NF-kappaB, and IRF3 pathways. J Virol 2009; 83:6757-68; PMID:19369349; http://dx.doi.org/10.1128/JVI.02570-08.

85. Deng L, Dai P, Parikh T, Cao H, Bhoj V, Sun Q, et al. Vaccinia virus subverts a mitochondrial antiviral signaling protein-dependent innate immune response in keratinocytes through its double-stranded RNA binding protein, E3. J Virol 2008; 82:10735-46; PMID:18715932; http://dx.doi.org/10.1128/JVI.01305-08.

86. Smith EJ, Marie I, Prakash A, Garcia-Sastre A, Levy DE. IRF3 and IRF7 phosphorylation in virus-infected cells does not require double-stranded RNA-dependent protein kinase R or Ikappa B kinase but is blocked by Vaccinia virus E3L protein. J Biol Chem 2001; 276:8951-7; PMID:11124948; http://dx.doi.org/10.1074/jbc.M008717200.

87. Marq JB, Hausmann S, Luban J, Kolakofsky D, Garcin D. The double-stranded RNA binding domain of the vaccinia virus E3L protein inhibits both RNA- and DNA-induced activation of interferon beta. J Biol Chem 2009; 284:25471-8; PMID:19584049; http://dx.doi.org/10.1074/jbc.M109.018895.

88. Valentine R, Smith GL. Inhibition of the RNA polymerase III-mediated dsDNA-sensing pathway of innate immunity by vaccinia virus protein E3. J Gen Virol 2010; 91:2221-9; PMID:20519457; http://dx.doi.org/10.1099/vir.0.021998-0.

89. Chang HW, Watson JC, Jacobs BL. The E3L gene of vaccinia virus encodes an inhibitor of the interferon-induced, double-stranded RNA-dependent protein kinase. Proc Natl Acad Sci USA 1992; 89:4825-9; PMID:1350676; http://dx.doi.org/10.1073/pnas.89.11.4825.

90. Beattie E, Denzler KL, Tartaglia J, Perkus ME, Paoletti E, Jacobs BL. Reversal of the interferon-sensitive phenotype of a vaccinia virus lacking E3L by expression of the reovirus S4 gene. J Virol 1995; 69:499-505; PMID:7527085.

91. Romano PR, Zhang F, Tan SL, Garcia-Barrio MT, Katze MG, Dever TE, et al. Inhibition of double-stranded RNA-dependent protein kinase PKR by vaccinia virus E3: role of complex formation and the E3 N-terminal domain. Mol Cell Biol 1998; 18:7304-16; PMID:9819417.

92. Sharp TV, Moonan F, Romashko A, Joshi B, Barber GN, Jagus R. The vaccinia virus E3L gene product interacts with both the regulatory and the substrate binding regions of PKR: implications for PKR autoregulation. Virology 1998; 250:302-15; PMID:9792841; http://dx.doi.org/10.1006/viro.1998.9365.

93. Zhang P, Jacobs BL, Samuel CE. Loss of protein kinase PKR expression in human HeLa cells complements the vaccinia virus E3L deletion mutant phenotype by restoration of viral protein synthesis. J Virol 2008; 82:840-8; PMID:17959656; http://dx.doi.org/10.1128/JVI.01891-07.

94. Xiang Y, Condit RC, Vijaysri S, Jacobs B, Williams BRG, Silverman RH. Blockade of Interferon Induction and Action by the E3L Double-Stranded RNA Binding Proteins of Vaccinia Virus. J Virol 2002; 76:5251-9; PMID:11967338; http://dx.doi.org/10.1128/JVI.76.10.5251-5259.2002.
95. Guerra S, Caceres A, Knobeloch KP, Horak I, Esteban M. Vaccinia virus E3 protein prevents the antiviral action of ISG15. PLoS Pathog 2008; 4:e1000096; PMID:18604270; http://dx.doi.org/10.1371/journal.ppat.1000096.
96. Skaug B, Chen ZJ. Emerging role of ISG15 in antiviral immunity. Cell 2010; 143:187-90; PMID:20946978; http://dx.doi.org/10.1016/j.cell.2010.09.033.
97. Beattie E, Kauffman EB, Martinez H, Perkus ME, Jacobs BL, Paoletti E, et al. Host-range restriction of vaccinia virus E3L-specific deletion mutants. Virus Genes 1996; 12:89-94; PMID:8879125; http://dx.doi.org/10.1007/BF00370005.
98. Brandt TA, Jacobs BL. Both carboxy- and amino-terminal domains of the vaccinia virus interferon resistance gene, E3L, are required for pathogenesis in a mouse model. J Virol 2001; 75:850-6; PMID:11134298; http://dx.doi.org/10.1128/JVI.75.2.850-856.2001.
99. Chang HW, Uribe LH, Jacobs BL. Rescue of vaccinia virus lacking the E3L gene by mutants of E3L. J Virol 1995; 69:6605-8; PMID:7666567.
100. Kahmann JD, Wecking DA, Putter V, Lowenhaupt K, Kim YG, Schmieder P, et al. The solution structure of the N-terminal domain of E3L shows a tyrosine conformation that may explain its reduced affinity to Z-DNA in vitro. Proc Natl Acad Sci USA 2004; 101:2712-7; PMID:14981270; http://dx.doi.org/10.1073/pnas.0308612100.
101. Ha SC, Lokanath NK, Van Quyen D, Wu CA, Lowenhaupt K, Rich A, et al. A poxvirus protein forms a complex with left-handed Z-DNA: crystal structure of a Yatapoxvirus Zalpha bound to DNA. Proc Natl Acad Sci USA 2004; 101:14367-72; PMID:15448208; http://dx.doi.org/10.1073/pnas.0405586101.
102. Kim YG, Lowenhaupt K, Oh DB, Kim KK, Rich A. Evidence that vaccinia virulence factor E3L binds to Z-DNA in vivo: Implications for development of a therapy for poxvirus infection. Proc Natl Acad Sci USA 2004; 101:1514-8; PMID:14757814; http://dx.doi.org/10.1073/pnas.0308260100.
103. Liu Y, Wolff KC, Jacobs BL, Samuel CE. Vaccinia virus E3L interferon resistance protein inhibits the interferon-induced adenosine deaminase A-to-I editing activity. Virology 2001; 289:378-87; PMID:11689059; http://dx.doi.org/10.1006/viro.2001.1154.
104. Beattie E, Tartaglia J, Paoletti E. Vaccinia virus-encoded eIF-2 alpha homolog abrogates the antiviral effect of interferon. Virology 1991; 183:419-22; PMID:1711259; http://dx.doi.org/10.1016/0042-6822(91)90158-8.
105. Davies MV, Chang HW, Jacobs BL, Kaufman RJ. The E3L and K3L vaccinia virus gene products stimulate translation through inhibition of the double-stranded RNA-dependent protein kinase by different mechanisms. J Virol 1993; 67:1688-92; PMID:8094759.
106. Davies MV, Elroy-Stein O, Jagus R, Moss B, Kaufman RJ. The vaccinia virus K3L gene product potentiates translation by inhibiting double-stranded-RNA-activated protein kinase and phosphorylation of the alpha subunit of eukaryotic initiation factor 2. J Virol 1992; 66:1943-50; PMID:1347793.
107. Jagus R, Gray MM. Proteins that interact with PKR. Biochimie 1994; 76:779-91; PMID:7893827; http://dx.doi.org/10.1016/0300-9084(94)90082-5.
108. Carroll K, Elroy-Stein O, Moss B, Jagus R. Recombinant vaccinia virus K3L gene product prevents activation of double-stranded RNA-dependent, initiation factor 2 alpha-specific protein kinase. J Biol Chem 1993; 268:12837-42; PMID:8099586.
109. Beattie E, Paoletti E, Tartaglia J. Distinct patterns of IFN sensitivity observed in cells infected with vaccinia K3L- and E3L- mutant viruses. Virology 1995; 210:254-63; PMID:7542414; http://dx.doi.org/10.1006/viro.1995.1342.
110. Langland JO, Jacobs BL. The role of the PKR-inhibitory genes, E3L and K3L, in determining vaccinia virus host range. Virology 2002; 299:133-41; PMID:12167348; http://dx.doi.org/10.1006/viro.2002.1479.
111. Rice AD, Turner PC, Embury JE, Moldawer LL, Baker HV, Moyer RW. Roles of vaccinia virus genes E3L and K3L and host genes PKR and RNase L during intratracheal infection of C57BL/6 mice. J Virol 2011; 85:550-67; PMID:20943971; http://dx.doi.org/10.1128/JVI.00254-10.
112. Dar AC, Sicheri F. X-ray crystal structure and functional analysis of vaccinia virus K3L reveals molecular determinants for PKR subversion and substrate recognition. Mol Cell 2002; 10:295-305; PMID:12191475; http://dx.doi.org/10.1016/S1097-2765(02)00590-7.
113. Dar AC, Dever TE, Sicheri F. Higher-order substrate recognition of eIF2alpha by the RNA-dependent protein kinase PKR. Cell 2005; 122:887-900; PMID:16179258; http://dx.doi.org/10.1016/j.cell.2005.06.044.
114. Kawagishi-Kobayashi M, Silverman JB, Ung TL, Dever TE. Regulation of the protein kinase PKR by the vaccinia virus pseudosubstrate inhibitor K3L is dependent on residues conserved between the K3L protein and the PKR substrate eIF2alpha. Mol Cell Biol 1997; 17:4146-58; PMID:9199350.

115. Rothenburg S, Seo EJ, Gibbs JS, Dever TE, Dittmar K. Rapid evolution of protein kinase PKR alters sensitivity to viral inhibitors. Nat Struct Mol Biol 2009; 16:63-70; PMID:19043413; http://dx.doi.org/10.1038/nsmb.1529.
116. Elde NC, Child SJ, Geballe AP, Malik HS. Protein kinase R reveals an evolutionary model for defeating viral mimicry. Nature 2009; 457:485-9; PMID:19043403; http://dx.doi.org/10.1038/nature07529.
117. Meng X, Jiang C, Arsenio J, Dick K, Cao J, Xiang Y. Vaccinia virus K1L and C7L inhibit antiviral activities induced by type I interferons. J Virol 2009; 83:10627-36; PMID:19656868; http://dx.doi.org/10.1128/JVI.01260-09.
118. Meng X, Chao J, Xiang Y. Identification from diverse mammalian poxviruses of host-range regulatory genes functioning equivalently to vaccinia virus C7L. Virology 2008; 372:372-83; PMID:18054061; http://dx.doi.org/10.1016/j.virol.2007.10.023.
119. Gillard S, Spehner D, Drillien R, Kirn A. Localization and sequence of a vaccinia virus gene required for multiplication in human cells. Proc Natl Acad Sci USA 1986; 83:5573-7; PMID:3461450; http://dx.doi.org/10.1073/pnas.83.15.5573.
120. Perkus ME, Goebel SJ, Davis SW, et al. Vaccinia virus host range genes. Virology 1990; 179:276-86; PMID:2171207; http://dx.doi.org/10.1016/0042-6822(90)90296-4.
121. Li Y, Meng X, Xiang Y, Deng J. Structure function studies of vaccinia virus host range protein k1 reveal a novel functional surface for ankyrin repeat proteins. J Virol 2010; 84:3331-8; PMID:20089642; http://dx.doi.org/10.1128/JVI.02332-09.
122. Sedgwick SG, Smerdon SJ. The ankyrin repeat: a diversity of interactions on a common structural framework. Trends Biochem Sci 1999; 24:311-6; PMID:10431175; http://dx.doi.org/10.1016/S0968-0004(99)01426-7.
123. Binz HK, Amstutz P, Kohl A, Stumpp MT, Briand C, Forrer P, et al. High-affinity binders selected from designed ankyrin repeat protein libraries. Nat Biotechnol 2004; 22:575-82; PMID:15097997; http://dx.doi.org/10.1038/nbt962.
124. Mosavi LK, Cammett TJ, Desrosiers DC, Peng ZY. The ankyrin repeat as molecular architecture for protein recognition. Protein Sci 2004; 13:1435-48; PMID:15152081; http://dx.doi.org/10.1110/ps.03554604.
125. Li J, Mahajan A, Tsai MD. Ankyrin repeat: a unique motif mediating protein-protein interactions. Biochemistry 2006; 45:15168-78; PMID:17176038; http://dx.doi.org/10.1021/bi062188q.
126. Bradley RR, Terajima M. Vaccinia virus K1L protein mediates host-range function in RK-13 cells via ankyrin repeat and may interact with a cellular GTPase-activating protein. Virus Res 2005; 114:104-12; PMID:16039000; http://dx.doi.org/10.1016/j.virusres.2005.06.003.
127. Meng X, Xiang Y. Vaccinia virus K1L protein supports viral replication in human and rabbit cells through a cell-type-specific set of its ankyrin repeat residues that are distinct from its binding site for ACAP2. Virology 2006; 353:220-33; PMID:16806385; http://dx.doi.org/10.1016/j.virol.2006.05.032.
128. Bowie A, Kiss-Toth E, Symons JA, Smith GL, Dower SK, O'Neill LA. A46R and A52R from vaccinia virus are antagonists of host IL-1 and toll-like receptor signaling. Proc Natl Acad Sci USA 2000; 97:10162-7; PMID:10920188; http://dx.doi.org/10.1073/pnas.160027697.

CHAPTER 10

Innate Immune Evasion Strategies of HCV and HIV:
Common Themes for Chronic Viral Infection

Brian P. Doehle and Michael Gale Jr.*

Abstract

The infections caused by Human Immunodeficiency Virus (HIV) and Hepatitis C Virus (HCV) rank as two of the most important public health problems worldwide. Hundreds of millions of people are infected with either HIV or HCV, and co-infection with both viruses represents a growing concern that dramatically complicates patient treatment and infection outcome. HCV and HIV are very different viruses but both cause chronic infection leading to lifelong and debilitating disease. Viral persistence in immune-competent hosts is supported by virus-directed innate immune-evasion programs that allow each virus to avoid the immediate host defenses designed to detect and clear pathogens from infected cells and tissues. Understanding the nature and mechanisms of these evasion strategies has the potential to uncover new targets for therapeutic intervention, as well as inform rational vaccine and adjuvant development aimed at protecting against infection by these devastating viruses.

Introduction

Non-self recognition of an invading microbial pathogen is a first and critical step in programming the host immune system for control of infection. Mammalian cells recognize microbial invaders through the actions of a wide variety of pathogen recognition receptor (PRR) molecules. PRRs serve to distinguish self from non-self by virtue of their recognition of and interaction with pathogen-specific macromolecules, termed pathogen associated molecular patterns (PAMPs).[1] Human cells variably express a variety of PRRs, including the RIG-I like receptors (RLRs), Toll-like receptors (TLRs), NOD-like receptors (NLRs), as well as other less defined sensors (such as those responsible for sensing cytoplasmic DNA, specific carbohydrates, and certain lipids).[1-4] Differential compartmentalization of PRRs, as well as their cell-specific expression, creates a comprehensive and complex network for PAMP sensing dedicated to immune signaling. PAMPs encompass a wide range of moieties, including protein, nucleic acids, lipids, and certain carbohydrates or combinations of each, that harbor structural signatures of a particular pathogen or group of pathogens. These molecules differ from host cell macromolecules sufficiently in structure, location, and/or interactions such that they are discriminated as non-self through PRR interaction. Non-self recognition and PAMP binding by PRRs leads to the rapid engagement of downstream intracellular signaling cascades that activate a variety of host transcription factors. This process lead to alteration of host cell gene expression and induction of intracellular immune defenses termed the innate immune response. In terms of virus infection, this response drives the expression of a variety of genes

*University of Washington, Department of Immunology, Seattle, Washington, USA.
 Corresponding Author: Michael Gale Jr.—Email: mgale@uw.edu

Nucleic Acid Sensors and Antiviral Immunity, edited by Suryaprakash Sambhara and Takashi Fujita.
©2013 Landes Bioscience.

directly induced by PRR signaling and indirectly induced by secreted product from the infected cell. These immediate response genes encode a variety of antiviral products, proinflammatory cytokines and chemokines that that respectively function to directly limit virus replication and to induce antiviral innate immune responses while attracting and modulating adaptive immune cells to the site of infection. Type 1 interferon (IFN) is a major product of PRR signaling and is produced and secreted from the infected cell. IFN binds to its receptor in autocrine and paracrine fashion to drive the expression of hundreds of interferon-stimulated genes (ISGs) within the infected cell and in the surrounding tissue. ISG products mediate antiviral, immunomodulatory, metabolic, and proapoptotic actions that suppress virus infection and stimulate the adaptive immune response[2,5]to mediate a systemic antiviral state.[2,6]

Prompt and specific signaling of these cell-intrinsic innate immune defenses serves the host by clearing viral infection and promoting lasting immunity to secondary challenges. However, viruses have evolved sophisticated programs of their own to subvert and prevent innate immune defenses from interfering with productive infection and dissemination within and among hosts. In this chapter we will discuss the current understanding of how HCV and HIV target and control cell intrinsic innate immunity and how these viral programs lead to persistent infection and disease. While the development of a tissue culture system for the growth and propagation of HCV has only recently occurred, a major understanding of the virus-host interactions that regulate innate immunity against HCV was gained largely prior to the development of HCV cell culture systems and without the aid of robust animal models. By comparison, the study of cell-intrinsic innate immune regulation by HIV has only recently become a major focus despite this large field having enjoyed the use of robust cell culture and nonhuman primate models of infection for nearly 25 years. We will address and compare the current understanding and commonalities of how these different viruses trigger and evade innate immune actions of host cells to mediate chronic infection and support distinct but shared global epidemics.

HCV Structure and Infection

HCV is a positive-sense, single stranded, hepatotropic RNA virus belonging to the Hepacivirus genus of the family *flaviviridae*. The HCV genomic RNA molecule is approximately 9.6 kb in length with heavily structured 5' and 3' non-coding region (NCR). The viral RNA is translated into a single poly-protein, which is cleaved into the mature viral structural and nonstructural proteins by host peptidases and viral-encoded proteases (Fig. 1A). HCV is parenterally transmitted and is nearly endemic within intravenous drug users.[7] The virus replicates with robust efficiency in vivo, and like other RNA viruses it lacks proofreading function. HCV thus generates an estimated 10^{12} virions per day that are present as a variety of genetically distinct variants or quasispecies.[8] HCV primarily infects hepatocytes but is reported to transiently infect or mediate low level persistent infection in certain lymphocytes and myeloid cells. About 200 million people worldwide are persistently infected with HCV, with an estimated 4 million new infections each year. Roughly 25 percent of people acutely infected with the virus will clear the infection without intervention. This leaves the majority of cases, which progress to a persistent chronic infection. These long-term infections associate with persistent liver inflammation, eventually precipitating liver fibrosis and cirrhosis.[9] HCV is the primary cause of liver transplantation as well as a leading cause of the development of hepatocellular carcinoma,[10] and is the third leading cause of cancer death worldwide. Importantly, HCV is now the leading cause of non-AIDS related death in individuals with HIV co-infection.[11]

There is no vaccine available for preventing HCV infection, and the current treatment for those chronically infected is a combination of ribavirin and pegylated IFN.[12] Unfortunately this is only effective in half of those treated, and treatment is complicated by a long drug regimen as well as undesirable side effects.[12] Recent work has lead to the development of new classes of direct antiviral drugs for the treatment of HCV that are soon to be in the clinic (see below). These antiviral drugs will be applied as combination therapy with IFN, at least in the near future, in an effort to avoid emergence of drug-resistance HCV variants. Thus, there is a great need to continue development of antiviral drugs to combat HCV infection.

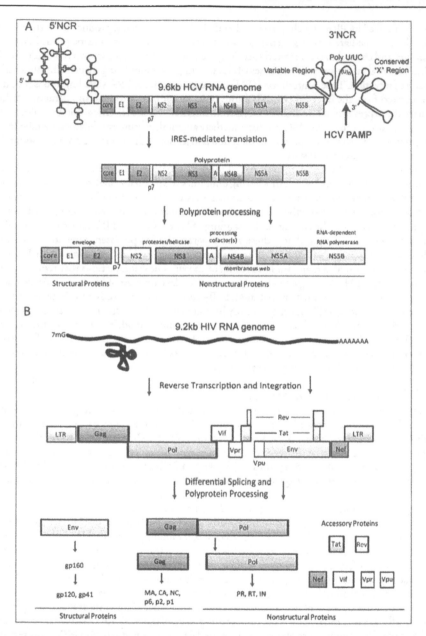

Figure 1. The genomic structure and processing of HCV and HIV. A) The 9.6 kb positive strand RNA genome of HCV is illustrated with secondary structure of the 5' and 3' noncoding regions (NCR). The 3' NCR contains several domains, including a single-stranded poly U/UC region (medium gray/red box) in which the minimal HCV PAMP resides. HCV proteins are generated via IRES-mediated translation to a single long polyprotein that is processed into the mature structural and nonstructural HCV proteins. B) Schematic of the 9.2 kb HIV RNA genome which is capped and poly-adenylated. After reverse transcription and integration of the proviral DNA molecule into the host genome, HIV RNA transcripts are produced via differential splicing, yielding a number of proteins and polyproteins that are processed to their mature forms. A color version of this figure is available online at www.landesbioscience.com/curie.

Recognition of HCV Infection

Work on HCV has uncovered roles for both the RLR and TLR pathways, including RIG-I, TLR2 and TLR3 in the recognition of viral infection. In hepatocytes, the major target cell of HCV infection, RIG-I is the major PRR that recognizes HCV and triggers the antiviral immune response. Studies have shown that HCV RNA can potently induce IFN production from hepatocytes through RIG-I signaling,[13,14] and this has been effectively modeled in chimeric mouse and chimpanzees models of HCV infection that demonstrate HCV triggering of ISG expression during acute infection.[15,16] Studies of human hepatoma cells and hepatocytes in culture has revealed a major role for RIG-I in PRR function against HCV, and demonstrate that defective RIG-I signaling confers increased cellular permissiveness for HCV growth.[14,17] More recent work from our laboratory has defined the HCV PAMP recognized by RIG-I as a combination of 5′ triphosphate on the genomic RNA along with the presence of poly-uridine within the viral RNA 3′ NCR (Fig. 1A).[18] These motifs confer a non-self signature that is bound by RIG-I and triggers the signaling cascade that imparts innate immunity.[18]

The role of TLRs in sensing HCV infection and promoting antiviral immunity is less clear than that of RIG-I. TLRs are most highly expressed in specialized immune cells such as dendritic cells, macrophages, B cells, and some types of T cells, although TLR3 exhibits wider expression patterns that include non-immune cells.[19,20] TLRs are found either on the cell surface or within endosomes, and they generally sense extracellular PAMPs or those that have been internalized by phagocytosis. Hepatocytes have been reported to be deficient in TLR signaling,[21] but HCV core and NS3 proteins have been shown to activate TLR2 signaling in cultured cells.[22-24] Evidence of TLR3 activation of by HCV RNA has recently been reported using cell systems that ectopically express TLR3, and there are reports that HCV may antagonize this pathway (see below).[20] Taken together, TLR responses may play a role in sensing HCV within infected cells, possibly amplifying IFN production and responses and driving inflammatory signaling within the infected liver.

RIG-I sensing of HCV PAMPs leads to the downstream phosphorylation and activation of the transcription factor IRF-3, which then translocates from its resting state in the cytosol into the nucleus where it directly binds its target genes to drive RNA expression.[13,14,18] IRF-3 target genes include a wide range of antiviral effectors, including IFN-β.[1,2] During acute HCV infection IFN-β is secreted by the infected hepatocyte and directs the local and tissue wide induction of ISG expression (ISGs).[2,6,25] Several ISGs have been reported to have direct anti-HCV action, including PKR, ISG56, ISG20, ADAR1, and viperin, and they act through a variety of mechanisms to disrupt the viral life cycle.[26] Indeed, treatment of HCV target cells with type I IFN potently blocks HCV infection,[27,28] and is the hallmark feature of the current therapeutic use of IFN for HCV patients.

HCV Antagonism of Innate Immune Signaling Pathways

Despite the recognition and signaling of HCV by RIG-I during acute infection, most patients will continue on to a chronic infection state. Moreover, those who receive IFN and ribavirin treatment often fail to respond to the therapy. These seemingly contradictory facts that IFN induces antiviral ISG actions but can fail to clear HCV infection have been reconciled by studies that uncovered the highly successfully evasion strategies employed by HCV to modulate the innate immune response. HCV blocks the production of type I IFN by antagonizing the upstream signaling pathways, as well as directly antagonizing the actions of specific ISG products (Fig. 2). This suppression of the host intracellular innate immune response allows for viral persistence, and supports development of a chronic infection.

RIG-I signaling of IRF-3 activation relies on an adaptor molecule called IPS-1 (also referred to as Cardif, MAVS, and VISA). IPS-1 mediates downstream signaling through recruitment and effector actions of a multiprotein signaling complex, or signalosome.[14,17,29] Engagement of a PAMP ligand by RIG-I causes its conformational change to release its repressor domain from auto inhibition of its Caspase Activation and Recruitment Domains (CARDs) that mediate downstream signaling.[30,31] This process allows for oligomerization of RIG-I molecules through interactions between opposing CARDs.[13] This process imposes an active conformation that

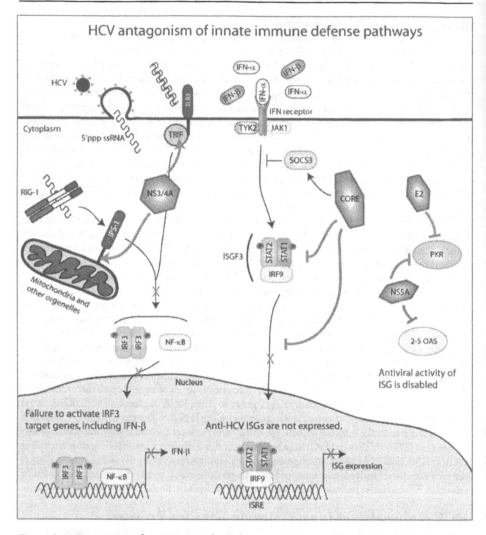

Figure 2. HCV strategies for evasion and antagonism of the innate immune defense pathways. Recognition of HCV PAMPs by RIG-I or TLR PRRs can lead to strong activation of antiviral genes and effector molecules. HCV has evolved a number of strategies to promote persistence and viral growth, including direct targeting of IPS-1, antagonism of the JAK/STAT signaling program, as well as inhibiting direct antiviral molecules. See text for details. Figure modified from reference 29.

permits RIG-I interactions with IPS-1 and stimulation of signalosome actions from location on the mitochondria-associated memebranes.[13,32]

While activated IRF-3 is observed at early times post infection with HCV and during cell to spread of infection, it is rapidly shut down through active antagonism of innate pathways by the replicating virus in vitro and in HCV patient liver.[17,25] To accomplish this innate immune suppression, HCV targets IPS-1 through its serine protease NS3/4A to cleave and inactivate the IPS-1-bound signalosome. NS3/4A is also responsible for processing the HCV polyprotein into mature viral non-structural proteins, and both of these activities are facilitated through NS3/4A anchoring into intracellular membranes.[26] In addition, NS3/4A has been shown to be capable of cleaving TRIF (Toll/interleukin-1 receptor/resistance domain-containing adaptor inducing IFN), an essential adaptor molecule required for TLR3 signaling.[33] The NS3 protein alone has also been reported to directly bind TBK1, blocking IRF3 engagement and activation.[34] However, the molecular features of how NS3/4A targets TRIF or TBK1 for proteolysis within endosome-associated signaling complexes or signalosomes has not been defined and a role for HCV regulation of TLR3 signaling has not been demonstrated.

HCV has also been reported to antagonize and attenuate IFN signaling by targeting the Jak/STAT pathways that lead to ISG expression. The HCV core protein can block Jak/STAT signaling when overexpressed alone in cells, and does this by directly binding to STAT1 and preventing its phosporlyation by upstream protein kinases.[35] Additionally, it has been shown that Core can induce the expression of suppressor of cytokine signaling-3 (SOCS3) which is a negative regulator of the JAK-STAT pathway.[36] This regulation has the effect of decreasing STAT1 activation, and lowering ISG induction in the face of IFN stimulation of cells. Expression of the HCV polyprotein has also been shown to stimulate the expression and effector function of protein phosphatase 2A (PP2A),[37] which decreases STAT1 activation and prevents ISGF3 dependent transcription of ISGs.[38-41] However, the role for each of these virus-host interactions in IFN response regulation in HCV patients has not been defined.

Other HCV proteins have also been shown to have direct anti-ISG activities. The NS5A protein is involved in HCV particle assembly and RNA replication, but has been shown to directly interact with 2'-5'-OAS, blocking its antiviral effects,[42] and can induce the secretion of IL-8, resulting in decreased ISG expression.[43] NS5A was more recently shown to bind the TLR adaptor molecule MyD88 to inhibit signaling in response to TLR ligands, although the significance of these findings is yet unclear.[44] NS5A also has a defined role for inhibiting PKR activation, an antiviral protein kinase. This event was shown to increase HCV replication through enhancement of viral RNA translation[45,46] but this process of regulation varies among NS5A sequences and its function in vivo in HCV patients has not been ascertained. HCV E2 protein also has been shown to antagonize PKR by direct binding that decreases PKR activity.[47] Again however, these observations have not been validated in vivo.

Human Immunodeficiency Virus

Thirty years of research has yielded a vast amount of information regarding the pathogenesis, structure, and immunobiology of HIV. From this knowledge has come the development of effective drugs for managing the disease, but a cure for those infected, or a vaccine to prevent infection in the first place, continues to be elusive. Until recently only little was known about the innate mechanisms employed to sense HIV and regulate viral growth, as well as understanding how the virus overcomes these host restrictions. Here we will discuss the current understanding of HIV interaction with the cell intrinsic innate immune sensing pathways, as well as highlight unresolved questions of interest for future study.

HIV Structure and Infection

HIV is a retrovirus, from the family *lentiviridae*. It is very closely related to simian immunodeficiency viruses (SIV) which specifically infects species of old world monkeys. The virus consists of an enveloped capsid structure containing a variety of viral and host proteins, as well as two RNA copies of the viral genome. After engaging its cognate receptors and co-receptors on target cells, the viral envelope proteins undergo structural changes leading to fusion of the viral envelope with the membrane of the target cell, resulting in release of the viral core and its contents into the host. The HIV RNA genome undergoes reverse transcription shortly after release into the cell, leading to the production of a proviral DNA copy which then translocates across the nuclear membrane into the nucleus where the now double-stranded genetic material is inserted into the host genome. This inserted DNA then becomes the template for production of viral RNA from the viral Long-terminal Repeat (LTR) promoter, generating RNA molecules to be translated into viral proteins, as well as the source of full length genomic RNA species which will eventually be packaged into new progeny virus.[48]

Transcription of HIV proviral DNA gives rise to a number of different RNA transcripts of various lengths, which lead to the production of nine different gene products. These proteins account for the structural and enzymatic properties of the virus, as well as several accessory gene products which are responsible for modulating the host environment to benefit the virus and promote replication and viral growth (Fig. 1B). HIV has a very distinct cellular tropism, determined by the expression of the HIV receptor CD4, as well as the expression of co-receptors, primarily CCR5 and CXCR4. Expression of these molecules is exclusive to specific myeloid cell and lymphocyte subsets, which directs HIV infection to the major immune cell compartment, to devastating effect. Spread of the virus occurs from the site of infection through the blood stream and from person to person through bodily fluid contact, most prevalently through sexual contact and intravenous drug usage. This puts the virus in contact with a number of target cells of infection.[48,49]

Infection with HIV is characterized by an initial acute phase of infection, during which time the virus replicates very high levels, mostly infecting CD4+ lymphocytes. This phase of disease is also characterized by an increase in turnover of CD4+ lymphocytes. Thus, the stage of peak viral infection contains waves of newly synthesized HIV infecting fresh CD4+ lymphocytes, which then produce more virus, and are rapidly killed or cleared. Eventually HIV-specific immune responses are induced and begin to control the level of viremia. These responses consist of both cytotoxic CD8+ T-lymphocyte (CTL) and CD4+ T-helper-mediated humoral responses. Adaptive immune responses are eventually insufficient to control infection, and patients will typically progress to AIDS, characterized by CD4+ T-cell depletion and degradation of the immune compartment leading to immunodeficiency and opportunistic infections.[48-50]

Initial Stages of Infection: Exposure, Eclipse, and Acute

The earliest events in HIV-1 infection remain somewhat obscure, as they cannot be studied in vivo in humans. Much information has been gleaned from a number of model systems, including human vaginal explant systems and SIV vaginal challenge models, and can be used to inform our understanding of HIV-1 infection and pathogenesis.[51] After the initial exposure of the virus to the mucosa, there appears to be a "seeding" of the infection in susceptible cells. In high dose SIV models, this seems to involve infection of a small (~50 cells) population of founder cells.[52,53] Data strongly suggests that these cells are resting CD4+ cells in HIV-1 infection and the founder infection is mostly initiated by a single virus.[54-56] This relatively small number of infected cells gives rise to virus which expands to a larger population of infected cells in the local environment, eventually leading to wide spread systemic infection of CD4+ lymphocytes. During this process, virus is not detected in the blood, and this has been termed the eclipse phase of infection.[50,51] The timing of this period from exposure to viral detection in the blood has been followed carefully in SIV models, and lasts approximately 7 days.[51,52] Estimates for HIV infection suggest that the eclipse phase may last slightly longer, at an estimate of 10 days post exposure and infection.[50] Once virus is detected in the blood, viral titers increase exponentially over time, and are accompanied by measurable innate immune responses, starting the acute phase of infection. While exceptionally difficult to study, especially in HIV-1 infected individuals, the period of time preceding exposure to the beginning of acute infection represents one of the best opportunities for meaningful therapeutic intervention.

Sensing of HIV by Cell Intrinsic Innate Immune Pathways

In contrast to other aspects of HIV biology and infection, understanding how HIV is sensed by a target cell through PRR programs is poorly understood. It has been long recognized that HIV infection elicits systemic IFN production and the initiation of humoral responses during the stage of acute viremia. Recently, however, studies have started to focus on defining the cell intrinsic mechanisms of HIV detection, and how the virus actively combats these defenses for its own benefit to mediate persistent infection (Fig. 3).

A number of studies have reported the production of IFN-α in patients during acute HIV infection as well as in healthy long-term non-progressing patients.[57-59] IFN production in this case has largely been attributed to a specific subset of dendritic cells, plasmacytoid dendritic cells

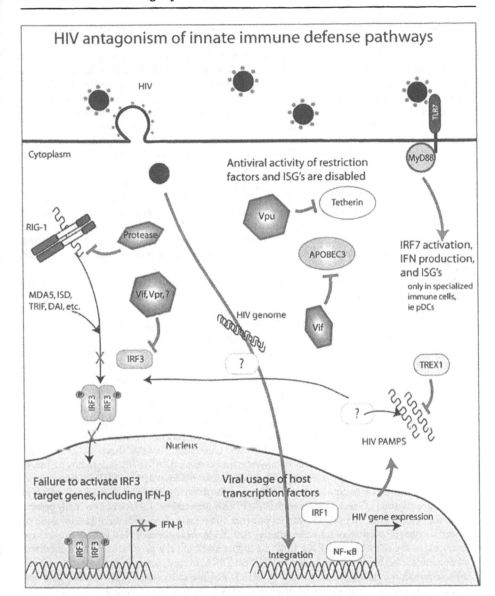

Figure 3. HIV interaction and antagonism of host innate immune defense pathways. HIV can be recognized by both TLR and less defined cell intrinsic pathways. HIV targeting of retroviral restriction factors (also characterized as ISGs) has been well established. Emerging evidence suggests robust antagonism of the signaling programs required for the induction of IFN and innate immune effector genes. See text for details.

(pDCs), as these cells are specialized to produce high levels of IFN-α.[60] pDCs are the primary producer of IFN-α during a number of viral infections, and the production of IFN is important for downstream adaptive immune responses to infection.[25,61] While pDCs are not a target of HIV infection they constitutively express a range of surface and endocytic PRRs that detect a wide range of PAMPs, likely including HIV products, and produce large amounts of systemic IFN and set up a systemic anti-viral state. Indeed, loss of IFN-producing cells has been associated with higher HIV RNA levels and advancement to AIDS.[57]

The actual PAMPs sensed by pDCs in response to HIV infection are not fully defined. Several lines of evidence suggest that pDCs sense HIV via a TLR dependent mechanism. Initial studies that measured ISG promoter expression in 293 cells overexpressing TLR7 and exposed to HIV derived RNA sequences, as well as studies that stimulated pDCs or macrophages with such sequences, revealed that HCV RNA can stimulate IFN-α.[62] Exposure to HIV infected cells, endocytosis of HIV-1 virions, and interaction of viral nucleic acids with TLRs, also has been shown to cause pDC production of IFN-α,[63,64] and this occurs in a manner dependent on MyD88, a critical TLR signaling adaptor protein.[65] Additionally, work within macaque models of SIV infection has also implicated TLR7 in particular, as necessary for pDC recognition of infection.[66] Collectively these data suggest that pDCs can sense HIV, possibly via nucleic acid recognition of either free virus or from sampling of HIV infected cells. Recently, data has emerged suggesting that TLR7 dependent sensing of HIV-1 is much more robust when infected cells are provided to dendritic cells, as opposed to free HIV-1 virons.[67] The authors of this study also demonstrated that there is a cell intrinsic cytoplasmic component to this process, which drives IRF-3 activation independent of TLR7 recognition. Further work is necessary to conclusively determine the exact nature of both the PAMP(s) and the PRR(s) required for pDC recognition of HIV.

A cell intrinsic sensing capability to detect HIV within conventional dendritic cells (DC) has been recently uncovered.[68] This DC population is not normally infected by HIV due to a cell-specific block of infection,[69] and therefore the investigators of this work utilized a model system featuring DC expression of the SIV Vpx protein. Importantly, some SIV isolates are able to overcome this block via the action of the SIV-specific Vpx protein, which when ectopically expressed in cells confers increased permissiveness for HIV infection.[70,71] While the exact nature of this cell regulation by Vpx is not clear, HIV does not encode its own ortholog of Vpx, thereby possibly explaining why human DCs restrict HIV infection. Indeed, expression of Vpx within human DCs has now been shown to release the restriction on HIV infection.[68] Interestingly, Vpx expression also appears to allow for presentation/recognition of a HIV PAMP and the ensuing cell-intrinsic activation of intracellular innate antiviral immunity. While these observations suggest that the SIV Vpx protein can regulate innate immune signaling processes in human DCs the overall relevance of these observations to actual HIV infection is not clear. However these studies reveal the Vpx-expressing DC model as a robust in vitro system for examining PAMP/PRR signaling pathways and defining their components that trigger innate immune defenses against HIV infection.

Studies of the DNA endonuclease TREX1 also points to the intrinsic ability of T cells and PBMCs to recognize HIV infection through PAMP/PRR interactions. DNA is not normally present within the cytoplasmic environment but its presence there marks a possible microbial invasion or nuclear damage.[72,73] New studies have examined TREX1 in the context of HIV infection, and have shown that in the absence of TREX1, there are higher levels of HIV proviral DNA intermediates that accumulate in the cytoplasm of the cells.[74] This DNA, in turn, activates a potent cytoplasmic DNA response, including the activation of IRF-3, and the induction of downstream antiviral signaling. Thus, TREX1 appears to be promoting HIV infection, by preventing the accumulation of these intermediates, and suppressing the antiviral response. Further studies to examine TREX1 as a possible target for anti-HIV treatment should reveal its role in governing infection outcome and immunity, as the physiological ramifications of this process are unclear.

From an evolutionary standpoint, TREX1 may have evolved to deal with DNA intermediates from a variety of sources, including endogenous retroviruses or retro-elements.[72] This process may be acting to dampen or regulate recognition of DNA in the cytoplasm, which while not a true "self" signature, may have been prevalent enough to no longer want to elicit a full signaling response every time encountered. Thus TREX1 may exist to "clean up" DNA that has become nearly self (retro-elements), while still allowing the recognition of similar types of PAMPs when an acute infectious event pushes the amounts of PAMP above a threshold level. Potentially consistent with this idea, a recent report suggests that a reverse-transcribed DNA intermediate may be recognized in the cytoplasm of abortively infected T cells that are presumably TREX1 competent.[75]

In addition to nucleic acid PAMPs, there is growing evidence that the retroviral capsid structures may also provide a potent PAMP that can lead to host innate immune signaling. TRIM5 has been extensively described as a retroviral restriction factor targeting and destabilizing incoming retroviral capsid structures.[76] However, several recent reports have suggested a signaling role, in addition to this passive restriction.[77-79] Recent work has further delineated this signaling component, and has described a potent activation of both AP-1 and NFκB signaling, suggesting that TRIM5 also acts as a PRR recognizing the capsid lattice of invading retroviruses.[80] More work is needed to carefully define the HIV PAMP(s) presented in target cells of infection.

Interferon and ISGs vs. HIV

IFN has been shown suppress acute HIV infection and to increase the ability of the adaptive immune system to recognize HIV infected cells by increasing MHC class I and other molecules.[81-87] The mechanism by which IFN promote these actions is only beginning to be understood (see below), and appears to have cell-specific component of actions which are not yet defined.[88]

While IFN signaling through the Jak-STAT pathway drives ISG expression, only a small percentage of the hundreds of known ISGs have been studies in functional detail. Such studies have revealed that some ISG products have either wide-ranging antiviral activities while others are known to act against specific viruses or virus classes. Several ISGs have been reported to have direct anti-HIV effects, including PKR, RNaseL, Trim22, ISG15, ISG20, Viperin, and the IFITM proteins. PKR can inhibit HIV by suppressing protein translation,[89] and RNaseL can degrade HIV RNA.[90] ISG15 is a small ubiquitin-like molecule, which can be directly conjugated to viral and cellular molecules. While the mechanism of action is not well understood, this "ISGylation" activity has been shown to directly affect HIV assembly, through conjugation with HIV Gag.[91] TRIM22 is an ISG that has also been shown to interfere with Gag assembly.[92] ISG20 and Viperin have also both been shown to be capable of inhibiting HIV infection and/or growth in in vitro systems, but the specificity and antiviral mechanism of action are currently unknown.[93,94] Recent work has also shown that HIV can be blocked largely at the entry level by the transmembrane IFITM proteins constituting a sub-family of related ISGs.[95]

Many studies have been directed at understanding the function and roles of a number of HIV restriction factors, including the APOBECs, TRIM5, and Tetherin/BST-2. The importance of these molecules for retroviral infection and evolution has been shown very clearly in a significant amount of work over the past decade.[76] Interestingly, all of these molecules expression can be induced too much higher levels in response to IFN treatment, characterizing them as ISGs. Thus, driving an innate immune signaling response through PAMP recognition or IFN production/ stimulation can induce all of the known anti-HIV molecules, and set up a specific anti-HIV state. This is most evident with the induction of BST-2 expression, as interferon treatment of cells was often associated with increased levels of cell-bound HIV particles,[76,96] which has been now shown to be a result of BST-2 mediated block of viral egress.[97] As only a handful of all recognized ISGs have defined anti-viral characteristics, the number of ISGs with direct or indirect anti-HIV effects is surely to grow with further investigation.

Viral Countermeasures: HIV Strikes Back

All viruses have to evade innate immune defenses in order to replicate and spread, and innate immune evasion strategies are linked with viral pathogenesis.[3] Studies from a wide range of viral pathogenesis models have found a plethora of viral mechanisms for blunting these responses or co-opting pathways for the benefit of the virus. However, despite some of the most robust culture systems and a tremendous number of high quality reagents for study, very little is known about HIV countermeasures to the innate immune signaling pathways in target cells. Recent findings in this area, along with some long recognized data, suggest the presence of sophisticated HIV programs for countering the earliest host defenses in response to infection.

Sequencing of the HIV genome uncovered the presence of a number of cellular transcription factor binding sites in the LTR promoter in addition to viral protein specific binding sites. This list includes NF-kB, NFAT-1, AP-1, IRF-1 and others which are needed to efficiently drive transcription of HIV RNA within the cellular environment.[48,98,99] NF-kB activation is required for the transcription of genes associated with a wide range of cellular processes, and in response to PAMP activation and inflammatory signals. In addition AP-1, NFAT-1, Sp1, and IRF-1 are all important for various pro-inflammatory, cytokine, and/or immune cell activation signals. This co-opting of transcription factors to help drive viral gene expression has a number of functional consequences for HIV. First, this process coordinately induces viral gene expression during the growth and division of CD4+ T cells. In the case of inflammatory or anti-viral signaling, the virus has generated a method for also upregulating its expression, potentially allowing for viral directed evasion mechanisms in the face of host antagonism. This principle has been experimentally shown recently in a system that activates NF-κB signaling in response to cytosolic DNA, thus increasing HIV expression.[100]

Several recent studies have begun to uncover viral directed antagonism of the innate immune signaling cascade by HIV. Of note is that these strategies appear to be highly analogous to evasion strategies already well-characterized for HCV. Many of the HIV sensing pathways described previously have in common the activation of the cellular transcription factor IRF-3, which is also essential for host defense against HCV infection.[17,101] Our recent studies, as well as those from other groups, have uncovered a robust antagonism of IRF-3 during acute HIV infection.[102,103] Upon infection of T cells or macrophages by HIV, there is little or no induction of IFN or ISGs, despite the fact that these cells are highly inducible in this manner by a variety of RNA or DNA viruses and other stimuli. IRF-3 is one of the master transcription factors activated after PRR recognition of a variety of PAMPs, and signaling by TLRs or RLRs, as well as stimulation with cytosolic interferon stimulatory DNA (ISD) all lead to a potent activation of IRF-3.[2] Infection with HIV of a wide range of target cells results in a potent down modulation of IRF-3 physical protein levels, and this leaves the cells unable to mount an effective signaling response, even in the face of strong secondary viral challenges.[102] The exact viral mechanism underlying this IRF-3 protein depletion has not been well-understood but is the topic of on-going studies.

Additional work has indicated that HIV may be directing the sequestration of RIG-I in an HIV protease dependent fashion.[104] RIG-I is known to recognize specific types of PAMP RNA ligands, and there is evidence that some types of in vitro derived HIV RNA species can trigger RIG-I-specific signaling in vitro. It is currently unclear what types of RNA species would be produced during HIV in vivo that would be recognized as non-self by RIG-I, as HIV RNA transcripts are capped and poly-adenylated, and look like host mRNA molecules and are thus not marked as canonical RIG-I ligands.

The Innate Immune Activation: Paradox or Dysregulation?

Recent studies have uncovered a variety of evidence to indicate that innate immune activation may actually have pathogenic consequences for HIV infection, and that HIV-1 may actually benefit from our immune system attempting to control and clear infection. First, activation of innate defenses and the stimulation of inflammation drives the infiltration of many more target cells into the infection site, thus supporting HIV expansion into these incoming CD4+ cells.[51] This paradox is at the heart of HIV infection. Additionally, there is powerful evidence that the initial systemic breakout of the virus during acute infection is accompanied by very high levels of IFN, cytokines, and chemokines.[59] This "cytokine storm" is present without imparting control of the virus via traditional cell-mediated innate mechanisms.[50,59] Of note is that TLR agonists have also been applied to macaques in an SIV infection model in which these compounds were expected to drive innate immune activation and suppression of the infection but instead they actually resulted in a major increase in the efficiency and spread of the acute infection.[105] Finally, several studies comparing "pathogenic" and non-pathogenic SIV infections in non-human primate models have demonstrated a protracted, less controlled innate immune response in the pathogenic infections, suggesting that too much innate immune activation is at least partially responsible for pathogenesis of infection.[106-109]

Importantly, there is a substantial amount of evidence that innate immune signaling can control HIV infection, and that the virus is actively modulating the host environment to control these defenses. IFN can inhibit HIV growth, and there are many ISGs with known anti-HIV properties (see above for detail). Many of the well characterized HIV restriction factors have been shown to be under strong evolutionary pressure, again supporting the importance of these factors, and work has shown that HIV has evolved specific mechanisms for antagonizing the cell intrinsic innate signaling pathways to avoid the anti-viral state.[76] So what should be taken away from these seemingly contradictory observations of innate immunity regulation, immune activation, and pathogenesis of HIV infection?

First, all innate immune responses are not created equal, and that the appropriate activity to protect the host from infection is most likely highly context dependent. Work with various vaccine and agonist systems have elegantly shown that very different immune responses can be driven by different stimuli, and that the most appropriate response is dependent on the pathogen.[100,101] For example, TLR7/9 agonists are inappropriate as antivirals or vaccine adjuvants unless it is shown that they impart the innate immune response similar to that naturally induced by non-pathogenic lentiviruses or by HIV variants that have lost ability to antagonize innate immune defenses. We currently do not understand what constitutes a successful innate immune response against HIV and what immune parameters successfully mediate protection from future HIV challenge. Obviously, more research is needed to inform agonist and vaccine design strategies but it is likely that innate immune stimulation and regulation strategies will be at the heart of any immune therapy design. We also have little insight into the viral host interactions that govern immunity during the HIV during the eclipse phase, a potentially vital time for overcoming infection. Studies aimed at defining HIV replication stage-specific innate immune programming may reveal new insights of immune regulation over the entire course of infection. Second, the data from in vivo infection studies must be viewed in the light of innate immune dysregulation, quite possibly due to direct viral antagonism of early innate immune defense pathways. The dysregulation of the immune system which is the hallmark of HIV infection can be compared with several other model systems where innate antagonism/ perturbations cause dramatic immune dysfunction. A significant amount of work with high quality mouse models of RNA virus infection have shown for instance that changes in innate signaling early in infection not only cause higher viral titers during infection, but cause major defects in downstream adaptive immune responses.[61,110-114] In fact, that removal of just the cell intrinsic signaling component of the innate immune defenses elicits major innate and adaptive immune defects, both at the cell and whole animal level and involves a dysregulation of production of proinflammatory cytokines, altered antibody profiles, altered T regulatory cell function, and increased inflammation analogous to the HIV cytokine storm and systemic immune activation.[61] Thus, virus and host governance of the innate immune response must be considered in any future immune modifying therapy to treat HIV infection.

Conclusions—Is Innate Immune Targeting a Path for Future Therapeutics and Vaccines?

The delineation of the innate immune signaling pathways important in the recognition and signaling of HCV, and the viral mediated antagonism of these pathways by NS3/4A has now provided hope for increasing the effectiveness of clinical HCV treatment. Several HCV protease inhibitors are showing promise during clinical trials, and should be coming to market in the near future. Remarkably, these drugs offer the capacity to suppress HCV replication while inhibiting the viral protease ability to cleave IPS-1, thereby providing a therapy to restore the RIG-I pathway and innate immunity against HCV infection. However exciting these drugs are for HCV treatment, there still is no current HCV vaccine, and vaccine adjuvants for HCV have not been investigated. Therefore much work remains to push protective vaccine immunity against HCV infection. In addition to generating targets for new therapeutic disruption of the virus life cycle, the study of innate immune signaling pathways in response to HCV has provided a wealth of knowledge about the types of ligands that act as PAMPs for recognition by RIG-I. This allows for the possibility of exploiting the RLR pathway for either therapeutic intervention or as a means of adjuvanting possible vaccine candidates in the future.

While there are effective antiviral therapeutics for the control of HIV infection, understanding how the virus interacts and modulates this host response may provide additional targets for therapeutics, and help improve therapy. The HIV field has an overall poor understanding of the nature of the HIV PAMP that triggers innate immunity and the immune response to infection. Studies comparing pathogenic and non-pathogenic models of SIV infection are beginning to unveil innate responses that yield at least host control of lentiviral infection, and these observations will serve to provide the first glimpse into the type of innate immune programming that we should be aiming for to control HIV infection and augment vaccine designs.

To date, the most effective vaccines against viral infection have been those that elicit both strong innate and adaptive responses utilizing the host's natural innate immune response pathways of combating the specific type of infection being vaccinated against. There is a significant amount of emerging data suggesting that not all adjuvants and vaccine components are created equal, and even robust stimuli of one PRR may yield little effective downstream protection if it is inappropriate or taken out of the natural context of infection. Approaches that embrace functional genomics and systems biology approaches, coupled with classical virologic and biochemical analyses now provide a unique opportunity to define the full and complex nature of a successful virus-specific innate immune response and to understand how this response impacts the outcome of infection and immunity.

Acknowledgments

The authors would like to thank Stacy M. Horner and Arjun Rustagi for helpful conversation and critical reading of the manuscript. BD is a Ruth L. Kirschstein (NRSA) Postdoctoral Fellow. Work in the Gale laboratory is supported by funds from the State of Washington, National Institutes of Health, and by the Burroughs-Wellcome Fund.

About the Authors

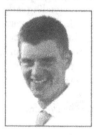

Brian Doehle is currently a Senior Fellow in the Department of Immunology at the University of Washington Medical Center in Seattle, Washington. Dr. Doehle received both a BS and MS in Biological Sciences from Ohio University in Athens, OH. He received his PhD in Molecular Genetics and Microbiology from Duke University in 2006. During his graduate education Dr. Doehle studied HIV and retroviral cellular tropism and virus host interactions focusing on the APOBEC family of proteins, under the direction of Dr. Bryan Cullen. In 2006 Dr. Doehle joined the Gale laboratory focusing efforts on developing novel programs studying into HIV modulation of innate immune signaling pathways including the degradation of IRF-3 by HIV-1.

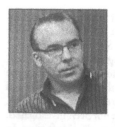

Michael Gale Jr. is a Professor in the Department of Immunology at the University of Washington Medical Center in Seattle, Washington. Dr. Gale received his PhD in 1994 from the University of Washington studying in the laboratory of Dr. Marilyn Parsons. From 1994-1999 he studied HCV pathogensisis, mechanisms of translational control, interferon biology, and viral host interactions in the laboratory of Dr. Michael Katze as postdoctoral fellow. Dr. Gale started his own research group as a faculty member at the University of Texas Southwestern Medical Center in 1999 as an Endowed Scholar, working to better understand the control of host responses to HCV and other RNA virus infections. Dr. Gale moved to University of Washington in 2007, and has been Professor in the Department of Immunology since 2010, and has adjunct appointments in the Department of Microbiology, Department of Global Health, and at the Fred Hutchinson Cancer Research Center.

References

1. Wilkins C, Gale M Jr. Recognition of viruses by cytoplasmic sensors. Curr Opin Immunol 2010; 22:41-7; PMID:20061127; http://dx.doi.org/10.1016/j.coi.2009.12.003.
2. Stetson DB, Medzhitov R. Type I interferons in host defense. Immunity 2006; 25:373-81; PMID:16979569; http://dx.doi.org/10.1016/j.immuni.2006.08.007.
3. Loo YM, Gale M. Viral regulation and evasion of the host response. Interferon: the 50Th Anniversary. 2007;316:295-313.
4. Kawai T, Akira S. The role of pattern-recognition receptors in innate immunity: update on Toll-like receptors. Nat Immunol 2010; 11:373-84; PMID:20404851; http://dx.doi.org/10.1038/ni.1863.
5. Pasare C, Medzhitov R. Toll-like receptors: linking innate and adaptive immunity. Microbes Infect 2004; 6:1382-7; PMID:15596124; http://dx.doi.org/10.1016/j.micinf.2004.08.018.
6. de Veer MJ, Holko M, Frevel M, Walker E, Der S, Paranjape JM, et al. Functional classification of interferon-stimulated genes identified using microarrays. J Leukoc Biol 2001; 69:912-20; PMID:11404376.
7. Williams IT, Bell BP, Kuhnert W, Alter MJ. Incidence and transmission patterns of acute hepatitis C in the United States, 1982-2006. Arch Intern Med 2011; 171:242-8; PMID:21325115; http://dx.doi.org/10.1001/archinternmed.2010.511.
8. Neumann AU, Lam NP, Dahari H, Gretch DR, Wiley TE, Layden TJ et al. Hepatitis C viral dynamics in vivo and the antiviral efficacy of interferon-alpha therapy. Science 1998; 282:103-7; PMID:9756471; http://dx.doi.org/10.1126/science.282.5386.103.
9. Bosch FX, Ribes J, Borras J. Epidemiology of primary liver cancer. Semin Liver Dis 1999; 19:271-85; PMID:10518307; http://dx.doi.org/10.1055/s-2007-1007117.
10. Sharma P, Lok A. Viral hepatitis and liver transplantation. Semin Liver Dis 2006; 26:285-97; PMID:16850378; http://dx.doi.org/10.1055/s-2006-947298.
11. Pineda JA, Garcia-Garcia JA, Aguilar-Guisado M, Ríos-Villegas MJ, Ruiz-Morales J, Rivero A, et al. Clinical progression of hepatitis C virus-related chronic liver disease in human immunodeficiency virus-infected patients undergoing highly active antiretroviral therapy. Hepatology 2007; 46:622-30; PMID:17659577; http://dx.doi.org/10.1002/hep.21757.
12. Soriano V, Peters MG, Zeuzem S. New therapies for hepatitis C virus infection. Clin Infect Dis 2009; 48:313-20; PMID:19123867; http://dx.doi.org/10.1086/595848.
13. Saito T, Hirai R, Loo YM, Owen D, Johnson CL, Sinha SC, et al. Regulation of innate antiviral defenses through a shared repressor domain in RIG-I and LGP2. Proc Natl Acad Sci USA 2007; 104:582-7; PMID:17190814; http://dx.doi.org/10.1073/pnas.0606699104.
14. Sumpter R, Loo YM, Foy E, Li K, Yoneyama M, Fujita T, et al. Regulating intracellular antiviral defense and permissiveness to hepatitis C virus RNA replication through a cellular RNA helicase, RIG-I. J Virol 2005; 79:2689-99; PMID:15708988; http://dx.doi.org/10.1128/JVL79.5.2689-2699.2005
15. Walters KA, Joyce MA, Thompson JC, Smith MW, Yeh MM, Proll S, et al. Host-specific response to HCV infection in the chimeric SCID-beige/Alb-uPA mouse model: role of the innate antiviral immune response. PLoS Pathog 2006; 2:e59; PMID:16789836; http://dx.doi.org/10.1371/journal.ppat.0020059.
16. Su AI, Pezacki JP, Wodicka L, Brideau AD, Supekova L, Thimme R, et al. Genomic analysis of the host response to hepatitis C virus infection. Proc Natl Acad Sci USA 2002; 99:15669-74; PMID:12441396; http://dx.doi.org/10.1073/pnas.202608199.
17. Loo YM, Owen DM, Li K, Erickson AK, Johnson CL, Fish PM, et al. Viral and therapeutic control of IFN-beta promoter stimulator 1 during hepatitis C virus infection. Proc Natl Acad Sci USA 2006; 103:6001-6; PMID:16585524; http://dx.doi.org/10.1073/pnas.0601523103.
18. Saito T, Owen DM, Jiang FG, Marcotrigiano J, Gale M. Innate immunity induced by composition-dependent RIG-I recognition of hepatitis C virus RNA. Nature 2008; 454:523-7; PMID:18548002; http://dx.doi.org/10.1038/nature07106.
19. Eisenächer K, Steinberg C, Reindl W, Krug A. The role of viral nucleic acid recognition in dendritic cells for innate and adaptive antiviral immunity. Immunobiology 2007; 212:701-14; PMID:18086372; http://dx.doi.org/10.1016/j.imbio.2007.09.007.
20. Wang N, Liang Y, Devaraj S, Wang J, Lemon SM, Li K. Toll-like receptor 3 mediates establishment of an antiviral state against hepatitis C virus in hepatoma cells. J Virol 2009; 83:9824-34; PMID:19625408; http://dx.doi.org/10.1128/JVL01125-09.
21. Seki E, Brenner DA. Toll-like receptors and adaptor molecules in liver disease: update. Hepatology 2008; 48:322-35; PMID:18506843; http://dx.doi.org/10.1002/hep.22306.
22. Dolganiuc A, Oak S, Kodys K, Golenbock DT, Finberg RW, Kurt-Jones E, et al. Hepatitis C core and nonstructural 3 proteins trigger toll-like receptor 2-mediated pathways and inflammatory activation. Gastroenterology 2004; 127:1513-24; PMID:15521019; http://dx.doi.org/10.1053/j.gastro.2004.08.067.

23. Chang S, Dolganiuc A, Szabo G. Toll-like receptors 1 and 6 are involved in TLR2-mediated macrophage activation by hepatitis C virus core and NS3 proteins. J Leukoc Biol 2007; 82:479-87; PMID:17595379; http://dx.doi.org/10.1189/jlb.0207128.

24. Tu Z, Pierce RH, Kurtis J, Kuroki Y, Crispe IN, Orloff MS. Hepatitis C virus core protein subverts the antiviral activities of human Kupffer cells. Gastroenterology 2010; 138:305-14; PMID:19769973; http://dx.doi.org/10.1053/j.gastro.2009.09.009.

25. Lau DT, Fish PM, Sinha M, Owen DM, Lemon SM, Gale M Jr. Interferon regulatory factor-3 activation, hepatic interferon-stimulated gene expression, and immune cell infiltration in hepatitis C virus patients. Hepatology 2008; 47:799-809; PMID:18203148; http://dx.doi.org/10.1002/hep.22076.

26. Horner SM, Gale M Jr. Intracellular innate immune cascades and interferon defenses that control hepatitis C virus. J Interferon Cytokine Res 2009; 29:489-98; PMID:19708811; http://dx.doi.org/10.1089/jir.2009.0063.

27. Guo JT, Bichko VV, Seeger C. Effect of alpha interferon on the hepatitis C virus replicon. J Virol 2001; 75:8516-23; PMID:11507197; http://dx.doi.org/10.1128/JVI.75.18.8516-8523.2001.

28. Pawlotsky JM. The nature of interferon-alpha resistance in hepatitis C virus infection. Curr Opin Infect Dis 2003; 16:587-92; PMID:14624110; http://dx.doi.org/10.1097/00001432-200312000-00012.

29. Loo YM, Fornek J, Crochet N, Bajwa G, Perwitasari O, Martinez-Sobrido L, et al. Distinct RIG-I and MDA5 signaling by RNA viruses in innate immunity. J Virol 2008; 82:335-45; PMID:17942531; http://dx.doi.org/10.1128/JVI.01080-07.

30. Saito T, Gale M. Principles of intracellular viral recognition. Curr Opin Immunol 2007; 19:17-23; PMID:17118636; http://dx.doi.org/10.1016/j.coi.2006.11.003.

31. Gee P, Chua PK, Gevorkyan J, Klumpp K, Najera I, Swinney DC, et al. Essential role of the N-terminal domain in the regulation of RIG-I ATPase activity. J Biol Chem 2008; 283:9488-96; PMID:18268020; http://dx.doi.org/10.1074/jbc.M706777200.

32. Cui S, Eisenacher K, Kirchhofer A, Brzózka K, Lammens A, Lammens K, et al. The C-terminal regulatory domain is the RNA 5′-triphosphate sensor of RIG-I. Mol Cell 2008; 29:169-79; PMID:18243112; http://dx.doi.org/10.1016/j.molcel.2007.10.032.

33. Li K, Foy E, Ferreon· JC, Ferreon AC, Ikeda M, Ray SC, et al. Immune evasion by hepatitis C virus NS3/4A protease-mediated cleavage of the Toll-like receptor 3 adaptor protein TRIF. Proc Natl Acad Sci USA 2005; 102:2992-7; PMID:15710891; http://dx.doi.org/10.1073/pnas.0408824102.

34. Otsuka M, Kato N, Moriyama M, Taniguchi H, Wang Y, Dharel N, et al. Interaction between the HCV NS3 protein and the host TBK1 protein leads to inhibition of cellular antiviral responses. Hepatology 2005; 41:1004-12; PMID:15841462; http://dx.doi.org/10.1002/hep.20666.

35. Lin W, Kim SS, Yeung E, Kamegaya Y, Blackard JT, Kim KA, et al. Hepatitis C virus core protein blocks interferon signaling by interaction with the STAT1 SH2 domain. J Virol 2006; 80:9226-35; PMID:16940534; http://dx.doi.org/10.1128/JVI.00459-06.

36. Bode JG, Ludwig S, Ehrhardt C, Albrecht U, Erhardt A, Schaper F, et al. IFN-alpha antagonistic activity of HCV core protein involves induction of suppressor of cytokine signaling-3. FASEB J 2003; 17:488-90; PMID:12551851.

37. Heim MH, Moradpour D, Blum HE. Expression of hepatitis C virus proteins inhibits signal transduction through the Jak-STAT pathway. J Virol 1999; 73:8469-75; PMID:10482599.

38. Blindenbacher A, Duong FH, Hunziker L, Stutvoet ST, Wang X, Terracciano L, et al. Expression of hepatitis C virus proteins inhibits interferon a signaling in the liver of transgenic mice. Gastroenterology 2003; 124:1465-75; PMID:12730885; http://dx.doi.org/10.1016/S0016-5085(03)00290-7.

39. Duong FHT, Filipowicz M, Tripodi M, La Monica N, Heim MH. Hepatitis C virus inhibits interferon signaling through up-regulation of protein phosphatase 2A. Gastroenterology 2004; 126:263-77; PMID:14699505; http://dx.doi.org/10.1053/j.gastro.2003.10.076.

40. de Lucas S, Bartolome J, Carreno V. Hepatitis C virus core protein down-regulates transcription of interferon-induced antiviral genes. J Infect Dis 2005; 191:93-9; PMID:15593009; http://dx.doi.org/10.1086/426509.

41. Melén K, Fagerlund R, Nyqvist M, Keskinen P, Julkunen I. Expression of hepatitis C virus core protein inhibits interferon-induced nuclear import of STATs. J Med Virol 2004; 73:536-47; PMID:15221897; http://dx.doi.org/10.1002/jmv.20123.

42. Taguchi T, Nagano-Fujii M, Akutsu M, Kadoya H, Ohgimoto S, Ishido S, et al. Hepatitis C virus NS5A protein interacts with 2 ′,5 ′-oligoadenylate synthetase and inhibits antiviral activity of IFN in an IFN sensitivity-determining region-independent manner. J Gen Virol 2004; 85:959-69; PMID:15039538; http://dx.doi.org/10.1099/vir.0.19513-0.

43. Polyak SJ, Khabar KSA, Paschal DM, Ezelle HJ, Duverlie G, Barber GN, et al. Hepatitis C virus nonstructural 5A protein induces interleukin-8, leading to partial inhibition of the interferon-induced antiviral response. J Virol 2001; 75:6095-106; PMID:11390611; http://dx.doi.org/10.1128/JVI.75.13.6095-6106.2001.

44. Abe T, Kaname Y, Hamamoto I, Tsuda Y, Wen X, Taguwa S, et al. Hepatitis C virus nonstructural protein 5A modulates the toll-like receptor-MyD88-dependent signaling pathway in macrophage cell lines. J Virol 2007; 81:8953-66; PMID:17567694; http://dx.doi.org/10.1128/JVI.00649-07.

45. Gale M, Blakely CM, Kwieciszewski B, Tan SL, Dossett M, Tang NM, et al. Control of PKR protein kinase by hepatitis C virus nonstructural 5A protein: Molecular mechanisms of kinase regulation. Mol Cell Biol 1998; 18:5208-18; PMID:9710605.

46. Pflugheber J, Fredericksen B, Sumpter R, Wang C, Ware F, Sodora DL, et al. Regulation of PKR and IRF-1 during hepatitis C virus RNA replication. Proc Natl Acad Sci USA 2002; 99:4650-5; PMID:11904369; http://dx.doi.org/10.1073/pnas.062055699.

47. Taylor DR, Shi ST, Romano PR, Barber GN, Lai MMC. Inhibition of the interferon-inducible protein kinase PKR by HCV E2 protein. Science 1999; 285:107-10; PMID:10390359; http://dx.doi.org/10.1126/science.285.5424.107.

48. Cherry E, Wainberg MA. The Structure and Biology of HIV-1: Introduction. In: Emini EA, ed. The Human Immunodeficiency Virus: Biology, Immunology and Therapy: Princeton University Press; 2002:1-43.

49. Anderson JP, Rain M, Shriner D, et al. The Genetics of HIV-1. In: Emini EA, ed. The Human Immunodeficiency Virus: Biology, Immunology, and Therapy: Princeton University Press; 2002:44-99.

50. McMichael AJ, Borrow P, Tomaras GD, Goonetilleke N, Haynes BF. The immune response during acute HIV-1 infection: clues for vaccine development. Nat Rev Immunol 2010; 10:11-23; PMID:20010788; http://dx.doi.org/10.1038/nri2674.

51. Haase AT. Early events in sexual transmission of HIV and SIV and opportunities for interventions. Annu Rev Med 2011; 62:127-39; PMID:21054171; http://dx.doi.org/10.1146/annurev-med-080709-124959.

52. Miller CJ, Li Q, Abel K, Kim EY, Ma ZM, Wietgrefe S, et al. Propagation and dissemination of infection after vaginal transmission of simian immunodeficiency virus. J Virol 2005; 79:9217-27; PMID:15994816; http://dx.doi.org/10.1128/JVI.79.14.9217-9227.2005.

53. Zhang Z, Schuler T, Zupancic M, Wietgrefe S, Staskus KA, Reimann KA, et al. Sexual transmission and propagation of SIV and HIV in resting and activated CD4+ T cells. Science 1999; 286:1353-7; PMID:10558989; http://dx.doi.org/10.1126/science.286.5443.1353.

54. Keele BF, Giorgi EE, Salazar-Gonzalez JF, Decker JM, Pham KT, Salazar MG, et al. Identification and characterization of transmitted and early founder virus envelopes in primary HIV-1 infection. Proc Natl Acad Sci USA 2008; 105:7552-7; PMID:18490657; http://dx.doi.org/10.1073/pnas.0802203105.

55. Abrahams MR, Anderson JA, Giorgi EE, Seoighe C, Mlisana K, Ping LH, et al. Quantitating the multiplicity of infection with human immunodeficiency virus type 1 subtype C reveals a non-poisson distribution of transmitted variants. J Virol 2009; 83:3556-67; PMID:19193811; http://dx.doi.org/10.1128/JVI.02132-08.

56. Salazar-Gonzalez JF, Salazar MG, Keele BF, Learn GH, Giorgi EE, Li H, et al. Genetic identity, biological phenotype, and evolutionary pathways of transmitted/founder viruses in acute and early HIV-1 infection. J Exp Med 2009; 206:1273-89; PMID:19487424; http://dx.doi.org/10.1084/jem.20090378.

57. Soumelis V, Scott I, Gheyas F, Bouhour D, Cozon G, Cotte L, et al. Depletion of circulating natural type I interferon-producing cells in HIV-infected AIDS patients. Blood 2001; 98:906-12; PMID:11493432; http://dx.doi.org/10.1182/blood.V98.4.906.

58. von Sydow M, Sonnerborg A, Gaines H, Strannegard O. Interferon-alpha and tumor necrosis factor-alpha in serum of patients in various stages of HIV-1 infection. AIDS Res Hum Retroviruses 1991; 7:375-80; PMID:1906289; http://dx.doi.org/10.1089/aid.1991.7.375.

59. Stacey AR, Norris PJ, Qin L, Haygreen EA, Taylor E, Heitman J, et al. Induction of a striking systemic cytokine cascade prior to peak viremia in acute human immunodeficiency virus type 1 infection, in contrast to more modest and delayed responses in acute hepatitis B and C virus infections. J Virol 2009; 83:3719-33; PMID:19176632; http://dx.doi.org/10.1128/JVI.01844-08.

60. Siegal FP, Kadowaki N, Shodell M, Fitzgerald-Bocarsly PA, Shah K, Ho S, et al. The nature of the principal type 1 interferon-producing cells in human blood. Science 1999; 284:1835-7; PMID:10364556; http://dx.doi.org/10.1126/science.284.5421.1835.

61. Suthar MS, Ma DY, Thomas S, Lund JM, Zhang N, Daffis S, et al. IPS-1 is essential for the control of West Nile virus infection and immunity. PLoS Pathog 2010; 6:e1000757; PMID:20140199; http://dx.doi.org/10.1371/journal.ppat.1000757.

62. Heil F, Hemmi H, Hochrein H, Ampenberger F, Kirschning C, Akira S, et al. Species-specific recognition of single-stranded RNA via toll-like receptor 7 and 8. Science 2004; 303:1526-9; PMID:14976262; http://dx.doi.org/10.1126/science.1093620.

63. Beignon AS, McKenna K, Skoberne M, Manches O, DaSilva I, Kavanagh DG, et al. Endocytosis of HIV-1 activates plasmacytoid dendritic cells via toll-like receptor-viral RNA interactions. J Clin Invest 2005; 115:3265-75; PMID:16224540; http://dx.doi.org/10.1172/JCI26032.

64. Schmidt B, Ashlock BM, Foster H, Fujimura SH, Levy JA. HIV-infected cells are major inducers of plasmacytoid dendritic cell interferon production, maturation, and migration. Virology 2005; 343:256-66; PMID:16278001; http://dx.doi.org/10.1016/j.virol.2005.09.059.

65. Meier A, Alter G, Frahm N, Sidhu H, Li B, Bagchi A, et al. MyD88-dependent immune activation mediated by human immunodeficiency virus type 1-encoded toll-like receptor ligands. J Virol 2007; 81:8180-91; PMID:17507480; http://dx.doi.org/10.1128/JVI.00421-07.

66. Mandl JN, Barry AP, Vanderford TH, Kozyr N, Chavan R, Klucking S, et al. Divergent TLR7 and TLR9 signaling and type I interferon production distinguish pathogenic and nonpathogenic AIDS virus infections. Nat Med 2008; 14:1077-87; PMID:18806803; http://dx.doi.org/10.1038/nm.1871.

67. Lepelley A, Louis S, Sourisseau M, Law HK, Pothlichet J, Schilte C, et al. Innate Sensing of HIV-Infected Cells. PLoS Pathog 2011; 7:e1001284; PMID:21379343; http://dx.doi.org/10.1371/journal.ppat.1001284.

68. Manel N, Hogstad B, Wang Y, Levy DE, Unutmaz D, Littman DR. A cryptic sensor for HIV-1 activates antiviral innate immunity in dendritic cells. Nature 2010; 467:214-7; PMID:20829794; http://dx.doi.org/10.1038/nature09337.

69. Nègre D, Mangeot PE, Duisit G, Blanchard S, Vidalain PO, Leissner P, et al. Characterization of novel safe lentiviral vectors derived from simian immunodeficiency virus (SIVmac251) that efficiently transduce mature human dendritic cells. Gene Ther 2000; 7:1613-23; PMID:11083469; http://dx.doi.org/10.1038/sj.gt.3301292.

70. Mangeot PE, Duperrier K, Negre D, Boson B, Rigal D, Cosset FL, et al. High levels of transduction of human dendritic cells with optimized SIV vectors. Mol Ther 2002; 5:283-90; PMID:11863418; http://dx.doi.org/10.1006/mthe.2002.0541.

71. Goujon C, Jarrosson-Wuilleme L, Bernaud J, Rigal D, Darlix JL, Cimarelli A. With a little help from a friend: increasing HIV transduction of monocyte-derived dendritic cells with virion-like particles of SIV(MAC). Gene Ther 2006; 13:991-4; PMID:16525481; http://dx.doi.org/10.1038/sj.gt.3302753.

72. Stetson DB, Ko JS, Heidmann T, Medzhitov R. Trex1 prevents cell-intrinsic initiation of autoimmunity. Cell 2008; 134:587-98; PMID:18724932; http://dx.doi.org/10.1016/j.cell.2008.06.032.

73. Stetson DB, Medzhitov R. Recognition of cytosolic DNA activates an IRF3-dependent innate immune response. Immunity 2006; 24:93-103; PMID:16413926; http://dx.doi.org/10.1016/j.immuni.2005.12.003.

74. Yan N, Regalado-Magdos AD, Stiggelbout B, Lee-Kirsch MA, Lieberman J. The cytosolic exonuclease TREX1 inhibits the innate immune response to human immunodeficiency virus type 1. Nat Immunol 2010; 11:1005-13; PMID:20871604; http://dx.doi.org/10.1038/ni.1941.

75. Doitsh G, Cavrois M, Lassen KG, Zepeda O, Yang Z, Santiago ML, et al. Abortive HIV infection mediates CD4 T cell depletion and inflammation in human lymphoid tissue. Cell 2010; 143:789-801; PMID:21111238; http://dx.doi.org/10.1016/j.cell.2010.11.001.

76. Neil S, Bieniasz P. Human immunodeficiency virus, restriction factors, and interferon. J Interferon Cytokine Res 2009; 29:569-80; PMID:19694548; http://dx.doi.org/10.1089/jir.2009.0077.

77. Berthoux L, Towers GJ, Gurer C, Salomoni P, Pandolfi PP, Luban J. As(2)O(3) enhances retroviral reverse transcription and counteracts Ref1 antiviral activity. J Virol 2003; 77:3167-80; PMID:12584341; http://dx.doi.org/10.1128/JVI.77.5.3167-3180.2003.

78. Shi M, Deng W, Bi E, Mao K, Ji Y, Lin G, et al. TRIM30 alpha negatively regulates TLR-mediated NF-kappa B activation by targeting TAB2 and TAB3 for degradation. Nat Immunol 2008; 9:369-77; PMID:18345001; http://dx.doi.org/10.1038/ni1577.

79. Tareen SU, Emerman M. Human Trim5alpha has additional activities that are uncoupled from retroviral capsid recognition. Virology 2011; 409:113-20; PMID:21035162; http://dx.doi.org/10.1016/j.virol.2010.09.018.

80. Pertel T, Hausmann S, Morger D, Züger S, Guerra J, Lascano J, et al. TRIM5 is an innate immune sensor for the retrovirus capsid lattice. Nature 2011; 472:361-5; PMID:21512573; http://dx.doi.org/10.1038/nature09976.

81. Bogdan C. The function of type I interferons in antimicrobial immunity. Curr Opin Immunol 2000; 12:419-24; PMID:10899033; http://dx.doi.org/10.1016/S0952-7915(00)00111-4.

82. Pomerantz RJ, Hirsch MS. Interferon and human immunodeficiency virus infection. Interferon 1987; 9:113-27; PMID:2445692.

83. Poli G, Orenstein JM, Kinter A, Folks TM, Fauci AS. Interferon-alpha but not AZT suppresses HIV expression in chronically infected cell lines. Science 1989; 244:575-7; PMID:2470148; http://dx.doi.org/10.1126/science.2470148.

84. Shirazi Y, Pitha PM. Alpha interferon inhibits early stages of the human immunodeficiency virus type 1 replication cycle. J Virol 1992; 66:1321-8; PMID:1738192.

85. Agy MB, Acker RL, Sherbert CH, Katze MG. Interferon treatment inhibits virus replication in HIV-1- and SIV-infected CD4+ T-cell lines by distinct mechanisms: evidence for decreased stability and aberrant processing of HIV-1 proteins. Virology 1995; 214:379-86; PMID:8553538; http://dx.doi.org/10.1006/viro.1995.0047.

86. Korth MJ, Taylor MD, Katze MG. Interferon inhibits the replication of HIV-1, SIV, and SHIV chimeric viruses by distinct mechanisms. Virology 1998; 247:265-73; PMID:9705919; http://dx.doi.org/10.1006/viro.1998.9249.

87. Taylor MD, Korth MJ, Katze MG. Interferon treatment inhibits the replication of simian immunodeficiency virus at an early stage: evidence for a block between attachment and reverse transcription. Virology 1998; 241:156-62; PMID:9454726; http://dx.doi.org/10.1006/viro.1997.8964.

88. Goujon C, Malim MH. Characterization of the alpha interferon-induced postentry block to HIV-1 infection in primary human macrophages and T cells. J Virol 2010; 84:9254-66; PMID:20610724; http://dx.doi.org/10.1128/JVI.00854-10.

89. Nagai K, Wong AH, Li S, Tam WN, Cuddihy AR, Sonenberg N, et al. Induction of CD4 expression and human immunodeficiency virus type 1 replication by mutants of the interferon-inducible protein kinase PKR. J Virol 1997; 71:1718-25; PMID:8995707.

90. Maitra RK, Silverman RH. Regulation of human immunodeficiency virus replication by 2',5'-oligoadenylate-dependent RNase L. J Virol 1998; 72:1146-52; PMID:9445011.

91. Okumura A, Lu GS, Pitha-Rowe I, Pitha PM. Innate antiviral response targets HIV-1 release by the induction of ubiquitin-like protein ISG15. Proc Natl Acad Sci USA 2006; 103:1440-5; PMID:16434471; http://dx.doi.org/10.1073/pnas.0510518103.

92. Barr SD, Smiley JR, Bushman FD. The interferon response inhibits HIV particle production by induction of TRIM22. PLoS Pathog 2008; 4:e1000007; PMID:18389079; http://dx.doi.org/10.1371/journal.ppat.1000007.

93. Espert L, Degols G, Lin YL, Vincent T, Benkirane M, Mechti N. Interferon-induced exonuclease ISG20 exhibits an antiviral activity against human immunodeficiency virus type 1. J Gen Virol 2005; 86:2221-9; PMID:16033969; http://dx.doi.org/10.1099/vir.0.81074-0.

94. Rivieccio MA, Suh HS, Zhao Y, Zhao ML, Chin KC, Lee SC, et al. TLR3 Ligation Activates an Antiviral Response in Human Fetal Astrocytes: A Role for Viperin/cig5. J Immunol 2006; 177:4735-41.

95. Lu J, Pan Q, Rong L, Liu SL, Liang C. The IFITM proteins inhibit HIV-1 infection. J Virol 2011; 85:2126-37; PMID:21177806; http://dx.doi.org/10.1128/JVI.01531-10.

96. Neil SJ, Sandrin V, Sundquist WI, Bieniasz PD. An interferon-alpha-induced tethering mechanism inhibits HIV-1 and Ebola virus particle release but is counteracted by the HIV-1 Vpu protein. Cell Host Microbe 2007; 2:193-203; PMID:18005734; http://dx.doi.org/10.1016/j.chom.2007.08.001.

97. Neil SJ, Zang T, Bieniasz PD. Tetherin inhibits retrovirus release and is antagonized by HIV-1 Vpu. Nature 2008; 451:425-30; PMID:18200009; http://dx.doi.org/10.1038/nature06553.

98. Battistini A, Marsili G, Sgarbanti M, Ensoli B, Hiscott J. IRF regulation of HIV-1 long terminal repeat activity. J Interferon Cytokine Res 2002; 22:27-37; PMID:11846973; http://dx.doi.org/10.1089/107999002753452638.

99. Sgarbanti M, Borsetti A, Moscufo N, Bellocchi MC, Ridolfi B, Nappi F, et al. Modulation of human immunodeficiency virus 1 replication by interferon regulatory factors. J Exp Med 2002; 195:1359-70; PMID:12021315; http://dx.doi.org/10.1084/jem.20010753.

100. Hayashi T, Nishitsuji H, Takamori A, Hasegawa A, Masuda T, Kannagi M. DNA-dependent activator of IFN-regulatory factors enhances the transcription of HIV-1 through NF-kappaB. Microbes Infect 2010; 12:937-47; PMID:20599623; http://dx.doi.org/10.1016/j.micinf.2010.06.003.

101. Foy E, Li K, Wang CF, Sumpter R Jr, Ikeda M, Lemon SM, et al. Regulation of interferon regulatory factor-3 by the hepatitis C virus serine protease. Science 2003; 300:1145-8; PMID:12702807; http://dx.doi.org/10.1126/science.1082604.

102. Doehle BP, Hladik F, McNevin JP, McElrath MJ, Gale M Jr. Human immunodeficiency virus type 1 mediates global disruption of innate antiviral signaling and immune defenses within infected cells. J Virol 2009; 83:10395-405; PMID:19706707; http://dx.doi.org/10.1128/JVI.00849-09.

103. Okumura A, Alce T, Lubyova B, Ezelle H, Strebel K, Pitha PM. HIV-1 accessory proteins VPR and Vif modulate antiviral response by targeting IRF-3 for degradation. Virology 2008; 373:85-97; PMID:18082865; http://dx.doi.org/10.1016/j.virol.2007.10.042.

104. Solis M, Nakhaei P, Jalalirad M, Lacoste J, Douville R, Arguello M, et al. RIG-I-mediated antiviral signaling is inhibited in HIV-1 infection by a protease-mediated sequestration of RIG-I. J Virol 2011; 85:1224-36; PMID:21084468; http://dx.doi.org/10.1128/JVI.01635-10.

105. Wang Y, Abel K, Lantz K, Krieg AM, McChesney MB, Miller CJ. The Toll-like receptor 7 (TLR7) agonist, imiquimod, and the TLR9 agonist, CpG ODN, induce antiviral cytokines and chemokines but do not prevent vaginal transmission of simian immunodeficiency virus when applied intravaginally to rhesus macaques. J Virol 2005; 79:14355-70; PMID:16254370; http://dx.doi.org/10.1128/JVI.79.22.14355-14370.2005.

106. Bosinger SE, Li Q, Gordon SN, Klatt NR, Duan L, Xu L, et al. Global genomic analysis reveals rapid control of a robust innate response in SIV-infected sooty mangabeys. J Clin Invest 2009; 119:3556-72; PMID:19959874.
107. Harris LD, Tabb B, Sodora DL, Paiardini M, Klatt NR, Douek DC, et al. Downregulation of robust acute type I interferon responses distinguishes nonpathogenic simian immunodeficiency virus (SIV) infection of natural hosts from pathogenic SIV infection of rhesus macaques. J Virol 2010; 84:7886-91; PMID:20484518; http://dx.doi.org/10.1128/JVI.02612-09.
108. Jacquelin B, Mayau V, Targat B, Liovat AS, Kunkel D, Petitjean G, et al. Nonpathogenic SIV infection of African green monkeys induces a strong but rapidly controlled type I IFN response. J Clin Invest 2009; 119:3544-55; PMID:19959873.
109. Silvestri G, Sodora DL, Koup RA, Paiardini M, O'Neil SP, McClure HM, et al. Nonpathogenic SIV infection of sooty mangabeys is characterized by limited bystander immunopathology despite chronic high-level viremia. Immunity 2003; 18:441-52; PMID:12648460; http://dx.doi.org/10.1016/S1074-7613(03)00060-8.
110. Zuniga EI, Liou LY, Mack L, Mendoza M, Oldstone MBA. Persistent Virus Infection Inhibits Type I Interferon Production by Plasmacytoid Dendritic Cells to Facilitate Opportunistic Infections. Cell Host Microbe 2008; 4:374-86; PMID:18854241; http://dx.doi.org/10.1016/j.chom.2008.08.016.
111. Zhao Y, De Trez C, Flynn R, Ware CF, Croft M, Salek-Ardakani S. The adaptor molecule MyD88 directly promotes CD8 T cell responses to vaccinia virus. J Immunol 2009; 182:6278-86; PMID:19414781; http://dx.doi.org/10.4049/jimmunol.0803682.
112. LaRosa DF, Stumhofer JS, Gelman AE, Rahman AH, Taylor DK, Hunter CA, et al. T cell expression of MyD88 is required for resistance to Toxoplasma gondii. Proc Natl Acad Sci USA 2008; 105:3855-60; PMID:18308927; http://dx.doi.org/10.1073/pnas.0706663105.
113. Rahman AH, Cui W, Larosa DF, Taylor DK, Zhang J, Goldstein DR, et al. MyD88 plays a critical T cell-intrinsic role in supporting CD8 T cell expansion during acute lymphocytic choriomeningitis virus infection. J Immunol 2008; 181:3804-10; PMID:18768833.
114. Quigley M, Martinez J, Huang X, Yang Y. A critical role for direct TLR2-MyD88 signaling in CD8 T-cell clonal expansion and memory formation following vaccinia viral infection. Blood 2009; 113:2256-64; PMID:18948575; http://dx.doi.org/10.1182/blood-2008-03-148809.

CHAPTER 11

Innate Immune Evasion Strategies of Influenza A Virus

Alesha Grant and Adolfo García-Sastre*

Abstract

Vertebrates possess a highly sophisticated sensing machinery to detect RNA viruses, including influenza A viruses, resulting in induction of interferon and antiviral responses. However, influenza A viruses, similar to other viruses, have acquired inhibitory activities of the sensing and interferon mediated antiviral activities of their hosts, facilitating viral replication. In the last years, a complex picture of these activities has emerged, that includes multiple mechanisms by which influenza A viruses evade the antiviral host innate response. While the NS1 protein of the virus is dedicated to antagonize the interferon response at multiple levels, other viral proteins, such as PB1-F2 and the polymerase complex, also appear to contribute to immune evasion. After briefly describing how the interferon response is induced by influenza A, we discuss the multiple interferon evasion strategies encoded by the virus and their possible implications in virulence and host tropism.

Introduction

Influenza A virus (IAV) is a negative-sense, single-stranded, segmented RNA virus belonging to the family *Orthomyxoviridae*. IAVs circulate worldwide and cause disease that is often associated with high economic burden and high mortality and morbidity rates, especially in the event of a pandemic. Wild aquatic birds are the main reservoir of IAVs, albeit infection and transmission among multiple animal species is a frequent and common occurrence. Consequently, reassortant viruses, possibly having undergone antigenic shift as well, are produced and often a more virulent phenotype is exhibited.[1-4] The recent novel quadruple reassortant pandemic 2009 H1N1 S-OIV is an example of this complex, ill-understood phenomenon.[5,6] These viruses can pose a great threat to global health and economics due to their ability to more readily overcome and/or modulate the host's innate and adaptive immune responses. Defining the gene segments and specific mutations that contribute to increased pathogenesis and host tropism is of invaluable measure. Furthermore, elucidating the mechanism of action behind the corresponding viral proteins will provide considerable insight for the development of vaccines and antiviral therapeutics.

In order to establish an infection, the invading pathogen must first subvert the host's innate immune responses. IAVs, along with any other pathogenic virus, have developed various mechanisms to accomplish this feat. The type I interferon (IFNβ and IFNα) system is paramount in generating an initial antiviral state and coordinating the appropriate adaptive immune response necessary to clear the virus. The signaling cascades that lead to the secretion of type I IFNs have been well studied and characterized. Fittingly, several proteins encoded by IAVs are capable of

*Department of Microbiology, Department of Medicine, and Global Health and Emerging Pathogens Institute, Mount Sinai School of Medicine, New York, New York, USA.
Corresponding Author: Adolfo García-Sastre—Email: adolfo.garcia-sastre@mssm.edu

Nucleic Acid Sensors and Antiviral Immunity, edited by Suryaprakash Sambhara and Takashi Fujita.
©2013 Landes Bioscience.

interfering with the IFN system at multiple levels and through various mechanisms. This review will detail how cells first recognize IAV, how the IFN signaling cascade is induced and propagated and finally how IAV proteins, specifically NS1, the polymerase (PA, PB1, PB2) and PB1-F2, can overcome the host's type I IFN response.

Recognition of IAV

IAV attaches to cells through the interaction of the viral hemagglutinin (HA) protein and sialic acid residues, specifically N-acetylneuraminic acid for human cells.[7,8] IAV then enters cells through a dynamin-dependent, clathrin-mediated endosomal pathway.[9] Recently, macropinocytosis was proposed as an alternative mechanism of entry.[10] The first step in the successful elimination of any pathogen is the detection of its presence in infected cells. Toll-like receptors (TLRs) and retinoic inducible gene I (RIG-I)-like receptors (RLRs) constitute two classes of germ-line encoded pattern-recognition receptors (PRRs) that recognize a variety of pathogen-associated molecular patterns (PAMPs).[11] Recognition of PAMPs results in a signaling cascade that leads to the production of type I IFN, cytokines, chemokines and interferon stimulated genes (ISGs) that initiate the process of clearing the pathogen. In the event of an IAV infection, endosomal TLR3, 7 and 8 signaling can become activated, however, research has demonstrated that RIG-I is the main PRR utilized in epithelial cells, the main target cell for IAV infection.[12-14]

RIG-I contains a C-terminal RNA-binding repressor domain (RD), an ATP-dependent RNA helicase domain and two N-terminal caspase associated recruitment domains (CARDs).[15-17] In IAV infected cells, RIG-I binds to viral RNA that contains a 5′ triphosphate and a partial dsRNA structure formed by the complementarity of the 5′ and 3′ RNA ends, characteristics associated with RIG-I sensing.[18,19] The binding of viral RNA to the RD activates the helicase activity of RIG-I and triggers a conformational change exposing the two CARDs. E3 ubiquitin ligases, such as TRIM25 and RIPLET, ubiquitinate the CARDs promoting interaction with the downstream adaptor molecule mitochondrial anti-viral signaling protein (MAVS).[20-22] The RIG-I/MAVS interaction triggers a complex signaling cascade that results in the activation of transcription factors that lead to the secretion of type I IFNs.

Induction and Propagation of Type I IFN

MAVS serves as a pivotal scaffolding protein that facilitates the interaction with numerous proteins necessary for proper IFN signaling,[23] although the complicated mechanism by which this process occurs remains largely enigmatic. Four independent laboratories simultaneously discovered MAVS in 2004.[22,24-26] It was identified as a novel RLR adaptor molecule that activates nuclear factor-κB (NF-κB) and interferon regulatory factor 3 and 7 (IRF3 and IRF7) signaling cascades resulting in the production of type I IFN and pro-inflammatory cytokines. MAVS contains an N-terminal CARD, a proline-rich region and a C-terminal transmembrane domain that localizes the protein to the mitochondrial outer membrane. Without mitochondrial localization, type I IFN production is severely abrogated.[27] MAVS dimerization or oligomerization is also necessary for optimal IRF3 phosphorylation and type I IFN production.[27-29] Additionally, the CARD domain of MAVS is crucial for proper IFN induction.[22,30] Finally, it has been demonstrated that without proper mitochondrial fusion and mitochondrial membrane potential, MAVS-mediated anti-viral signaling is dramatically reduced.[31]

The induction and propagation of type I IFN is highlighted in Figure 1. First, following RIG-I activation, the CARDs of RIG-I interact with the CARD of MAVS. This triggers the activation and binding of multiple tumor necrosis factor receptor-associated factor (TRAF) family members to MAVS. TRAF2, 3, 5 and 6 and TNFR1-associated death domain protein (TRADD) complexes have been implicated in MAVS binding and subsequent activation of downstream effector molecules.[24,25,32-35] In short, TRAF3 complexes lead to the activation of kinases such as IKKε and TBK1 that phosphorylate IRF3/IRF7 resulting in dimerization and nuclear transloca-tion. TRAF6/TRADD complexes activate canonical NF-κB signaling through the activation of the IKK complex, which then leads to the degradation of the inhibitory IκBα subunit, allowing

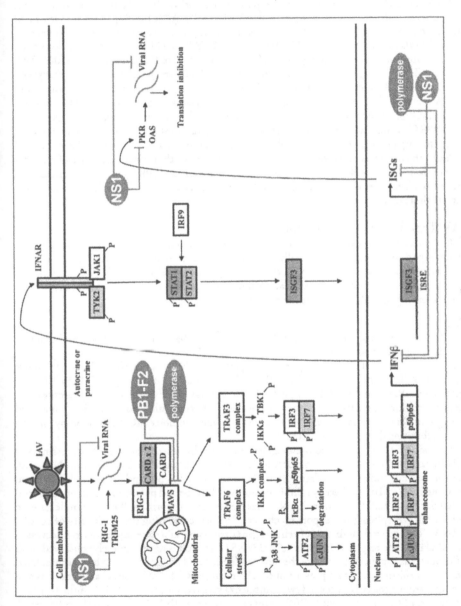

Figure 1. Induction and evasion of interferon responses by influenza A viruses.

the p50 and p65 subunits of NF-κB to freely translocate into the nucleus. Finally, cellular stress or TRAF6 complexes lead to the activation of p38 kinase and c-JUN N-terminal kinase (JNK), which then phosphorylate and activate ATF-2 and c-JUN.

Activation of the IFNβ gene requires the cooperative binding of specific transcription factors, ATF-2/c-Jun, IRF3/IRF7, and the p50 and p65 subunits of NFκB, to the IFNβ enhancer[36]; this complex is deemed the enhanceosome. Following the subsequent binding of co-activators and chromatin remodeling proteins to the INFβ promoter, INFβ is then secreted from infected cells where it binds the heterodimeric IFNα/β receptor (IFNAR) in either an endocrine or paracrine manner. This initiates the signaling cascade for the production of IFNα through the JAK/STAT pathway.[37] The receptor-associated Janus tyrosine kinases TYK2 and JAK1 become phosphorylated and the activated kinases then phosphorylate signal transducer and activator of transcription 1 and 2 (STAT1 and STAT2). STAT heterodimers form and association with IRF9 occurs. This complex, termed ISGF3, translocates into the nucleus and binds to the interferon-stimulated response element (ISRE), which induces the transcription of hundreds of ISGs.[38,39] These ISGs are involved in eliminating the virus from infected cells, maintaining an antiviral state in non-infected cells and initiating the necessary adaptive immune response needed for the ultimate clearance of the virus from the host. For example, as detailed by Figure 1, protein kinase R (PKR) and 2'5'-oligoadenylate synthetase (OAS), cellular enzymes activated by viral dsRNA, are two ISGs that translationally impede viral and cellular protein synthesis.

IAV Type I IFN Antagonists

Given the intricate evolutionary design of the innate immune response, it is remarkable that viruses have developed their own equally complex mechanisms to overcome this countermeasure. IAVs encode the IFN antagonists NS1, the viral polymerase and PB1-F2, which ultimately provide a window for successful viral replication and transmission. The points of inhibition by these proteins during the IFN cascade are illustrated in Figure 1.

NS1

NS1 is a remarkably multi-functional virulence factor that can inhibit IFNβ production at both the pre- and post-transcriptional level.[40] First, NS1 contains a dimerization-dependent N-terminal RNA binding domain (RBD) that preferentially binds dsRNA molecules.[41,42] Since activation of RIG-I, protein kinase R (PKR) and 2'5'-oligoadenylate synthetase (OAS)/RNase L depend on dsRNA binding, NS1 competes for RNA binding, with OAS to the greatest extent, thereby inhibiting the activation of these molecules.[43,44] Further inhibition of PKR is maintained through the direct binding of NS1[45,46] and NS1 efficiently inhibits RIG-I activation by binding to and inhibiting the activity of TRIM25.[47]

Second, NS1 can localize to the nucleus where it inhibits cellular mRNA processing and mRNA export. Cellular mRNA processing is disrupted through the interaction of NS1 with cellular cleavage and polyadenylation specific factor 30 (CPSF30) and polyadenylation binding protein II (PABPII), thereby inhibiting normal cleavage and polyadenylation of the 3' end of cellular mRNAs.[48,49] Additionally, NS1 has been shown to form inhibitory complexes with cellular mRNA splicing and export machinery,[50-53] further limiting the availability of cellular mRNAs. This general inhibition of cellular gene expression subsequently results in a decreased anti-viral immune response. Interestingly, this NS1 function is not completely conserved in all influenza virus strains, as the NS1 of the new pandemic H1N1 virus appears to have accumulated amino acid substitutions that prevent optimal binding to CPSF30.[54] This characteristic is also common among the NS1 of several swine influenza virus strains, of early H5N1 influenza virus strains and of the mouse adapted PR8 strain of influenza H1N1 virus.[55,56] On the other hand, the NS1 of human H3N2 viruses appears to have acquired yet an additional mechanism how to inhibit cellular gene expression. The NS1 of these viruses contains a motif at the very C-terminal that mimics the N-terminal histone tails, allowing the interaction of NS1 with histone modifying enzymes, such as histone acetylases and methylases, and with components of the cellular chromatin remodeling machinery. These interactions interfere with transcriptional elongation of genes involved in antiviral responses, resulting in evasion of the antiviral response.[57] It is attractive to speculate that by using multiple mechanisms to evade innate immune responses, the NS1 of IAV contributes to the highly zoonotic potential of IAV, as this might allow IAV a broader capability to inhibit IFN responses in multiple hosts.

Finally, NS1 can preferentially mediate the enhancement of IAV replication and translation, further exacerbating the antiviral properties of NS1. NS1 can bind to the p85-β regulatory subunit of phosphatidylinositol-3-kinase (PI3K), which increases PI3K signaling and allows for the formation of a favorable IAV replication environment.[58,59] NS1 can also bind eukaryotic translation initiation factor eIF4GI and polyadenylation binding protein I (PABI) forming a trimeric complex that enhances the translational initiation of viral mRNAs in a 5' UTR dependent manner.[60,61] It has also been suggested that the interaction between NS1 and human Staufen protein, which normally functions to direct microtubule transport of cellular mRNAs toward polysomes, may contribute to the mechanism of enhanced viral mRNA translation.[62] Collectively, NS1 depicts an exhaustively clever viral strategy designed to impede and overcome the host's immune response.

The Viral Polymerase

Studies using UV irradiation, yeast two-hybrid systems and systems biology approaches have implicated the importance of the IAV RNA polymerase in regards to IFN antagonism.[63,64] In addition to its previously described nuclear localization, PB2 has been shown to localize to the mitochondria.[65-67] Further investigation into the functional significance of this phenotype revealed that PB2 could interact with MAVS and inhibit MAVS-mediated IFNβ production.[68] An additional group has reported this same finding for not only the PB2 but also the PB1 and PA subunits of the viral polymerase.[69] Since the viral polymerase is responsible for the cellular cap-snatching activity,[70] it has been hypothesized that the viral polymerase confers an overall decrease in cellular gene expression, potentially supporting its anti-IFN phenotype. It is evident that much work is needed to fully investigate the significance of the viral polymerase anti-IFN phenotype and its contribution to virulence.

PB1-F2

First identified in 2001, PB1-F2 is a short, multifunctional polypeptide that is encoded from the +1 open reading frame of the PB1 gene of some IAV strains.[71] Initial characterization revealed that PB1-F2 could localize to the mitochondria where it could disrupt inner mitochondrial membrane potential and induce apoptosis, possibly through interactions with mitochondrial voltage-dependent anion channel 1 (VDAC1) and adenine nucleotide translocator 3 (ANT3).[71-73] It has also been proposed that PB1-F2 can permeate and destabilize mitochondrial membranes through the formation of an α-helical apoptotic pore.[74-76] In vivo studies suggest that PB1-F2 mediated apoptosis may be specific to immune cells and contributes to increased pathogenesis in the mouse model.[71,77,78] Additionally, a single amino acid substitution at position 66, an asparagine to serine, conferred dramatically increased viral pathogenicity and secondary bacterial infection[79,80] and inhibited early IFN responses in vivo.[81] Further mechanistic characterization revealed that PB1-F2 antagonizes IFNβ induction at the level of MAVS and this phenotype was further exacerbated by the N66S mutation.[82,83]

Overall, PB1-F2 exhibits a broad array of functions and is implicated with increased viral pathogenesis; therefore, further investigation into PB1-F2's mechanism of action is warranted. For instance, PB1-F2 sequences vary greatly depending on the isolate,[84] the dominate population being 57 and 90 amino acids in length. The functional significance, if any, of the majority of the sequences has not been determined. The new pandemic H1N1 IAV contains a truncated form of PB1-F2,[85] which is thought to contribute to its low virulence when compared with other pandemic strains.[86] However, when the virus was engineered to express full length PB1-F2, with and without the N66S mutation, an increase in virulence was not observed in either the mouse or ferret model.[87]

Conclusion

Many advances have been made on the mechanisms through which IAV induce and evade IFN responses, and it is now clear that innate immune responses generated during IAV infection are the result of multiple cellular and viral factors that interact at different levels. How the integration of these complex interactions contributes to the virulence and host tropism of IAV is still unclear. It is critical to note that not every viral protein function mentioned above is conserved in all IAV strains, so many of these functions are dispensable for IAV survival.[55,88-96] Nevertheless, they may contribute to enhanced virulence by promoting unimpeded viral replication[97] or enhanced immunopathology.[98] The need for further research addressing these concerns is imperative, as this may allow for further advancement in current vaccines and antiviral therapeutics.

Acknowledgments

Work in the García-Sastre lab is supported by NIAID grants and by the Center for Research on Influenza Pathogenesis (CRIP), and NIAID funded Center of Excellence for Influenza Research and Surveillance (CEIRS).

About the Authors

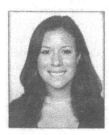
Alesha Grant is PhD student in the Department of Microbiology at the Mount Sinai School of Medicine in New York. She graduated in 2009 with a Bachelor's of Science in Biochemistry from the University of Nevada, Reno. Currently, her research interests involve characterizing RNA virus interferon antagonists and elucidating their mechanisms of action.

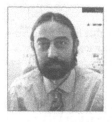
Adolfo García-Sastre is a Professor in the Departments of Microbiology and of Medicine at the Mount Sinai School of Medicine in New York. Dr. García-Sastre received his PhD in 1990 from the University of Salamanca where he focused on the characterization of the neuraminidase activity of influenza and Newcastle disease viruses. From 1991 to 1994 he studied influenza virus molecular biology as a postdoc in the laboratory of Dr. Peter Palese, at Mount Sinai School of Medicine in New York. He then established his own group in Mount Sinai School of Medicine, where he characterized for the first time that the NS1 protein of influenza virus is a virulence factor involved in inhibiting the host interferon response, and, in collaboration with Dr. Peter Palese, established reverse genetics techniques to generate influenza viruses from plasmid DNA. During the last years, his research has been focused on the molecular pathogenesis and immunity of influenza virus, on the characterization of the induction and inhibition of interferon responses by RNA viruses, and on the use of this information for the generation of novel vaccines and antivirals. Since 1997, Adolfo García-Sastre is also the Director of the Global Health and Emerging Pathogens Institute at Mount Sinai School of Medicine.

References

1. Morens DM, Taubenberger JK, Fauci AS. The persistent legacy of the 1918 influenza virus. N Engl J Med 2009; 361:225-9; PMID:19564629; http://dx.doi.org/10.1056/NEJMp0904819.
2. Zimmer SM, Burke DS. Historical perspective--Emergence of influenza A (H1N1) viruses. N Engl J Med 2009; 361:279-85; PMID:19564632; http://dx.doi.org/10.1056/NEJMra0904322.
3. Dong C, Ying L, Yuan D. Detecting transmission and reassortment events for influenza A viruses with genotype profile method. Virol J 2011; 8:395; PMID:21824442; http://dx.doi.org/10.1186/1743-422X-8-395.

4. Nelson MI, Viboud C, Simonsen L, Bennett RT, Griesemer SB, St George K, et al. Multiple reassortment events in the evolutionary history of H1N1 influenza A virus since 1918. PLoS Pathog 2008; 4:e1000012; PMID:18463694; http://dx.doi.org/10.1371/journal.ppat.1000012.
5. Dawood FS, Jain S, Finelli L, Shaw MW, Lindstrom S, Garten RJ, et al.; Novel Swine-Origin Influenza A (H1N1) Virus Investigation Team. Emergence of a novel swine-origin influenza A (H1N1) virus in humans. N Engl J Med 2009; 360:2605-15; PMID:19423869; http://dx.doi.org/10.1056/NEJMoa0903810.
6. Smith GJD, Vijaykrishna D, Bahl J, Lycett SJ, Worobey M, Pybus OG, et al. Origins and evolutionary genomics of the 2009 swine-origin H1N1 influenza A epidemic. Nature 2009; 459:1122-5; PMID:19516283; http://dx.doi.org/10.1038/nature08182.
7. Skehel JJ, Wiley DC. Receptor binding and membrane fusion in virus entry: the influenza hemagglutinin. Annu Rev Biochem 2000; 69:531-69; PMID:10966468; http://dx.doi.org/10.1146/annurev.biochem.69.1.531.
8. Suzuki Y, Ito T, Suzuki T, Holland RE Jr., Chambers TM, Kiso M, et al. Sialic acid species as a determinant of the host range of influenza A viruses. J Virol 2000; 74:11825-31; PMID:11090182; http://dx.doi.org/10.1128/JVI.74.24.11825-11831.2000.
9. Luo M. Influenza Virus Entry Viral Molecular Machines. Vol. 726 (eds. Rossmann, M.G. & Rao, V.B.) 201-221 (Springer US, 2012).
10. de Vries E, Tscherne DM, Wienholts MJ, Cobos-Jiménez V, Scholte F, García-Sastre A, et al. Dissection of the influenza A virus endocytic routes reveals macropinocytosis as an alternative entry pathway. PLoS Pathog 2011; 7:e1001329; PMID:21483486; http://dx.doi.org/10.1371/journal.ppat.1001329.
11. Akira S, Uematsu S, Takeuchi O. Pathogen recognition and innate immunity. Cell 2006; 124:783-801; PMID:16497588; http://dx.doi.org/10.1016/j.cell.2006.02.015.
12. Lund JM, Alexopoulou L, Sato A, Karow M, Adams NC, Gale NW, et al. Recognition of single-stranded RNA viruses by Toll-like receptor 7. Proc Natl Acad Sci U S A 2004; 101:5598-603; PMID:15034168; http://dx.doi.org/10.1073/pnas.0400937101.
13. Le Goffic R, Pothlichet J, Vitour D, Fujita T, Meurs E, Chignard M, et al. Cutting Edge: Influenza A virus activates TLR3-dependent inflammatory and RIG-I-dependent antiviral responses in human lung epithelial cells. J Immunol 2007; 178:3368-72; PMID:17339430.
14. Kato H, Takeuchi O, Sato S, Yoneyama M, Yamamoto M, Matsui K, et al. Differential roles of MDA5 and RIG-I helicases in the recognition of RNA viruses. Nature 2006; 441:101-5; PMID:16625202; http://dx.doi.org/10.1038/nature04734.
15. Cui S, Eisenächer K, Kirchhofer A, Brzózka K, Lammens A, Lammens K, et al. The C-terminal regulatory domain is the RNA 5'-triphosphate sensor of RIG-I. Mol Cell 2008; 29:169-79; PMID:18243112; http://dx.doi.org/10.1016/j.molcel.2007.10.032.
16. Yoneyama M, Kikuchi M, Natsukawa T, Shinobu N, Imaizumi T, Miyagishi M, et al. The RNA helicase RIG-I has an essential function in double-stranded RNA-induced innate antiviral responses. Nat Immunol 2004; 5:730-7; PMID:15208624; http://dx.doi.org/10.1038/ni1087.
17. Myong S, Cui S, Cornish PV, Kirchhofer A, Gack MU, Jung JU, et al. Cytosolic viral sensor RIG-I is a 5'-triphosphate-dependent translocase on double-stranded RNA. Science 2009; 323:1070-4; PMID:19119185; http://dx.doi.org/10.1126/science.1168352.
18. Baum A, Sachidanandam R, García-Sastre A. Preference of RIG-I for short viral RNA molecules in infected cells revealed by next-generation sequencing. Proc Natl Acad Sci U S A 2010; 107:16303-8; PMID:20805493; http://dx.doi.org/10.1073/pnas.1005077107.
19. Rehwinkel J, Tan CP, Goubau D, Schulz O, Pichlmair A, Bier K, et al. RIG-I detects viral genomic RNA during negative-strand RNA virus infection. Cell 2010; 140:397-408; PMID:20144762; http://dx.doi.org/10.1016/j.cell.2010.01.020.
20. Oshiumi H, Miyashita M, Inoue N, Okabe M, Matsumoto M, Seya T. The ubiquitin ligase Riplet is essential for RIG-I-dependent innate immune responses to RNA virus infection. Cell Host Microbe 2010; 8:496-509; PMID:21147464; http://dx.doi.org/10.1016/j.chom.2010.11.008.
21. Gack MU, Shin YC, Joo CH, Urano T, Liang C, Sun L, et al. TRIM25 RING-finger E3 ubiquitin ligase is essential for RIG-I-mediated antiviral activity. Nature 2007; 446:916-20; PMID:17392790; http://dx.doi.org/10.1038/nature05732.
22. Kawai T, Takahashi K, Sato S, Coban C, Kumar H, Kato H, et al. IPS-1, an adaptor triggering RIG-I- and Mda5-mediated type I interferon induction. Nat Immunol 2005; 6:981-8; PMID:16127453; http://dx.doi.org/10.1038/ni1243.
23. West AP, Shadel GS, Ghosh S. Mitochondria in innate immune responses. Nat Rev Immunol 2011; 11:389-402; PMID:21597473; http://dx.doi.org/10.1038/nri2975.
24. Xu L-G, Wang YY, Han KJ, Li LY, Zhai Z, Shu HB. VISA is an adapter protein required for virus-triggered IFN-β signaling. Mol Cell 2005; 19:727-40; PMID:16153868; http://dx.doi.org/10.1016/j.molcel.2005.08.014.

25. Seth RB, Sun L, Ea C-K, Chen ZJ. Identification and characterization of MAVS, a mitochondrial antiviral signaling protein that activates NF-kappaB and IRF 3. Cell 2005; 122:669-82; PMID:16125763; http://dx.doi.org/10.1016/j.cell.2005.08.012.
26. Meylan E, Curran J, Hofmann K, Moradpour D, Binder M, Bartenschlager R, et al. Cardif is an adaptor protein in the RIG-I antiviral pathway and is targeted by hepatitis C virus. Nature 2005; 437:1167-72; PMID:16177806; http://dx.doi.org/10.1038/nature04193.
27. Tang ED, Wang C-Y. MAVS self-association mediates antiviral innate immune signaling. J Virol 2009; 83:3420-8; PMID:19193783; http://dx.doi.org/10.1128/JVI.02623-08.
28. Hou F, Sun L, Zheng H, Skaug B, Jiang QX, Chen ZJ. MAVS forms functional prion-like aggregates to activate and propagate antiviral innate immune response. Cell 2011; 146:448-61; PMID:21782231; http://dx.doi.org/10.1016/j.cell.2011.06.041.
29. Baril M, Racine M-E, Penin F, Lamarre D. MAVS dimer is a crucial signaling component of innate immunity and the target of hepatitis C virus NS3/4A protease. J Virol 2009; 83:1299-311; PMID:19036819; http://dx.doi.org/10.1128/JVI.01659-08.
30. Sun QM, Sun L, Liu HH, Chen X, Seth RB, Forman J, et al. The specific and essential role of MAVS in antiviral innate immune responses. Immunity 2006; 24:633-42; PMID:16713980; http://dx.doi.org/10.1016/j.immuni.2006.04.004.
31. Koshiba, T., Yasukawa, K., Yanagi, Y. & Kawabata, S.-i. Mitochondrial Membrane Potential Is Required for MAVS-Mediated Antiviral Signaling. Sci. Signal. 4, ra7- (2011).
32. Saha SK, Pietras EM, He JQ, Kang JR, Liu SY, Oganesyan G, et al. Regulation of antiviral responses by a direct and specific interaction between TRAF3 and Cardif. EMBO J 2006; 25:3257-63; PMID:16858409; http://dx.doi.org/10.1038/sj.emboj.7601220.
33. Tang ED, Wang C-Y. TRAF5 is a downstream target of MAVS in antiviral innate immune signaling. PLoS One 2010; 5:e9172; PMID:20161788; http://dx.doi.org/10.1371/journal.pone.0009172.
34. Michallet MC, Meylan E, Ermolaeva MA, Vazquez J, Rebsamen M, Curran J, et al. TRADD protein is an essential component of the RIG-like helicase antiviral pathway. Immunity 2008; 28:651-61; PMID:18439848; http://dx.doi.org/10.1016/j.immuni.2008.03.013.
35. Honda K, Takaoka A, Taniguchi T, Type I interferon [corrected] gene induction by the interferon regulatory factor family of transcription factors. Immunity 2006; 25:349-60; PMID:16979567; http://dx.doi.org/10.1016/j.immuni.2006.08.009.
36. Panne D, Maniatis T, Harrison SC. An atomic model of the interferon-β enhanceosome. Cell 2007; 129:1111-23; PMID:17574024; http://dx.doi.org/10.1016/j.cell.2007.05.019.
37. Fensterl V, Sen GC. Interferons and viral infections. Biofactors 2009; 35:14-20; PMID:19319841; http://dx.doi.org/10.1002/biof.6.
38. Der SD, Zhou A, Williams BRG, Silverman RH. Identification of genes differentially regulated by interferon α, β, or γ using oligonucleotide arrays. Proc Natl Acad Sci U S A 1998; 95:15623-8; PMID:9861020; http://dx.doi.org/10.1073/pnas.95.26.15623.
39. Platanias LC. Mechanisms of type-I- and type-II-interferon-mediated signalling. Nat Rev Immunol 2005; 5:375-86; PMID:15864272; http://dx.doi.org/10.1038/nri1604.
40. Hale BG, Albrecht RA, García-Sastre A. Innate immune evasion strategies of influenza viruses. Future Microbiol 2010; 5:23-41; PMID:20020828; http://dx.doi.org/10.2217/fmb.09.108.
41. Liu J, Lynch PA, Chien CY, Montelione GT, Krug RM, Berman HM. Crystal structure of the unique RNA-binding domain of the influenza virus NS1 protein. Nat Struct Biol 1997; 4:896-9; PMID:9360602; http://dx.doi.org/10.1038/nsb1197-896.
42. Wang W, Riedel K, Lynch P, Chien CY, Montelione GT, Krug RM. RNA binding by the novel helical domain of the influenza virus NS1 protein requires its dimer structure and a small number of specific basic amino acids. RNA 1999; 5:195-205; PMID:10024172; http://dx.doi.org/10.1017/S1355838299981621.
43. Floyd-Smith G, Slattery E, Lengyel P. Interferon action: RNA cleavage pattern of a (2'-5')oligoadenylate--dependent endonuclease. Science 1981; 212:1030-2; PMID:6165080; http://dx.doi.org/10.1126/science.6165080.
44. Min J-Y, Krug RM. The primary function of RNA binding by the influenza A virus NS1 protein in infected cells: Inhibiting the 2'-5' oligo (A) synthetase/RNase L pathway. Proc Natl Acad Sci U S A 2006; 103:7100-5; PMID:16627618; http://dx.doi.org/10.1073/pnas.0602184103.
45. Li S, Min J-Y, Krug RM, Sen GC. Binding of the influenza A virus NS1 protein to PKR mediates the inhibition of its activation by either PACT or double-stranded RNA. Virology 2006; 349:13-21; PMID:16466763; http://dx.doi.org/10.1016/j.virol.2006.01.005.
46. Min J-Y, Li S, Sen GC, Krug RM. A site on the influenza A virus NS1 protein mediates both inhibition of PKR activation and temporal regulation of viral RNA synthesis. Virology 2007; 363:236-43; PMID:17320139; http://dx.doi.org/10.1016/j.virol.2007.01.038.

47. Gack MU, Albrecht RA, Urano T, Inn KS, Huang IC, Carnero E, et al. Influenza A virus NS1 targets the ubiquitin ligase TRIM25 to evade recognition by the host viral RNA sensor RIG-I. Cell Host Microbe 2009; 5:439-49; PMID:19454348; http://dx.doi.org/10.1016/j.chom.2009.04.006.
48. Nemeroff ME, Barabino SML, Li Y, Keller W, Krug RM. Influenza virus NS1 protein interacts with the cellular 30 kDa subunit of CPSF and inhibits 3′end formation of cellular pre-mRNAs. Mol Cell 1998; 1:991-1000; PMID:9651582; http://dx.doi.org/10.1016/S1097-2765(00)80099-4.
49. Chen Z, Li Y, Krug RM. Influenza A virus NS1 protein targets poly(A)-binding protein II of the cellular 3′-end processing machinery. EMBO J 1999; 18:2273-83; PMID:10205180; http://dx.doi.org/10.1093/emboj/18.8.2273.
50. Fortes P, Beloso A, Ortín J. Influenza virus NS1 protein inhibits pre-mRNA splicing and blocks mRNA nucleocytoplasmic transport. EMBO J 1994; 13:704-12; PMID:8313914.
51. Fortes P, Lamond AI, Ortín J. Influenza virus NS1 protein alters the subnuclear localization of cellular splicing components. J Gen Virol 1995; 76:1001-7; PMID:9049349; http://dx.doi.org/10.1099/0022-1317-76-4-1001.
52. Qiu Y, Nemeroff M, Krug RM. The influenza virus NS1 protein binds to a specific region in human U6 snRNA and inhibits U6-U2 and U6-U4 snRNA interactions during splicing. RNA 1995; 1:304-16; PMID:7489502.
53. Satterly N, Tsai PL, van Deursen J, Nussenzveig DR, Wang Y, Faria PA, et al. Influenza virus targets the mRNA export machinery and the nuclear pore complex. Proc Natl Acad Sci U S A 2007; 104:1853-8; PMID:17267598; http://dx.doi.org/10.1073/pnas.0610977104.
54. Hale BG, Steel J, Medina RA, Manicassamy B, Ye J, Hickman D, et al. Inefficient control of host gene expression by the 2009 pandemic H1N1 influenza A virus NS1 protein. J Virol 2010; 84:6909-22; PMID:20444891; http://dx.doi.org/10.1128/JVI.00081-10.
55. Kochs G, García-Sastre A, Martínez-Sobrido L. Multiple anti-interferon actions of the influenza A virus NS1 protein. J Virol 2007; 81:7011-21; PMID:17442719; http://dx.doi.org/10.1128/JVI.02581-06.
56. Spesock A, Malur M, Hossain MJ, Chen LM, Njaa BL, Davis CT, et al. The virulence of 1997 H5N1 influenza viruses in the mouse model is increased by correcting a defect in their NS1 proteins. J Virol 2011; 85:7048-58; PMID:21593152; http://dx.doi.org/10.1128/JVI.00417-11.
57. Marazzi I, Ho JS, Kim J, Manicassamy B, Dewell S, Albrecht RA, et al. Suppression of the antiviral response by an influenza histone mimic. Nature 2012; 483:428-33; PMID:22419161; http://dx.doi.org/10.1038/nature10892.
58. Hale BG, Jackson D, Chen Y-H, Lamb RA, Randall RE. Influenza A virus NS1 protein binds p85β and activates phosphatidylinositol-3-kinase signaling. Proc Natl Acad Sci U S A 2006; 103:14194-9; PMID:16963558; http://dx.doi.org/10.1073/pnas.0606109103.
59. Cooray S. The pivotal role of phosphatidylinositol 3-kinase-Akt signal transduction in virus survival. J Gen Virol 2004; 85:1065-76; PMID:15105524; http://dx.doi.org/10.1099/vir.0.19771-0.
60. Burgui I, Aragón Ts, Ortín J, Nieto A. PABP1 and eIF4GI associate with influenza virus NS1 protein in viral mRNA translation initiation complexes. J Gen Virol 2003; 84:3263-74; PMID:14645908; http://dx.doi.org/10.1099/vir.0.19487-0.
61. de la Luna S, Fortes P, Beloso A, Ortín J. Influenza virus NS1 protein enhances the rate of translation initiation of viral mRNAs. J Virol 1995; 69:2427-33; PMID:7884890.
62. Falcón AM, Fortes P, Marión RM, Beloso A, Ortín J. Interaction of influenza virus NS1 protein and the human homologue of Staufen in vivo and in vitro. Nucleic Acids Res 1999; 27:2241-7; PMID:10325410; http://dx.doi.org/10.1093/nar/27.11.2241.
63. Marcus PI, Rojek JM, Sekellick MJ. Interferon induction and/or production and its suppression by influenza A viruses. J Virol 2005; 79:2880-90; PMID:15709007; http://dx.doi.org/10.1128/JVI.79.5.2880-2890.2005.
64. Shapira SD, Gat-Viks I, Shum BO, Dricot A, de Grace MM, Wu L, et al. A physical and regulatory map of host-influenza interactions reveals pathways in H1N1 infection. Cell 2009; 139:1255-67; PMID:20064372; http://dx.doi.org/10.1016/j.cell.2009.12.018.
65. Woodfin BM, Kazim AL. Interaction of the amino-terminus of an influenza virus protein with mitochondria. Arch Biochem Biophys 1993; 306:427-30; PMID:8215446; http://dx.doi.org/10.1006/abbi.1993.1533.
66. Fodor E, Smith M. The PA subunit is required for efficient nuclear accumulation of the PB1 subunit of the influenza A virus RNA polymerase complex. J Virol 2004; 78:9144-53; PMID:15308710; http://dx.doi.org/10.1128/JVI.78.17.9144-9153.2004.
67. Carr SM, Carnero E, García-Sastre A, Brownlee GG, Fodor E. Characterization of a mitochondrial-targeting signal in the PB2 protein of influenza viruses. Virology 2006; 344:492-508; PMID:16242167; http://dx.doi.org/10.1016/j.virol.2005.08.041.

68. Graef KM, Vreede FT, Lau YF, McCall AW, Carr SM, Subbarao K, et al. The PB2 subunit of the influenza virus RNA polymerase affects virulence by interacting with the mitochondrial antiviral signaling protein and inhibiting expression of beta interferon. J Virol 2010; 84:8433-45; PMID:20538852; http://dx.doi.org/10.1128/JVI.00879-10.

69. Iwai A, Shiozaki T, Kawai T, Akira S, Kawaoka Y, Takada A, et al. Influenza A virus polymerase inhibits type I interferon induction by binding to interferon β promoter stimulator 1. J Biol Chem 2010; 285:32064-74; PMID:20699220; http://dx.doi.org/10.1074/jbc.M110.112458.

70. Plotch SJ, Bouloy M, Ulmanen I, Krug RM. A unique cap(m7GpppXm)-dependent influenza virion endonuclease cleaves capped RNAs to generate the primers that initiate viral RNA transcription. Cell 1981; 23:847-58; PMID:6261960; http://dx.doi.org/10.1016/0092-8674(81)90449-9.

71. Chen W, Calvo PA, Malide D, Gibbs J, Schubert U, Bacik I, et al. A novel influenza A virus mitochondrial protein that induces cell death. Nat Med 2001; 7:1306-12; PMID:11726970; http://dx.doi.org/10.1038/nm1201-1306.

72. Zamarin D, García-Sastre A, Xiao X, Wang R, Palese P. Influenza virus PB1-F2 protein induces cell death through mitochondrial ANT3 and VDAC1. PLoS Pathog 2005; 1:e4; PMID:16201016; http://dx.doi.org/10.1371/journal.ppat.0010004.

73. Yamada H, Chounan R, Higashi Y, Kurihara N, Kido H. Mitochondrial targeting sequence of the influenza A virus PB1-F2 protein and its function in mitochondria. FEBS Lett 2004; 578:331-6; PMID:15589841; http://dx.doi.org/10.1016/j.febslet.2004.11.017.

74. Chanturiya AN, Basañez G, Schubert U, Henklein P, Yewdell JW, Zimmerberg J. PB1-F2, an influenza A virus-encoded proapoptotic mitochondrial protein, creates variably sized pores in planar lipid membranes. J Virol 2004; 78:6304-12; PMID:15163724; http://dx.doi.org/10.1128/JVI.78.12.6304-6312.2004.

75. Gibbs JS, Malide D, Hornung F, Bennink JR, Yewdell JW. The influenza A virus PB1-F2 protein targets the inner mitochondrial membrane via a predicted basic amphipathic helix that disrupts mitochondrial function. J Virol 2003; 77:7214-24; PMID:12805420; http://dx.doi.org/10.1128/JVI.77.13.7214-7224.2003.

76. Bruns K, Studtrucker N, Sharma A, Fossen T, Mitzner D, Eissmann A, et al. Structural characterization and oligomerization of PB1-F2, a proapoptotic influenza A virus protein. J Biol Chem 2007; 282:353-63; PMID:17052982; http://dx.doi.org/10.1074/jbc.M606494200.

77. Zamarin D, Ortigoza MB, Palese P. Influenza A virus PB1-F2 protein contributes to viral pathogenesis in mice. J Virol 2006; 80:7976-83; PMID:16873254; http://dx.doi.org/10.1128/JVI.00415-06.

78. McAuley JL, Chipuk JE, Boyd KL, Van De Velde N, Green DR, McCullers JA. PB1-F2 proteins from H5N1 and 20 century pandemic influenza viruses cause immunopathology. PLoS Pathog 2010; 6:e1001014; PMID:20661425; http://dx.doi.org/10.1371/journal.ppat.1001014.

79. Conenello GM, Zamarin D, Perrone LA, Tumpey T, Palese P. A single mutation in the PB1-F2 of H5N1 (HK/97) and 1918 influenza A viruses contributes to increased virulence. PLoS Pathog 2007; 3:1414-21; PMID:17922571; http://dx.doi.org/10.1371/journal.ppat.0030141.

80. McAuley JL, Hornung F, Boyd KL, Smith AM, McKeon R, Bennink J, et al. Expression of the 1918 influenza A virus PB1-F2 enhances the pathogenesis of viral and secondary bacterial pneumonia. Cell Host Microbe 2007; 2:240-9; PMID:18005742; http://dx.doi.org/10.1016/j.chom.2007.09.001.

81. Conenello GM, Tisoncik JR, Rosenzweig E, Varga ZT, Palese P, Katze MG. A single N66S mutation in the PB1-F2 protein of influenza A virus increases virulence by inhibiting the early interferon response in vivo. J Virol 2011; 85:652-62; PMID:21084483; http://dx.doi.org/10.1128/JVI.01987-10.

82. Varga ZT, Ramos I, Hai R, Schmolke M, García-Sastre A, Fernandez-Sesma A, et al. The influenza virus protein PB1-F2 inhibits the induction of type I interferon at the level of the MAVS adaptor protein. PLoS Pathog 2011; 7:e1002067; PMID:21695240; http://dx.doi.org/10.1371/journal.ppat.1002067.

83. Dudek SE, Wixler L, Nordhoff C, Nordmann A, Anhlan D, Wixler V, et al. The influenza virus PB1-F2 protein has interferon antagonistic activity. Biol Chem 2011; 392:1135-44; PMID:22050228; http://dx.doi.org/10.1515/BC.2011.174.

84. DeLuca DS, Keskin DB, Zhang GL, Reinherz EL, Brusic V. PB1-F2 Finder: scanning influenza sequences for PB1-F2 encoding RNA segments. BMC Bioinformatics 2011; 12(Suppl 13):S6; PMID:22373288; http://dx.doi.org/10.1186/1471-2105-12-S13-S6.

85. Trifonov V, Racaniello V, Rabadan R. The Contribution of the PB1-F2 protein to the fitness of Influenza A viruses and its recent evolution in the 2009 Influenza A (H1N1) pandemic virus. PLoS Curr 2009; 1:RRN1006; PMID:20029605; http://dx.doi.org/10.1371/currents.RRN1006.

86. Wang TT, Palese P. Unraveling the mystery of swine influenza virus. Cell 2009; 137:983-5; PMID:19524497; http://dx.doi.org/10.1016/j.cell.2009.05.032.

87. Hai R, Schmolke M, Varga ZT, Manicassamy B, Wang TT, Belser JA, et al. PB1-F2 expression by the 2009 pandemic H1N1 influenza virus has minimal impact on virulence in animal models. J Virol 2010; 84:4442-50; PMID:20181699; http://dx.doi.org/10.1128/JVI.02717-09.

88. Suarez DL, Perdue ML. Multiple alignment comparison of the non-structural genes of influenza A viruses. Virus Res 1998; 54:59-69; PMID:9660072; http://dx.doi.org/10.1016/S0168-1702(98)00011-2.
89. Melén K, Kinnunen L, Fagerlund R, Ikonen N, Twu KY, Krug RM, et al. Nuclear and nucleolar targeting of influenza A virus NS1 protein: striking differences between different virus subtypes. J Virol 2007; 81:5995-6006; PMID:17376915; http://dx.doi.org/10.1128/JVI.01714-06.
90. Petri T, Patterson S, Dimmock NJ. Polymorphism of the NS1 proteins of type A influenza virus. J Gen Virol 1982; 61:217-31; PMID:6214614; http://dx.doi.org/10.1099/0022-1317-61-2-217.
91. Quinlivan M, Zamarin D, García-Sastre A, Cullinane A, Chambers T, Palese P. Attenuation of equine influenza viruses through truncations of the NS1 protein. J Virol 2005; 79:8431-9; PMID:15956587; http://dx.doi.org/10.1128/JVI.79.13.8431-8439.2005.
92. Billharz R, Zeng H, Proll SC, Korth MJ, Lederer S, Albrecht R, et al. The NS1 protein of the 1918 pandemic influenza virus blocks host interferon and lipid metabolism pathways. J Virol 2009; 83:10557-70; PMID:19706713; http://dx.doi.org/10.1128/JVI.00330-09.
93. Jackson D, Hossain MJ, Hickman D, Perez DR, Lamb RA. A new influenza virus virulence determinant: the NS1 protein four C-terminal residues modulate pathogenicity. Proc Natl Acad Sci U S A 2008; 105:4381-6; PMID:18334632; http://dx.doi.org/10.1073/pnas.0800482105.
94. Hayman A, Comely S, Lackenby A, Murphy S, McCauley J, Goodbourn S, et al. Variation in the ability of human influenza A viruses to induce and inhibit the IFN-β pathway. Virology 2006; 347:52-64; PMID:16378631; http://dx.doi.org/10.1016/j.virol.2005.11.024.
95. Hatta M, Gao P, Halfmann P, Kawaoka Y. Molecular basis for high virulence of Hong Kong H5N1 influenza A viruses. Science 2001; 293:1840-2; PMID:11546875; http://dx.doi.org/10.1126/science.1062882.
96. Bradel-Tretheway BG, Kelley Z, Chakraborty-Sett S, Takimoto T, Kim B, Dewhurst S. The human H5N1 influenza A virus polymerase complex is active in vitro over a broad range of temperatures, in contrast to the WSN complex, and this property can be attributed to the PB2 subunit. J Gen Virol 2008; 89:2923-32; PMID:19008377; http://dx.doi.org/10.1099/vir.0.2008/006254-0.
97. Grimm D, Staeheli P, Hufbauer M, Koerner I, Martínez-Sobrido L, Solórzano A, et al. Replication fitness determines high virulence of influenza A virus in mice carrying functional Mx1 resistance gene. Proc Natl Acad Sci U S A 2007; 104:6806-11; PMID:17426143; http://dx.doi.org/10.1073/pnas.0701849104.
98. Kobasa D, Jones SM, Shinya K, Kash JC, Copps J, Ebihara H, et al. Aberrant innate immune response in lethal infection of macaques with the 1918 influenza virus. Nature 2007; 445:319-23; PMID:17230189; http://dx.doi.org/10.1038/nature05495.

CHAPTER 12

Autophagy in Antiviral Immunity

Brian Yordy and Akiko Iwasaki*

Abstract

Autophagy is an evolutionary ancient pathway by which cells maintain cell-autonomous homeostasis by removing intracellular material through lysosomal degradation. In addition to its homeostatic function, autophagy is also utilized by infected cells to remove intracellular pathogens, and likely represents one of the earliest forms of eukaryotic defense against intracellular pathogens. However, the autophagy pathway is not merely a one way ticket to the lysosome, but rather, an adaptable system capable of performing a diverse set of functions within cells. The vertebrate immune system utilizes autophagy not only to degrade intracellular pathogens, but also employs the autophagic machinery to enhance and precisely regulate innate and adaptive antiviral immune responses. However, in many cases, the autophagy pathway and its machinery are targeted by viral pathogens to either counter host viral restriction or to achieve maximal viral replication by subversion of autophagy pathway. Herein, we aim to summarize this rapidly expanding field, highlighting the diverse contribution of the autophagy pathway to antiviral immunity.

Introduction

Autophagy is a highly conserved catabolic pathway whose classical induction occurs under metabolic stress. Recent studies have demonstrated that autophagy is active in all tissues[1] and is critical not only in stress response but also in maintaining basal turnover of bulk cellular components.[2] Autophagy's central role in metabolism and stress response places it at the crossroads of many key signaling pathways. It is therefore not surprising that the autophagy machinery has been established as a key regulator of such diverse processes as aging, cancer, neurodegenerative disorders, and numerous immunological functions.[3] The term "autophagy" has been used inclusively to refer to intracellular degradation that occurs through the lysosomal pathway. This pathway now includes several distinct forms of lysosomal degradation including macroautophagy, chaperone-mediated autophagy and microautophagy (reviewed by refs. 4 and 5).

Macroautophagy (hereafter referred to as autophagy) involves the formation of double membrane structures that engulfs bulk cytoplasmic components including proteins, lipids, and entire organelles. Autophagosome formation is dependent on the precise coordination of a series of AuTophaGy (ATG) proteins that are evolutionary conserved from yeast to man. Autophagosome formation begins with the initiation complex involving Beclin-1 (ATG6) and the class III phosphoinositide 3-kinase (PI3K), Vps34, which initiate membrane formation from an intracellular source[6] of controversial origin (Fig. 1). Upon initiation, two different ubiquitin-like protein conjugation systems are required for the elongation of the autophagosome membrane.[7] The ATG5-ATG12 conjugation system begins with the conjugation of ATG12

*Department of Immunobiology, Yale University School of Medicine, New Haven, Connecticut, USA.
 Corresponding Author: Akiko Iwasaki—Email: akiko.iwasaki@yale.edu

Nucleic Acid Sensors and Antiviral Immunity, edited by Suryaprakash Sambhara and Takashi Fujita.
©2013 Landes Bioscience.

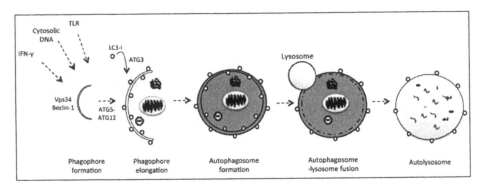

Figure 1. Induction of autophagy after viral infection. Autophagosome formation begins with the initiation complex involving Beclin-1 and the class III phosphoinositide 3-kinase Vps34, which initiate membrane formation. Two ubiquitin-like protein conjugation systems are required for the elongation of the autophagosome membrane. The ATG5-ATG12 conjugation system begins with the conjugation of ATG12 to ATG7—an E1 like enzyme that activates ATG12, resulting in the transfer of ATG12 to ATG10. After transfer of ATG12 to ATG10, ATG12 is transferred to ATG5. The ATG5-ATG12 complex is stabilized by ATG16, and this complex plays a critical role in elongation of the autophagosome membrane. The second conjugation system is initiated with the cleavage of cytosolic LC3 by ATG4 to LC3 I. Cleaved LC3 I is then bound and activated by ATG7 and transferred to ATG3. This association allows for LC3 I to be covalently linked to the lipid phosphatidylethanolamine (PE). LC3-PE (LC3 II) is subsequently incorporated into both cytoplasmic and luminal faces of the elongating autophagosomal membrane. Upon completion of membrane formation, autophagosomes can fuse with endosomes (amphisome) or lysosomes (autolysosome). Autophagy is induced in many different contexts, including viral infection. Autophagy can be induced by cellular stress associated with viral infection, several different cytokines, and through innate recognition.

to ATG7—an E1 like enzyme that activates ATG12, resulting in the transfer of ATG12 to ATG10. After transfer of ATG12 to ATG10, ATG 12 is transferred to ATG5, this time through a covalent bond. The ATG5-ATG12 complex is stabilized by ATG16, and this complex plays a critical role in elongation of the autophagosome membrane. The second conjugation system is initiated with the cleavage of LC3 (mammalian ortholog of yeast ATG8) by ATG4 to LC3 I. Cleaved LC3 I is then bound and activated by ATG7 and transferred to ATG3. This association allows for LC3 I to be covalently linked to the lipid phosphatidylethanolamine (PE). LC3-PE (LC3 II) is subsequently incorporated into both cytoplasmic and luminal faces of the elongating autophagosomal membrane.[6] Upon completion of membrane formation, autophagosomes can fuse with endosomes (called amphisome) or lysosomes (called autolysosome), resulting in the degradation of autophagosome contents in the latter.

It is now clear that ATG proteins contribute to a diverse array of immunological processes critical in antiviral immunity.[8] These processes span the entire spectrum of vertebrate antiviral immune responses including direct viral degradation, innate recognition, and antigen presentation. However, it is likely a misnomer to refer to all the processes in which the ATG proteins have been implicated in as "autophagy." ATG proteins contribute to antiviral immunological processes by at least three mechanistically distinct processes: (1) delivery of intracellular material to the lysosome for degradation or to specialized endosomes (i.e., classical autophagy), (2) delivery of extracellular material by the ATG machinery to specialized endosomal compartments (i.e., use of autophagic machinery), and (3) regulation of cellular operations by ATG proteins independent of autophagic process or machinery (i.e., individual Atg protein function) (Fig. 2).[9] Moreover, autophagy is essential for maintaining homeostasis in metazoans, thereby indirectly affecting nearly every aspect of the immune response.[10] Here, we focus on the direct contribution of the three distinct processes involving Atg system to antiviral defense.

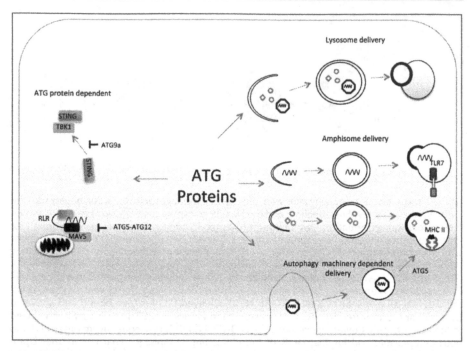

Figure 2. Atg regulation of antiviral immunity. Left) Several cellular operations are regulated by ATG proteins independent of autophagic process or machinery (i.e., Atg protein dependent). Atg proteins and complexes block signalling downstream of pattern recognition receptors. Atg9a can block STING from interacting with TBK1, while Atg5-Atg12 conjugate blocks MAVS-RLR interaction. Right) Autophagy aids in the delivery of intracellular pathogens to the lysosome for degradation (lysosome delivery) or to specialized endosomes (amphisome delivery). Autophagy proteins also contribute to delivery of extracellular microbes, as the ATG machinery to is utilized to transport extracellular material to specialized endosomal compartments (i.e., use of autophagic machinery).

Autophagy Induction after Virus Infection

Autophagy is a dynamic process that cells constantly fine-tune in response to both external and internal stimuli. The classic case of inducible autophagy is the starvation response. Cells that are either deprived of growth factors or amino acids rapidly induce autophagy through signaling pathways involving the mTOR complex and class III PI3Ks.[11,12] Autophagy provides the cells with the necessary nutrients for survival by degrading pre-existing cytosolic components. In the context of viral infection, at least two competing interests affect the autophagy status of the cell: the desire of the host cell to induce autophagy to remove virus and/or maintain homeostasis, and the desire of the virus to maintain an anabolic state to propagate viral replication (thus indirectly inhibiting autophagy). Viruses must maintain an anabolic state to build the macromolecular components required for replication, and maintenance of this anabolic state can inhibit autophagy.[13] In response to virus infection, the host induces autophagy by at least two distinct mechanisms. First, viral-induced cellular stress including unfolded protein response can induce autophagy. Second, viral replication also results in the production of pathogen associated molecular patterns (PAMPs). Detection of PAMPs through pattern recognition receptors (PRRs) can induce autophagy in either a cell intrinsic manner or in bystander cells. Rather than providing a comprehensive list of literature, in this section we aim to summarize key findings and highlight themes that have emerged from recent findings.

Innate Immune Signaling Induces Autophagy

The innate immune response relies on pathogen recognition to initiate a rapid, non-specific protective response as well as to prime a pathogen specific adaptive response.[14] Recent reports identify a link between TLR signaling and the induction of autophagy.[15,16] Initial studies revealed that autophagy is induced by TLR engagement in the RAW 264.7 macrophage cell line.[16] TLR signaling enhances the interaction of MyD88 and TRIF with Beclin-1, and reduces the binding of Beclin-1 to Bcl-2.[17] Later, the same group showed that TRAF6, an E3 ligase activated by TLR stimulation, is able to modify Beclin-1 in the BH3 domain with K63 linked ubiquitination. This ubiquitination abrogates Belcin-1-Bcl2 interaction, freeing Beclin-1 to initiate autophagy.[18] However, in other studies, induction of autophagy was not observed following stimulation with a diverse panel of TLR agonists in primary fetal-liver derived macrophages[19] or in plasmacytoid dendritic cells after TLR7 stimulation.[20] In addition, in intestinal epithelial cells, TLR stimulation, while inducing innate signals, did not induce significant autophagy.[21] Therefore, TLR-induction of autophagy appears to be cell-type dependent.

In addition to TLRs, other PRRs including NOD-like receptors (NLR), RIG-I like receptors (RLRs) and other cytosolic sensors have been implicated in autophagy induction. The first evidence that innate PRR sensing links pathogen recognition to selective autophagic destruction of pathogens came from a study in *Drosophila,* in which sensing of *Listeria monocytogenes* infection by peptidoglycan-recognition protein (PGRP) led to induction of autophagy.[22] PGRP, but not Toll or IMD pathways, was required for resistance to *L. monocytogenes* infection, and this process depended on PRGP-induction of autophagic removal of the bacteria. In mammals, NOD1 and NOD2 are among the PRRs that recognize peptidoglycan components in the cytosol. Both NOD1 and NOD2 recruit the autophagy protein ATG16L1 to the plasma membrane at the bacterial entry site, and promoted autophagosomal engulfment of *Shigella flexneri*.[23] Similarly, NOD2 stimulation induced autophagy, which promoted bacterial handling and antigen presentation.[24] Thus, both invertebrates and vertebrates utilize peptidoglycan sensing to specifically target intracellular bacteria for autophagic destruction. RLR signaling can also lead to autophagy induction. Transfection of melanoma cells with poly I:C, which engages MDA-5, resulted in enhanced autophagy and cell death.[25] Recent data showed that infection with HSV-1 and CMV (dsDNA viruses) induces autophagy in a manner independent of viral replication and de novo protein synthesis.[26] Electroporation of DNA, but not RNA, induced autophagy in human skin fibroblast, suggesting that cytosolic DNA sensors can induce autophagy. Therefore, autophagy process serves as an important effector mechanism downstream of multiple PRRs, linking innate sensing pathways to inducible autophagy. Virus-induced autophagy may be utilized for the purposes of pathogen containment, degradation, and antigen presentation to T cells as described below.

Cytokine Influence on Autophagy

Recently, a paradigm has emerged in which Th1 cytokines induce autophagy while Th2 cytokines inhibit autophagy. In CD4 T cells, IFN-γ induces autophagy-dependent cell death in the absence of Irgm1.[27] In contrast, the Th2 cytokines have been shown to functionally reduce autophagy.[28] This is an appealing paradigm, as both autophagy and Th1 responses are critical against in defense against numerous intracellular pathogens.[29] Coupling Th1 signaling to autophagy induction provides an additional mechanism by which Th1 signals can prime cells for defense against intracellular pathogens.[30] In addition to classical Th1 /Th2 cytokines, other inflammatory cytokines have been shown to induce autophagy. For example, TNF-α induced autophagy in skeletal muscle cells and enhanced antigen presentation on MHC class II.[31] However, whether cytokines alone are sufficient to induce autophagy may be cell type dependent. Aside from cytokine receptors, other immune receptors such as CD40[32] and B-cell receptor[33] have been linked to the induction of autophagy. The molecules and mechanisms involved in linking receptor signaling to autophagy induction require future investigation.

Virus Induced Autophagy May Be Unique

As discussed above, virus infection often results in autophagy induction. Whether or not autophagy induced during viral infection is distinct from canonical starvation-induced autophagy is an important question that requires further investigation. In this regard, a genome-wide siRNA screening revealed that under normal nutrient conditions, upregulation of autophagy requires the type III PI3 kinase, but not inhibition of mTORC1, the essential negative regulator of starvation-induced autophagy.[34] These data indicated that there are multiple pathways to trigger autophagy, and that starvation induced autophagy (involving mTORC1, elicited also by rapamycin) is only one such pathway. More importantly, this study highlighted the possibility that virus induced autophagy might employ distinct initiation pathways.

Autophagosomes induced during both Sindbis and herpes simplex virus (HSV) type 1 infection contain both viral particles and host components, indicating it is unlikely that induced autophagy is specific to viral particles. However, autophagosomes induced during HSV-1 infection appear to localize near the nucleus and may be morphologically distinct from starvation or rapamycin induced autophagosomes.[35] Thus, autophagy induced by HSV-1 infection may differ at the level of induction or subcellular localization. These findings suggest a model in which autophagy may target either viral replication within the nucleus or immediate viral nuclear egress. However, the molecular link(s) that would enable such selective autophagy for viruses are only beginning to be elucidated. To this end, exciting recent evidence suggests that virus-specific autophagy may be mediated by sequestasome-1 (p62). Following Sindbis virus infection, p62 interacts with the Sindbis capsid protein and targets it for degradation in autophagosomes.[36]

Studies with intracellular bacteria have demonstrated that intracellular pathogens can be directly targeted to autophagosomes by interacting with p62-like molecules following ubiquitination.[10] It is interesting to speculate whether or not eukaryotic hosts have evolved mechanisms, in addition to p62, to specifically recognize and eliminate viral pathogens via autophagy. Virally infected cells undergoing productive replication synthesize vast amounts of often a limited subset of proteins, mainly the viral proteins. In this regard, it is interesting to draw a parallel to host retrovirus restriction mechanisms. Retroviruses are recognized by host antiviral molecules, including TRIM-5α and cyclophilin A, that bind to capsid proteins.[37] It is possible that yet identified receptors for viral capsid or other conserved motifs within viral components exists that can be used to target them to autophagosomes. Alternatively, viral infection may induce generalized autophagy induction by triggering cellular stress / unfolded protein response that can induce autophagy. By utilizing a set of adaptors that recognize common protein sequences and ubiquitination, autophagy may serve as regulation system that recognizes and eliminates excess proteins, irrespective of origin. Thus, in this case, the "pattern" recognized by autophagy may be related to production volume and conserved motifs rather than unique molecular signatures. Future studies are needed to unravel the molecules involved in linking virus infection to autophagy, and whether viruses can be specifically selected for autophagic engulfment through the use of specific adaptors.

Autophagy Machinery as a "Delivery" Mechanism for Innate and Adaptive Antiviral Systems

At its core, the ATG machinery is a delivery system, engulfing cytoplasmic components and delivering them to the lysosome for degradation. However, the ATG machinery is not restricted to lysosomal delivery. Indeed, the ATG machinery can be utilized to delivery cytoplasmic material to endosomes at various stages of maturation (making structure called amphisomes). Thus, the ATG machinery is not a one-way to ticket to the lysosome, but rather, an adaptable delivery system capable of performing a variety of intracellular functions. Recently, it has become clear that this delivery system is utilized by both the innate and adaptive immune systems for optimal antiviral defense.

Autophagy in Innate Viral Recognition

Toll-like receptors (TLRs) recognize a variety of pathogens through their ability to bind PAMPs derived from viruses, bacteria, fungi and parasites. Viruses are recognized by TLRs that access the endosomes, namely, TLR3, TLR7, TLR8 and TLR9.[38] Plasmacytoid dendritic cells (pDCs) are specialized type I IFN producing cells that detect viral infection primarily through Toll-like receptors (TLRs) expressed in endosomal signaling compartments. Efficient innate recognition of viral pathogens via TLRs requires viral PAMP to reach specific endosomal compartments, yet viral replication intermediates are primarily found within the cytosolic and nuclear compartments of the cell. Several well-defined mechanisms exist to ensure viral PAMP to reach the TLRs in the endosomes, foremost of which is phagocytosis / endocytosis of viral particles in infected cells. However, viral genomic nucleic acid associated with the virions is insufficient to trigger TLR for certain viral pathogens. In this context, autophagy is utilized to deliver cytoplasmic viral replication intermediates to endosomes containing TLRs. Genetic deletion of host *Atg5* resulted in the absence of TLR-7 dependent cytokine production in pDCs infected with VSV.[20] Similarly, TLR7 stimulation by a paramyxovirus, simian virus 5, requires access to the cytoplasm and autophagic sampling of cytoplasmic contents.[39] This study found that UV-irradiation of simian virus 5 did not impair TLR7-dependent recognition, indicating that the active viral replication is not required to generate viral PAMPs capable of TLR7 activation. Of note, another paramyxovirus, Sendai virus, only has partial dependency on viral replication for TLR7-dependent recognition by pDCs, in a process that requires autophagy.[20] These data likely reflect a putative difference in the nature of PAMP recognized by TLR7 following autophagic delivery. It is also interesting to note that no examples exist in which the recognition of a DNA virus requires autophagic delivery of viral PAMPs to TLR9 compartment. Instead, as discussed below, Atg5 is required for IRF-7, but not NF-kB, dependent signaling downstream of TLR9.[20]

Autophagy in Antigen Presentation

Activation of naïve T cells requires activation signals from antigen presenting cells. Proper trafficking, processing, and presentation of viral antigens on MHC molecules within the antigen presenting cells are necessary to accomplish this goal. The autophagic process has been shown to enhance processing and presentation of both extracellular and intracellular antigens on MHC II.

The role of Atg proteins in MHC class II presentation in dendritic cells (DC), was investigated in vivo using a DC-selective knockout of *Atg5*.[40] This study revealed a critical role for autophagic machinery in presentation of extracellular viral antigens on MHC II (Fig. 3). Mice with DC-specific deletion in *Atg5*, ATG5[flox/flox] CD11c-Cre, were impaired in their ability to present viral antigen on MHC II and activate CD4[+] T cells following intravaginal infection with HSV-2. The requirement for Atg5 only applied to extracellular phagocytosed antigens containing PAMPs. Importantly, induction of canonical autophagy by rapamycin treatment did not increase antigen presentation / processing, and no double-membrane structure was observed at the phagosomal membrane. In addition, siRNA knockdown of *Atg12* and *Atg7* phenocopied the *Atg5*[-/-] DCs in their ability to present exogenous antigens on MHC class II. These data strongly imply that distinct components of the ATG machinery, and not canonical autophagy, were responsible for the observed phenotype. Thus, ATG machinery is utilized by dendritic cells to deliver microbial antigens to MHC II loading compartments. A subsequent study demonstrated a similar requirement for autophagic machinery in promoting exogenous antigen presentation on MHC II for HIV-1 antigens by dendritic cells.[41] In macrophages, phagosomes containing TLR ligands utilize autophagic machinery to facilitate phagosome fusion with lysosomes, leading to rapid acidification and enhanced killing of the ingested organism.[42] Thus, macrophages and DCs utilize autophagic machinery for optimal phagosomal maturation for pathogen degradation and antigen processing for MHC class II, respectively. Importantly, this strategy is not countered by viral measures, as it occurs in uninfected phagocytes.

As discussed above, classical presentation of peptides on MHC II occurs through uptake of exogenous antigens, transport of antigens to MHC II loading compartment, and transport

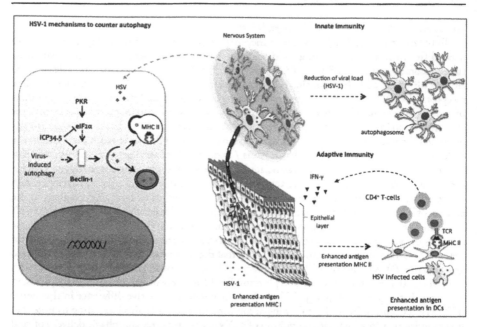

Figure 3. Role of autophagy in herpes simplex virus infection. HSV-1 encodes a neurovirulence factor, ICP34.5, which inhibits autophagy via PKR and Beclin-1 dependent mechanisms. Removal of the Beclin-1 binding domain of HSV-1 ICP34.5 resulted in a mutant virus with impaired ability to inhibit host autophagy induced during HSV-1 infection. This mutant virus has a markedly decreased viral replication and pathogenesis following intracranial infection. Additionally, intraocular infection with this HSV-1 mutant incapable of inhibiting host autophagy resulted in increased activation of CD4+ T cells, likely via enhanced antigen presentation in a productively infected cell type. Autophagy machinery is also utilized by dendritic cells to deliver phagocytosed HSV-2 antigens to MHC II loading compartments and activate CD4+ T-cell responses. Importantly, this strategy is not countered by viral measures, as it occurs primarily in uninfected phagocytes. Autophagy has also been reported to temporarily increase presentation of HSV-1 antigens on MHC I in macrophage cell lines.

of MHC II-peptide complexes to the cell surface for presentation to CD4+ T cells.[43] Although this pathway is efficient for presenting exogenous antigens, it does not allow for antigens from intracellular pathogens to be presented to CD4+ T cells. The discovery that cytosolic antigens are in fact presented on MHC II implied that alternative pathways are involved in bringing antigens to MHC II loading compartments.[44,45] Autophagy has been identified as one such pathway that is important in facilitating intracellular antigens to be presented on MHC II.[46] Autophagy facilitates MHC II presentation of cytosolic viral,[47] bacterial,[48] and self[49,50] antigens on MHC II. Furthermore, autophagy has been demonstrated to play an important role in MHC II antigen presentation of cytosolic viral antigens in professional antigen presenting cells by constitutive fusion of autophagosomes with MHC II loading compartments.[51] This mechanism of autophagy-dependent antigen presentation is important in antiviral defense in vivo. Intraocular infection with a HSV-1 mutant impaired in its ability to inhibit host autophagy resulted in decreased mortality and increased activation of CD4+ T cells, presumably via enhanced antigen presentation in a productively infected cell type.[52] Additionally, autophagy has also been reported to temporarily increase presentation of HSV-1 antigens on MHC I in macrophage cell lines.[35] However, no defects in MHC I presentation pathway were observed in *Atg*-deficient DCs,[40,41] suggesting that the requirement for autophagy in MHC I presentation may depend on the cell type.

Autophagy and ATG Proteins Regulate Innate Signaling

Autophagy and ATG proteins have recently been identified as playing key roles in the regulation of several distinct innate receptor and cytokine signaling pathways.

Autophagy Regulation of TLR and Cytokine Signaling

Genetic deletion of *Atg5* within pDCs results in abrogated TLR-9 dependent type I IFN production, but not NF-κB dependent pro-inflammatory cytokine production.[20] These data indicate that Atg5 plays a critical role in IRF-7 dependent signaling independent of TLR-9 ligand delivery. In this case, the autophagy machinery may play an important role in directing the IRF-7 signaling complex to the necessary signaling compartment. Alternatively, Atg5 may aid IRF-7 signaling independent of other components of the autophagy machinery. Another study indicated that siRNA knockdown of *LC3* or *Atg5* led to a decrease in TNF-α induction following TLR4 or TLR8 stimulation of human DCs.[41] Moreover, *Atg7* gene expression silencing led to downregulation of TLR-mediated IL-8 expression in intestinal epithelial cells.[53] These data indicate that certain TLRs employ Atg proteins for optimal signaling in a variety of cells.

In contrast to the supportive role of autophagy in TLR signaling, other reports indicate the importance of autophagy in negatively regulating innate signaling pathways. The autophagy adaptor protein p62 is specifically degraded by autophagy, and accumulation of p62 can lead to the activation of NF-κB dependent signaling.[54,55] Therefore, autophagy indirectly regulates NF-κB signaling by maintaining p62 at homeostatic levels. Additionally, several recent reports have demonstrated that genetic deletion or functional reduction of ATG16L results in increased production of the pro-inflammatory cytokines IL-1β and IL-17.[56-58]

Autophagy is also involved in signaling through cytokine receptors. *Atg5*$^{-/-}$ or *Atg7*$^{-/-}$ MEFs are unable to activate Jak2-STAT1 downstream of IFN-γR, which suggests that autophagy is important for IFN-gamma signal transduction.[59] Therefore, autophagy or components of autophagic machinery appear to be required for optimal stimulation and signaling through multiple immune receptors.

Cytosolic Innate Viral Recognition Pathways

Unlike the TLRs, RIG-I-like receptors (RLR) recognize signatures of viral RNA in the cytosol of infected cells.[60] Autophagy and ATG proteins have been shown to negatively regulate components of the cytosolic innate recognition pathway via two distinct, but not necessarily exclusive mechanisms. In the cytosol, Atg5 and Atg12 constitutively form conjugate as a result of the actions of Atg7 (E1-like protein) and Atg10 (E2-like protein).[7] Jounai et al. showed that the Atg5-Atg12 conjugate inhibits RLR signaling by binding to and functionally inhibiting the RLR adaptor protein, MAVS.[61] The second mechanism involves constitutive autophagy. In cells genetically deficient in *Atg5*, increased cellular levels of MAVS and increased reactive species produced by damaged mitochondria synergize to amplify RLR signaling.[62] ATG proteins have also been shown to negatively regulate the DNA sensor pathway. ATG9a associates with STING, preventing it from localizing to TBK1 signaling complexes required for signaling.[19] Thus, autophagy 'polices' the cytosolic viral recognition pathway both indirectly by maintaining cell homeostasis and directly via ATG protein-protein interaction with cytosolic innate signaling components. At first glance, this role of autophagy could be interpreted as a pro-viral function, as reduced cytokine responses in the absence of autophagy and ATG proteins have been demonstrated to increase viral replication in vitro. However, neither autophagy nor ATG proteins functionally abrogate cytokine production. Rather, the role of autophagy and ATG proteins is likely to effectively safeguard cytokine responses, helping restore order at both the cellular and organism level.

Autophagy in Cell-Autonomous Antiviral Defense

Prior to the evolution of the type I interferon system, eukaryotes relied mostly on cell autonomous antiviral defense mechanisms. Autophagy provided our eukaryotic ancestors with a means of sequestering and degrading intracellular pathogens such as viruses and intracellular bacteria. This process, termed xenophagy,[63] likely represents a primitive form of eukaryotic defense against intracellular pathogens. Several studies within the past decade have revealed that metazoans have retained this role of autophagy in antiviral defense. However, as these studies illustrate, the contribution of autophagy to antiviral defense in the context of complex vertebrate immune responses likely extends beyond degradation of infectious virions. In addition, the role of autophagy in viral clearance appears to be both cell-type and host species dependent.

Neurotropic Viruses—Sindbis Virus and HSV-1

The first evidence for the role of autophagy proteins in antiviral defense came from studies with the neurotropic Sindbis virus. Overexpression of the host ATG protein Beclin-1 (mammalian ortholog of yeast ATG6) resulted in decreased cell death and decreased mortality following intracranial infection in neonatal mice.[64] Recently, the same group showed that genetic deletion of host ATG5 or ATG7 results in increased neuron death and increased mortality following intracranial infection of neonatal mice with Sindbis virus.[36] Interestingly, viral replication was identical in WT and ATG5 deficient hosts both in vivo and in vitro. However, cells genetically deficient in ATG proteins were incapable of clearing the overwhelming amounts of proteins that accumulate during Sindbis virus infection. Importantly, as discussed above, Sindbis viral proteins were cleared via specific p62-mediated targeting to autophagosomes. Thus, Sindbis viral proteins appear to be recognized and directly targeted to autophagosomes by p62 for degradation.

Autophagy is also critical in herpes simplex virus 1 (HSV-1) antiviral defense. HSV-1 encodes a neurovirulence factor, ICP34.5, which inhibits autophagy via PKR and Beclin-1 dependent mechanisms (discussed in detail below). Removal of the Beclin-1 binding domain of HSV-1 ICP34.5 resulted in a mutant virus with impaired ability to inhibit host autophagy induced during HSV-1 infection. This mutant virus has a markedly decreased viral replication and pathogenesis following intracranial infection.[65] Ultrastructural analysis revealed that HSV-1 virions localized to autophagosomes in a *pkr* dependent mechanism,[66] indicating xenophagic degradation of host virions is likely at least partially responsible for the observed phenotype.

Of note, Sindbis virus and HSV-1 are both neurotropic viruses that infect neurons. Although HSV-1 virions and Sindbis viral proteins are localized to autophagosomes in mitotic cell lines in vitro, genetic deletion of host *Atg* genes has minimal effect on viral replication or outcome in cell lines in vitro. In contrast, the absence of autophagy results in a dramatic difference in host morbidity and mortality due to neuropathogenesis in vivo. These studies highlight several emerging themes of the role of autophagy in antiviral defense. First, studies in cell lines in vitro, although informative, appear to be insufficient to fully elucidate the role of autophagy in antiviral defense in the context of the whole organism. Second, these findings reveal that viruses encode factors that antagonize autophagy. Identification and mutation / removal of these viral factors is often necessary to reveal the contribution of autophagy to antiviral defense. Finally, the role of autophagy in antiviral defense appears to be influenced by the cell type in which viral replication is occurring. Further studies are necessary to define and understand the mechanisms responsible for the cell type specific requirement of autophagy in antiviral defense.

Vesicular Stomatitis Virus—Xenophagy Requirement Is Host Dependent

Autophagy has also been shown to play an important role in defense against intracellular pathogens in multiple model organisms including *Drosophila*[67] and *C. elegans*.[68] These systems provide a genetically tractable model to evaluate the role of autophagy in the absence of adaptive immune system. Deletion of multiple host *Atg* genes in *Drosophila* resulted in increased VSV replication both in vitro and increased replication and mortality in vivo.[67] Interestingly, overexpression of PTEN phosphatase, which blocks the PI3K-Akt signaling pathway, resulted in induction of autophagy and further reduction of VSV replication. These data suggest that canonical induction of autophagy through the nutrient pathway can be employed as an effective antiviral strategy. Conversely, autophagy and ATG proteins increase VSV replication in murine cells via negative regulation of type I IFN production in vitro,[61,62] and no role for autophagy has been reported in VSV antiviral defense in vertebrates in vivo. These contrasting findings lead to an emerging theme in the relationship between autophagy and the vertebrate immune system; although the autophagy machinery is remarkably conserved from yeast to man, it has been functionally integrated into numerous components and regulatory mechanisms of vertebrate antiviral defense. These "modern" functions appear to often supersede the evolutionary ancient role of degrading intracellular pathogens in the vertebrate immune system.

Human Immunodeficiency Virus 1—Role of Autophagy Depends on Cell Types and Infection Status

Autophagy has also been shown to play an important role in cell autonomous antiviral defense during HIV infection. However, the precise role of autophagy during HIV infection appears to be quite complex, varying significantly among cell types. Autophagy was initially shown to play a role in inducing death of bystander CD4 T cells.[69] HIV env engagement induced Beclin-1 accumulation and autophagy induction in CD4 T cells. Pharmacological inhibition of autophagy or siRNA knockdown of ATG proteins resulted in decreased apoptosis of bystander CD4 T cells. Moreover, pharmacological inhibition of apoptosis resulted in death of bystander CD4+ T cells by "autophagic cell death." However, it is important to note that autophagy is regarded a pro-survival pathway, and the concept of "autophagic death" remains controversial.[70] Furthermore, the role of autophagy appears to be quite different during acute infection of CD4 T cells, as HIV infection inhibits autophagy by markedly decreasing both mRNA and protein levels of Beclin-1 and LC3 II.[71]

A complex relationship also exists between HIV-1 and host autophagy in macrophages. Autophagy proteins associate with HIV-1 gag and promote the processing of gag within productively infected macrophages.[72] Conversely, autophagy is capable of interfering with HIV-1 replication by xenophagic degradation of HIV virions and viral proteins.[68] However, HIV-1 abrogates this antiviral function through HIV-1 nef-dependent blockade of autophagosome maturation.[68] Thus, in macrophages, autophagy functions in a cell-autonomous anti-HIV-1 capacity, but HIV-1 has evolved countermeasures to both inhibit and subvert autophagy. Recently, HIV-1 was also shown to contribute to numerous antiviral processes within infected dendritic cells (DCs). HIV-1 interaction with DCs triggers the activation of the metabolic sensor mTOR, resulting in the inhibition of autophagy.[41] HIV-dependent inhibition of autophagy increased viral protein accumulation and trans-infection of CD4 T cells. In addition, HIV-inhibition of negatively affected autophagy several DC functions key in anti-HIV immunity, including antigen presentation and TLR signaling. Thus, autophagy is capable of performing numerous antiviral functions within HIV-1 infected DCs but is countered by upstream HIV-1 inhibitory mechanisms.

Gamma Herpes Viruses—Autophagy in Infected Cells Restricts Chronic Infection

Gamma herpes virus 68 (γHV68) encodes a virulence factor, vBcl-2 (also known as M11), which inhibits apoptosis through its interaction with pro-apoptotic family members, Bax and Bak. Recently, it was revealed that vBcl-2 also inhibits autophagy through binding and inhibiting Beclin-1.[73] Structural analysis of vBcl-2 revealed that the Bax/Bak binding domain (antiapoptotic) and Beclin-1 binding domain of vBcl-2 are distinct.[74,75] Deletion of the Beclin-1 binding domain of vBcl-2 resulted in a mutant fully capable of inhibiting apoptosis but incapable of inhibiting autophagy. Infection of splenocytes in vitro and intranasal in vivo infection with this mutant revealed that the viral blockade of autophagy is important in the maintenance of γHV68 chronic infection.[75] In contrast, in vivo infection with γHV68 expressing vBcl-2 mutant that is unable to block apoptosis but is intact for autophagy blockade had impaired ex vivo reactivation from latency.

Viral Evasion Mechanisms

Autophagy is targeted by numerous viral pathogens at multiple levels, underscoring the importance of autophagy in antiviral defense. Although autophagy primarily directs cytosolic components to lysosomal degradation, evidence exists that the ATG machinery is an adaptable system that performs a diverse set of functions within metazoan cells. This inherent adaptability may represent a vulnerability capable of exploitation by viral pathogens. Indeed, the ATG machinery appears to be exploited by several classes of viruses to achieve maximal viral replication in vitro.

Viral Inhibition of Autophagy through Metabolic Pathways

Viral replication requires the large-scale synthesis of numerous macromolecules. To this end, viruses regulate multiples aspects of the host cells metabolism in order to maintain a net anabolic state. The serine/threonine protein kinase mammalian target of rapamycin (mTOR) regulates cellular and organismal homeostasis by coordinating anabolic and catabolic processes with nutrient, energy, and oxygen availability and growth factor signaling.[76] Viruses often utilize the mTOR signaling pathway to achieve optimal replication. For example, HSV-1 encodes Us3, an Akt mimic that induces mTORC1 activation, which is critical in maintaining translation and viral replication.[77] In contrast, autophagy is a catabolic process, and anabolic pathways negatively regulate autophagy through several pathways, including the mTOR signaling node. Therefore, it is important to note that upstream modulation of autophagy alone is insufficient evidence to conclude that a given virus has evolved mechanisms to counter host autophagy per se. However, in several of the viruses discussed below, it is clear that autophagy functions in an antiviral capacity during viral infection. Thus, by manipulating metabolic pathways upstream of autophagy, viral pathogens may effectively modify multiple cellular functions to maximize viral fitness.

Although multiple metabolic pathways regulate autophagy, current reports of upstream viral inhibition of autophagy have primarily been limited to signaling through the mTOR pathway. Human cytomegalovirus (HCMV) inhibits autophagy in a yet to be identified mechanism through the mTOR signaling pathway in human fibroblasts.[78] Analogously, HIV-1 env inhibits autophagy by inducing mTOR signaling in HIV-1-infected dendritic cells.[41] Inhibition of autophagy reduces numerous antiviral functions of DCs, including TLR signaling and antigen presentation. Interestingly, lowering intracellular inositol and myo-inositol-1,4,5-triphosphate ($Ins(1,4,5)P_3$) levels[79,80] induces autophagy in an mTOR-independent pathway. Whether viruses target this pathway to block autophagy is unknown, but remains an interesting possibility.

Direct Inhibition of ATG Proteins

As discussed above, inhibition of autophagy by viral infection antagonism of upstream signaling pathways is insufficient evidence to conclude that autophagy has a direct role in antiviral defense, as this strategy also interferes with many other downstream signaling pathways. However, direct inhibition of host autophagy via viral protein interactions with host ATG proteins provides strong evidence for such a relationship. A landmark study by Levine and colleagues revealed that viral pathogens encode virulence factors that directly inhibit host autophagy.[52] Herpes simplex virus 1 encodes a virulence factor, ICP34.5, which abrogates several key host immune processes. ICP34.5 antagonizes the effects of the host interferon stimulatory gene (ISG), RNA-dependent Protein Kinase (PKR), by dephosphorylating the transcription factor eIF2α.[81,82] Recently, it has also been shown that ICP34.5 inhibits autophagy by two distinct mechanisms, (1) ICP34.5 inhibits PKR-dependent autophagy induction, and (2) ICP34.5 abrogates autophagy induction by binding to and inhibiting the host ATG protein Beclin-1.[52,83] Importantly, removal of the Beclin-1 binding domain of ICP34.5 resulted in decreased viral replication and decreased mortality following intracranial infection. Thus, these studies provided the first definitive evidence that viruses encode virulence factors that specifically inhibit autophagy, and removal of this viral inhibition results in decreased viral pathogenesis.

Gamma herpes viruses also antagonize host autophagy by directly inhibiting ATG proteins. All members of the γ-herpesvirus family express orthologs of Bcl-2, the cellular inhibitor of apoptosis. In addition to modulating apoptosis, these viral Bcl-2s (vBcl-2) bind to Beclin-1 and prevent it from binding to PI3 kinase complexes and initiating autophagy.[75] Kaposi's sarcoma associated herpes virus (KSHV) and gamma herpes virus 68 (γHV68) both contain Bcl-2 homologs that can interact with Beclin-1. Interestingly, the γHV68 vBcl-2 orthologoue, M11, binds to Beclin-1 significantly more strongly than KSHV vbcl2 or mammalian Bcl-2.[73] This interaction between γHV68 M11 and Beclin-1 was subsequently shown to prevent Beclin-1 from initiating de novo

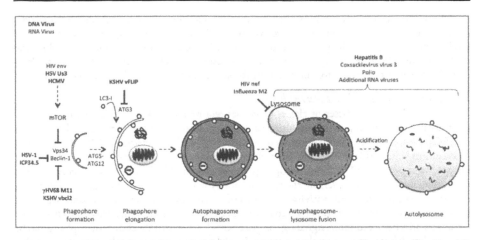

Figure 4. Autophagy inhibition by viral pathogens. HCMV and HIV env activate signaling through the negative regulator of autophagy mTOR, thus reducing HSV autophagy initiation. HSV Us3 also activates mTOR, but a role in autophagy initiation has not yet been elucidated. Several viral proteins have been shown to directly inhibit the host autophagy machinery via interacting with host ATG proteins. HSV-1 encodes a virulence factor ICP34.5, which inhibits autophagy by binding to and inhibiting beclin 1; ICP34.5 inhibits host *pkr*-dependent autophagy initiation as well. M11 (vbcl2) of γHV68 and vbcl2 of KHSV also inhibit autophagosome formation by interacting with Beclin-1 and vFLIP of KHSV antagonizes autophagy by binding to Atg3 and preventing it from modifying LC3 during autophagosome formation. Additionally, multiples viruses antagonize host autophagy via preventing autophagosome maturation and / or delivery. HIV nef and Influenza M2 block autophagosome fusion with lysosomes. Coxsackievirus 3, polio, and hepatitis B have strategies to interfere with autophagosome maturation and trafficking.

autophagosome formation in vitro and is important in maintaining chronic γHV68 infection in vivo. Moreover, some gamma herpesiviruses encode additional factors to ensure blockade of autophagy in infected cells. KSHV, Herpesvirus saimiri (HVS), and Molluscum contagiosum virus (MCV) all encode vFLIP, a homolog of cellular FLICE-like inhibitor protein (cFLIP), that blocks autophagy.[84] Interestingly, both cFLIP and vFLIPs bind to Atg3 and suppress autophagy by preventing Atg3 from binding and modifying LC3 during autophagosome formation (Fig. 4). Paradoxically, autophagy is induced during lytic re-activation of KSHV.[85] RTA (replication and transcription activator), an essential viral protein for KSHV lytic reactivation, is able to enhance autophagy, which somehow facilitates KSHV lytic replication. Thus, the relationship between autophagy and KSHV appears to be intimately linked to the replication stage of KSHV.

Blockade of Autophagosome-to-Lysosome Fusion

Several viral pathogens have evolved mechanisms to antagonize destruction by blocking autophagosome-to-lysosome fusion. Coxsackie virus B3 inhibits autophagosome maturation by a yet to be elucidated mechanism.[86] Moreover, HIV-1 nef inhibits autophagosome maturation in macrophages[72] and influenza M2 inhibits autophagosome-lysosome fusion in influenza infected fibroblasts.[87] Intriguingly, both HIV-1 nef and influenza M2 interact with Beclin-1, yet neither nef nor M2 interfere with autophagosome initiation. Recent studies shed light on the possible mechanism behind these observations. It is now known that Beclin-1 exists in at least three distinct complexes; Atg14L/ Beclin-1/Vps34/Vps15, UVRAG/ Beclin-1/Vps34/Vps15, Rubicon/UVRAG/ Beclin-1/Vps34/Vps15; and one that involves UVRAG/Vps34/Vps15 has been shown to mediate autophagosome-to-lysosome fusion.[88,89] Thus, nef and M2 may inhibit autophagosome-to-lysosome fusion via functionally blocking this specific Beclin-1 complex. Inhibition of the autophagy pathway significantly increases apoptosis in influenza virus-infected cells, but this was not correlated with any change in viral titer.[87]

Of note, many of the viruses known to counter host autophagy via preventing autophagosome maturation are RNA viruses which undergo cytosolic replication. It is currently unclear whether these viral mechanisms specifically prevent autophagosome-lysosome fusion or ubiquitously block the ATG machinery from delivering viral components to other intracellular compartments. In the later case, this viral evasion strategy would effectively abrogate all known antiviral functions of autophagy.

Viral Subversion of Host Autophagy

Intriguingly, several classes of classes of viruses require autophagy to achieve maximal viral replication in vitro. In the past decade, pharmacological inhibition of autophagy and / or knockdown of ATG proteins has been also demonstrated to reduce viral yields of Hepatitis C,[90-92] foot and mouth disease virus,[93] Hepatitis B,[94] dengue fever virus,[95] adenoviruses,[96] Coxsackie virus 3,[97] Coxsackie virus 4,[98] and poliovirus.[99,100] Thus, autophagy can be exploited by RNA viruses to enhance viral replication. Less clear, however, are the mechanisms by which these viruses utilize the autophagy machinery without initiating antiviral functions of autophagy. In some cases, distinct set of Atg proteins may be exploited to aid viral replication in a manner that prevents delivery to lysosomes or innate and adaptive immune signaling compartments.[86] Alternatively, classical autophagy may be induced, but delivery to lysosomal or immune signaling compartments may be restricted by either novel mechanisms or mechanisms analogous to those discussed in the previous section.

Viruses also use autophagy to indirectly enhance viral replication and / or survival. Oncogenic viruses must ensure survival of cells within large tumor mass, which often experience insufficient supply of oxygen and nutrients. Simian virus 40 small T antigen activates AMPK and triggers autophagy to protect cancer cells from nutrient deprivation.[101] Analogously, viruses have evolved strategies to utilize autophagy to ensure that the infected cells' energy needs are met during viral replication. Supplementation of Dengue virus infected cells with fatty acids increased viral replication, and this increase was abrogated by inhibiting autophagy.[102] Thus, autophagy can be exploited to ensure the energy requirements required for continued cell survival and viral replication will be met.

The mechanism by which subversion of the autophagy aids replication of several classes of viruses is under investigation. Several non-mutually exclusive models have been proposed. Double membrane structures initiated by the autophagy machinery may serve as viral replication scaffolds, increasing the efficiency of viral replication by keeping viral components in close proximity. Autophagy machinery may also be utilized in facilitating viral egress. Alternatively, replication within autophagosome-like structures may reduce detection by cytosolic innate recognition receptors by sequestering viral PAMP in membrane enclosed compartments.

Conclusion

Innate antiviral immunity is mediated through multiple different effector mechanisms. In our early eukaryotic ancestors, antiviral defense consisted of cell autonomous defense mechanisms including xenophagy and RNA interference. In the context of vertebrate antiviral defense, these ancient defense mechanisms are often superseded by type I interferon and numerous interferon-inducible genes dedicated to antiviral defense. However, careful analysis has begun to reveal that autophagy has retained a critical role in antiviral defense at multiple levels, including viral clearance, innate receptor signaling, and antigen presentation. Complementing these findings, recent studies have revealed a multitude of ways in which viruses evade autophagy-dependent degradation, innate sensing, and antigen presentation through blockade / subverting of the autophagy machinery. In many cases, such subversion of host autophagy has been shown to enhance viral replication in vitro.

One of the outstanding questions in this regard is the mechanism by which viruses or viral components are targeted to autophagosomes. Whether virus specific adaptor(s) exist that enable targeting of these components to autophagosomes remains to be determined. We have seen evidence for this in bacterial system, through PGRP and NODs. Additionally, recent data has indicated that Sendai viral capsid protein is targeted to autophagosomes via p62. Another critical question is to understand why autophagy is required in certain cell types to restrict virus replication. In particular, in vivo evidence point toward neurons as a cell type that heavily relies on autophagy for viral defense, and consequently, virulence factors that allow viruses to replicate in neurons appear to target autophagy. In addition to these basic questions, our understanding of the relevant role of autophagy in both supporting and blocking virus replication will potentially enable us to specifically design interventions for viral diseases. Current drugs that inhibit or promote autophagy do so non-specifically, targeting either the mTORC1 pathway or the inositol pathway. Rapamycin induces autophagy by blocking mTORC1 while mood-stabilizing drugs such as lithium chloride, carbamazepine (CBZ) and valproic acid (VPA), are known to induce autophagy by depleting intracellular inositol levels[79] and through oxidative stress.[103] However, these agents also affect other downstream signaling pathways. Therefore, development of pharmaceutical agents that enable selective regulation of autophagy is of high priority.

Acknowledgements

This work was supported by National Institutes of Health (NIH) (AI054359, AI062428, AI064705 and AI083242 to A.I.). A.I. holds an Investigators in Pathogenesis of Infectious Disease Award from the Burroughs Wellcome Fund. B.Y. was supported, in part, by Predoctoral Virology Training grant number T32 AI055403 from the NIH. The content is solely the responsibility of the authors and does not necessarily represent the official views of the NIH. Authors declare no conflicts of interest.

About the Authors

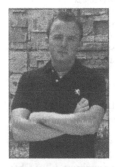

Brian Yordy received a Bachelors of Science in Biochemistry from the University of Notre Dame in 2006. He is currently a graduate student at Yale University, where is pursuing a PhD in Immunobiology in the laboratory of Dr. Akiko Iwasaki. Brian's thesis work is focused on understanding the tissue specific mechanisms utilized by the innate immune system to control neurotropic viruses.

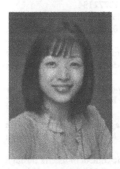

Akiko Iwasaki, received her PhD from the University of Toronto, and her postdoctoral training from the National Institutes of Health. She joined Yale University as a faculty member in 2000, and currently is a Professor of Immunobiology. Dr. Iwasaki's main interest is in understanding the mechanisms by which viruses are recognized by the host innate immune system, and how such recognition pathways lead to the generation of adaptive immunity. Her research has identified the role and mechanisms by which Toll-like receptors (TLR) recognize DNA and RNA viruses within the endosomes. Her research program has also provided key molecular insights into the intracellular mechanisms involved in TLR-mediated viral recognition, by identifying the role of autophagy and adaptor proteins in trafficking of viral ligand and receptors to the appropriate endosomes. Her research has also led to the identification of tissue dendritic subsets that orchestrate various aspects of adaptive immune responses to viruses including herpes simplex virus and influenza. In addition, Dr. Iwasaki's research shed light on the role of NOD-like receptors (NLR) in linking innate viral recognition to adaptive immune response against influenza virus infection. This process is aided by endogenous microbiota, which trigger priming signals for NLR-dependent cytokine responses.

References

1. Mizushima N, Yamamoto A, Matsui M, Yoshimori T, Ohsumi Y. In vivo analysis of autophagy in response to nutrient starvation using transgenic mice expressing a fluorescent autophagosome marker. Mol Biol Cell 2004; 15:1101-11; http://dx.doi.org/10.1091/mbc.E03-09-0704; PMID:14699058.
2. Klionsky DJ, Emr SD. Autophagy as a regulated pathway of cellular degradation. Science 2000; 290:1717-21; http://dx.doi.org/10.1126/science.290.5497.1717; PMID:11099404.
3. Shintani T, Klionsky DJ. Autophagy in health and disease: A double-edged sword. Science 2004; 306:990-5; http://dx.doi.org/10.1126/science.1099993; PMID:15528435.
4. Majeski AE. Fred Dice J. Mechanisms of chaperone-mediated autophagy. Int J Biochem Cell Biol 2004; 36:2435-44; http://dx.doi.org/10.1016/j.biocel.2004.02.013; PMID:15325583.
5. Santambrogio L, Cuervo AM. Chasing the elusive mammalian microautophagy. Autophagy 2011; 7:652-4; http://dx.doi.org/10.4161/auto.7.6.15287; PMID:21460618.
6. Meijer AJ, Codogno P. Regulation and role of autophagy in mammalian cells. Int J Biochem Cell Biol 2004; 36:2445-62; http://dx.doi.org/10.1016/j.biocel.2004.02.002; PMID:15325584.
7. Mizushima N, Noda T, Yoshimori T, Tanaka Y, Ishii T, George MD, et al. A protein conjugation system essential for autophagy. Nature 1998; 395:395-8; http://dx.doi.org/10.1038/26506; PMID:9759731.
8. Virgin HW, Levine B. Autophagy genes in immunity. Nat Immunol 2009; 10:461-70; PMID:19381141; http://dx.doi.org/10.1038/ni.1726.
9. Levine B, Mizushima N, Virgin HW. Autophagy in immunity and inflammation. Nature 2011; 469:323-35; http://dx.doi.org/10.1038/nature09782; PMID:21248839.
10. Deretic V. Autophagy in immunity and cell-autonomous defense against intracellular microbes. Immunol Rev 2011; 240:92-104; http://dx.doi.org/10.1111/j.1600-065X.2010.00995.x; PMID:21349088.
11. Nobukuni T, Joaquin M, Roccio M, Dann SG, Kim SY, Gulati P, et al. Amino acids mediate mTOR/raptor signaling through activation of class 3 phosphatidylinositol 3OH-kinase. Proc Natl Acad Sci USA 2005; 102:14238-43; http://dx.doi.org/10.1073/pnas.0506925102; PMID:16176982.
12. Nobukuni T, Kozma SC, Thomas G. hvps34, an ancient player, enters a growing game: MTOR Complex1/S6K1 signaling. Curr Opin Cell Biol 2007; 19:135-41; http://dx.doi.org/10.1016/j.ceb.2007.02.019; PMID:17321123.
13. Buchkovich NJ, Yu Y, Zampieri CA, Alwine JC. The TORrid affairs of viruses: Effects of mammalian DNA viruses on the PI3K-akt-mTOR signalling pathway. Nat Rev Microbiol 2008; 6:266-75; http://dx.doi.org/10.1038/nrmicro1855; PMID:18311165.
14. Iwasaki A, Medzhitov R. Toll-like receptor control of the adaptive immune responses. Nat Immunol 2004; 5:987-95; http://dx.doi.org/10.1038/ni1112; PMID:15454922.
15. Xu Y, Jagannath C, Liu X. -, Sharafkhaneh A, Kolodziejska KE, Eissa NT. Toll-like receptor 4 is a sensor for autophagy associated with innate immunity. Immunity 2007; 27:135-44; http://dx.doi.org/10.1016/j.immuni.2007.05.022; PMID:17658277.
16. Delgado MA, Elmaoued RA, Davis AS, Kyei G, Deretic V. Toll-like receptors control autophagy. EMBO J 2008; 27:1110-21; http://dx.doi.org/10.1038/emboj.2008.31; PMID:18337753.
17. Shi CS. -, Kehrl JH. MyD88 and trif target beclin 1 to trigger autophagy in macrophages. J Biol Chem 2008; 283:33175-82; http://dx.doi.org/10.1074/jbc.M804478200; PMID:18772134.
18. Shi CS. -, Kehrl JH. TRAF6 and A20 regulate lysine 63-linked ubiquitination of beclin-1 to control TLR4-induced autophagy. Sci Signal 2010; 3: http://dx.doi.org/10.1126/scisignal.2000751; PMID:20501938.
19. Saitoh T, Fujita N, Hayashi T, Takahara K, Satoh T, Lee H, et al. Atg9a controls dsDNA-driven dynamic translocation of STING and the innate immune response. Proc Natl Acad Sci USA 2009; 106:20842-6; PMID:19926846; http://dx.doi.org/10.1073/pnas.0911267106.
20. Lee HK, Lund JM, Ramanathan B, Mizushima N, Iwasaki A. Autophagy-dependent viral recognition by plasmacytoid dendritic cells. Science 2007; 315:1398-401; PMID:17272685; http://dx.doi.org/10.1126/science.1136880.
21. Li YY, Ishihara S, Aziz MM, Oka A, Kusunoki R, Tada Y, et al. Autophagy is required for toll-like receptor-mediated interleukin-8 production in intestinal epithelial cells. Int J Mol Med 2011; 27:337-44; http://dx.doi.org/10.3892/ijmm.2011.596; PMID:21225224.
22. Yano T, Mita S, Ohmori H, Oshima Y, Fujimoto Y, Ueda R, et al. Autophagic control of listeria through intracellular innate immune recognition in drosophila. Nat Immunol 2008; 9:908-16; http://dx.doi.org/10.1038/ni.1634; PMID:18604211.
23. Travassos LH, Carneiro LAM, Ramjeet M, Hussey S, Kim Y, Magalhães JG, et al. Nod1 and Nod2 direct autophagy by recruiting ATG16L1 to the plasma membrane at the site of bacterial entry. Nat Immunol 2010; 11:55-62; http://dx.doi.org/10.1038/ni.1823; PMID:19898471.
24. Cooney R, Baker J, Brain O, Danis B, Pichulik T, Allan P, et al. NOD2 stimulation induces autophagy in dendritic cells influencing bacterial handling and antigen presentation. Nat Med 2010; 16:90-7; http://dx.doi.org/10.1038/nm.2069; PMID:19966812.

25. Tormo D, Checińska A, Alonso-Curbelo D, Pérez-Guijarro E, Cañón E, Riveiro-Falkenbach E, et al. Targeted activation of innate immunity for therapeutic induction of autophagy and apoptosis in melanoma cells. Cancer Cell 2009; 16:103-14; http://dx.doi.org/10.1016/j.ccr.2009.07.004; PMID:19647221.

26. McFarlane S, Aitken J, Sutherland JS, Nicholl MJ, Preston VG, Preston CM. Early induction of autophagy in human fibroblasts after infection with human cytomegalovirus or herpes simplex virus 1. J Virol 2011; 85:4212-21; http://dx.doi.org/10.1128/JVI.02435-10; PMID:21325419.

27. Feng CG, Zheng L, Jankovic D, Báfica A, Cannons JL, Watford WT, et al. The immunity-related GTPase Irgm1 promotes the expansion of activated CD4+ T cell populations by preventing interferon-γ-induced cell death. Nat Immunol 2008; 9:1279-87; http://dx.doi.org/10.1038/ni.1653; PMID:18806793.

28. Harris J, De Haro SA, Master SS, Keane J, Roberts EA, Delgado M, et al. T helper 2 cytokines inhibit autophagic control of intracellular mycobacterium tuberculosis. Immunity 2007; 27:505-17; http://dx.doi.org/10.1016/j.immuni.2007.07.022; PMID:17892853.

29. Delgado M, Singh S, De Haro S, Master S, Ponpuak M, Dinkins C, et al. Autophagy and pattern recognition receptors in innate immunity. Immunol Rev 2009; 227:189-202; http://dx.doi.org/10.1111/j.1600-065X.2008.00725.x; PMID:19120485.

30. Gutierrez MG, Master SS, Singh SB, Taylor GA, Colombo MI, Deretic V. Autophagy is a defense mechanism inhibiting BCG and mycobacterium tuberculosis survival in infected macrophages. Cell 2004; 119:753-66; http://dx.doi.org/10.1016/j.cell.2004.11.038; PMID:15607973.

31. Keller CW, Fokken C, Turville SG, Lünemann A, Schmidt J, Münz C, et al. TNF-α induces macroautophagy and regulates MHC class II expression in human skeletal muscle cells. J Biol Chem 2011; 286:3970-80; http://dx.doi.org/10.1074/jbc.M110.159392; PMID:20980264.

32. Andrade RM, Wessendarp M, Gubbels M. -, Striepen B, Subauste CS. CD40 induces macrophage anti-toxoplasma gondii activity by triggering autophagy-dependent fusion of pathogen-containing vacuoles and lysosomes. J Clin Invest 2006; 116:2366-77; http://dx.doi.org/10.1172/JCI28796; PMID:16955139.

33. Chaturvedi A, Dorward D, Pierce SK. The B cell receptor governs the subcellular location of toll-like receptor 9 leading to hyperresponses to DNA-containing antigens. Immunity 2008; 28:799-809; http://dx.doi.org/10.1016/j.immuni.2008.03.019; PMID:18513998.

34. Lipinski MM, Hoffman G, Ng A, Zhou W, Py BF, Hsu E, et al. A genome-wide siRNA screen reveals multiple mTORC1 independent signaling pathways regulating autophagy under normal nutritional conditions. Dev Cell 2010; 18:1041-52; PMID:20627085; http://dx.doi.org/10.1016/j.devcel.2010.05.005.

35. English L, Chemali M, Duron J, Rondeau C, Laplante A, Gingras D, et al. Autophagy enhances the presentation of endogenous viral antigens on MHC class I molecules during HSV-1 infection. Nat Immunol 2009; 10:480-7; PMID:19305394; http://dx.doi.org/10.1038/ni.1720.

36. Orvedahl A, MacPherson S, Sumpter R Jr., Tallóczy Z, Zou Z, Levine B. Autophagy protects against sindbis virus infection of the central nervous system. Cell Host Microbe 2010; 7:115-27; PMID:20159618; http://dx.doi.org/10.1016/j.chom.2010.01.007.

37. Pertel T, Hausmann S, Morger D, Züger S, Guerra J, Lascano J, et al. TRIM5 is an innate immune sensor for the retrovirus capsid lattice. Nature 2011; 472:361-5; http://dx.doi.org/10.1038/nature09976; PMID:21512573.

38. Takeda K, Kaisho T, Akira S. Toll-like receptors. Annu Rev Immunol 2003; 21:335-76; http://dx.doi.org/10.1146/annurev.immunol.21.120601.141126; PMID:12524386.

39. Manuse MJ, Briggs CM, Parks GD. Replication-independent activation of human plasmacytoid dendritic cells by the paramyxovirus SV5 requires TLR7 and autophagy pathways. Virology 2010; 405:383-9; http://dx.doi.org/10.1016/j.virol.2010.06.023; PMID:20605567.

40. Lee HK, Mattei LM, Steinberg BE, Alberts P, Lee YH, Chervonsky A, et al. In vivo requirement for Atg5 in antigen presentation by dendritic cells. Immunity 2010; 32:227-39; PMID:20171125; http://dx.doi.org/10.1016/j.immuni.2009.12.006.

41. Blanchet FP, Moris A, Nikolic DS, Lehmann M, Cardinaud S, Stalder R, et al. Human immunodeficiency virus-1 inhibition of immunoamphisomes in dendritic cells impairs early innate and adaptive immune responses. Immunity 2010; 32:654-69; PMID:20451412; http://dx.doi.org/10.1016/j.immuni.2010.04.011.

42. Sanjuan MA, Dillon CP, Tait SWG, Moshiach S, Dorsey F, Connell S, et al. Toll-like receptor signalling in macrophages links the autophagy pathway to phagocytosis. Nature 2007; 450:1253-7; PMID:18097414; http://dx.doi.org/10.1038/nature06421.

43. Cresswell P. Assembly, transport, and function of MHC class II molecules. Annu Rev Immunol 1994; 12:259-93; PMID:8011283; http://dx.doi.org/10.1146/annurev.iy.12.040194.001355.

44. Jaraquemada D, Marti M, Long EO. An endogenous processing pathway in vaccinia virus-infected cells for presentation of cytoplasmic antigens to class II-restricted T cells. J Exp Med 1990; 172:947-54; http://dx.doi.org/10.1084/jem.172.3.947; PMID:2388037.

45. Nuchtern JG, Biddison WE, Klausner RD. Class II MHC molecules can use the endogenous pathway of antigen presentation. Nature 1990; 343:74-6; http://dx.doi.org/10.1038/343074a0; PMID:1967486.

46. Crotzer VL, Blum JS. Cytosol to lysosome transport of intracellular antigens during immune surveillance. Traffic 2008; 9:10-6; http://dx.doi.org/10.1111/j.1600-0854.2007.00664.x; PMID:17916226.
47. Paludan C, Schmid D, Landthaler M, Vockerodt M, Kube D, Tuschl T, et al. Endogenous MHC class II processing of a viral nuclear antigen after autophagy. Science 2005; 307:593-6; PMID:15591165; http://dx.doi.org/10.1126/science.1104904.
48. Nimmerjahn F, Milosevic S, Behrends U, Jaffee EM, Pardoll DM, Bornkamm GW, et al. Major histocompatibility complex class II-restricted presentation of a cytosolic antigen by autophagy. Eur J Immunol 2003; 33:1250-9; http://dx.doi.org/10.1002/eji.200323730; PMID:12731050.
49. Dörfel D, Appel S, Grünebach F, Weck MM, Müller MR, Heine A, et al. Processing and presentation of HLA class I and II epitopes by dendritic cells after transfection with in vitro-transcribed MUC1 RNA. Blood 2005; 105:3199-205; http://dx.doi.org/10.1182/blood-2004-09-3556; PMID:15618468.
50. Brazil MI, Weiß S, Stockinger B. Excessive degradation of intracellular protein in macrophages prevents presentation in the context of major histocompatibility complex class II molecules. Eur J Immunol 1997; 27:1506-14; http://dx.doi.org/10.1002/eji.1830270629; PMID:9209504.
51. Schmid D, Pypaert M, Münz C. Antigen-loading compartments for major histocompatibility complex class II molecules continuously receive input from autophagosomes. Immunity 2007; 26:79-92; PMID:17182262; http://dx.doi.org/10.1016/j.immuni.2006.10.018.
52. Leib DA, Alexander DE, Cox D, Yin J, Ferguson TA. Interaction of ICP34.5 with beclin 1 modulates herpes simplex virus type 1 pathogenesis through control of CD4+ T-cell responses. J Virol 2009; 83:12164-71; PMID:19759141; http://dx.doi.org/10.1128/JVI.01676-09.
53. Li YY, Ishihara S, Aziz MM, Oka A, Kusunoki R, Tada Y, et al. Autophagy is required for toll-like receptor-mediated interleukin-8 production in intestinal epithelial cells. Int J Mol Med 2011; 27:337-44; http://dx.doi.org/10.3892/ijmm.2011.596; PMID:21225224.
54. Sanz L, Diaz-Meco MT, Nakano H, Moscat J. The atypical PKC-interacting protein p62 channels NF-κB activation by the IL-1-TRAF6 pathway. EMBO J 2000; 19:1576-86; PMID:10747026; http://dx.doi.org/10.1093/emboj/19.7.1576.
55. Moscat J, Diaz-Meco MT. p62 at the crossroads of autophagy, apoptosis and cancer. Cell 2009; 137:1001-4; PMID:19524504; http://dx.doi.org/10.1016/j.cell.2009.05.023.
56. Saitoh T, Fujita N, Jang MH, Uematsu S, Yang B, Satoh T, et al. Loss of the autophagy protein Atg16L1 enhances endotoxin-induced IL-1β production. Nature 2008; 456:264-8; PMID:18849965; http://dx.doi.org/10.1038/nature07383.
57. Cadwell K, Liu JY, Brown SL, Miyoshi H, Loh J, Lennerz JK, et al. A key role for autophagy and the autophagy gene Atg16l1 in mouse and human intestinal paneth cells. Nature 2008; 456:259-63; PMID:18849966; http://dx.doi.org/10.1038/nature07416.
58. Cadwell K, Patel KK, Maloney NS, Liu T, Ng ACY, Storer CE, et al. Virus-plus-susceptibility gene interaction determines crohn's disease gene Atg16L1 phenotypes in intestine. Cell 2010; 141:1135-45; PMID:20602997; http://dx.doi.org/10.1016/j.cell.2010.05.009.
59. Chang YP, Tsai CC, Huang WC, Wang CY, Chen CL, Lin YS, et al. Autophagy facilitates IFN-δ-induced Jak2-STAT1 activation and cellular inflammation. J Biol Chem 2010; 285:28715-22; http://dx.doi.org/10.1074/jbc.M110.133355; PMID:20592027.
60. Yoneyama M, Fujita T. RIG-I family RNA helicases: Cytoplasmic sensor for antiviral innate immunity. Cytokine Growth Factor Rev 2007; 18:545-51; http://dx.doi.org/10.1016/j.cytogfr.2007.06.023; PMID:17683970.
61. Jounai N, Takeshita F, Kobiyama K, Sawano A, Miyawaki A, Xin KQ, et al. The Atg5-Atg12 conjugate associates with innate antiviral immune responses. Proc Natl Acad Sci USA 2007; 104:14050-5; PMID:17709747; http://dx.doi.org/10.1073/pnas.0704014104.
62. Tal MC. Absence of autophagy results in reactive oxygen speciesdependent amplification of RLR signaling. Proc Natl Acad Sci USA 2009; 106:2770-5; PMID:19196953; http://dx.doi.org/10.1073/pnas.0807694106.
63. Levine B. Eating oneself and uninvited guests: Autophagy-related pathways in cellular defense. Cell 2005; 120:159-62; http://dx.doi.org/10.1016/S0092-8674(05)00043-7; PMID:15680321.
64. Liang XH, Kleeman LK, Jiang HH, Gordon G, Goldman JE, Berry G, et al. Protection against fatal sindbis virus encephalitis by beclin, a novel bcl-2-interacting protein. J Virol 1998; 72:8586-96; PMID:9765397.
65. Orvedahl A, Alexander D, Tallóczy Z, Sun Q, Wei Y, Zhang W, et al. HSV-1 ICP34.5 confers neurovirulence by targeting the beclin 1 autophagy protein. Cell Host Microbe 2007; 1:23-35; PMID:18005679; http://dx.doi.org/10.1016/j.chom.2006.12.001.
66. Tallóczy Z, Virgin HW IV, Levine B. PKR-dependent autophagic degradation of herpes simplex virus type 1. Autophagy 2006; 2:24-9; PMID:16874088.

67. Shelly S, Lukinova N, Bambina S, Berman A, Cherry S. Autophagy is an essential component of drosophila immunity against vesicular stomatitis virus. Immunity 2009; 30:588-98; PMID:19362021; http://dx.doi.org/10.1016/j.immuni.2009.02.009.

68. Jia K, Thomas C, Akbar M, Sun Q, Adams-Huet B, Gilpin C, et al. Autophagy genes protect against salmonella typhimurium infection and mediate insulin signaling-regulated pathogen resistance. Proc Natl Acad Sci USA 2009; 106:14564-9; PMID:19667176.

69. Espert L, Denizot M, Grimaldi M, Robert-Hebmann V, Gay B, Varbanov M, et al. Autophagy is involved in T cell death after binding of HIV-1 envelope proteins to CXCR4. J Clin Invest 2006; 116:2161-72; http://dx.doi.org/10.1172/JCI26185; PMID:16886061.

70. Levine B, Yuan J. Autophagy in cell death: An innocent convict? J Clin Invest 2005; 115:2679-88; http://dx.doi.org/10.1172/JCI26390; PMID:16200202.

71. Zhou D, Spector SA. Human immunodeficiency virus type-1 infection inhibits autophagy. AIDS 2008; 22:695-9; http://dx.doi.org/10.1097/QAD.0b013e3282f4a836; PMID:18356598.

72. Kyei GB, Dinkins C, Davis AS, Roberts E, Singh SB, Dong C, et al. Autophagy pathway intersects with HIV-1 biosynthesis and regulates viral yields in macrophages. J Cell Biol 2009; 186:255-68; PMID:19635843; http://dx.doi.org/10.1083/jcb.200903070.

73. Sinha S, Colbert CL, Becker N, Wei Y, Levine B. Molecular basis of the regulation of beclin 1-dependent autophagy by the γ-herpesvirus 68 bcl-2 homolog M11. Autophagy 2008; 4:989-97; PMID:18797192.

74. Ku B, Woo JS, Liang C, Lee KH, Hong HS, E X, et al. Structural and biochemical bases for the inhibition of autophagy and apoptosis by viral BCL-2 of murine γ-herpesvirus 68. PLoS Pathog 2008; 4: http://dx.doi.org/10.1371/journal.ppat.0040025; PMID:18248095.

75. E X, Hwang S, Oh S, Lee JS, Jeong JH, Gwack Y, et al. Viral bcl-2-mediated evasion of autophagy aids chronic infection of γherpesvirus 68. PLoS Pathog 2009; 10; PMID:19816569

76. Sengupta S, Peterson TR, Sabatini DM. Regulation of the mTOR complex 1 pathway by nutrients, growth factors, and stress. Mol Cell 2010; 40:310-22; http://dx.doi.org/10.1016/j.molcel.2010.09.026; PMID:20965424.

77. Chuluunbaatar U, Roller R, Feldman ME, Brown S, Shokat KM, Mohr I. Constitutive mTORC1 activation by a herpesvirus akt surrogate stimulates mRNA translation and viral replication. Genes Dev 2010; 24:2627-39; PMID:21123650; http://dx.doi.org/10.1101/gad.1978310.

78. Chaumorcel M, Souquère S, Pierron G, Codogno P, Esclatine A. Human cytomegalovirus controls a new autophagy-dependent cellular antiviral defense mechanism. Autophagy 2008; 4:46-53; PMID:18340111.

79. Sarkar S, Floto RA, Berger Z, Imarisio S, Cordenier A, Pasco M, et al. Lithium induces autophagy by inhibiting inositol monophosphatase. J Cell Biol 2005; 170:1101-11; http://dx.doi.org/10.1083/jcb.200504035; PMID:16186256.

80. Williams A, Sarkar S, Cuddon P, Ttofi EK, Saiki S, Siddiqi FH, et al. Novel targets for huntington's disease in an mTOR-independent autophagy pathway. Nat Chem Biol 2008; 4:295-305; http://dx.doi.org/10.1038/nchembio.79; PMID:18391949.

81. Clemens MJ, Elia A. The double-stranded RNA-dependent protein kinase PKR: Structure and function. J Interferon Cytokine Res 1997; 17:503-24; PMID:9335428; http://dx.doi.org/10.1089/jir.1997.17.503.

82. He B, Gross M, Roizman B. The γ134.5 protein of herpes simplex virus 1 complexes with protein phosphatase 1α to dephosphorylate the α subunit of the eukaryotic translation initiation factor 2 and preclude the shutoff of protein synthesis by double-stranded RNA-activated protein kinase. Proc Natl Acad Sci USA 1997; 94:843-8; PMID:9023344; http://dx.doi.org/10.1073/pnas.94.3.843.

83. Tallóczy Z, Jiang W, Virgin HW IV, Leib DA, Scheuner D, Kaufman RJ, et al. Regulation of starvation- and virus-induced autophagy by the eIF2α kinase signaling pathway. Proc Natl Acad Sci USA 2002; 99:190-5; http://dx.doi.org/10.1073/pnas.012485299; PMID:11756670.

84. Lee JS, Li Q, Lee JY, Lee SH, Jeong JH, Lee HR, et al. FLIP-mediated autophagy regulation in cell death control. Nat Cell Biol 2009; 11:1355-62; PMID:19838173; http://dx.doi.org/10.1038/ncb1980.

85. Wen HJ Yang Z, Zhou Y, Wood C. Enhancement of autophagy during lytic replication by the kaposi's sarcoma-associated herpesvirus replication and transcription activator. J Virol 2010; 84:7448-58; http://dx.doi.org/10.1128/JVI.00024-10; PMID:20484505.

86. Kemball CC, Alirezaei M, Flynn CT, Wood MR, Harkins S, Kiosses WB, et al. Coxsackievirus infection induces autophagy-like vesicles and megaphagosomes in pancreatic acinar cells in vivo. J Virol 2010; 84:12110-24; http://dx.doi.org/10.1128/JVI.01417-10; PMID:20861268.

87. Gannagé M, Dormann D, Albrecht R, Dengjel J, Torossi T, Rämer PC, et al. Matrix protein 2 of influenza A virus blocks autophagosome fusion with lysosomes. Cell Host Microbe 2009; 6:367-80; http://dx.doi.org/10.1016/j.chom.2009.09.005; PMID:19837376.

88. Zhong Y, Wang QJ, Li X, Yan Y, Backer JM, Chait BT, et al. Distinct regulation of autophagic activity by Atg14L and rubicon associated with beclin 1-phosphatidylinositol-3-kinase complex. Nat Cell Biol 2009; 11:468-76; http://dx.doi.org/10.1038/ncb1854; PMID:19270693.

89. Matsunaga K, Saitoh T, Tabata K, Omori H, Satoh T, Kurotori N, et al. Two beclin 1-binding proteins, Atg14L and rubicon, reciprocally regulate autophagy at different stages. Nat Cell Biol 2009; 11:385-96; http://dx.doi.org/10.1038/ncb1846; PMID:19270696.
90. Dreux M, Gastaminza P, Wieland SF, Chisari FV. The autophagy machinery is required to initiate hepatitis C virus replication. Proc Natl Acad Sci USA 2009; 106:14046-51; PMID:19666601; http://dx.doi.org/10.1073/pnas.0907344106.
91. Shrivastava S, Raychoudhuri A, Steele R, Ray R, Ray RB. Knockdown of autophagy enhances the innate immune response in hepatitis C virus-infected hepatocytes. Hepatology 2011; 53:406-14; http://dx.doi.org/10.1002/hep.24073; PMID:21274862.
92. Ke PY Chen SS. Activation of the unfolded protein response and autophagy after hepatitis C virus infection suppresses innate antiviral immunity in vitro. J Clin Invest 2011; 121:37-56; http://dx.doi.org/10.1172/JCI41474; PMID:21135505.
93. O'Donnell V, Pacheco JM, LaRocco M, Burrage T, Jackson W, Rodriguez LL, et al. Foot-and-mouth disease virus utilizes an autophagic pathway during viral replication. Virology 2011; 410:142-50; http://dx.doi.org/10,1016/j.virol.2010.10.042; PMID:21112602.
94. Sir D, Tian Y, Chen W. -, Ann DK, Yen T-B, Ou J-J. The early autophagic pathway is activated by hepatitis B virus and required for viral DNA replication. Proc Natl Acad Sci USA 2010; 107:4383-8; PMID:20142477; http://dx.doi.org/10.1073/pnas.0911373107.
95. Lee YR, Lei HY, Liu MT, Wang JR, Chen SH, Jiang-Shieh YF, et al. Autophagic machinery activated by dengue virus enhances virus replication. Virology 2008; 374:240-8; http://dx.doi.org/10.1016/j.virol.2008.02.016; PMID:18353420.
96. Rodriguez-Rocha H, Gomez-Gutierrez JG, Garcia-Garcia A, Rao XM, Chen L, McMasters KM, et al. Adenoviruses induce autophagy to promote virus replication and oncolysis. Virology 2011; 416:9-15; http://dx.doi.org/10.1016/j.virol.2011.04.017; PMID:21575980.
97. Wong J, Zhang J, Si X, Gao G, Mao I, McManus BM, et al. Autophagosome supports coxsackievirus B3 replication in host cells. J Virol 2008; 82:9143-53; http://dx.doi.org/10.1128/JVI.00641-08; PMID:18596087.
98. Yoon SY, Ha YE, Choi JE, Ahn J, Lee H, Kweon HS, et al. Coxsackievirus B4 uses autophagy for replication after calpain activation in rat primary neurons. J Virol 2008; 82:11976-8; http://dx.doi.org/10.1128/JVI.01028-08; PMID:18799585.
99. Suhy DA, Giddings THJ, Kirkegaard K. Remodeling the endoplasmic reticulum by poliovirus infection and by individual viral proteins: An autophagy-like origin for virus-induced vesicles. J Virol 2000; 74:8953-65; PMID:10982339; http://dx.doi.org/10.1128/JVI.74.19.8953-8965.2000.
100. Taylor MP, Kirkegaard K. Modification of cellular autophagy protein LC3 by poliovirus. J Virol 2007; 81:12543-53; PMID:17804493; http://dx.doi.org/10.1128/JVI.00755-07.
101. Kumar SH, Rangarajan A. Simian virus 40 small T antigen activates AMPK and triggers autophagy to protect cancer cells from nutrient deprivation. J Virol 2009; 83:8565-74; http://dx.doi.org/10.1128/JVI.00603-09; PMID:19515765.
102. Heaton NS, Randall G. Dengue virus-induced autophagy regulates lipid metabolism. Cell Host Microbe 2010; 8:422-32; http://dx.doi.org/10.1016/j.chom.2010.10.006; PMID:21075353.
103. Fu J, Shao CJ, Chen FR, Ng HK, Chen ZP. Autophagy induced by valproic acid is associated with oxidative stress in glioma cell lines. Neuro-oncol 2010; 12:328-40; http://dx.doi.org/10.1093/neuonc/nop005; PMID:20308311.

CHAPTER 13

Synthetic and Natural Ligands of RLR

Martin Schlee, Janos Ludwig, Christoph Coch, Jasper G. van den Boorn, Winfried Barchet and Gunther Hartmann*

Abstract

The innate immune system employs a limited number of germ line-encoded pattern recognition receptors (PRR) that sense molecular patterns such as microbial molecules and unphysiological concentrations or structures of self molecules. Sensing of molecular patterns leads to cell autonomous defense mechanisms and triggers innate and adaptive immune responses. The family of RIG-I (retinoic acid-inducible gene I) like receptors (RLR) comprises RIG-I, MDA5 and Lgp2 which control the immune recognition of most pathogenic RNA viruses. These highly specialized immunosensors are expressed in the cytosol of both immune cells and non-immune cells and sense viral nucleic acids. As viral RNA is located in the same cellular compartment as host RNA, RLRs must be equipped to discriminate between viral and self RNA. Specifications of RLR ligands include nucleic acid structure, backbone modifications, and unusual cellular locations of nucleic acids. Here we review the tremendous progress that has been made towards defining the molecular characteristics of RLR ligands.

Introduction

Innate sensor systems for bacteria, fungi or viruses detect highly conserved microbe-specific proteins, sugars, lipids or nucleic acids; the so-called microbe-associated molecular patterns (MAMPs).[1] Sensing of MAMPs leads to cell-autonomous defense mechanisms and to the induction of innate immune responses. Most of the highly pathogenic and newly emerging viruses are RNA genome-based, which give rise to zoonotic and epidemic diseases (Flu, Foot-and-mouth disease) or cause viral hemorrhagic fever including yellow fever, dengue, lassa fever and Ebola.[2] In innate immune cells the endosomal Toll-like receptors (TLR) 7, 8 and 9 recognize GU-rich RNA and CpG-containing DNA, and induce the secretion of type-I interferons (IFN), IL-12 and chemokines[3-9] as reviewed extensively before.[10-12] Unlike TLR7, 8 and 9, the fourth member of the nucleic acid-detecting Toll-like receptors, TLR3, is expressed more broadly (for example in endothelial cells, fibroblasts, astrocytes)[11,12] and is thought to recognize long double-stranded RNA.[13] In contrast to the TLRs, the RIG-I-like receptors (RLR) RIG-I, MDA5 and Lgp2 are expressed in the cytosol and found in all cell types. While TLR3, 7, 8, 9 contribute to antiviral immunity, RLRs control the immune recognition of most pathogenic RNA viruses and are essential for initiation of an effective antiviral immune response (Fig. 1).[14-19]

RIG-I (retinoic acid-inducible gene I) was discovered by screening a cDNA library for IFN-beta inducing genes.[14] The related proteins MDA5 (melanoma differentiation-associated gene-5) and Lgp2 (laboratory of genetics and physiology-2) were identified by database homology searches.[14] MDA5 and RIG-I are related DExD/H-box helicase family proteins, which are composed of a N-terminal tandem caspase activation and recruitment domain

*Institute of Clinical Chemistry and Clinical Pharmacology, University Hospital Bonn, Bonn, Germany.
Corresponding Author: Gunther Hartmann—Email: gunther.hartmann@ukb.uni-bonn.de

Nucleic Acid Sensors and Antiviral Immunity, edited by Suryaprakash Sambhara and Takashi Fujita.
©2013 Landes Bioscience.

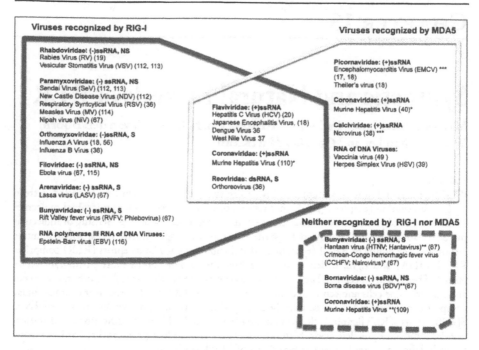

Figure 1. Viruses recognized by RIG-I and MDA5 and evading RIG-I/MDA5 recognition. S: segmented; NS: non-segmented; dsRNA: double-stranded RNA; ssRNA: single-stranded RNA; (-): negative strand genome; (+): positive strand genome; *no recognition by MDA5 or RIG-I in BM-DC or fibroblasts,[109] recognition by RIG-I and MDA5 in oligodendrocytes,[110] recognition by MDA5, not RIG-I in macrophages and microglia;[40] **Evasion of RIG-I recognition by monophosphate at the 5′ end of the viral genome due to viral nuclease cleavage;[67,111] ***Evasion of RIG-I recognition by Vpg protein at the 5′ end of the viral genome.[87-89]

(CARD) followed by a DExD/H-box helicase domain and the C-terminal "regulatory domain" (RD) with a Zinc coordination site.[20] Upon activation by viral RNA, RIG-I or MDA5 bind via their CARDs to the adaptor molecule MAVS (also known as IPS-1, Cardif or VISA[21-24]) leading to activation of TBK-1, which phosphorylates IRF3 to induce transcription of type-I IFN genes.[25-27] The current understanding is that the RD of RIG-I represents the viral sensor, mediating specificity for pathogenic RNA. Binding of viral RNA to the RD liberates the CARD domain to bind to MAVS, which in turn activates the signaling cascade leading to type-I IFN production.[20,28-31] The roles of the helicase domains in the activation of RIG-I and MDA5 are presently not entirely understood.[20] Lgp2 lacks a CARD domain, and thus initial reports suggested an immune suppressive function of Lgp2.[14,15,20] Later, studies on Lgp2 deficient mice revealed that absence of Lgp2 impairs the response to viruses that are recognized by MDA5, and can both enhance or impair RIG-I mediated antiviral responses.[16,32,33] The RD of Lgp2 shows some similarity to the RIG-I RD albeit with different ligand properties as discussed below.[33-35] Of all RLRs, most details are available on the RIG-I receptor ligand interaction. Therefore, the major focus of this review will be the current information on RIG-I-mediated recognition of synthetic and natural RNA.

MDA5

MDA5 was reported to recognize long double stranded RNA and to be involved in the detection of double stranded (dsRNA) and positive strand RNA [(+)ssRNA] viruses (Fig. 1).[17,18,36-40] MDA5 is essential for initiating innate immune responses against picornaviruses, like encephalo-myocarditis virus (EMCV) or Theiler's virus, or the Caliciviridae family member Norovirus which can not be sensed by RIG-I.[17,18,38] At first glance, MDA5 appears to recognize viruses belonging to families which produce substantial amounts of dsRNA during their replication cycle, including (+)ssRNA, dsRNA or DNA viruses.[38-42] However this concept seems incomplete. (-)ssRNA paramyxoviruses express the immune suppressive *V protein* which was found to target and inhibit MDA5 but not RIG-I, suggesting that also (-)ssRNA viruses (which do not produce long double stranded RNA[41]) generate MDA5 ligands.[43-45] Of note, many forms of double stranded RNA do not activate MDA-5. Thus far only one artifical, albeit enzymatically generated, MDA5-stimulating ligand (polyinosine-polycytidylic acid = poly I:C) has been described. It consists of annealed strands of long (>7000 nt) RNA polymers of inosins (polyI) and cytidines (polyC).[17,18,46] Most studies investigating the recognition of long double stranded RNA (dsRNA) in fact have used poly I:C. Importantly, poly I:C is a "dsRNA" originally reported to be the only co-polymer among many other artificial dsRNAs, which induced substantial amounts of type I IFN in mammalian cells.[47] The lack of well-defined MDA5 ligands hampers the understanding of MDA5 ligand-binding and activation. Although, the RD of MDA5 was reported to bind blunt-ended dsRNA,[48] MDA5 is not activated by short dsRNA and thus far no specific contribution for the RD for the recognition of RNA has been demonstrated.[20]

Although poly I:C also binds RIG-I and can stimulate it under certain conditions in vitro,[14,46] it is important understand that poly I:C actually fails to induce type I IFN when applied intravenously into MDA5-deficient mice or transfected in vitro into MDA5-deficient MEFs, peritoneal macrophages or dendritic cells.[17,18] By using poly I:C fragments of different size (generated by treatment of poly I:C with the dsRNA degrading RNase-III) Kato and colleagues found that MDA5 recognizes only long poly I:C fragments. However, another interpretation of these results is that treatment with RNase-III randomly destroys unusual secondary structures. It actually could be these secondary structures, which are recognized by MDA5. Pichlmair and colleagues suggested that not the property of doublestrandedness but other RNA structures in large complexes of RNA are responsible for MDA5 activation.[49] Recently, Luthra and colleagues identified a mRNA fragment from the ss(-)RNA parainfluenza virus 5 (PIV5) that activated type-I IFN expression through MDA5.[45] As type I IFN induction by this RNA also depended on presence of RNase L the authors suggested that RNase L recognized and processed viral mRNA into a MDA5 activating RNA form. In this work, the sequence critical for MDA5 recognition was mapped to a 432-nt-long region. However, no specific features of a minimal recognition motif for MDA5 were identified. Also, Züst and colleagues observed that deficiency of the viral 2'O-methylase in a type of corona virus (murine hepatitis virus; MHV) enables recognition of this MHV by MDA5 and TLR7.[50] This finding was interpreted as non-acceptance of capped RNA by MDA5, because of the 2'O-methylation at N_1 at the 5' end of viral RNA. However, binding assays confirming the interaction with MDA5 were not performed. In light of the finding that capped RNA (mRNA) transcripts are recognized by MDA5, made by Luthra and colleagues, it is more likely that indirect effects lead to the MDA5 activation observed by Züst and colleagues.

RIG-I

When RIG-I was first described as antiviral sensor in the seminal paper by the Fujita group,[14] the structural features of its RNA ligands were unclear. Overexpressed RIG-I was shown to bind to and be stimulated by *poly I:C*. Independently, the group of John Rossi, while developing siRNAs against HIV, observed that siRNAs generated by in vitro transcription with phage-polymerase[51] strongly induced type-I interferon in a variety of human cell lines (HEK293, HeLa, K562, CEM, Jurkat). Type I interferon was induced in an RNA sequence independent manner. Surprisingly, synthetic siRNAs did not show this immune stimulatory effect. DNA template-dependent RNA transcription occurs primer independently from the 5'- to the 3' end of RNA. Therefore de novo generated RNA transcripts of all known RNA polymerases including phage polymerase possess a triphosphate at the 5' end.[52] Kim and colleagues concluded that the 5'triphosphate likely was the type-I IFN-inducing structural element of in vitro transcribed RNAs. Indeed, removal of the triphosphate at the 5' end either by RNase T1 (removes the 5'end pppG) or phosphatase was sufficient to completely abrogate the type I IFN-inducing activity of the RNA.[51] This observation then prompted us to analyze the IFN-alpha inducing capacity of in vitro transcribed RNA with 5'-terminal triphosphate (pppRNA) in human blood cells.[19] Until then plasmacytoid dendritic cells (PDC) were considered to be the main type I IFN producing cells.[53,54] PDC express only two nucleic acid-sensing TLRs, TLR7 and 9, and produce large amounts of IFN-alpha upon stimulation of TLR7 with single or double stranded RNA[5] or with TLR9.[55] Although human monocytes also possess the RNA-sensing endosomal TLR8, stimulation of this TLR does not induce the secretion of IFN-alpha.[11] Surprisingly, pppRNA induced high amounts of IFN-alpha not only in PDC but also in primary human monocytes. Thus, pppRNA was found to be the first stimulus that induced IFN-alpha in human monocytes at similar quantities as in human PDC.[19] Removal of the triphosphate at the 5'end abolished IFN-alpha inducing activity of RNA in monocytes but not in PDC.[19] Incorporation of nucleotides with modified bases (pseudouridine, 2-thio-uridine) or backbone modifications (2'-O-methyl-uridine) abolished IFN-alpha inducing activity of pppRNA both in monocytes and PDC. Furthermore, RIG-I was identified to be the receptor responsible for IFN-alpha induction in myeloid immune cells, while TLR7 was responsible for IFN-alpha induction in PDC. At the same time, Pichlmair and colleagues observed 5'phosphate-dependent recognition of Influenza virus vRNA, which contained no dsRNA as concluded from experiments using a dsRNA specific antibody.[56] Saito and colleagues suggested that RIG-I recognizes (+) RNA viruses (e.g. HCV) in a sequence dependent manner.[57] In their study small domains of the HCV genome were generated by in vitro transcription, and analyzed for RIG-I binding and -activation. A 100 nt U- or A-rich region 8000 nt downstream of the 5' end was identified as a particular RIG-I inducing sequence. Interestingly, a poly-U elicited a similar IFN response as a polyA sequence. In their experiments RIG-I stimulation was strictly dependent on the presence of triphosphate at the 5'end. To demonstrate in vivo relevance of sequence-dependent RIG-I stimulation, a full length HCV genomic transcript was injected into mice and the IFN response compared with a transcript lacking its whole 3' non-translated region (3'NTR, 230 nt) including the proposed RIG-I stimulating sequence (NTR, 230 nt). Indeed, the genome lacking the 3'NTR did not stimulate RIG-I in vivo. However, it is important to note that transfected (+)ssRNA virus genomes are translated, and thus the RNA molecule represents a highly infectious agent. The effect of this deletion on virus translation and replication in vivo was not tested, which complicates interpretation of these results.

While aiming to produce phage-polymerase transcription-generated shRNA without RIG-I activating properties, Gondai and colleagues discovered that extension of the 5' end by more than one G abolished type I IFN induction.[58] The findings by Saito and Gondai suggested that a distinct 5' RNA sequence is preferred for the activation of RIG-I. However, experiments with defined synthetic RIG-I ligands indicate that the work of both groups needs to be revisited and their conclusions revised.

Synthetic dsRNA Ligands

Prior to the discovery of the 5'triphosphate RNA-motif for RIG-I activation, Marques and colleagues proposed that synthetic blunt ended dsRNA oligonucleotides can stimulate RIG-I (Fig. 2).[59] For this, the glioblastoma cell line T98G was transfected with blunt ended siRNAs or siRNA possessing 3'overhangs. The type I IFN response in these cells was not monitored directly, instead western blot analysis of p56 was performed to indicate upregulation of this type I IFN-induced protein. In contrast to siRNA with 3'overhangs, blunt ended dsRNA oligos induced substantial p56 upregulation. Similar effects were seen in MRC-5 cells. SiRNA-mediated knockdown of RIG-I in T98G indicated RIG-I to be involved in the signaling pathway mediating type I IFN induction. By contrast, HeLa cells and HT1080 cells were not responsive to blunt ended dsRNA, but showed p56 induction in response to in vitro transcribed RNA. In HT1080 cells the response to blunt dsRNA was restored by priming with type I IFN. Based on their results with T98G cells the RIG-I stimulation motif was defined as double blunt ended dsRNA longer

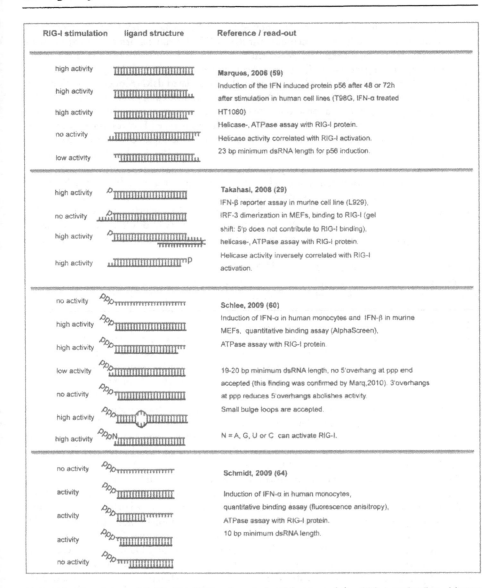

RIG-I stimulation	ligand structure	Reference / read-out
high activity		**Marques, 2006 (59)**
high activity		Induction of the IFN induced protein p56 after 48 or 72h
high activity		after stimulation in human cell lines (T98G, IFN-α treated
no activity		HT1080)
low activity		Helicase-, ATPase assay with RIG-I protein.
		Helicase activity correlated with RIG-I activation.
		23 bp minimum dsRNA length for p56 induction.
high activity		**Takahasi, 2008 (29)**
no activity		IFN-β reporter assay in murine cell line (L929),
high activity		IRF-3 dimerization in MEFs, binding to RIG-I (gel
high activity		shift: 5'p does not contribute to RIG-I binding),
		helicase-, ATPase assay with RIG-I protein.
		Helicase activity inversely correlated with RIG-I
		activation.
no activity		**Schlee, 2009 (60)**
high activity		Induction of IFN-α in human monocytes and IFN-β in murine
high activity		MEFs, quantitative binding assay (AlphaScreen),
low activity		ATPase assay with RIG-I protein.
no activity		19-20 bp minimum dsRNA length, no 5'overhang at ppp end
high activity		accepted (this finding was confirmed by Marq,2010). 3'overhangs
high activity		at ppp reduces 5'overhangs abolishes activity.
		Small bulge loops are accepted.
		N = A, G, U or C can activate RIG-I.
no activity		**Schmidt, 2009 (64)**
activity		Induction of IFN-α in human monocytes,
activity		quantitative binding assay (fluorescence anisitropy),
activity		ATPase assay with RIG-I protein.
no activity		10 bp minimum dsRNA length.

Figure 2. Structures of synthetic RNA oligonucleotides tested for RIG-I activation. Upper strands are in 5'-3' direction, lower strands in 3'-5' direction. p = 5' or 3'monophosphate; ppp = 5'triphosphate

than 23bp. Double blunt ended dsRNA was more active than single blunt ended; and 5'overhangs still exhibited detectable activity after 72 hours of stimulation while 3'overhangs did not (Fig. 2).

Further studies investigated the physical interaction of synthetic blunt ended dsRNA or in vitro transcribed pppRNA with recombinant full-length RIG-I or CARD- or RD domain deletion mutants.[28] For several of these mutants, the ATPase activity of synthetic blunt ended dsRNA and in vitro transcribed ssRNA (*ivt*ppp-ssRNA) was compared. The data demonstrated that full length RIG-I is highly activated by *ivt*ppp-ssRNA while synthetic non-phosphorylated dsRNA was much less active. By contrast, for RIG-I lacking the CARD domain, dsRNA and *ivt*ppp-RNA showed the same degree of ATPase activity. Interaction studies using fluorescence anisotropy with recombinant RIG-I protein or the recombinant RIG-I RD domain confirmed the requirement of the 5'triphosphate for substantial interaction.[28]

Interestingly, during their work Takahasi and colleagues observed a RIG-I-dependent response to synthetic 5'monophosphorylated and 3'monophosphorylated dsRNA oligonucleotides in a IFN-beta-treated murine cell line and in IFN-beta-treated mouse embryonic fibroblasts (MEF), as monitored by IRF-3 dimerization and IFNbeta promoter reporter assays (Fig. 2).[29] In contrast to previous reports[59] non-modified dsRNA did not induce any type I IFN response.[29] Similar to earlier work by Marques and co-workers,[59] 3'-overhangs at the 5'monophosphorylated end were not tolerated, while 5'overhangs were actually not tested (Fig. 2).[29] For 3'monophosphorylated dsRNA 2nt 3'overhangs induced a type-I IFN response but no other end structures were analyzed (blunt, 5'overhang). The authors found that monophosphorylation did not enhance binding of dsRNA to RIG-I protein but did serve to increase RNA stability in the cell. Therefore they proposed that the increased RNA stability is responsible for the elevated RIG-I activity which was observed.[29] Unlike the studies of Marques and colleagues[59] the immunologic activity of dsRNA with 3' overhangs at the 5'monophosporylated end was inversely correlated with the helicase activity for RIG-I.

Synthetic Triphosphorylated dsRNA Ligands

The 5'triphosphorylated end sequence of phage polymerase in vitro transcribed RNA is restricted to a conserved starting nucleotide G (or A followed by G). Therefore, in vitro transcription is not appropriate for comparing sequence variations at the 5'end of triphosphorylated oligonucleotides. Our group generated synthetic well-defined triphosphorylated RNAs[60] based on modifications of a previously described protocol.[61] In contrast to all previous studies using in vitro transcribed RNA, synthetic single stranded triphosphorylated RNA (ppp-ssRNA) did not induce type-I IFN in human monocytes, while the "same" RNA sequence generated by in vitro transcription (*ivt*ppp-ssRNA) was a profound RIG-I activator. Cloning and sequencing of *ivt*ppp-ssRNA transcription products revealed the presence of double stranded hairpin species and complementary sequences, generated by template-dependent RNA transcription, a phenomenon that had been described earlier.[62,63] This suggested, that RIG-I was not activated by the intended ssRNA transcript but rather by aberrant side products. Indeed, transcription reaction conditions that did not permit synthesis of complementary RNA abolished RIG-I activation by in vitro transcribed ssRNA.[60] Consequently, addition of a complementary ssRNA strand to synthetic ppp-ssRNA reestablished RIG-I stimulation. Furthermore, we could show that base pairing of the nucleoside carrying the 5'triphosphate was strictly required, since 5'overhangs of the triphosphorylated end were not tolerated. Optimal RIG-I agonists appeared to be blunt ended, and 2nt 3'overhangs at the 5'triphosphate end impaired RIG-I activation by more than 70% (Fig. 2). The structure at the non-phosphorylated end had no substantial impact on RIG-I activation, as long as the dsRNA encompassed at least 19 bp. Similarly, small (3 nt) bulge loops were well tolerated. All four nucleotides were able to form active triphosphorylated 5'ends of the RIG-I ligand. While activity of pppA, pppG and pppU differed only slightly (A=G>U), pppC induced around 50% less type I IFN. However, this sequence dependency of RIG-I stimulation has so far been tested with only one dsRNA sequence (NACACACACACACACACACACUUU). Most genomic viral RNAs (vRNA) start with pppA, and to our knowledge no vRNA starting with pppC has been described. Using synthetic ppp-ssRNA Schmidt and colleagues (Fig. 2) confirmed the importance of dsRNA.[64] In contrast to our results they observed that RIG-I tolerates a 1 nt 5'overhang at the 5'-ppp and concluded from their experiments that longer (more than 1nt) 5'-triphosphate overhangs in hairpin RNAs are tolerated. However, this interpretation is misleading since these specific experiments were performed using again in vitro transcribed ppp-RNA without ensuring the identity of the obtained sequences by mass spectrometry. Therefore, contamination with completely double stranded material cannot be excluded as one-time size fractionation is not sufficient to exclude contamination of transcripts with small size differences. Moreover, Schmidt et al. also reported a minimum double stranded stretch of only 10bp for RIG-I activation. However, only three different sizes of ppp-dsRNA (15, 10 and 5 bp, blunt at the ppp-end) were tested and a 10mer ppp-dsRNA elicited a stronger type-I IFN response than a 15mer, and a direct comparison of the full 19mer duplex ppp-RNA to hybridizations with the 15mer and 10mer has not been performed.[64] Therefore, it remains unclear whether RIG-I activation by a 10mer duplex represents a general feature. It has to be noted that due to the possibility of G-U wobbles and further non canonical base pairings, ssRNA has ample opportunities to hybridize into double stranded regions, all of which have to be considered when determining a dsRNA structure and when claiming RNA structures to be single stranded.

So far only a limited number of synthetic ppp-dsRNA sequences have been tested (seven in our work,[60] one in the work of Schmidt et al.[64]). It might be possible that the composition of nucleotides next to the 5'-ppp end contribute to a tolerance of 1nt 5'-ppp-overhangs. Independent experiments with highly purified in vitro transcribed ppp-RNA from arenavirus sequences confirmed that the 5'-ppp end of dsRNA needs to be base paired for RIG-I activation.[65] Therefore, it was suggested that some arenaviruses and bunyaviruses use a so-called *prime and realign* mechanism to initiate genome synthesis, which generates 5'overhangs in order to avoid RIG-I mediated recognition.[65]

The requirement of a base paired end at the 5'triphosphate-bearing side of dsRNA was confirmed by crystallization of the RIG-I RD with ppp-dsRNA.[30,31] As will be discussed in detail below, base pairing enables an essential stacking interaction with a conserved phenylalanine residue in the RNA binding cleft of the RD with the terminal nucleotides ppp-dsRNA (Fig. 3A).

In contrast to previous results using type-I IFN-primed murine cells,[29] no substantial type I IFN induction could be detected when human monocytes were stimulated with 5'monophosphorylated and non-phosphorylated dsRNAs.[60,64] Nonetheless Schmidt and colleagues tested the same sequences, which were previously reported to induce type I IFN in type I IFN-primed MEFs.[29,64] However, in both studies monophosphorylated and non-phosphorylated dsRNA promoted a substantial ATPase activity of recombinant RIG-I protein at higher RNA doses.[60,64] It is conceivable that RIG-I activation observed by Marques[59] and Takahasi[29] are caused by relatively high local RNA concentrations in the cytosol of highly RIG-I responsive cell lines (T98G) or murine cells combined with long incubation times (48-72h[59]), pre-activation by priming with type I IFN[59] and sensitive detection methods (p56 western blot, IFN-beta reporter assay, IRF-3 dimerization[29,59]). By crystallization of RIG-I RD with 5'OH-dsRNA Lu and colleagues confirmed that binding of dsRNA is possible in principle.[60] Although the binding site for dsRNA appeared to be the same as 5'ppp-dsRNA and 5'OH-dsRNA, the crystal exhibited that 5'OH-dsRNA bound in a different angle, and with other amino acid positions.

Habjan and colleagues observed that Hantaan virus (HTNV), Crimean-Congo hemorrhagic fever virus (CCHTV) and Borna disease virus (BDV) can prevent RIG-I-mediated detection by the prime and realign mechanism including cleavage of the 5' terminal base of their genomic RNA to obtain their characteristic monophosphorylated 5'ends.[67] They observed that in contrast to 5'ppp end bearing genomic RNA, the genomic RNAs of HTNV, BDV or CCHTV with 5'monophosphate ends were not able to bind recombinant RIG-I or to stimulate endogenous RIG-I when transfected into HEK293 cells. Although HEK293 cells are not a sensitive detection system for RIG-I mediated responses, this relatively complicated mechanism of (-)ssRNA viruses to circumvent RIG-I recognition by introduction of monophosphates at the 5'end of genomes does not support the concept that 5'mono-phosphorylated RNA is a preferred ligand structure for RIG-I during viral infection.

The generation of aberrant dsRNA during in vitro transcription challenges the conclusions from earlier studies, which aimed to define RIG-I recognition sequences based on experiments using this in vitro transcribed RNA. In this respect, the observations of Gondai and colleagues allow an interesting interpretation.[58] When the authors constructed shRNAs with 3'UU hairpin RNA with base paired 5'ppp-ends and a UU 3'-overhang, RIG-I activation was observed. Introduction of extra Gs at the 5'-ppp end instead established single stranded or mismatched 5'ppp ends, which did not stimulate RIG-I. Therefore, the inhibition of RIG-I activity may not be due to the sequence but due to the structure formed by the 5'ppp end of the RNA hairpin. The finding of Saito and colleagues that both

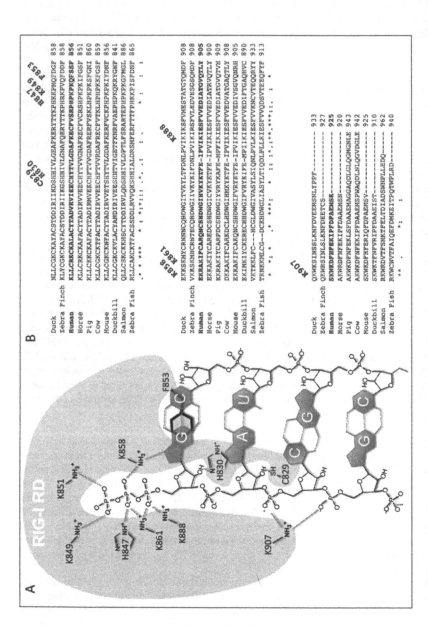

Figure 3. Interaction of the RIG-I regulatory domain with double-stranded triphosphorylated RNA. A) Data from crystal structures: K858, K851, K849, H847, K861, K888 form a basic binding cleft for binding of 5′triphosphate. K907 binds backbone phosphates. B) Alignment of RIG-I regulatory domains of the indicated species. Amino acids which are crucial for ligand binding, are identical or at least functionally related in all vertebrate RIG-I species. Figure continued on following page.

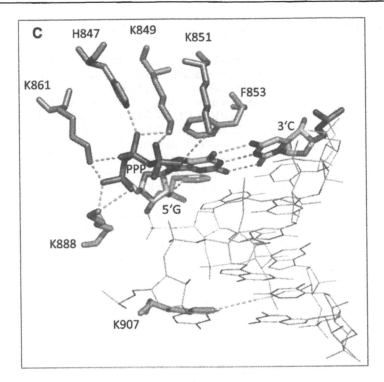

Figure 3, continued from previous page. C) Stereoview of RIG-I RD amino acids interacting with ppp-dsRNA.

poly A as well as poly U rich ppp-ssRNAs elicited a more potent RIG-I response can then be explained by the fact that both complementary RNA species are formed in the phage-polymerase transcription reaction that was intended to produce only one ssRNA species.[57] In fact, by using the same template as used by Saito and colleagues for phage-polymerase mediated production of the reportedly RIG-I stimulating poly A rich sequence Schmidt and colleagues did not obtain any RIG-I stimulating activity when no UTP or CTP (both are not required for the synthesis of a poly A sequence) was present in the transcription mix.[57,64] Conversely, inclusion of UTP and CTP re-established RIG-I-activating capacity.[64] This strongly points to recognition of a double stranded polyA rich sequence. High RIG-I stimulation by this structure can be explained by the fact, that poly A and poly U represent highly repetitive sequences, which form weak or no secondary structures. It is conceivable that hybridization of complementary non-structured RNAs to dsRNA is facilitated in comparison to mixed G/C containing sequences. With regard to the work of Saito and colleagues[57] it is important to note that subgenomic (single stranded) RNAs of HCV carry 5′monophosphorylated ends.[68] As RIG-I activation by polyU was described to strictly depend on the presence of 5′triphosphate,[57] triphosphate-dependent RIG-I activation can only occur in the context of recognition of double stranded replicative RNA intermediates, which are generated during replication.[42]

Thus far, evidence for a sequence dependent recognition by RIG-I is scarce. Our own results suggest a slight preference for A, G and U with lower acceptance of C at the 5′ppp end in perfect blunt ended ppp-dsRNA. However, this needs to be confirmed for other sequence contexts. Most likely, recognition sequences are more important in the context of imperfect secondary RNA structures, however this requires more scrutiny, using well-defined synthetic RIG-I ligands in the future. Another key question is whether RIG-I evolved to preferentially recognize viral structures, and whether viruses evolved mechanisms or structures to escape RIG-I recognition.

Structural and Functional Insights into RNA Recognition by RIG-I Like Helicases

From its crystal structure, a triphosphate binding site in the RD domain (amino acids 802-925) of RIG-I was predicted.[28] Structure-guided mutational analysis of RIG-I function in HEK293 cells suggested a positively charged grove as the likely 5'-triphosphate binding site, in which K858 is essential for mediating RIG-I activation upon binding to 5'triphosphate RNA. Alternatively, a residual ATPase activity of the isolated RIG-I-DECH domain with synthetic dsRNA pointed to a dsRNA interacting site in the DECH domain.[28] Takahasi and colleagues applied a NMR approach to analyze the structure of the RIG-I RD domain and its interaction with dsRNA and *ivt*ppp-ssRNA in solution.[29] NMR titration experiments exhibited a positively charged "cleft", which is involved in binding of both RNA ligand types. Mutational analysis of RIG-I function in RIG-I deficient MEFs revealed that K858 together with K861 (KK858/861AA double mutant) is crucial for both dsRNA and *ivt*ppp-ssRNA induced type I IFN induction. Using well defined synthetic triphosphorylated RNA the crystal structure of the RIG-I RD bound to a 12mer ppp-dsRNA palindromic sequence was resolved.[30] The crystal exhibited a basic binding cleft with specific amino acids involved in binding of the triphosphate itself, the 5'terminal base pair and the backbone phosphate (Fig. 3A). K849 and K851 are in contact with the gamma phosphate of the triphosphate. However, conservative K849A and K851A mutations impaired RIG-I activation only at very low ligand concentrations.[30] K858, H847 and K861were found to bind to the beta phosphate of the triphosphate. Single substitution of K861, which is also in contact with alpha phosphate, to alanine (A) and double substitution of H847 and K858 to A abolished RIG-I activation by ppp-dsRNA. Also substitution of K888, being in contact with the alpha phosphate group, inhibited recognition of ppp-dsRNA by RIG-I. K907 is in proximity to the backbone phosphate between N2 and N3[30] or N3 and N4.[31] As substitution of K907 to A abolishes RIG-I activity completely[30] this interaction appears critical for recognition of the ribose backbone of a dsRNA structure. Interaction of K907 with the phosphate between N2 and N3[30] or N3 and N4, as found in another RIG-I crystal-structure study,[31] may either depend on the individual oligonucleotide sequence (pppGACGCUAGCGUC[30] or pppGGCGCGCGCGCGCC[31]), the crystal packaging or the interpretation of the data. In summary, both studies provide very similar RNA structures as ligands for binding to the RIG-I RD domain.

Importantly, the amino acids involved in RNA ligand binding, being H847, K858, K861, K888 and K907 are 100% conserved in RIG-I of birds mammals and fish (Fig. 3B). This underscores the importance of these positions for RIG-I-mediated RNA-virus recognition. Interestingly, F853 is involved in a stacking interaction with the 5'terminal base pair (Fig. 3A/C). This particular stacking interaction is only stable when N_1 is base paired, validating the observed need of base pairing at the triphosphate-bearing end of dsRNA to stimulate RIG-I. This is confirmed by the observation that the F853A RIG-I mutant does not respond to ppp-dsRNA. According to RIG-I RD species sequence alignment (Fig. 3B), F853 can only be substituted by the functionally related tyrosine (Y). This confirms the crystal data to reflect the recognition of ppp-dsRNA by RIG-I in the cytosol.

The finding by Lu and colleagues that RIG-I can bind, and simultaneously be stimulated by single-stranded ppp-RNA is misleading, since in vitro transcribed RNA was used for stimulation of cells.[31] As noted before, this usually contains ppp-dsRNA species. Although interaction of RIG-I RD appears to be restricted to the ppp bearing RNA strand, helix formation still is essential for proper interaction of the RNA with the amino acid residues H853, K907, H830 and C829. Marq and colleagues observed that inactive ligands can bind RIG-I with similar affinity as active ligands suggesting the existence of stimulatory ("productive") and non-stimulatory ("non-productive") ligand binding modes to RIG-I.[69] This indicates that interaction with RIG-I is necessary but not sufficient for *activation* of RIG-I. Additionally, the involvement of the helicase domain and CARD in selective recognition of dsRNA and 5'triphosphate was suggested.[28]

The RD of the RIG-I inhibiting helicase Lgp2 was found to resemble the RIG-I RD.[33,34] Similar to RIG-I, Lgp2 binds preferentially to blunt ended dsRNA.[33-35] In contrast to RIG-I, Lgp2 binds dsRNA in a 5'triphosphate independent manner.[33] Interestingly, the amino acids mediating the interaction with the 5′ terminal base pair and the ribose backbone (H830, F853, K907) are highly conserved between RIG-I and the Lgp2 RD, while triphosphate interacting amino acids (H847, K849, K858 and K861) are missing in the Lgp2 RD. Accordingly, H830, F853 and K907 were found to be involved in dsRNA binding of the Lgp2 RD.[34] Conversely, the binding mode of OH-dsRNA to Lgp2 differed considerably from the binding mode of ppp-dsRNA. Mutation of the amino acids in the Lgp2 RD corresponding to K888 and K907 in the RIG-I RD led to loss of RNA binding but did not impair Lgp2-mediated inhibition of RIG-I activation.[34]

Based on the crystallization of RIG-I RD with 5′OH-dsRNA Lu and colleagues confirmed that binding of dsRNA is possible.[66] Although the binding site for dsRNA appeared to be the same for 5′ppp-dsRNA and 5′OH-dsRNA, the crystal showed that 5′OH-dsRNA binds in a different angle, using different amino acid contacts, in particular at the antisense (non-triphosphorylated) strand.[66]

RNase Cleavage Products

Interestingly, the above results are in contrast to the initial finding that RIG-I can be activated by poly I:C,[14] a dsRNA polymer with monophosphates at the 5′ end.[70] Aiming to dissect recognition patterns differentiating MDA5 and RIG-I recognition, Kato and colleagues fractionated poly I:C digested with RNAse-II (resulting in 5′monophosphates and 2nt 3′overhangs), and observed that high molecular weight poly I:C (7 kb) was preferentially recognized by MDA5 while fractions equal to 300 bp or smaller were exclusively recognized by RIG-I.[46] A similar conclusion was drawn by Pichlmair et al.[49] Malathi and colleagues[71] reported, that activation of the antiviral endoribonuclease RNase L by 2′,5′-linked oligoadenylate produces small RNA cleavage products from self-RNA that initiate type I IFN production.[71] Interestingly, both, MDA5 and RIG-I were observed to be involved in recognition of small (<200 nt) RNase L cleavage products of total cellular RNA. The type I IFN-induced RNase L cleaves single-stranded RNA resulting in RNA products containing 5′-OH and 3′-monophosphate groups.

In a follow-up paper Malathi and colleagues identified HCV genome sequence-derived RNase-L cleavage products that bind to RIG-I by reverse sequencing.[72] Among 15 RIG-I binding sequences one structure was found to significantly stimulate RIG-I in a 3′monophosphate dependent but 5′triphosphate independent manner. The sequence was predicted to contain long (>20 bp) dsRNA regions but also long (>5 nt) single stranded 5′ and 3′ ends. As the sequence was derived from in vitro transcription and the identity was not revealed by mass spectrometry, it is unclear whether the intended structure is responsible for RIG-I stimulation. Nevertheless, this finding demonstrates the existence of special RNA structures being able to activate RIG-I in a 3′monophosphate dependent manner and that such structures can originate from RNase L dependent cleavage of RNA virus genomes.

In Vivo RNA Polymerase III Transcripts of Exogenous DNA

The groups of Akira and Medzhitov described a TLR9 independent type I IFN response when dsDNA was transfected into the cytosol of cells.[73,74] SiRNA-mediated knock-down of MAVS in 293T cells led to reduction of the dsDNA induced type I IFN response suggesting a MAVS dependent pathway of dsDNA recognition.[73] However, murine MAVS deficient cells were still able to respond to dsDNA.[75] Of note, in the above-mentioned experiments the heteropolymer dAdT (a polymer of the alternating sequence AT) was used as a "synthetic" dsDNA analog. Cheng and colleagues realized that human cell lines (Huh7, HEK293) raise a MAVS and RIG-I dependent type I IFN response after transfection of dAdT but not plasmid DNA.[76] The initially confusing result was later clarified by two independent groups.[77,78] Ablasser and colleagues and Chiu and colleagues found that dAdT serves as a template for the endogenous RNA polymerase III, which transcribes 5′triphosphorylated self-complementary AU-polymers, forming an excellent target structure for RIG-I-mediated recognition.

Unlike murine cell lines and human monocytic cells, most other human cell lines tested were not stimulated by dsDNAs (e.g. PCR products or plasmid DNA) other than dAdT, probably due to the absence of a receptor in the cytosol which can sense DNA directly.[76,77] For those cells the

Polymerase III – RIG-I pathway represents the only way to detect cytosolic dsDNA. Because some DNA viruses and intracellular bacteria raised a MAVS or RIG-I-dependent type I IFN response in non-immune cells it was proposed that in these cells the innate immune response to intracellular dsDNA-containing pathogens generally occurs via activation of RIG-I by pathogen-derived polymerase III transcripts.[77,78]

Detection of Bacterial RNA

All enzymatically transcribed RNAs start with a 5′triphosphorylated nucleotide. In eukaryotes, subsequent 5′ processing and modifications like capping are key features of the regulation of mRNA translation. By contrast, in *E. coli* one third of mRNA remains 5′triphosphorylated[79] which is expected to also apply other bacteria species. The 5′phosphorylation status of bacterial mRNA is regulated by the pyrophosphatase RppH[80] which determines mRNA decay.[81] In this context, the 5′triphosphate moiety protects bacterial mRNA from decay by RNase-E.[81] Interestingly, the pyrophosphatase RppH was shown to strongly prefer single-stranded triphosphorylated 5′nucleotides as substrate over base paired ends.[80] This finding is consistent with the observation that bacterial RNAs can be stabilized by a 5′-terminal stem-loop.[82,83] Therefore, the occurrence of base paired triphosphorylated RNA appears to be characteristic for bacteria, and this structure represents a ligand for RIG-I.

Using siRNAs Opitz and colleagues identified that *Legionella pneumophilae*, a Gram-negative facultative intracellular bacterium with type IV secretion system, induced a MAVS-dependent but RIG-I- or MDA5-independent type-I IFN response in a human endothelial cell line (A549).[84] This MAVS-dependency was later confirmed using MAVS- and MDA5-deficient, anti-RIG-I shRNA-expressing bone marrow-derived macrophage cell lines.[85] In contrast to Opitz and colleagues,[84] this study suggested a role for MDA5 and RIG-I.[85] Although knock-down of RIG-I completely abolished the response to purified bacterial RNA, it remains unclear whether *Legionella*-derived RNA can indeed gain access to host cell cytosol during infection. Since MDA5 was apparently not involved in direct sensing of bacterial RNA, the authors proposed an alternative mechanism indirectly leading to induction of RIG-I and MDA5. Recognition of bacterial RNA by RIG-I was also observed for the bacterium *Helicobacter pylori*.[86] By contrast, DNA from *Legionella pneumophilae* was interestingly shown to lack type-I IFN induction in HEK293 cells.[85] This excludes its direct recognition and RIG-I-mediated recognition following polymerase-III transcription[78] in the host cell.

Detection of Viral RNA by RIG-I

As mentioned above, not only dsRNA viruses but also positive single-strand RNA [(+)ssRNA] viruses produce copious amounts of cytosolic dsRNA during their replication.[41,42] This is in agreement with the dsRNA-requirement for RIG-I recognition (Fig. 2). Exceptions are picornaviruses and caliciviruses (Fig. 1), which evade RIG-I recognition by replacing the 5′ppp in their RNA genomes with a peptide (Vpg) linked via a tyrosine residue to the monophosphate at the 5′end.[87-89] The Vpg peptide has an additional function in the initiation of ribosomal translation of the viral RNA.

RIG-I is responsible for the detection of many (-)ssRNA viruses, which were initially reported *not* to produce double-stranded RNA during infection.[41,56] This discrepancy is explained by the fact that the antibody used in these earlier studies only binds dsRNA longer than 40 bases.[90]

The Influenza virus genome consists of 8 genomic (-)ssRNA segments containing highly complementary 5′and 3′sequences[91] that form a short (about 15 bp) double stranded, perfect blunt ended structure, the so called *panhandle*, during Influenza virus replication (Fig. 4).[92] The Influenza virus *panhandle* structure serves as the RNA transcription-initiation site for the viral RNA polymerase complex in the nucleus of the host cell.[93] By their small 15 bp size, these short panhandle structures can not be detected by the dsRNA specific antibody. Nonetheless, they do meet the requirements for RIG-I activation as dictated by the synthetic model of ppp-dsRNA structures. Accordingly, they contain a triphosphorylated, blunt ended stretch of double stranded RNA and hence are recognized by RIG-I (Figs. 1, 2 and 4).[60]

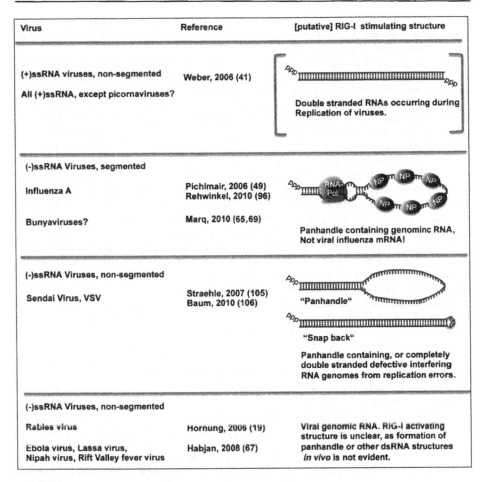

Figure 4. Predicted or established RIG-I-stimulating viral RNA structures.

Recently, Dauber et al. demonstrated that after export from the nucleus the Influenza panhandle is accessible for the antiviral double-stranded RNA-dependent protein kinase (PKR) in the cytosol of the host cell.[94] Given that PKR and RIG-I apparently bind similar RNA structures – short triphosphorylated dsRNA,[60,95] it is conceivable that RIG-I is also able to access and recognize the Influenza panhandle structure. However, this hypothesis still needs to be verified using well-defined RIG-I ligands. By using mutated Influenza RNA polymerases which either selectively produce replicative genomic RNA or viral mRNA, Rehwinkel and colleagues confirmed that Influenza genomic RNA contributed to RIG-I mediated type I IFN induction rather than Influenza mRNA.[96] Indeed, purification of RIG-I-bound viral RNA from cells infected with Influenza virus revealed that only 5'triphosphorylated viral genomic RNA bound RIG-I.

So far only one (-)ssRNA virus replicating in the cytosol (La Crosse Virus; LACV) was monitored for production of dsRNA using the 40bp dsRNA specific antibody.[41] In general, the genomes of all (-)ssRNA viruses have the potential to form panhandle structures due to complementary 5'and 3' terminal sequences. For Bunyaviridae including LACV it was shown by electron microscopy and psoralen-crosslinking that 5'- and 3'- end of the viral genome form a panhandle structure in vivo.[97,98] The panhandles of LACV constist of a 24-27bp dsRNA stretch with few mismatched sites,[98] thereby meeting virtually all requirements for optimal RIG-I recognition.[60]

As mentioned before, Marq and colleages suggested that some arenaviruses and bunyaviruses perform the *prime and realign* mechanism to escape RIG-I activation by thus generating their typical 5'overhangs in their genome.[65]

By contrast, viral particles of Sendai Virus (SeV) and Measles Virus (MeV) contain predominantly linear nucleocapsids, suggesting that formation of a panhandle is prevented by encapsidation with structural proteins.[99,100] On the other hand SeV and VSV are known to produce defective interfering (DI) viral genomes during their life cycle (Fig. 4).[101-103] Three types of DI genomes were classified: DI genomes with internal deletions, 5'promoter duplications leading to completely complementary 5'-3' ends (Fig. 4, "Panhandle"), and "snap back", hairpin DI genomes, consisting of a completely dsRNA hairpin of 100-1000bp (Fig. 4; Snap Back). At least the "snap back" and the "panhandle" DI RNAs should represent excellent RIG-I ligands. Indeed, Strahle et al. correlated activation of RIG-I by Sendai virus with the presence of snap back DI genomes (DI-H4) which occur during infection and do not show encapsidation and therefore can form panhandle structures in infected cells.[104,105] Additionally, by applying a deep sequencing approach after purification of RIG-I bound RNA from Sendai virus infected cells, Baum and colleagues demonstrated that RIG-I preferred binding of such DI genomes.[106]

It is assumed that the genomic RNA of RNA viruses should be the preferred target structure for RIG-I. Indeed, purified genomic RNA from most analyzed (-)ssRNA viruses including Rabies virus,[19] Rift Valley fever virus, Lassa virus, Nipah virus[67] induced RIG-I activation. However, genomic RNA purification by standard methods strips the RNA from interacting viral nuclear proteins, and thereby misleadingly enables the formation of secondary RIG-I activating structures in the viral RNA which actually do not occur during their replication cycle. Therefore it is unclear if these viral genomes would activate RIG-I during infection. By contrast, viruses possess mechanisms to cap their mRNA either by viral encoded capping enzymes or cap-snatching mechanisms[107] leading to loss of, or masking of the 5'triphosphate. The fact that (-)ssRNA viruses modify their 5'end to avoid RIG-I recognition[65,67] clearly indicates that dsRNA structures occurring at the 5'end of viral genomes are critical. In principle, recognition of panhandle structures is a clever adaptation of an antiviral innate immune receptor to detect (-)ssRNA viruses since replication of (-)ssRNA viruses requires a highly conserved promoter at both ends of the genome resulting in self-complementary 5' and 3' ends. For VSV it was shown that during replication, artificially introduced extra nucleotides at the 5'end of the VSV (-)ssRNA genome are eliminated while extra nucleotides at the 3'end are not tolerated at all.[108] Thus, the formation of short double-stranded and blunt ended 5'triphosphate RNA, the consequence of the requirement of two conserved promoters, represents a negative strand virus-associated molecular pattern detected by RIG-I.

So far, only panhandle structures of Arenavirus RNA genomes which possess relatively long dsRNA stretches, were studied using clearly defined RNAs and were found to stimulate RIG-I.[65] Possibly, during the evolution of viruses, selective pressures have forced an adaptation of bulge loops in panhandle structures of some viruses to circumvent RIG-I recognition, when viral genomes are properly made. If this was the case, it would imply that for those viruses RIG-I detects the errors of viral RNA polymerases as it is the case for phage RNA-polymerase in vitro transcripts.[60,64]

Conclusion and Outlook

Taken together, the members of the RLR family are the central and ubiquitous alarm switches of the innate immune system for the detection of non-self RNA molecules in the cytosol of host cells. Their activation triggers cell autonomous and cytokine responses, which in turn recruit and activate additional innate immune cells in the vicinity of the site of infection, and in secondary lymphoid organs assist in priming adaptive immune responses essential to achieve full clearance of viral infections and via immunological memory prevent their recurrence. While our understanding of MDA5 and Lgp2 is still incomplete, a large body of data now exists for RIG-I. From these – albeit slowly - an almost clear picture on RIG-I function emerges. When defined synthetic RNA structures were not yet available, poorly defined enzymatic products including in vitro transcribed RNAs or poly I:C have clouded the conclusions drawn from numerous early studies. Here we attempted to carefully reassess the studies carried out thus far, and conclude that the spectrum of sources of RNAs detected by RIG-I is broader than initially thought. RIG-I not only detects viral triphosphate RNA directly but is also able to detect pathogen DNA via RNA products transcribed by polymerase-III; moreover RNA sensing by RIG-I is not limited to viruses but may additionally mediate the detection of intracellular bacteria.

The work reported so far invites further scrutiny into the full function of RIG-I, as well as MDA5 and Lgp2. It appears that RLRs are promising targets for interventions in certain viral- and bacterial infections, and may be successfully employed in anti-tumor immunotherapy.

About the Authors

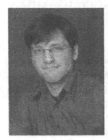

Martin Schlee is group leader at the Institute of Clinical Chemistry and Clinical Pharmacology at the University Hospital in Bonn. He studied Biochemistry at the University of Bielefeld. During his PhD thesis from 1999 to 2003 and early post doc time he worked in the group of Prof. Georg W. Bornkamm (Institute of Clinical Molecular Biology and Tumor Genetics, German Research Center for Environmental Health, Munich) on the immunogenicity of Epstein-Barr virus and c-myc transformed B cells (Burkitt's lymphoma) and its impact on pathogenesis. In 2005 he joined the group of Gunther Hartmann. His team explores cytosolic immunorecognition of nucleic acids especially by RIG-I.

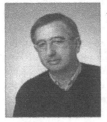

Janos Ludwig is nucleic acid chemist. His most widely recognized scientific accomplishment is the development of novel phosphorylation techniques for the synthesis for nucleoside triphoshates and their analogs. He worked in leading laboratories of RNA chemistry: First as post doc with Fritz Eckstein at the Max Planck Institute for Experimentelle Medizin in Göttingen, Germany and later with Tom Tuschl in the Laboratory of RNA Biochemisry at the Rockefeller University in New York. From here he joined the team of Gunther Hartmann. His synhtetic methods for pppRNA served as the basis for understanding the correct structure of the RIG-I ligand.

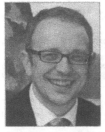

Since 2007 Christoph Coch is head of the clinical study unit of the Institute of Clinical Chemistry and Clinical Pharmacology at the University Hospital in Bonn. He studied Medicine at the University of Cologne and Freiburg and received his MD in 2005. He joined G. Hartmanns group in 2006 to study immunorecognition of nucleic acid, specifically ligands for RIG-I, MDA-5 and the TLR in vitro and in vivo in disease models and to translate the findings into concepts for clinical development.

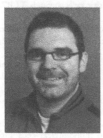

Jasper G. van den Boorn joined the Institute of Clinical Chemistry and Clinical Pharmacology of the University Hospital in Bonn, Germany, in 2011. He received his PhD doctorate from the University of Amsterdam, The Netherlands, in 2010. He performed his dissertation research under guidance of Prof. J.D. Bos, Prof. C. Melief, and Dr. R. Luiten. He developed an effective new melanoma immunotherapy regimen based upon the active induction of vitiligo by monobenzone which lead to the initiation of a phase 2a clinical trial in Amsterdam.

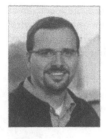

Since 2006 Winfried Barchet is an independent research group leader funded by the DFG Emmy Noether-programme „Immune Recognition of Viral Nucleic Acids in the Cytosol". He studied Biochemistry at the FU Berlin and at the ETH Zürich, Switzerland. He worked in the laboratory of Hans Hengartner and Rolf Zinkernagel. He then joined Ulrich Kalinke and Klaus Rajewsky at EMBL Mouse Biology Programme, Monterotondo, Italy, to study the role of plasmacytoid dendritic cells (PDC) in the type I IFN response to viral infection, and received his PhD in 2002 from the University of Cologne, Germany. As postdoc he joined the laboratory of Marco Colonna at Washington University in St. Louis, USA. The current focus of his group is developing RNA ligand structures that selectively engage TLRs 7 and 8, as well as RIG-I and MDA-5, towards their therapeutic use to promote antiviral and anti-tumor immunity.

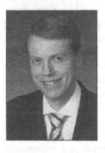

Since 2007 Gunther Hartmann is director of the Institute of Clinical Chemistry and Clinical Pharmacology at the University Hospital in Bonn. He studied Medicine at the University of Ulm where he received his MD in 1993. In 1994 he moved to the University of Munich for training in Internal Medicine and Clinical Pharmacology, and to perform research in the laboratory of Prof. Stefan Endres on antisense and immunorecognition of nucleic acids. From 1998 to 1999 he joined Art Krieg at the University of Iowa studying CpG. From 2000 to 2004 he established the group Therapeutic Oligonucleotides at the Division of Clinical Pharmacology (Stefan Endres) in Munich. In 2005 he moved to Bonn to become professor of Clinical Pharmacology. Gunther Hartmann gained scientific reputation in the field of immunorecognition of nucleic acids, and its intersection with RNA interference. Besides contributions to TLR9 and CpG DNA the group found that short interfering RNA molecules (siRNA) activate TLR7, defined the structural requirements for the detection of RNA by TLR7 and TLR8, identified the RNA ligand for RIG-I, analyzed the signaling pathways of RIG-I, and resolved the crystal structure or RIG-I bound to its ligand 5'-triphosphate RNA. The group applies immunostimulatory nucleic acids and siRNA for immunotherapy of cancer and viral infection.

References

1. Takeuchi O, Akira S. Pattern recognition receptors and inflammation. Cell 2010; 140:805-20; PMID:20303872; http://dx.doi.org/10.1016/j.cell.2010.01.022.
2. Bray M. Highly pathogenic RNA viral infections: challenges for antiviral research. Antiviral Res 2008; 78:1-8; PMID:18243346; http://dx.doi.org/10.1016/j.antiviral.2007.12.007.
3. Heil F, Hemmi H, Hochrein H, Ampenberger F, Kirschning C, Akira S, et al. Species-specific recognition of single-stranded RNA via toll-like receptor 7 and 8. Science 2004; 303:1526-9; PMID:14976262; http://dx.doi.org/10.1126/science.1093620.
4. Diebold SS, Montoya M, Unger H, Alexopoulou L, Roy P, Haswell LE, et al. Viral infection switches non-plasmacytoid dendritic cells into high interferon producers. Nature 2003; 424:324-8; PMID:12819664; http://dx.doi.org/10.1038/nature01783.
5. Hornung V, Guenthner-Biller M, Bourquin C, Ablasser A, Schlee M, Uematsu S, et al. Sequence-specific potent induction of IFN-alpha by short interfering RNA in plasmacytoid dendritic cells through TLR7. Nat Med 2005; 11:263-70; PMID:15723075; http://dx.doi.org/10.1038/nm1191.
6. Judge AD, Sood V, Shaw JR, Fang D, McClintock K, MacLachlan I. Sequence-dependent stimulation of the mammalian innate immune response by synthetic siRNA. Nat Biotechnol 2005; 23:457-62; PMID:15778705; http://dx.doi.org/10.1038/nbt1081.
7. Krieg AM, Yi AK, Matson S, Waldschmidt TJ, Bishop GA, Teasdale R, et al. CpG motifs in bacterial DNA trigger direct B-cell activation. Nature 1995; 374:546-9; PMID:7700380; http://dx.doi.org/10.1038/374546a0.
8. Hemmi H, Takeuchi O, Kawai T, Kaisho T, Sato S, Sanjo H, et al. A Toll-like receptor recognizes bacterial DNA. Nature 2000; 408:740-5; PMID:11130078; http://dx.doi.org/10.1038/35047123.
9. Hornung V, Rothenfusser S, Britsch S, Krug A, Jahrsdorfer B, Giese T, et al. Quantitative expression of toll-like receptor 1-10 mRNA in cellular subsets of human peripheral blood mononuclear cells and sensitivity to CpG oligodeoxynucleotides. J Immunol 2002; 168:4531-7; PMID:11970999.

10. Schlee M, Hornung V, Hartmann G. siRNA and isRNA: two edges of one sword. Mol Ther 2006; 14:463-70; PMID:16877044; http://dx.doi.org/10.1016/j.ymthe.2006.06.001.
11. Barchet W, Wimmenauer V, Schlee M, Hartmann G. Accessing the therapeutic potential of immuno-stimulatory nucleic acids. Curr Opin Immunol 2008; 20:389-95; PMID:18652893; http://dx.doi.org/10.1016/j.coi.2008.07.007.
12. Schlee M, Barchet W, Hornung V, Hartmann G. Beyond double-stranded RNA-type I IFN induction by 3pRNA and other viral nucleic acids. Curr Top Microbiol Immunol 2007; 316:207-30; PMID:17969450; http://dx.doi.org/10.1007/978-3-540-71329-6_11.
13. Alexopoulou L, Holt AC, Medzhitov R, Flavell RA. Recognition of double-stranded RNA and activation of NF-kappaB by Toll-like receptor 3. Nature 2001; 413:732-8; PMID:11607032; http://dx.doi.org/10.1038/35099560.
14. Yoneyama M, Kikuchi M, Natsukawa T, Shinobu N, Imaizumi T, Miyagishi M, et al. The RNA helicase RIG-I has an essential function in double-stranded RNA-induced innate antiviral responses. Nat Immunol 2004; 5:730-7; PMID:15208624; http://dx.doi.org/10.1038/ni1087.
15. Rothenfusser S, Goutagny N, DiPerna G, Gong M, Monks BG, Schoenemeyer A, et al. The RNA helicase Lgp2 inhibits TLR-independent sensing of viral replication by retinoic acid-inducible gene-I. J Immunol 2005; 175:5260-8; PMID:16210631.
16. Venkataraman T, Valdes M, Elsby R, Kakuta S, Caceres G, Saijo S, et al. Loss of DExD/H box RNA helicase LGP2 manifests disparate antiviral responses. J Immunol 2007; 178:6444-55; PMID:17475874.
17. Gitlin L, Barchet W, Gilfillan S, Cella M, Beutler B, Flavell RA, et al. Essential role of mda-5 in type I IFN responses to polyriboinosinic:polyribocytidylic acid and encephalomyocarditis picornavirus. Proc Natl Acad Sci USA 2006; 103:8459-64; PMID:16714379; http://dx.doi.org/10.1073/pnas.0603082103.
18. Kato H, Takeuchi O, Sato S, Yoneyama M, Yamamoto M, Matsui K, et al. Differential roles of MDA5 and RIG-I helicases in the recognition of RNA viruses. Nature 2006; 441:101-5; PMID:16625202; http://dx.doi.org/10.1038/nature04734.
19. Hornung V, Ellegast J, Kim S, Brzozka K, Jung A, Kato H, et al. 5'-Triphosphate RNA is the ligand for RIG-I. Science 2006; 314:994-7; PMID:17038590; http://dx.doi.org/10.1126/science.1132505.
20. Saito T, Hirai R, Loo YM, Owen D, Johnson CL, Sinha SC, et al. Regulation of innate antiviral defenses through a shared repressor domain in RIG-I and LGP2. Proc Natl Acad Sci USA 2007; 104:582-7; PMID:17190814; http://dx.doi.org/10.1073/pnas.0606699104.
21. Kawai T, Takahashi K, Sato S, Coban C, Kumar H, Kato H, et al. IPS-1, an adaptor triggering RIG-I- and Mda5-mediated type I interferon induction. Nat Immunol 2005; 6:981-8; PMID:16127453; http://dx.doi.org/10.1038/ni1243.
22. Meylan E, Curran J, Hofmann K, Moradpour D, Binder M, Bartenschlager R, et al. Cardif is an adaptor protein in the RIG-I antiviral pathway and is targeted by hepatitis C virus. Nature 2005; 437:1167-72; PMID:16177806; http://dx.doi.org/10.1038/nature04193.
23. Seth RB, Sun L, Ea CK, Chen ZJ. Identification and characterization of MAVS, a mitochondrial antiviral signaling protein that activates NF-kappaB and IRF 3. Cell 2005; 122:669-82; PMID:16125763; http://dx.doi.org/10.1016/j.cell.2005.08.012.
24. Xu LG, Wang YY, Han KJ, Li LY, Zhai Z, Shu HB. VISA is an adapter protein required for virus-triggered IFN-beta signaling. Mol Cell 2005; 19:727-40; PMID:16153868; http://dx.doi.org/10.1016/j.molcel.2005.08.014.
25. Doyle S, Vaidya S, O'Connell R, Dadgostar H, Dempsey P, Wu T, et al. IRF3 mediates a TLR3/TLR4-specific antiviral gene program. Immunity 2002; 17:251-63; PMID:12354379; http://dx.doi.org/10.1016/S1074-7613(02)00390-4.
26. Fitzgerald KA, Rowe DC, Barnes BJ, Caffrey DR, Visintin A, Latz E, et al. LPS-TLR4 signaling to IRF-3/7 and NF-kappaB involves the toll adapters TRAM and TRIF. J Exp Med 2003; 198:1043-55; PMID:14517278; http://dx.doi.org/10.1084/jem.20031023.
27. Sharma S, tenOever BR, Grandvaux N, Zhou GP, Lin R, Hiscott J. Triggering the interferon antiviral response through an IKK-related pathway. Science 2003; 300:1148-51; PMID:12702806; http://dx.doi.org/10.1126/science.1081315.
28. Cui S, Eisenacher K, Kirchhofer A, Brzozka K, Lammens A, Lammens K, et al. The C-terminal regulatory domain is the RNA 5'-triphosphate sensor of RIG-I. Mol Cell 2008; 29:169-79; PMID:18243112; http://dx.doi.org/10.1016/j.molcel.2007.10.032.
29. Takahasi K, Yoneyama M, Nishihori T, Hirai R, Kumeta H, Narita R, et al. Nonself RNA-sensing mechanism of RIG-I helicase and activation of antiviral immune responses. Mol Cell 2008; 29:428-40; PMID:18242112; http://dx.doi.org/10.1016/j.molcel.2007.11.028.
30. Wang Y, Ludwig J, Schuberth C, Goldeck M, Schlee M, Li H, et al. Structural and functional insights into 5'-ppp RNA pattern recognition by the innate immune receptor RIG-I. Nat Struct Mol Biol 2010; 17:781-7; PMID:20581823; http://dx.doi.org/10.1038/nsmb.1863.

31. Lu C, Xu H, Ranjith-Kumar CT, Brooks MT, Hou TY, Hu F, et al. The Structural Basis of 5' Triphosphate Double-Stranded RNA Recognition by RIG-I C-Terminal Domain. Structure 2010; 18:1032-43; PMID:20637642; http://dx.doi.org/10.1016/j.str.2010.05.007.

32. Satoh T, Kato H, Kumagai Y, Yoneyama M, Sato S, Matsushita K, et al. LGP2 is a positive regulator of RIG-I- and MDA5-mediated antiviral responses. Proc Natl Acad Sci USA 2010; 107:1512-7; PMID:20080593; http://dx.doi.org/10.1073/pnas.0912986107.

33. Pippig DA, Hellmuth JC, Cui S, Kirchhofer A, Lammens K, Lammens A, et al. The regulatory domain of the RIG-I family ATPase LGP2 senses double-stranded RNA. Nucleic Acids Res 2009; 37:2014-25; PMID:19208642; http://dx.doi.org/10.1093/nar/gkp059.

34. Li X, Ranjith-Kumar CT, Brooks MT, Dharmaiah S, Herr AB, Kao C, et al. The RIG-I-like receptor LGP2 recognizes the termini of double-stranded RNA. J Biol Chem 2009; 284:13881-91; PMID:19278996; http://dx.doi.org/10.1074/jbc.M900818200.

35. Murali A, Li X, Ranjith-Kumar CT, Bhardwaj K, Holzenburg A, Li P, et al. Structure and function of LGP2, a DEX(D/H) helicase that regulates the innate immunity response. J Biol Chem 2008; 283:15825-33; PMID:18411269; http://dx.doi.org/10.1074/jbc.M800542200.

36. Loo YM, Fornek J, Crochet N, Bajwa G, Perwitasari O, Martinez-Sobrido L, et al. Distinct RIG-I and MDA5 signaling by RNA viruses in innate immunity. J Virol 2008; 82:335-45; PMID:17942531; http://dx.doi.org/10.1128/JVI.01080-07.

37. Fredericksen BL, Keller BC, Fornek J, Katze MG, Gale M Jr. Establishment and maintenance of the innate antiviral response to West Nile Virus involves both RIG-I and MDA5 signaling through IPS-1. J Virol 2008; 82:609-16; PMID:17977974; http://dx.doi.org/10.1128/JVI.01305-07.

38. McCartney SA, Thackray LB, Gitlin L, Gilfillan S, Virgin HW, Colonna M. MDA-5 recognition of a murine norovirus. PLoS Pathog 2008; 4:e1000108; PMID:18636103; http://dx.doi.org/10.1371/journal.ppat.1000108.

39. Melchjorsen J, Rintahaka J, Soby S, Horan KA, Poltajainen A, Ostergaard L, et al. Early innate recognition of herpes simplex virus in human primary macrophages is mediated via the MDA5/MAVS-dependent and MDA5/MAVS/RNA polymerase III-independent pathways. J Virol 2010; 84:11350-8; PMID:20739519; http://dx.doi.org/10.1128/JVI.01106-10.

40. Roth-Cross JK, Bender SJ, Weiss SR. Murine coronavirus mouse hepatitis virus is recognized by MDA5 and induces type I interferon in brain macrophages/microglia. J Virol 2008; 82:9829-38; PMID:18667505; http://dx.doi.org/10.1128/JVI.01199-08.

41. Weber F, Wagner V, Rasmussen SB, Hartmann R, Paludan SR. Double-stranded RNA is produced by positive-strand RNA viruses and DNA viruses but not in detectable amounts by negative-strand RNA viruses. J Virol 2006; 80:5059-64; PMID:16641297; http://dx.doi.org/10.1128/JVI.80.10.5059-5064.2006.

42. Targett-Adams P, Boulant S, McLauchlan J. Visualization of double-stranded RNA in cells supporting hepatitis C virus RNA replication. J Virol 2008; 82:2182-95; PMID:18094154; http://dx.doi.org/10.1128/JVI.01565-07.

43. Poole E, He B, Lamb RA, Randall RE, Goodbourn S. The V proteins of simian virus 5 and other paramyxoviruses inhibit induction of interferon-beta. Virology 2002; 303:33-46; PMID:12482656; http://dx.doi.org/10.1006/viro.2002.1737.

44. Andrejeva J, Childs KS, Young DF, Carlos TS, Stock N, Goodbourn S, et al. The V proteins of paramyxoviruses bind the IFN-inducible RNA helicase, mda-5, and inhibit its activation of the IFN-beta promoter. Proc Natl Acad Sci USA 2004; 101:17264-9; PMID:15563593; http://dx.doi.org/10.1073/pnas.0407639101.

45. Luthra P, Sun D, Silverman RH, He B. Activation of IFN-β expression by a viral mRNA through RNase L and MDA5. Proc Natl Acad Sci USA 2011; 108:2118-23; PMID:21245317; http://dx.doi.org/10.1073/pnas.1012409108.

46. Kato H, Takeuchi O, Mikamo-Satoh E, Hirai R, Kawai T, Matsushita K, et al. Length-dependent recognition of double-stranded ribonucleic acids by retinoic acid-inducible gene-I and melanoma differentiation-associated gene 5. J Exp Med 2008; 205:1601-10; PMID:18591409; http://dx.doi.org/10.1084/jem.20080091.

47. Field AK, Tytell AA, Lampson GP, Hilleman MR. Inducers of interferon and host resistance. II. Multistranded synthetic polynucleotide complexes. Proc Natl Acad Sci USA 1967; 58:1004-10; PMID:5233831; http://dx.doi.org/10.1073/pnas.58.3.1004.

48. Li X, Lu C, Stewart M, Xu H, Strong RK, Igumenova T, et al. Structural basis of double-stranded RNA recognition by the RIG-I like receptor MDA5. Arch Biochem Biophys 2009; 488:23-33; PMID:19531363; http://dx.doi.org/10.1016/j.abb.2009.06.008.

49. Pichlmair A, Schulz O, Tan CP, Rehwinkel J, Kato H, Takeuchi O, Akira S, Way M, Schiavo G, Reis ESC. Activation of MDA5 requires higher order RNA structures generated during virus infection. J Virol 2009.

50. Züst R, Cervantes-Barragan L, Habjan M, Maier R, Neuman BW, Ziebuhr J, et al. Ribose 2'-O-methylation provides a molecular signature for the distinction of self and non-self mRNA dependent on the RNA sensor Mda5. Nat Immunol 2011; 12:137-43; PMID:21217758; http://dx.doi.org/10.1038/ni.1979.

51. Kim DH, Longo M, Han Y, Lundberg P, Cantin E, Rossi JJ. Interferon induction by siRNAs and ssRNAs synthesized by phage polymerase. Nat Biotechnol 2004; 22:321-5; PMID:14990954; http://dx.doi.org/10.1038/nbt940.

52. Banerjee AK. 5'-terminal cap structure in eucaryotic messenger ribonucleic acids. Microbiol Rev 1980; 44:175-205; PMID:6247631.

53. Cella M, Jarrossay D, Facchetti F, Alebardi O, Nakajima H, Lanzavecchia A, et al. Plasmacytoid monocytes migrate to inflamed lymph nodes and produce large amounts of type I interferon. Nat Med 1999; 5:919-23; PMID:10426316; http://dx.doi.org/10.1038/11360.

54. Siegal FP, Kadowaki N, Shodell M, Fitzgerald-Bocarsly PA, Shah K, Ho S, et al. The nature of the principal type 1 interferon-producing cells in human blood. Science 1999; 284:1835-7; PMID:10364556; http://dx.doi.org/10.1126/science.284.5421.1835.

55. Krug A, Rothenfusser S, Hornung V, Jahrsdorfer B, Blackwell S, Ballas ZK, et al. Identification of CpG oligonucleotide sequences with high induction of IFN-alpha/beta in plasmacytoid dendritic cells. Eur J Immunol 2001; 31:2154-63; PMID:11449369; http://dx.doi.org/10.1002/1521-4141(200107)31:7<2154::AID-IMMU2154>3.0.CO;2-U.

56. Pichlmair A, Schulz O, Tan CP, Naslund TI, Liljestrom P, Weber F, et al. RIG-I-mediated antiviral responses to single-stranded RNA bearing 5'-phosphates. Science 2006; 314:997-1001; PMID:17038589; http://dx.doi.org/10.1126/science.1132998.

57. Saito T, Owen DM, Jiang F, Marcotrigiano J, Gale M. Innate immunity induced by composition-dependent RIG-I recognition of hepatitis C virus RNA. Nature 2008.

58. Gondai T, Yamaguchi K, Miyano-Kurosaki N, Habu Y, Takaku H. Short-hairpin RNAs synthesized by T7 phage polymerase do not induce interferon. Nucleic Acids Res 2008; 36:e18; PMID:18208841; http://dx.doi.org/10.1093/nar/gkm1043.

59. Marques JT, Devosse T, Wang D, Zamanian-Daryoush M, Serbinowski P, Hartmann R, et al. A structural basis for discriminating between self and nonself double-stranded RNAs in mammalian cells. Nat Biotechnol 2006; 24:559-65; PMID:16648842; http://dx.doi.org/10.1038/nbt1205.

60. Schlee M, Roth A, Hornung V, Hagmann CA, Wimmenauer V, Barchet W, et al. Recognition of 5' triphosphate by RIG-I helicase requires short blunt double-stranded RNA as contained in panhandle of negative-strand virus. Immunity 2009; 31:25-34; PMID:19576794; http://dx.doi.org/10.1016/j.immuni.2009.05.008.

61. Ludwig J, Eckstein F. Rapid and Efficient Synthesis of Nucleoside 5'-0 - (1-Thiotriphosphates), 5'-Triphosphates and 2',3'-Cyclophosphorothioates Using 2-Chloro-4H- 1,3,2-benzodioxaphosphorin-4-one. J Org Chem 1989; 54:631-5; http://dx.doi.org/10.1021/jo00264a024.

62. Cazenave C, Uhlenbeck OC. RNA template-directed RNA synthesis by T7 RNA polymerase. Proc Natl Acad Sci USA 1994; 91:6972-6; PMID:7518923; http://dx.doi.org/10.1073/pnas.91.15.6972.

63. Triana-Alonso FJ, Dabrowski M, Wadzack J, Nierhaus KH. Self-coded 3'-extension of run-off transcripts produces aberrant products during in vitro transcription with T7 RNA polymerase. J Biol Chem 1995; 270:6298-307; PMID:7534310; http://dx.doi.org/10.1074/jbc.270.11.6298.

64. Schmidt A, Schwerd T, Hamm W, Hellmuth JC, Cui S, Wenzel M, et al. 5'-triphosphate RNA requires base-paired structures to activate antiviral signaling via RIG-I. Proc Natl Acad Sci USA 2009; 106:12067-72; PMID:19574455; http://dx.doi.org/10.1073/pnas.0900971106.

65. Marq JB, Kolakofsky D, Garcin D. Unpaired 5' ppp-nucleotides, as found in arenavirus double-stranded RNA panhandles, are not recognized by RIG-I. J Biol Chem 2010; 285:18208-16; PMID:20400512; http://dx.doi.org/10.1074/jbc.M109.089425.

66. Lu C, Ranjith-Kumar CT, Hao L, Kao CC, Li P. Crystal structure of RIG-I C-terminal domain bound to blunt-ended double-strand RNA without 5' triphosphate. Nucleic Acids Res 2011; 39:1565-75; PMID:20961956; http://dx.doi.org/10.1093/nar/gkq974.

67. Habjan M, Andersson I, Klingstrom J, Schumann M, Martin A, Zimmermann P, et al. Processing of genome 5' termini as a strategy of negative-strand RNA viruses to avoid RIG-I-dependent interferon induction. PLoS ONE 2008; 3:e2032; PMID:18446221; http://dx.doi.org/10.1371/journal.pone.0002032.

68. Takahashi H, Yamaji M, Hosaka M, Kishine H, Hijikata M, Shimotohno K. Analysis of the 5' end structure of HCV subgenomic RNA replicated in a Huh7 cell line. Intervirology 2005; 48:104-11; PMID:15812182; http://dx.doi.org/10.1159/000081736.

69. Marq JB, Hausmann S, Veillard N, Kolakofsky D, Garcin D. Short dsRNAs with an overhanging 5 prime ppp-nucleotide, as found in arenavirus genomes, act as RIG-I decoys. J Biol Chem 2010.

70. Grunberg-Manago M. Polynucleotide phosphorylase: structure and mechanism of action. Biochem J 1967; 103:62P; PMID:4292833.

71. Malathi K, Dong B, Gale M Jr., Silverman RH. Small self-RNA generated by RNase L amplifies antiviral innate immunity. Nature 2007; 448:816-9; PMID:17653195; http://dx.doi.org/10.1038/nature06042.

72. Malathi K, Saito T, Crochet N, Barton DJ, Gale M Jr., Silverman RH. RNase L releases a small RNA from HCV RNA that refolds into a potent PAMP. RNA 2010; 16:2108-19; PMID:20833746; http://dx.doi.org/10.1261/rna.2244210.

73. Ishii KJ, Coban C, Kato H, Takahashi K, Torii Y, Takeshita F, et al. A Toll-like receptor-independent antiviral response induced by double-stranded B-form DNA. Nat Immunol 2006; 7:40-8; PMID:16286919; http://dx.doi.org/10.1038/ni1282.

74. Stetson DB, Medzhitov R. Recognition of cytosolic DNA activates an IRF3-dependent innate immune response. Immunity 2006; 24:93-103; PMID:16413926; http://dx.doi.org/10.1016/j.immuni.2005.12.003.

75. Sun Q, Sun L, Liu HH, Chen X, Seth RB, Forman J, et al. The specific and essential role of MAVS in antiviral innate immune responses. Immunity 2006; 24:633-42; PMID:16713980; http://dx.doi.org/10.1016/j.immuni.2006.04.004.

76. Cheng G, Zhong J, Chung J, Chisari FV. Double-stranded DNA and double-stranded RNA induce a common antiviral signaling pathway in human cells. Proc Natl Acad Sci USA 2007; 104:9035-40; PMID:17517627; http://dx.doi.org/10.1073/pnas.0703285104.

77. Ablasser A, Bauernfeind F, Hartmann G, Latz E, Fitzgerald KA, Hornung V. RIG-I-dependent sensing of poly(dA:dT) through the induction of an RNA polymerase III-transcribed RNA intermediate. Nat Immunol 2009.

78. Chiu YH, Macmillan JB, Chen ZJ. RNA polymerase III detects cytosolic DNA and induces type I interferons through the RIG-I pathway. Cell 2009; 138:576-91; PMID:19631370; http://dx.doi.org/10.1016/j.cell.2009.06.015.

79. Bieger CD, Nierlich DP. Distribution of 5'-triphosphate termini on the mRNA of Escherichia coli. J Bacteriol 1989; 171:141-7; PMID:2464575.

80. Deana A, Celesnik H, Belasco JG. The bacterial enzyme RppH triggers messenger RNA degradation by 5' pyrophosphate removal. Nature 2008; 451:355-8; PMID:18202662; http://dx.doi.org/10.1038/nature06475.

81. Celesnik H, Deana A, Belasco JG. Initiation of RNA decay in Escherichia coli by 5' pyrophosphate removal. Mol Cell 2007; 27:79-90; PMID:17612492; http://dx.doi.org/10.1016/j.molcel.2007.05.038.

82. Emory SA, Bouvet P, Belasco JG. A 5'-terminal stem-loop structure can stabilize mRNA in Escherichia coli. Genes Dev 1992; 6:135-48; PMID:1370426; http://dx.doi.org/10.1101/gad.6.1.135.

83. Mackie GA. Stabilization of circular rpsT mRNA demonstrates the 5'-end dependence of RNase E action in vivo. J Biol Chem 2000; 275:25069-72; PMID:10871599; http://dx.doi.org/10.1074/jbc.C000363200.

84. Opitz B, Vinzing M, van Laak V, Schmeck B, Heine G, Gunther S, et al. Legionella pneumophila induces IFNbeta in lung epithelial cells via IPS-1 and IRF3, which also control bacterial replication. J Biol Chem 2006; 281:36173-9; PMID:16984921; http://dx.doi.org/10.1074/jbc.M604638200.

85. Monroe KM, McWhirter SM, Vance RE. Identification of host cytosolic sensors and bacterial factors regulating the type I interferon response to Legionella pneumophila. PLoS Pathog 2009; 5:e1000665; PMID:19936053; http://dx.doi.org/10.1371/journal.ppat.1000665.

86. Rad R, Ballhorn W, Voland P, Eisenacher K, Mages J, Rad L, et al. Extracellular and intracellular pattern recognition receptors cooperate in the recognition of Helicobacter pylori. Gastroenterology 2009; 136:2247-57; PMID:19272387; http://dx.doi.org/10.1053/j.gastro.2009.02.066.

87. Hruby DE, Roberts WK. Encephalomyocarditis virus RNA. III. Presence of a genome-associated protein. J Virol 1978; 25:413-5; PMID:202751.

88. Lee YF, Nomoto A, Detjen BM, Wimmer E. A protein covalently linked to poliovirus genome RNA. Proc Natl Acad Sci USA 1977; 74:59-63; PMID:189316; http://dx.doi.org/10.1073/pnas.74.1.59.

89. Rohayem J, Robel I, Jager K, Scheffler U, Rudolph W. Protein-primed and de novo initiation of RNA synthesis by norovirus 3Dpol. J Virol 2006; 80:7060-9; PMID:16809311; http://dx.doi.org/10.1128/JVI.02195-05.

90. Bonin M, Oberstrass J, Lukacs N, Ewert K, Oesterschulze E, Kassing R, et al. Determination of preferential binding sites for anti-dsRNA antibodies on double-stranded RNA by scanning force microscopy. RNA 2000; 6:563-70; PMID:10786847; http://dx.doi.org/10.1017/S1355838200992318.

91. Desselberger U, Racaniello VR, Zazra JJ, Palese P. The 3' and 5'-terminal sequences of influenza A, B and C virus RNA segments are highly conserved and show partial inverted complementarity. Gene 1980; 8:315-28; PMID:7358274; http://dx.doi.org/10.1016/0378-1119(80)90007-4.

92. Hsu MT, Parvin JD, Gupta S, Krystal M, Palese P. Genomic RNAs of influenza viruses are held in a circular conformation in virions and in infected cells by a terminal panhandle. Proc Natl Acad Sci USA 1987; 84:8140-4; PMID:2446318; http://dx.doi.org/10.1073/pnas.84.22.8140.

93. Portela A, Digard P. The influenza virus nucleoprotein: a multifunctional RNA-binding protein pivotal to virus replication. J Gen Virol 2002; 83:723-34; PMID:11907320.

94. Dauber B, Martinez-Sobrido L, Schneider J, Hai R, Waibler Z, Kalinke U, et al. Influenza B virus ribonucleoprotein is a potent activator of the antiviral kinase PKR. PLoS Pathog 2009; 5:e1000473; PMID:19521506; http://dx.doi.org/10.1371/journal.ppat.1000473.

95. Nallagatla SR, Hwang J, Toroney R, Zheng X, Cameron CE, Bevilacqua PC. 5'-triphosphate-dependent activation of PKR by RNAs with short stem-loops. Science 2007; 318:1455-8; PMID:18048689; http://dx.doi.org/10.1126/science.1147347.

96. Rehwinkel J, Tan CP, Goubau D, Schulz O, Pichlmair A, Bier K, et al. RIG-I Detects Viral Genomic RNA during Negative-Strand RNA Virus Infection. Cell 2010; 140:397-408; PMID:20144762; http://dx.doi.org/10.1016/j.cell.2010.01.020.
97. Hewlett MJ, Pettersson RF, Baltimore D. Circular forms of Uukuniemi virion RNA: an electron microscopic study. J Virol 1977; 21:1085-93; PMID:850304.
98. Raju R, Kolakofsky D. The ends of La Crosse virus genome and antigenome RNAs within nucleocapsids are base paired. J Virol 1989; 63:122-8; PMID:2908922.
99. Bhella D, Ralph A, Yeo RP. Conformational flexibility in recombinant measles virus nucleocapsids visualised by cryo-negative stain electron microscopy and real-space helical reconstruction. J Mol Biol 2004; 340:319-31; PMID:15201055; http://dx.doi.org/10.1016/j.jmb.2004.05.015.
100. Loney C, Mottet-Osman G, Roux L, Bhella D. Paramyxovirus ultrastructure and genome packaging: cryo-electron tomography of sendai virus. J Virol 2009; 83:8191-7; PMID:19493999; http://dx.doi.org/10.1128/JVI.00693-09.
101. Kolakofsky D. Isolation and characterization of Sendai virus DI-RNAs. Cell 1976; 8:547-55; PMID:182384; http://dx.doi.org/10.1016/0092-8674(76)90223-3.
102. Perrault J, Leavitt RW. Inverted complementary terminal sequences in single-stranded RNAs and snap-back RNAs from vesicular stomatitis defective interfering particles. J Gen Virol 1978; 38:35-50; PMID:202671; http://dx.doi.org/10.1099/0022-1317-38-1-35.
103. Lazzarini RA, Keene JD, Schubert M. The origins of defective interfering particles of the negative-strand RNA viruses. Cell 1981; 26:145-54; PMID:7037195; http://dx.doi.org/10.1016/0092-8674(81)90298-1.
104. Strahle L, Garcin D, Kolakofsky D. Sendai virus defective-interfering genomes and the activation of interferon-beta. Virology 2006; 351:101-11; PMID:16631220; http://dx.doi.org/10.1016/j.virol.2006.03.022.
105. Strähle L, Marq JB, Brini A, Hausmann S, Kolakofsky D, Garcin D. Activation of the beta interferon promoter by unnatural Sendai virus infection requires RIG-I and is inhibited by viral C proteins. J Virol 2007; 81:12227-37; PMID:17804509; http://dx.doi.org/10.1128/JVI.01300-07.
106. Baum A, Sachidanandam R, Garcia-Sastre A. Preference of RIG-I for short viral RNA molecules in infected cells revealed by next-generation sequencing. Proc Natl Acad Sci USA 2010; 107:16303-8; PMID:20805493; http://dx.doi.org/10.1073/pnas.1005077107.
107. Fechter P, Brownlee GG. Recognition of mRNA cap structures by viral and cellular proteins. J Gen Virol 2005; 86:1239-49; PMID:15831934; http://dx.doi.org/10.1099/vir.0.80755-0.
108. Pattnaik AK, Ball LA, LeGrone AW, Wertz GW. Infectious defective interfering particles of VSV from transcripts of a cDNA clone. Cell 1992; 69:1011-20; PMID:1318785; http://dx.doi.org/10.1016/0092-8674(92)90619-N.
109. Zhou H, Perlman S. Mouse hepatitis virus does not induce Beta interferon synthesis and does not inhibit its induction by double-stranded RNA. J Virol 2007; 81:568-74; PMID:17079305; http://dx.doi.org/10.1128/JVI.01512-06.
110. Li J, Liu Y, Zhang X. Murine coronavirus induces type I interferon in oligodendrocytes through recognition by RIG-I and MDA5. J Virol 2010; 84:6472-82; PMID:20427526; http://dx.doi.org/10.1128/JVI.00016-10.
111. Garcin D, Lezzi M, Dobbs M, Elliott RM, Schmaljohn C, Kang CY, et al. The 5' ends of Hantaan virus (Bunyaviridae) RNAs suggest a prime-and-realign mechanism for the initiation of RNA synthesis. J Virol 1995; 69:5754-62; PMID:7637020.
112. Kato H, Sato S, Yoneyama M, Yamamoto M, Uematsu S, Matsui K, et al. Cell type-specific involvement of RIG-I in antiviral response. Immunity 2005; 23:19-28; PMID:16039576; http://dx.doi.org/10.1016/j.immuni.2005.04.010.
113. Yoneyama M, Kikuchi M, Matsumoto K, Imaizumi T, Miyagishi M, Taira K, et al. Shared and unique functions of the DExD/H-box helicases RIG-I, MDA5, and LGP2 in antiviral innate immunity. J Immunol 2005; 175:2851-8; PMID:16116171.
114. Plumet S, Herschke F, Bourhis JM, Valentin H, Longhi S, Gerlier D. Cytosolic 5'-triphosphate ended viral leader transcript of measles virus as activator of the RIG I-mediated interferon response. PLoS ONE 2007; 2:e279; PMID:17356690; http://dx.doi.org/10.1371/journal.pone.0000279.
115. Cárdenas WB, Loo YM, Gale M Jr., Hartman AL, Kimberlin CR, Martinez-Sobrido L, et al. Ebola virus VP35 protein binds double-stranded RNA and inhibits alpha/beta interferon production induced by RIG-I signaling. J Virol 2006; 80:5168-78; PMID:16698997; http://dx.doi.org/10.1128/JVI.02199-05.
116. Samanta M, Iwakiri D, Takada K. Epstein-Barr virus-encoded small RNA induces IL-10 through RIG-I-mediated IRF-3 signaling. Oncogene 2008; 27:4150-60; PMID:18362887; http://dx.doi.org/10.1038/onc.2008.75.

CHAPTER 14

Antiviral Actions of Double-Stranded RNA

Saurabh Chattopadhyay, Michifumi Yamashita and Ganes C. Sen*

Abstract

The host responds to virus infection by triggering various antiviral defense mechanisms, many of which are initiated by double-stranded (ds) RNA, which is often produced in virus-infected cells. Surprisingly, similar responses are also triggered by cellular dsRNA produced by necrotic, or otherwise stressed, uninfected cells; in human and mouse, such responses have been genetically linked to protection against several diseases of non-viral etiology. Thus, dsRNA has a wide role in mediating host defense. DsRNA is recognized, in the cell, by a large family of dsRNA-binding proteins, some of which share similar structural motifs that mediate the binding. Functionally, some of these proteins are dsRNA-dependent enzymes while others are signaling receptors that trigger transcription of a cohort of cellular genes, many of which encode antiviral proteins.

Introduction

Cellular antiviral responses largely depend on the ability of the host cells to recognize viral components to induce innate and adaptive immune responses. DsRNA, often generated as a byproduct of viral replication, is a potent danger signal that the host cells can recognize to initiate the innate immune responses. A large number of cellular proteins specifically recognize dsRNA in a sequence-independent fashion, some of which share similar structural motifs that mediate the dsRNA-binding. Although the cellular and biochemical functions of many dsRNA-binding proteins are as yet unknown, this family of proteins appear to be of broad biological significance. Among the dsRNA-binding proteins of known functions, one family comprises of enzymes, such as dsRNA-dependent Protein Kinase (PKR), 2'-5' Oligoadenylate Synthetase (OAS) and Adenosine Deaminases Acting on RNA (ADAR), which mediate cellular antiviral responses.[1-3] Another family constitutes of pattern recognition receptors, e.g., the Toll Like Receptor 3 (TLR3) and RNA helicases such as, the retinoic acid-inducible gene I (RIG-I) like receptors (RLRs) and the DDX1 RNA helicases.[4] These receptors initiate cascades of signaling leading to the transcriptional induction of dsRNA-induced genes, many of which encode cytokines, such as interferon, and other antiviral proteins. However, all cellular effects of these signaling cascades are not mediated by induced proteins; as elaborated below, some effects do not require new gene expression. In this review, we discuss how dsRNA is recognized by specific proteins, the functional effects of these interactions and their physiological consequences, especially in the context of virus infection (Fig. 1).

*Department of Molecular Genetics, Lerner Research Institute, Cleveland Clinic, Cleveland, Ohio, USA.
Corresponding Author: Ganes C. Sen—Email: seng@ccf.org

Nucleic Acid Sensors and Antiviral Immunity, edited by Suryaprakash Sambhara and Takashi Fujita.
©2013 Landes Bioscience.

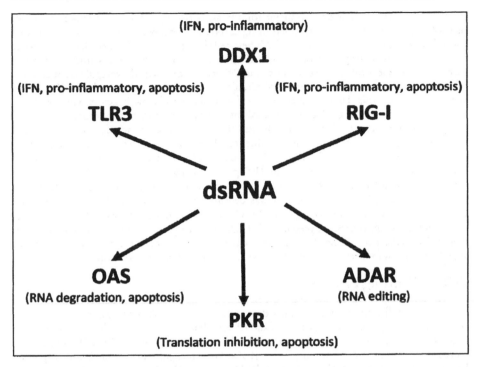

Figure 1. DsRNA-mediated antiviral effects. DsRNA, produced by virus infection is recognized by various dsRNA sensors to initiate the host defense processes. Some of the cellular dsRNA sensors and their mode of action are shown.

Sources of dsRNA

The most well characterized source of dsRNA in infected cells is viral dsRNA. For dsRNA viruses, the genome of infecting viruses can directly generate dsRNA inside the cells. The ssRNA viruses also generate dsRNA as replication intermediates. In addition, ssRNAs with extensive secondary structures such as hairpin loop formations are also effectively recognized by the receptors. The ssRNA virus populations, containing defective particles with ds defective genomes also serve as a source of dsRNA. For DNA viruses, complementary mRNAs are often produced; they are encoded by partially overlapping genes, located on the opposite strands of the viral genome. Recently, cytosolic RNA polymerase III has been shown to generate dsRNA from dsDNA, which are produced by DNA viruses and intracellular bacteria.[5] In addition to viral infections, extracellular RNA, generated by tissue damage or necrotic cells, has enough ds structures to serve as potential sources of dsRNA. Extracellular dsRNA is endocytosed and transported to endosomal lumen for presentation to dsRNA recognizing protein TLR3, whereas cytosolic dsRNA generated during viral replication is directly recognized by cytosolic RNA helicases such as RIG-I or MDA-5. A synthetic dsRNA, polyI.polyC, is often used as an experimental mimic to trigger host response to virus infection. An antibody raised against dsRNA has been successfully used to detect viral and other dsRNAs in cells and to identify the intracellular sites of accumulation of viral dsRNA.[6]

Genes Regulated by dsRNA

DsRNA, when added to, or transfected into cells, can rapidly trigger transcription of multiple genes, including interferons (IFN), or downregulate the expression of another set of genes. Many of the dsRNA-stimulated genes can also be induced by type I IFNs or virus infection. The common group of genes that is induced by viruses, IFN and dsRNA is called the viral stress-inducible genes (VSIG); their products play major roles in antiviral responses.[7] A systematic search of dsRNA-regulated genes was performed using cDNA microarray analyses of mRNA isolated form dsRNA-treated human glioma cells.[8] These cells lack the type I IFN gene locus and hence secondary regulation of gene expression by IFNs was also eliminated in this study. This study identified 175 genes, which were upregulated and 95 genes, which were downregulated by dsRNA. The dsRNA-stimulated genes include IFN-stimulated genes and genes involved in TNF-induced signaling and apoptosis. They also include genes for cytokines and growth factors, RNA synthesis, protein synthesis and degradation, metabolism and biosynthesis, transporters, cytoskeletal components and extracellular matrix. The dsRNA-repressed genes include genes involved in metabolism, cell cycle regulation, and cell adhesion. At least four families of transcription factors are activated by dsRNA: NF-κB, IRF-3, c-Jun and ATF2.[9] These factors can coordinately induce transcription of some genes, such as the IFN-β gene, or they can act individually to induce transcription of different sets of genes. A key difference between the requirements of induction of the same genes by dsRNA and Sendai virus was identified in HEK 293 cells.[10] Extracellular dsRNA cannot induce any genes unless exogenous TLR3 is expressed, but Sendai virus can induce genes equally well in the absence or the presence of TLR3. The two agents induce a set of common genes, in addition to the genes induced by one but not the other. These results strongly suggest that the signaling pathways activated by dsRNA and viruses are not completely overlapping.

dsRNA Binding Proteins

A large number of cellular and viral proteins have been identified for their ability to interact with dsRNA.[1] Gene disruption studies in mice demonstrate essential roles of several such mammalian proteins; for example, the absence of RIG-I and ADAR1 leads to embryonic lethality. A large family of these proteins, but not all, contains one or more dsRNA binding domains (DRBD), consisting of conserved 65–70 amino acid residues. The DRBDs do not recognize specific nucleotide sequences but interact primarily with the A-form of double-helical RNA. Biochemical evidence suggests that 11–16 bp of dsRNA can span a single DRBD. Three-dimensional models of DRBDs, from human PKR, Staufen (a Drosophila protein) and RNase III (a bacterial protein), show that the motif folds in a compact αβββα structure. Conserved hydrophobic residues in the α-helices pack along one side of the three-stranded anti-parallel β-sheet to maintain the overall structure, and the three RNA contact regions show high conservation of hydrophilic residues that support the DRBD-RNA interactions. Mutation of the most conserved residues within the consensus DRBD reduces or abolishes the binding of dsRNA.

Several other biologically important dsRNA-binding proteins do not contain the above DRBD motifs. Crystallographic and NMR-studies have been conducted to determine the structures of the dsRNA-binding regions of some of them, including TLR3, RIG-I and OAS1, key proteins involved in cellular antiviral functions. The crystal structure of TLR3 ectodomain (ECD) bound to dsRNA has been reported.[11] TLR3 ECD forms a horseshoe structure and is composed of 23 Leucine Rich Repeats (LRR). The dsRNA interacts with both N- and C-terminal on the lateral side of the concave surface of TLR3. The N-terminal interaction site is composed of LRR1–3 modules and the C-terminal site is composed of LRR19–21 modules. The positively charged residues of the termini of TLR3 make the major contributions to the interaction with sugar-phosphate backbones of the dsRNA ligand. Only a minor TLR3-TLR3 interaction is located near the C-terminus demonstrating that the ligand-protein interaction is the main driving force for TLR3 homodimerization. The ligand interaction sites are separated by a distance which accounts for a minimum length of 40–50 bp to stabilize the binding of dsRNA to TLR3. Similarly, the dsRNA binding to RIG-I has also been studied by structural analyses. Limited protease digestion of RIG-I-RNA complex has identified that a C-terminal domain (CTD) consisting of 792–925 amino acids (17 kDa) is sufficient for binding of dsRNA. The atomic structure of the CTD has been identified in solution and in crystal and essentially revealed a similar structure with respect to its dsRNA binding.[12,13] One side of the CTD exhibits a large cleft with positive surface charges, and the opposite side contains acidic patches. The structural studies suggest that the basic cleft is responsible for RNA recognition (both dsRNA and 5' ppp RNA). Consistent with the structural studies, mutagenesis of the basic cleft specifically reduced both RNA binding and signaling capacity of RIG-I. We have previously identified the RNA binding region of OAS1 protein using a combination of crystallographic and mutagenesis approaches.[14] Although, OAS1 does not have a well-defined dsRNA binding motif, the crystal structure revealed a positively charged groove at the interface of the N- and C-terminal domains.[14] Alignment analysis suggests that this groove is responsible for binding to dsRNA helix. Mutations of solvent-exposed positively charged residues, within the groove, result in a reduction or loss of RNA binding. The structural analysis also helps explain the two-step activation of OAS1, first by binding to dsRNA and second by a conformational change leading to the assembly of the active site.

Functions of Specific dsRNA-Binding Proteins

Toll-Like Receptor 3

Toll-like receptors (TLRs) are transmembrane signaling proteins that are expressed by cells of the innate immune system. They are designed to recognize, with high specificity, various proteins, lipids, carbohydrates and nucleic acids of invading microorganisms and activate signaling cascades in the cells that can trigger immune and inflammatory responses to combat the infectious agent.[15,16] In mammals, 11 members of this family have been identified so far. Although every member responds to a specific ligand, they all share strong similarities in their structures and properties. These proteins are located on either plasma membrane or internal membranes. Their cytoplasmic signaling domains are separated from the ligand-recognizing extracellular or luminal domains by a single membrane-spanning domain. The extracellular domain contains multiple repeats of a leucine-rich repeat (LRR), XXLXLXX. The 19–25 tandem copies of LRR are thought to provide the highly specific binding surface for the cognate ligand. The cytoplasmic domains of all TLRs and members of the IL-1 receptors family share a domain, called Toll/IL-1 receptor (TIR) domain, which extends to about 200 residues. The TIR domains serve as platforms for assembling multiple protein kinases and adaptor proteins that initiate the intracellular signaling process. Many of the adaptors proteins also contain TIR domains. The signaling proteins for different TLRs include the adaptor protein MyD88, the IL-1R-associated protein kinases (IRAKs), the TGF-β-activated kinase (TAK1), the TAK1 binding proteins TAB1 and TAB2, the TNF receptor associated factor 6 (TRAF6), the proteins Tollip and Pellino, the TIR-domain containing proteins TIRAP/MAL and TRIF/TICAM1.[4,17]

Among the mammalian TLRs, four are designed to recognize nucleic acids. TLR3 recognizes dsRNA, a by-product of replication of some viruses, whereas mouse TLR7 or human TLR8 recognizes viral single-stranded RNAs.[17,18] TLR9, on the other hand, recognizes DNA containing unmethylated CpG motifs common to both bacterial and viral genomes.[17] All of the nucleic acid-recognizing TLRs are expressed on endosomal membranes, rather than the plasma membrane, of cells; hence ligand-binding by the LRR motifs of these TLRs occurs in the lumen of the intracellular vesicles. Extracellular nucleic acids released from damaged tissues or cells, infected or uninfected, are endocytosed and presented to the internal TLRs.[19] Alternatively, nucleic acids from bacteria or viruses, multiplying within a cell, can be captured in membranous vesicles and brought to the TLRs in the endosomes. Activation of these TLRs leads to the induction of type I interferon (IFN) genes, among others.[9] IFN-α induction by TLR7, TLR8 and TLR9 requires the MyD88-dependent pathway, the transcription factor IRF-7 and the signaling proteins TRAF6 and IRAK4.[17] In contrast, as discussed in detail below, the MyD88-independent pathway activated by TLR3 uses the adaptor protein TRIF and the transcription factor IRF-3 to induce the type I IFN genes and other antiviral genes (Fig. 2).[20]

TLR3 consists of a large ectodomain, which is accessible in the endosomal lumen, a transmembrane domain and a cytoplasmic domain. TLR3 ectodomain contains 23 LRRs, which are 24-residue motifs with characteristically spaced hydrophobic residues. The majority of the LRRs present in TLR3 conform to the major consensus sequence, but LRRs 12, 14, 18 and 20

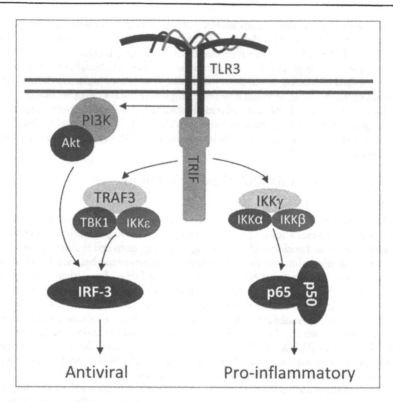

Figure 2. TLR3 mediated dsRNA signaling. DsRNA, recognized by endosomal TLR3 engages two distinct downstream signaling pathways using the adaptor protein TRIF, leading to transcriptional activation of IRF-3 and NF-κB to induce the expression of antiviral and pro-inflammatory genes.

belong to a variant class carrying insertions after residue 15. The ectodomain of TLR3 has recently been shown to be secreted into the medium and the secretion requires Unc93b1, an integral, endoplasmic reticulum-associated protein that also regulates TLR7 and TLR9 localization.[21] The cytoplasmic region of TLR3 (residues 726–904) consists of two functional domains: the Linker Region (LR) (726–753) and Toll/Interleukin-1 Receptor (TIR) domain (754–896). The LR regulates TLR3's subcellular localization. The TIR domain serves as a platform for the assembly of multiple protein kinases and adaptor proteins. TLR3 uses the adaptor protein TRIF, a TIR domain-containing protein, and specific TRAFs to enable the assembly of downstream signaling kinases that activates specific transcription factors.[20] When endosomal TLR3 is activated by dsRNA, TRIF transiently colocalizes with TLR3 and then dissociates from the receptor and forms speckled structures that colocalize with downstream signaling molecules.[22] TRIF consists of a proline-rich N-terminal region, a TIR domain, and a C-terminal region. The TIR domain of TRIF is essential for binding to the TIR domain of TLR3. The N-terminal region is crucial for TRIF-mediated IRF-3 activation via recruitment of IRF-3-activating kinases, TANK-binding kinase 1 (TBK1) and inhibitor of nuclear factor κB kinase ε (IKKε, also called IKKi).[23] The C-terminal region is involved in NF-κB activation by binding to the receptor interacting protein (RIP) 1 with the RIP homotypic-interacting motif (RHIM) domain.[24] Homo-oligomerization of TRIF, in which both the TIR and the C-terminal domain of TRIF are involved, has been shown to be critical for TRIF-mediated activation of NF-κB and IRF-3;[25] A splice variant of TRIF, TRIS, which lacks the TIR domain, can trigger some TLR3 signaling: knockdown of TRIS inhibits

TLR3 signaling, while overexpression of TRIS activates TLR3 signaling.[26] The cytoplasmic domain of TLR3 contains five tyrosine residues: Tyr733 in LR and Tyr756, Tyr759, Tyr764, and Tyr858 in TIR. Two of these five tyrosine residues, Tyr759 and Tyr733 or Tyr858, and their phosphorylation are essential for TLR3-mediated IRF-3 and NF-κB activation.[27,28] Moreover, TLR3 interacts with and activates PI3 kinase (PI3K), which is essential for the transcriptional activity of IRF-3.[27] TLR3 also associates with the proto-oncoprotein, c-Src, on endosomes and Src activity is required for the transcriptional activation of IRF-3 and NF-κB.[29] Microarray expression analyses revealed that TLR3 activation leads to induced expression of many cellular genes including many IFN-stimulated genes.[8]

Cellular Functions of TLR3

By inducing many antiviral proteins in a virus infected cell, TLR3 directly inhibits virus replication. In addition, TLR3 activation has major effects on other cellular properties, such as apoptosis and migration. In melanoma cells, TLR3-signaling induces apoptosis via TRIF-dependent activation of caspase-8; this process is controlled by inhibitors of apoptotic proteins (IAPs).[30] In human breast cancer cells, TLR3-induced apoptosis involves TRIF, and type I IFN autocrine signaling.[31] IFN-α sensitizes human umbilical vein endothelial cells (HUVECs) to apoptosis by dsRNA.[32] In HUVECs, TLR3-mediated apoptosis is triggered by the activation of both caspases-8 and caspase-9, indicating the involvement of both extrinsic and intrinsic apoptotic pathways. DsRNA upregulates TRAIL and its receptors, death receptors 4/5 (DR4/5), resulting in initiation of the extrinsic pathway; dsRNA downregulates the anti-apoptotic protein, Bcl-2, and upregulates Noxa, a pro-apoptotic protein, leading to activation of the intrinsic apoptotic pathway.[33] DsRNA can induce caspase-8-independent cellular apoptosis in a mouse model of cone-rod dystrophy, an inherited ocular disorder.[34]

Multiple roles of TLR3 signaling on cell migration have been reported. TLR3 signaling enhances skin wound closure and the recruitment of neutrophils and macrophages through chemokines, MIP-2/CXCL2, MIP-1α/CCL3, and MCP-1/CCL2.[35] On the other hand, a randomized clinical trial showed that the treatment with dsRNA reduces the risk of metastatic relapse, suggesting the suppression of cell migration, in TLR3-positive but not in TLR3-negative breast cancers; this effect is dependent on TLR3 and independent of type I IFN.[36] We have uncovered a new branch of TLR3 signaling which regulates cell migration through activation of Src; the effect is biphasic and independent of TRIF-mediated downstream signaling (unpublished data).

Role in Viral and Non-Viral Pathogenesis

In addition to cell-intrinsic antiviral role, TLR3 plays major roles in both innate and adaptive antiviral immune responses; dsRNA induces the maturation of DCs, boosting their ability to produce IFN and prime and expand antigen-specific T-cell responses.[37] It also promotes cross-priming of the cytotoxic T-cell response against viral infection.[38] Immunization with virus-infected cells or cells containing synthetic dsRNA leads to a striking increase in cytotoxic T-cell cross-priming against cell-associated antigens. Traditionally TLR3 has been viewed as the critical sensor of virus infection and the initiator of resultant innate immune response. TLR3 is expressed in the central nervous system (CNS) and plays important roles to control herpes simplex virus 1, which spreads from the epithelium to the CNS via cranial nerves.[39] In a subset of patients with HSV-1 encephalitis, a dominant-negative allele of TLR3 is expressed.[39] However, the role of TLR3 in mediating host response to virus infection is complex. TLR3 has been shown to be dispensable for viral pathogenesis and adaptive antiviral responses after LCMV, VSV, MCMV or reovirus infection. Although in many case TLR3 contributes to the host defense, it may also contribute to pathogenesis. TLR3-deficient mice have been shown to be more resistant to lethal infection and have a reduced incidence of liver disease associated with hepatotropic Punta Toro virus infection compared with Wt mice.[40] A recombinant-strain Western Reserve Vaccinia virus has been reported to be more deleterious to the Wt mice than TLR3−/− mice.[41] West Nile virus causes encephalitis and surprisingly TLR3−/− mice are more resistant to lethal infection by this virus than Wt mice.[42] Although in the absence of TLR3, virally induced cytokine production is impaired and peripheral viral load is higher, in the brains of TLR3–/– mice viral load, inflammation and neuropathology are reduced. The observed difference between Wt and TLR3–/– mice disappeared when the virus was administered not peripherally but intra-cranially. These results demonstrate that TLR3-dependent inflammatory response to West Nile virus infection is needed for efficient viral entry to the brain and consequent neuronal injury.

In addition to TLR3's role in antiviral host defense, TLR3 has also been shown to be important in the pathogenesis of several non-viral diseases. Activation of TLR3 protects against dextran sulfate sodium (DSS)-induced colitis. DSS-colitis is an acute model of inflammatory bowel diseases (IBD), primarily ulcerative colitis and Crohn's disease. IBD is characterized by cytokine imbalance and the production of inflammatory mediators, especially TNFα, have been linked to the pathology associated with experimental colitis and IBD in humans.[43] Subcutaneous injection of dsRNA to Wt mice has been shown to have a protective role against DSS-colitis; the effect is dependent on TLR3.[44]

TLR3 Leu412Phe variant has a protective role against age-related macular degeneration in human patients, probably by suppressing the death of retinal pigment epithelial (RPE) cells.[45] Age-related macular degeneration is the most common cause of irreversible visual impairment in the developing world. DsRNA induces cell death in primary human RPE cells or mouse RPE cells that are homozygous for the 412Leu (TLR3$^{412Leu/412Leu}$). In contrast, dsRNA did not reduce the viability of human RPE cells that are heterozygous for the TLR3 412 (TLR3$^{412Leu/412Phe}$) and TLR3–/– mouse RPE cells.[45]

The role of TLR3 signaling in suppression of angiogenesis has been shown in a clinical study as well as in an animal experiment.[46] Choroidal neovascularization (CNV), wherein the retina is invaded by choroidal vessels beneath the retinal epithelium, is an advanced stage of age-related macular degeneration that afflicts 30–50 million people globally. Originally, successful trials of small interfering RNA (siRNA) targeting vascular endothelial growth factor-A (VEGF-A) or its receptor VEGFR1 (also called FLT1) have been reported in animal experiments and in clinical trials.[47,48] However, as shown recently, the anti-angiogenic effect of the siRNA is TLR3-mediated, but not sequence dependent.[46] Subsequent genetic experiments using IRF3–/– or NFκB1–/– mice revealed that the observed anti-angiogenic effect is independent of IRF-3, but dependent on NF-κB.

A pathogenic role of TLR3, which is expressed in vascular endothelial cells, has been observed. Intravenous injection of poly(I:C) to ApoE–/– mice, a murine model of atherosclerosis, enhanced atherosclerosis, while there was no effect in TLR3–/–, ApoE–/– mice.[49]

TLR3 has been shown to have a protective role in type I diabetes mellitus. Type I diabetes is an autoimmune disease that is primarily caused by selective destruction of islet β cells secreting insulin.[50] Clinical and experimental studies have suggested that viral infections contribute to type I diabetes, particularly infections by members of the enterovirus family of RNA viruses.[51,52] Encephalomyocarditis virus strain D (EMCV-D) has preferential tropism for pancreatic β cells and can induce diabetes in some mouse strains, such as DBA/2.[53] C57Bl/6 mice are normally resistant to EMCV-D-induced diabetes. EMCV-D infection, however, caused diabetes in TLR3–/– C57Bl/6 mice due to β cell damage induced directly by virus rather than T-cell-mediated autoimmunity.[54] TLR3 in hematopoietic cells is essential to limit β cell infection. The chimeric mice containing TLR3–/– hematopoietic cells and WT stroma cells were sensitive to EMCV-D-induced diabetes, while the mice having WT hematopoietic cells and TLR3–/– stroma cells were resistant. Upon virus infection, TLR3-mediated type I IFN production from hematopoietic cells protects β cell infection and/or β cell death by infection.

RIG-I Like Receptors (RLRs)

Cytosolic dsRNA generated by replication of viruses can be recognized by cytoplasmic RNA helicases, RIG-I, MDA5 or LGP2.[4,55] RIG-I and MDA5 consist of two N-terminal caspase-recruitment domains (CARD), RNA helicase domain and C-terminal repressor domain (RD), whereas LGP2 lacks the CARD domain. The helicase domain and RD are responsible for the recognition of RNA, whereas the CARD domains are important for downstream signaling.

RLRs recognize viral dsRNA and RNA with 5'-triphosphate ends in the virus-infected cells. Cellular RNA normally does not contain dsRNA structures and their 5'-ends are typically capped and, therefore, escapes the recognition by the RLRs. LGP2, which lacks the CARD domains, was initially thought to be a repressor of the cytosolic RNA signaling; however, recent studies suggest that LGP2 may also act as a positive inducer of Type-I IFN. RIG-I and MDA-5 display selectivity regarding recognition of RNA viruses based on their ability to detect dsRNA. RIG-I plays an important role in recognizing paramyxoviruses, orthomyxoviruses and rhabdoviruses, whereas MDA-5 is responsible for recognition of the picornaviruses and reoviruses. Some viruses, such as West Nile virus (WNV) and dengue virus are recognized by both RIG-I and MDA-5. The specificity of viral recognition by RIG-I and MDA-5 is thought to be mediated at the RNA structural level. Although it has been shown that RIG-I preferentially recognizes short dsRNA while MDA-5 recognizes long dsRNA, additional RNA recognition patterns have been identified.[56] DNA viruses and bacteria can also be sensed by RIG-I after their DNA is transcribed into uncapped RNA by cytosolic RNA polymerase III.[5]

Both RIG-I and MDA-5 induce antiviral responses through the adaptor protein IPS-1 in a CARD-CARD-dependent manner. IPS-1 is expressed on the mitochondrial outer membrane and interaction with RIG-I and MDA-5 facilitates its dimerization.[57] IPS-1 subsequently recruits two IκB-related kinases, TBK1 and IKKε via TRAF3. These kinases phosphorylate IRF-3 and IRF-7, resulting in their translocation from cytoplasm to nucleus, which activates transcription of antiviral genes including interferons. In addition, IPS-1 activates NF-κB via FADD and caspase-8/10 dependent pathway to regulate the expression of pro-inflammatory genes. Although, the RLRs play a prominent role in triggering innate defenses in epithelial cells, myeloid cells and cells of central nervous system, their actions are not essential for induction of interferons in plasmacytoid dendritic cells, which specifically activate the TLR-dependent responses.[55]

RLR-Induced Apoptosis: The IRF-3/BAX Axis

In addition to the activation of transcriptional pathways (by inducing antiviral and pro-inflammatory genes), viral dsRNA recognized by RIG-I or MDA-5 efficiently triggers cellular apoptosis by different mechanisms. Apoptosis is premature cell death, by which the infected cells are eliminated from the host. Induction of apoptosis is therefore considered as a host defense mechanism against virus infection. Although the pro-apoptotic genes induced by RIG-I/MDA-5-dependent signaling processes are known to cause cellular apoptosis, our studies have identified a direct pro-apoptotic function of IRF-3 triggered by dsRNA-stimulated RIG-I signaling. The RIG-I/IRF-3 mediated apoptotic pathway contributes significantly to the host antiviral responses. Paramyxoviruses trigger efficient apoptosis in various cell types. We have demonstrated that Paramyxovirus-induced apoptosis requires the activation of RIG-I; this effect is independent of IFN and NF-κB signaling pathways, but IRF-3 plays an essential role.[58] IRF-3, activated by RIG-I signaling, exhibits its pro-apoptotic activity by a distinct mechanism that is independent of its role as a transcription factor.[59,60] IRF-3 mutants lacking transcriptional activity are capable of inducing apoptosis, demonstrating the existence of a distinct mechanism by which IRF-3 exhibits its apoptotic effect. Although RIG-I signaling is critical, the apoptotic pathway requires additional proteins, TRAF2 and TRAF6; they are specific for the IRF-3 mediated apoptotic, but not the transcriptional, signaling pathway (Fig. 3). The activated IRF-3 executes its direct apoptotic effect by interacting with a pro-apoptotic protein, Bax and translocating to the mitochondria. The interaction of IRF-3 and Bax followed by their translocation to the mitochondria triggers the intrinsic apoptotic pathway to release cytochrome C into the cytosol and subsequently activates caspase-9. Activation of Bax is achieved by its direct interaction with IRF-3, by a previously unrecognized BH3-like domain of IRF-3. Mutation of the BH3-like domain of IRF-3 leads to impaired Bax-interaction and loss of apoptosis. It is not clear at this stage how RIG-I signaling enables the interaction of IRF-3 with Bax; but it is possible that the 'activation' of IRF-3 in the apoptotic pathway is achieved by conformational

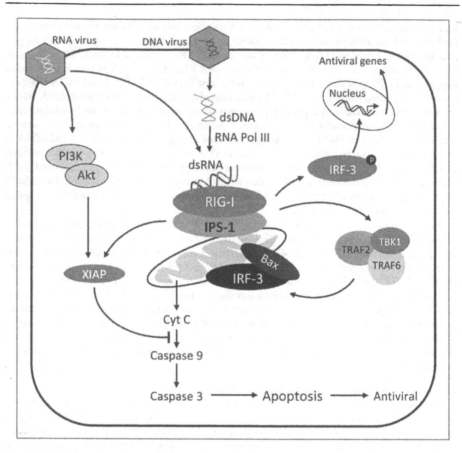

Figure 3. RIG-I mediated antiviral pathways. Cytosolic dsRNA produced by viral replication is recognized by RIG-I and triggers IRF-3 dependent signaling cascades leading to either antiviral gene induction or cellular apoptosis. The apoptotic pathway is temporally regulated by a PI3K/Akt/XIAP dependent mechanism.

changes that expose its BH3-domain. As expected, Bax deficiency prevents IRF-3-dependent apoptosis. Our subsequent study indicates that cytosolic dsDNA, generated by DNA-virus infection, also activates the mitochondrial apoptotic pathway mediated by RIG-I/IRF-3/Bax via an intermediate RNA Polymerase III-dependent step.[61] Therefore, RIG-I signaling, activated by both RNA and DNA viruses, plays a central role in triggering an IRF-3-dependent but transcription-independent cellular apoptosis. The IRF-3-induced apoptotic effect is temporally inhibited by PI3K/Akt-dependent stabilization of XIAP, a cellular inhibitor of apoptosis. Blocking the activity of PI3K accelerates the viral apoptosis, due to rapid degradation of XIAP.[62] IRF-3-dependent apoptosis contributes significantly to the innate immune responses against viral infection. The replication of a broad range of RNA and DNA viruses is enhanced in the absence of IRF-3-dependent apoptotic pathway. Absence of apoptosis, in cells deficient in IRF-3 or RIG-I leads to viral persistence caused by SeV; the persistently infected cells continuously produce progeny virus.[58] Viral replication is significantly enhanced in Bax−/− cells, due to deficiency in IRF-3-mediated apoptotic pathway. The IRF-3/Bax mediated apoptotic pathway also plays a protective role against viral pathogenesis; Bax−/− mice show greater morbidity and enhanced viral load upon challenge by EMCV, as compared with the Wt mice. The IRF-3/Bax apoptotic axis, activated by RIG-I signaling provides a defense mechanism by which the virus-infected cells are killed and the gene-induction independent apoptotic branch contributes considerably to the inhibition of viral replication and pathogenesis.[61]

Additional Mechanisms of RIG-I-Induced Cell Death

In addition to the IRF-3-dependent apoptotic response, RIG-I/IPS-1 complex can also trigger cell death by a variety of other mechanisms in a cell-type dependent manner. Distinct mechanisms of apoptotic induction have been reported for RIG-I signaling in melanoma cells, pancreatic β cells and macrophages. Although these effects are independent of IFN signaling, the induced pro-apoptotic proteins play major roles. In human melanoma cells, a pro-apoptotic signaling activated by RIG-I/IPS-1 is mediated by induced Puma; however, this effect is independent of IRF-3 and IFN.[63] Noxa, a BH3-domain containing pro-apoptotic protein, transcriptionally induced by IRF-1 and IRF-3, is involved in ssRNA virus-induced apoptosis.[64] RIG-I signaling also triggers efficient apoptosis in pancreatic β cells and macrophages by an IFN-independent mechanism.[65-67] In macrophages, RIG-I-induced apoptosis is dependent on cathepsin. Although the role of RIG-I is not clear, a signaling complex comprising of FADD/TRADD/caspase-8 mediates a dsRNA-induced apoptotic effect in HeLa cells.[68] RIG-I signaling pathway can also be activated by unrelated inducers such as, retinoic acid, which triggers efficient apoptosis in human melanoma cells.[69] DsRNA-induced apoptosis by RIG-I in uninfected cells, such as human melanoma cells, is being considered as a therapeutic potential against cancer.

Other Antiviral Functions of RLRs

The cellular antiviral response is a complex process involving multiple functions; cytosolic RLRs exhibit their cellular and antiviral functions by additional unexpected mechanisms. RIG-I signaling, in addition to activating the apoptotic caspases, can activate caspase-12 in WNV pathogenesis.[70] RIG-I activated caspase-12 is required for protection against WNV; caspase-12 deficient mice show greater morbidity after challenge with WNV, due to increased viral load. Viral infection often triggers pro-inflammatory responses; cytosolic dsRNA activates the pro-inflammatory caspase, caspase-1, for production of pro-inflammatory cytokine IL-1β.[67] A unique role of RIG-I has recently been demonstrated for the activation of the inflammasome. RIG-I, activated by cytosolic RNA can engage two signaling complexes, one involving IPS-1/CARD9/Bcl-10 to activate NF-κB responses and the second complex containing RIG-I/ASC/caspase-1 for the activation of inflammasome.[71] MDA-5, in addition to its pro-apoptotic role, is involved in the formation of autophagosome upon cytosolic dsRNA signaling in melanoma cells, although the mechanism behind this function remains unclear.[72]

DDX1 RNA Helicase

Although, TLR3 and RLRs play major roles in triggering antiviral responses, there are additional receptors with similar actions. A recent study demonstrated that DDX1 acts as a cytoplasmic dsRNA sensor in myeloid dendritic cells (mDCs).[73] DDX1 possesses an RNA helicase domain which recognizes cytosolic dsRNA to activate type I IFN and pro-inflammatory responses. Surprisingly, DDX1-mediated downstream signaling is not dependent on mitochondrial adaptor IPS-1. DDX1 forms a complex with two additional RNA helicases, DDX21 and DHX36, which interact with TRIF for activation of IRF-3 and NF-κB pathways. TRIF was originally thought to be a TLR3-specific adaptor protein and identification of DDX1-DDX21-DHX36-TRIF signaling pathway further broadens the antiviral function of TRIF in dendritic cells. Unlike RIG-I and MDA-5, DDX1 does not show any selectivity toward the length of poly(I:C) and is not upregulated by IFN signaling. The existence of DDX1-mediated type I IFN induction pathway is thought to be the first line of defense against viral infection in mDCs, which then can upregulate the expression of RIG-I and MDA-5 to further amplify the host antiviral responses. Redundancy of signaling pathways is a common feature in the innate immune responses and the existence of multiple dsRNA sensors provides multiple layers of regulation against viral antagonism.

dsRNA Dependent Protein Kinase (PKR)

PKR was discovered as an inhibitor of protein synthesis while studying cell-free translation systems made from IFN- and dsRNA-treated cells.[74] It belongs to a family of protein kinases which phosphorylate the α-subunit of eukaryotic initiation factor 2 (eIF-2). It is a serine/threonine kinase, with two distinct kinase activities: autophosphorylation, which is an activation step and the phosphorylation of eIF-2α, which impairs eIF-2 activity, resulting in inhibition of protein synthesis within the infected cells. In addition to eIF-2α, additional substrates of PKR have been identified to suggest broader roles of PKR phosphorylation in cellular antiviral functions. PKR phosphorylates and inhibits the function of RNA helicase A, a dsRNA binding protein, which is required for the replication of HIV-1.[75] A recent study further revealed that PKR phosphorylates two other dsRNA binding proteins NFAR (nuclear factor associated with dsRNA) 1 and NFAR2, causing their retention in the cytosol and association with viral transcripts, thereby inhibiting viral replication.[76] In addition to its translational regulatory function, PKR has roles in induction of cellular apoptosis and NF-κB signaling pathway.

PKR is expressed in all tissues at a basal level and is upregulated by type I and type III IFN. Under normal conditions, PKR is maintained as an inactive monomer, through steric hindrance of the kinase domain by its N-terminal dsRNA binding domain (Fig. 4). The N-terminal dsRNA binding domain of PKR has two dsRNA binding motifs of 70 amino acids each, dsRBM1 and dsRBM2, which are connected by a short 20 amino acid-linker. After binding to dsRNA, PKR undergoes a number of conformational changes to relieve the autoinhibitory interactions and allow substrate recognition. The conformational change results in homodimerization of PKR, which allows for autophosphorylation at Thr[446] and Thr[551] in the kinase domain. The autophosphorylation further stabilizes PKR dimers, which in turn increases the catalytic activity of the kinase. While viral dsRNA is the activator of PKR in virus-infected cells, a physiological activator of PKR, PACT, has been identified in uninfected cells.[77] PACT can directly bind to PKR and activate it, independent of dsRNA. PACT, like PKR, is a dsRNA binding protein, contains N-terminal dsRNA binding motifs and C-terminal PKR activation domain (also known as domain 3). Phosphorylation of PACT on specific Ser residues in domain 3 is required for activation of PKR.[78] The phosphorylation of PACT can be induced in response to a wide range of stress stimuli, indicating PACT as a mediator which links the cellular stress to PKR. PACT, which was discovered for activating PKR, has now been shown to have broader roles in host antiviral responses. A PKR-independent antiviral action of PACT has been identified, where it directly interacts with RIG-I and enhances the cellular antiviral effect by triggering IFN-β induction.[79]

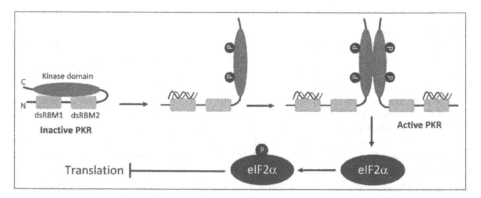

Figure 4. Activation of PKR by dsRNA. PKR exists in a closed inactive conformation; binding of dsRNA facilitates its dimerization and autophosphorylation on Thr-446 and Thr-451. Autophosphorylation activates PKR, allowing it to phosphorylate eIF2α, thereby inhibiting protein translation.

PKR has been implicated in the induction of cellular apoptosis in the absence or the presence of virus infection. A variety of viruses including vaccinia virus, influenza virus, and EMCV, induce PKR-dependent apoptosis in infected cells.[80] The role of PKR in apoptosis was reinforced by studies using PKR deficient MEFs or cells expressing a noncatalytic mutant of PKR. In the absence of virus infection, PKR-dependent apoptotic induction has been shown in response to dsRNA, inflammatory and stress stimuli; PKR deficient MEFs are more resistant than Wt MEFs to apoptosis induced by them. There are multiple mechanisms of PKR-induced apoptosis: studies suggest the role of eIF-2α as well as NF-κB-signaling in mediating PKR-induced apoptosis. PKR-induced apoptosis involves mainly the FADD/caspase-8 pathway, with lesser contribution from Apaf-1/caspase-9 pathway.[81] Although the major role of PKR has been studied in the context of induction of apoptosis and translation inhibition, a number of studies have proposed the involvement of PKR in cellular signal transduction by dsRNA. PKR deficient MEFs showed impaired NF-κB activity by dsRNA signaling, suggesting a function of PKR in activating NF-κB pathway. Subsequent analyses suggest PKR activates NF-κB signaling by interacting with IKK; however, the catalytic activity of PKR is not clear. PKR also regulates the activation of p53; PKR deficient cells show impaired function of p53. A subsequent study suggests that PKR interacts with and phosphorylates p53 on Ser^{392}.[82] Recent studies further indicate the involvement of PKR in activation of IRF-3 and induction of IFN by virus infection or cytosolic dsRNA.[83,84] The role of PKR in host antiviral response has been studied in greater detail by generating PKR deficient mice. Although PKR has been shown to be involved in apoptosis and cell growth, the PKR-null mice develop normally. PKR-null mice have impaired antiviral responses and show increased susceptibility to a wide range of viruses including VSV, reovirus, influenza virus and bunyamwera virus. In vitro studies using PKR deficient MEFs show that PKR is involved in protection against infection by RNA viruses, including HCV, WNV, HIV-1, Sindbis virus, as well as DNA viruses such as HSV-1.[2] NIH 3T3 cells expressing the noncatalytic mutant of PKR, are not able to inhibit the growth of EMCV, suggesting the catalytic activity of PKR in mediating its antiviral effects.

The biological importance of PKR function is further indicated by the existence of multiple cellular and viral regulators of PKR action. A number of cellular proteins are known to inhibit PKR activity. Cellular tar RNA binding protein, TRBP, inhibits PKR activity by competing for common RNA substrates. Viruses have evolved with elegant strategies to target PKR function and hence the PKR-dependent components of innate antiviral response of cells.[05,06] A wide range of viral inhibitors have been studied which have the potential to block PKR catalytic function. Adenovirus VAI and Epstein-Barr virus EBER are virally encoded RNAs that bind to the dsRBMs of PKR to inhibit its activation. The internal ribosome entry site (IRES) RNA of HCV genomic RNA also binds to PKR and prevents kinase autophoshorylation and activation.[87] Vaccinia virus encoded proteins, E3L and K3L interfere with PKR-mediated translational inhibition. E3L acts by sequestering dsRNA, while K3L works as a pseudosubstrate inhibitor. Influenza viral protein NS1 inhibits PKR function by activating P58^{IPK}, a cellular chaperone and inhibitor of PKR. The Us11 gene product of HSV-1 is an RNA binding protein and inhibits PKR activation by binding to its N-terminal half. HCV encoded proteins NS5A, E2 and KSHV encoded vIRF-2 protein, repress PKR activation through direct interaction with the kinase.[88]

2'-5' Oligoadenylate Synthetases (OAS)

OAS was discovered as one of the 'factors' responsible for the inhibition of cell-free protein synthesis by dsRNA.[89] It was initially purified from IFN-treated cells and found to be capable of synthesizing small 2'-5' linked oligomers of adenosine [2–5(A)] in the presence of dsRNA and ATP. The latent ribonuclease, RNase L, binds to trimeric or higher oligomers of 2–5(A)s, forms active dimers and degrades viral or cellular RNA (Fig. 5). Active RNase L prevents viral replication by degrading RNA replication intermediates of viral proteins. There are three structurally related classes of 2–5(A) OAS genes, these genes are present at low levels in host cells and induced by viral infection.[90] The OAS genes produce alternatively spliced mRNA encoding multiple isozymes with different carboxyl terminal regions. Three major forms of OAS genes in human cells encode

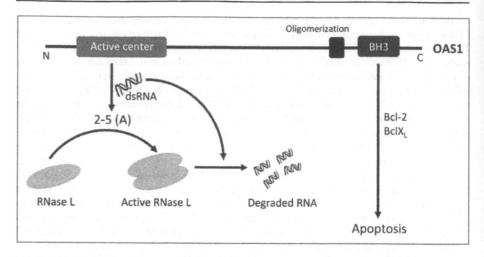

Figure 5. OAS1 mediated antiviral pathways. A schematic representation of various functional domains of OAS1 is shown. OAS1 catalyzes the formation of 2'-5' oligoadenylates and activate RNase L, which in turn degrades RNA. In addition, OAS1 also interacts with Bcl-2 and Bcl-xL via its BH3 domain to mediate apoptosis.

OAS1, the smaller 40–46 kDa isozyme, OAS2, the medium 69–71 kDa isozyme and OAS3, the 100 kDa larger isozyme. Oligomerization of OAS1 and OAS2 is necessary for their enzymatic activity. In the native form, OAS1 exists as tetramers, OAS2 forms dimers and OAS3 exists as a monomer. Some of these isozymes are post-translationally modified causing their translocation to different subcellular compartments.[91] In addition to the active OAS enzymes, OAS-like proteins induced by IFN were identified in human cells; however they lack catalytic activity.[92]

There are notable differences in enzymatic properties of the three classes of OAS. The OAS1 isozymes synthesize upto hexamers of 2–5(A) and the OAS2 isozyme can synthesize upto 30-mers of 2–5(A).[91] In contrast, OAS3 can make only dimeric 2–5(A), which are incapable of activating RNase L. Extensive structure-function studies of OAS1 and OAS2 have led to identification of their oligomerization site, the catalytic site and the substrate acceptor site. Dimerization of OAS2 P69 is essential for its enzymatic activity because of the crisscross nature of catalysis.[93] The donor bound to one subunit is covalently linked to the acceptor site of the other subunit, which also contains the catalytic site. A similar crisscross activity is suggested from the crystal structure of OAS1 isozyme. The structure of OAS1 sheds light on its mechanism of activation by dsRNA as well. Unlike other dsRNA-binding proteins, OAS proteins do not have any defined dsRNA binding motif; dsRNA alignment with the crystal structure revealed an RNA-binding region in OAS1. The crystal structure, mutagenesis and enzyme kinetic studies suggest that the activation is a two-step process. First, dsRNA binds to a positively charged groove of OAS, followed by a structural rearrangement that widens the active site cleft.[14]

Non-enzymatic role of OAS has also been apparent. The human 9–2/E17 isozyme of OAS1 gene has been shown to possess a Bcl-2 homology 3 (BH3) domain necessary for its interaction with Bcl2 family proteins for causing apoptosis (Fig. 5).[94] This action of E17 does not require oligomerization of the protein, the presence of dsRNA, the enzymatic activity or the presence of RNase L. Mutation of the BH3-domain of E17 causes a loss of its apoptotic activity. This study suggests that E17 is a dual function protein, with two mutually independent activities for synthesizing 2–5(A) and promoting apoptosis. The first action is dsRNA-dependent but the second is not.

The role of OAS proteins in the host defense has been studied for various viruses. The replication of EMCV is inhibited by the expression of OAS1 and OAS2 proteins. We have shown that OAS2 P69 isozyme specifically inhibits the replication of EMCV in a dose- and enzymatic activity-dependent manner.[95] OAS1 has also been shown to mediate a direct, RNase L-independent effect against some viruses. Extracellular OAS1 enters the cells and inhibits replication of EMCV, VSV and HSV-2. Recent studies suggest the antiviral roles of OAS3 against members of alphavirus family e.g., Chikungunya virus, Sindbis virus, and Semliki Forest virus.[96] An inactive OAS like protein, P59 OAS L, has been shown to confer antiviral activity against EMCV;[97] a mouse homolog of this protein has also been shown to be effective against WNV. Besides the demonstrated antiviral activities, polymorphisms in the human OAS gene are also associated with susceptibility against WNV, Hepatitis C virus and SARS coronavirus.[98-100] Antiviral effects of OAS proteins are targeted by viral proteins to antagonize the IFN action in the infected cells. Vaccinia viral protein E3, has been shown to inhibit the function of OAS by sequestering dsRNA from the enzyme. A human CMV ORF94 gene product has recently been shown to downregulate the expression of OAS and inhibits its enzymatic activity.[101] OAS activity is also targeted by Influenza viral protein NS1, which has been reported to out-compete OAS for interaction with dsRNA, thereby inhibiting its enzymatic activity. Given the role of RNase L in IFN-β induction, NS1-mediated inactivation of OAS might also contribute to the suppression of IFN synthesis by NS1.[102]

Adenosine Deaminases Acting on RNA (ADARs)

ADARs, RNA adenosine deaminases, catalyze hydrolytic C6 deamination of adenosine to produce inosine in RNA structures with double-stranded character.[3,103] This reaction is commonly referred to as A-to-I RNA editing (Fig. 6). ADAR genes were first identified in *Xenopus laevis* as DNA-unwinding enzymes, with human and mouse homologs subsequently identified. The deamination of adenosine in duplexes leads to destabilization of the dsRNA structure because I:U mismatch base pairs are less stable than A:U pairs. The common structural features of ADAR family proteins include a dsRNA-binding domain and a conserved deaminase domain at the C-terminus that contains highly conserved residues thought to be involved in its catalytic activity (Fig. 6). Depending on the location of A-to-I modification, this editing can lead to a codon change

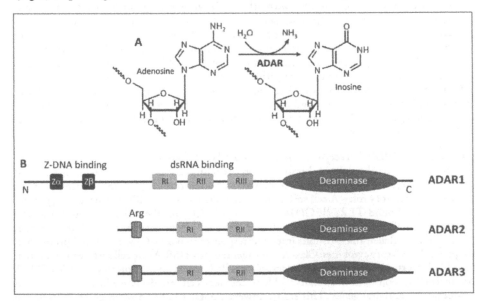

Figure 6. Structure and function of ADARs. A) ADAR mediated catalytic conversion of adenosine to inosine is shown; (B) The members of ADAR family and their functional domains are shown.

and alteration of protein functions. Major targets of ADAR-mediated RNA editing include viral RNAs, such as hepatitis delta virus antigenome RNA and kaposin K12 transcript of human herpes virus 8 and cellular RNAs, such as mammalian glutamate receptor R2 (GluR2), serotonin, and serotonin receptor mRNAs.[104] Different ADAR family members appear to bind particular targets, with specificity possibly mediated by differences in the number of and spacing between dsRNA-binding domains between family members.[105]

In vertebrates, three Adar genes, Adar1, Adar2, and Adar3, are present. Adar1 is constitutively expressed; however, its promoter contains an ISRE that mediates increased mRNA levels by IFN-α and IFN-γ treatment.[106] Two major protein species of ADAR1 are found: p150 is IFN-inducible and p110 is constitutively expressed. In contrast, Adar2 expression is controlled by CREB-binding protein elements present in the promoter, and the mechanism regulating Adar3 expression is currently unclear. Expression of ADAR1 and ADAR2 has been identified in many tissues including human heart, brain, lung, liver, skeletal muscles, kidney, pancreas, while expression of ADAR3 is restricted to the brain. Subcellular localization studies indicate that p150 form of ADAR1 exists in cytosol, whereas p110 form of ADAR1 and ADAR2 localize predominantly in the nucleus. ADAR3 protein does not display demonstrable deaminase catalytic activity with known A-to-I RNA editing substrates; it has been implicated as an inhibitor of both ADAR1 and ADAR2.[3]

The significance of A-to-I editing in normal physiology of uninfected cells and animals is illustrated by the striking phenotypes observed in the mouse model with either disruption of Adar genes or overexpression of ADAR proteins. Adar1 deficiency results in embryonic lethality, caused by apoptosis in many tissues, liver disintegration and defects in hematopoiesis.[107] In contrast, Adar2−/− mice are viable but display behavioral abnormalities including epileptic seizures.[108] On the other hand, transgenic overexpression of ADAR2 protein in mice leads to metabolic alterations characterized by hyperphagia and adult-onset obesity. ADARs play important roles during viral infections; they can have either proviral or antiviral consequences, depending on the virus-host combination.[3] A-to-I mutations attributed to the action of ADAR during lytic and persistent infections have been described for several different RNA viruses, initially with measles virus and then with other RNA viruses including human parainfluenza virus, respiratory syncytial virus, influenza virus, LCMV, Rift Valley fever virus, mumps virus and hepatitis C virus, and a DNA virus, mouse polyoma virus.[3,109] Adar1−/− MEFs displayed extensive syncytium formation and virus-induced cytotoxicity following infection with measles virus, and produced 3–4 log higher infectious virus, compared with Wt MEFs. Studies with influenza virus indicated enhanced virus-induced cytopathic effect in Adar1−/− MEFs, showing antiviral role of ADAR1 against influenza virus. A recent study reveals an antagonistic role of ADAR1 in dsRNA-induced IFN induction and apoptosis.[110] The study suggests that hyperedited dsRNA (IU-dsRNA) generated by ADAR1, binds specifically to RIG-I and MDA-5 and outcompete dsRNA from its receptors.

Additional dsRNA Receptors in Antiviral Host Defense

In addition to the dsRNA binding proteins which are directly involved in antiviral functions, there are indications of the presence of additional dsRNA recognizing proteins which play accessory roles. A cell surface protein, CD14 acts as a dsRNA transporting protein to endosome-bound TLR3.[111] CD14 binds to poly(I:C) on the cell surface and interacts directly with TLR3, to enhance the antiviral responses. Bone-marrow derived macrophages from CD14 deficient mice exhibits impaired responses to poly(I:C) and reduced production of pro-inflammatory cytokines. Class A scavanger receptors (SR-A) are cell surface proteins that can bind to extracellular dsRNA in macrophages.[112] A recent study indicates the role of SR-A in antiviral responses in fibroblasts.[113] SR-A deficient cells are defective in dsRNA-induced induction of antiviral genes. This study, however, doesn't indicate whether SR-A itself can activate any downstream antiviral signaling pathways, rather suggests that this might function in delivering the extracellular dsRNA to endosome-bound TLR3 for activation of IRF-3 and

NF-κB. A subsequent study suggests that high-mobility group box (HMGB) proteins play critical roles in recognizing immunogenic nucleic acids including dsRNA, for activating both TLR and RLR-dependent antiviral responses. Cells deficient in HMGB proteins fail to activate IRF-3 and NF-κB by dsRNA-induced signaling.[114] DDX60, a cytosolic RNA helicase, promotes RLR signaling by recognizing viral dsRNA.[115] DDX60 increases the association of dsRNA with RIG-I and MDA-5, but not TLR3.

Conclusion

DsRNA is a broad and potent regulator of cellular functions. Without doubt, it is a major component of host defense against virus infection; the same may be true for other infectious agents too. Its effects are mediated by dsRNA-binding proteins or receptor, some of which play important roles in specific non-viral diseases as well. Several dsRNA-binding proteins are essential or regulatory components of the machinery of microRNA biogenesis, thus bridging the fields of miRNA action and antiviral response, a connection that remains to be fully explored. One anticipates that future research on the diverse biological roles of dsRNA will produce exciting and novel results.

Acknowledgements

We acknowledge the helpful discussions with Volker Fensterl and other members of the Sen Laboratory. Our research is supported by National Institutes of Health grants AI 073303 and CA62220.

About the Authors

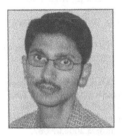

Saurabh Chattopadhyay is a Project Staff in the Department of Molecular Genetics at Lerner Research Institute, Cleveland Clinic. He received his PhD in 2002 from Indian Institute of Technology, Delhi, in Biotechnology. He worked as a Research Fellow in the Department of Molecular Cardiology at Lerner Research Institute. He joined the laboratory of Ganes Sen in 2005, when he started to work on the role of IRF-3 in mediating virus-induced apoptosis. His studies revealed new mechanisms of IRF-3 activation in virus-induced cell death. He is a recipient of Milstein Young Investigator Award in 2010 by ISICR and Boltzmann Award in 2008 by ISICR and ICS. In another area of research, he is studying the role of Angiotensin Converting Enzyme in blood pressure regulation and kidney functions in transgenic mouse models.

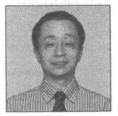

Michifumi Yamashita is a postdoctoral fellow in Ganes Sen's laboratory, Department of Molecular Genetics, Lerner Research Institute, Cleveland Clinic, since 2007. He is also an adjunct faculty member at Division of Nephrology, Juntendo University School of Medicine. Finished residency program and served as Chief Resident in internal medicine at Toranomon Hospital, Tokyo, in 2000, after received MD from Kagoshima University, Japan. Finished his PhD/nephrology fellow program in 2004 at Juntendo University, Tokyo, where he studied the mechanism of IgA nephropathy. During 2004-2007, he worked as a postdoctoral fellow in Steven Emancipator's laboratory, Department of Pathology, Case Western Reserve University, Cleveland, OH, where studied the effect of innate immunity on IgA nephropathy. In 2007, He joined in Sen's laboratory to pursue his PhD, working on Toll-like receptor 3 signaling and role of angiotensin-converting enzyme in polycystic kidney disease. From July 2011, he is a resident physician, Department of Pathology, University Hospitals Case Medical Center, Cleveland, OH.

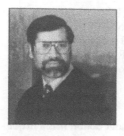

Ganes C. Sen received his PhD in Biochemistry from McMaster University, Canada. During his postdoctoral training with Peter Lengyel at Yale University, USA, he began investigating the interferon (IFN) system. He has continued and expanded his activities in this area of research in his own laboratory, first at the Memorial Sloan-Kettering Cancer Center, USA, and then at the Lerner Research Institute of The Cleveland Clinic, USA, where he nucleated the formation of a strong cytokine research group. He is currently the Chairman and Professor of Molecular Genetics at Cleveland Clinic. He has published extensively on the mechanism of actions of IFN-induced proteins and the mode of induction and actions of double-stranded RNA-stimulated genes. For his contributions to IFN research, he received the Milstein Award in 2002. In another line of research, Sen studies the physiological roles of angiotensin-converting enzyme in blood pressure regulation, male fertility and kidney functions. Sen is a consultant for the National Institutes of Health (NIH) and the American Foundation for AIDS Research. Currently, he is a Senior Editor of the *Journal of Virology* and Editor-in-Chief of the *Journal of Interferon and Cytokine Research*.

References

1. Saunders LR, Barber GN. The dsRNA binding protein family: critical roles, diverse cellular functions. FASEB J 2003; 17:961-83; PMID:12773480; http://dx.doi.org/10.1096/fj.02-0958rev.
2. Sadler AJ, Williams BR. Interferon-inducible antiviral effectors. Nat Rev Immunol 2008; 8:559-68; PMID:18575461; http://dx.doi.org/10.1038/nri2314.
3. Samuel CE. Adenosine deaminases acting on RNA (ADARs) are both antiviral and proviral. Virology 2011; 411:180-93; PMID:21211811; http://dx.doi.org/10.1016/j.virol.2010.12.004.
4. Kawai T, Akira S. Toll-like receptor and RIG-I-like receptor signaling. Ann N Y Acad Sci 2008; 1143:1-20; PMID:19076341; http://dx.doi.org/10.1196/annals.1443.020.
5. Chiu YH, Macmillan JB, Chen ZJ. RNA polymerase III detects cytosolic DNA and induces type I interferons through the RIG-I pathway. Cell 2009; 138:576-91; PMID:19631370; http://dx.doi.org/10.1016/j.cell.2009.06.015.
6. Weber F, Wagner V, Rasmussen SB, Hartmann R, Paludan SR. Double-stranded RNA is produced by positive-strand RNA viruses and DNA viruses but not in detectable amounts by negative-strand RNA viruses. J Virol 2006; 80:5059-64; PMID:16641297; http://dx.doi.org/10.1128/JVI.80.10.5059-5064.2006.
7. Sarkar SN, Sen GC. Novel functions of proteins encoded by viral stress-inducible genes. Pharmacol Ther 2004; 103:245-59; PMID:15464592; http://dx.doi.org/10.1016/j.pharmthera.2004.07.007.
8. Geiss G, Jin G, Guo J, Bumgarner R, Katze MG, Sen GC. A comprehensive view of regulation of gene expression by double-stranded RNA-mediated cell signaling. J Biol Chem 2001; 276:30178-82; PMID:11487589.
9. Sen GC, Sarkar SN. Transcriptional signaling by double-stranded RNA: role of TLR3. Cytokine Growth Factor Rev 2005; 16:1-14; PMID:15733829; http://dx.doi.org/10.1016/j.cytogfr.2005.01.006.
10. Elco CP, Guenther JM, Williams BR, Sen GC. Analysis of genes induced by Sendai virus infection of mutant cell lines reveals essential roles of interferon regulatory factor 3, NF-kappaB, and interferon but not toll-like receptor 3. J Virol 2005; 79:3920-9; PMID:15767394; http://dx.doi.org/10.1128/JVI.79.7.3920-3929.2005.
11. Choe J, Kelker MS, Wilson IA. Crystal structure of human toll-like receptor 3 (TLR3) ectodomain. Science 2005; 309:581-5; PMID:15961631; http://dx.doi.org/10.1126/science.1115253.
12. Cui S, Eisenacher K, Kirchhofer A, Brzozka K, Lammens A, Lammens K, et al. The C-terminal regulatory domain is the RNA 5'-triphosphate sensor of RIG-I. Mol Cell 2008; 29:169-79; PMID:18243112; http://dx.doi.org/10.1016/j.molcel.2007.10.032.
13. Takahasi K, Yoneyama M, Nishihori T, Hirai R, Kumeta H, Narita R, et al. Nonself RNA-sensing mechanism of RIG-I helicase and activation of antiviral immune responses. Mol Cell 2008; 29:428-40; PMID:18242112; http://dx.doi.org/10.1016/j.molcel.2007.11.028.
14. Hartmann R, Justesen J, Sarkar SN, Sen GC, Yee VC. Crystal structure of the 2'-specific and double-stranded RNA-activated interferon-induced antiviral protein 2'-5'-oligoadenylate synthetase. Mol Cell 2003; 12:1173-85; PMID:14636576; http://dx.doi.org/10.1016/S1097-2765(03)00433-7.

15. Janeway CA Jr., Medzhitov R. Innate immune recognition. Annu Rev Immunol 2002; 20:197-216; PMID:11861602; http://dx.doi.org/10.1146/annurev.immunol.20.083001.084359.

16. Beutler B. Toll-like receptors and their place in immunology. Where does the immune response to infection begin? Nat Rev Immunol 2004; 4:498; PMID:18293536; http://dx.doi.org/10.1038/nri1401.

17. Kawai T, Akira S. The role of pattern-recognition receptors in innate immunity: update on Toll-like receptors. Nat Immunol 2010; 11:373-84; PMID:20404851; http://dx.doi.org/10.1038/ni.1863.

18. Alexopoulou L, Holt AC, Medzhitov R, Flavell RA. Recognition of double-stranded RNA and activation of NF-kappaB by Toll-like receptor 3. Nature 2001; 413:732-8; PMID:11607032; http://dx.doi.org/10.1038/35099560.

19. Cavassani KA, Ishii M, Wen H, Schaller MA, Lincoln PM, Lukacs NW, et al. TLR3 is an endogenous sensor of tissue necrosis during acute inflammatory events. J Exp Med 2008; 205:2609-21; PMID:18838547; http://dx.doi.org/10.1084/jem.20081370.

20. Yamamoto M, Sato S, Hemmi H, Hoshino K, Kaisho T, Sanjo H, et al. Role of adaptor TRIF in the MyD88-independent toll-like receptor signaling pathway. Science 2003; 301:640-3; PMID:12855817; http://dx.doi.org/10.1126/science.1087262.

21. Qi R, Hoose S, Schreiter J, Sawant KV, Lamb R, Ranjith-Kumar CT, et al. Secretion of the human Toll-like receptor 3 ectodomain is affected by single nucleotide polymorphisms and regulated by Unc93b1. J Biol Chem 2010; 285:36635-44; PMID:20855885; http://dx.doi.org/10.1074/jbc.M110.144402.

22. Funami K, Sasai M, Ohba Y, Oshiumi H, Seya T, Matsumoto M. Spatiotemporal mobilization of Toll/IL-1 receptor domain-containing adaptor molecule-1 in response to dsRNA. J Immunol 2007; 179:6867-72; PMID:17982077.

23. Sato S, Sugiyama M, Yamamoto M, Watanabe Y, Kawai T, Takeda K, et al. Toll/IL-1 receptor domain-containing adaptor inducing IFN-beta (TRIF) associates with TNF receptor-associated factor 6 and TANK-binding kinase 1, and activates two distinct transcription factors, NF-kappa B and IFN-regulatory factor-3, in the Toll-like receptor signaling. J Immunol 2003; 171:4304-10; PMID:14530355.

24. Meylan E, Burns K, Hofmann K, Blancheteau V, Martinon F, Kelliher M, et al. RIP1 is an essential mediator of Toll-like receptor 3-induced NF-kappa B activation. Nat Immunol 2004; 5:503-7; PMID:15064760; http://dx.doi.org/10.1038/ni1061.

25. Funami K, Sasai M, Oshiumi H, Seya T, Matsumoto M. Homo-oligomerization is essential for Toll/interleukin-1 receptor domain-containing adaptor molecule-1-mediated NF-kappaB and interferon regulatory factor-3 activation. J Biol Chem 2008; 283:18283-91; PMID:18450748; http://dx.doi.org/10.1074/jbc.M801013200.

26. Han KJ, Yang Y, Xu LG, Shu HB. Analysis of a TIR-less splice variant of TRIF reveals an unexpected mechanism of TLR3-mediated signaling. J Biol Chem 2010; 285:12543-50; PMID:20200155; http://dx.doi.org/10.1074/jbc.M109.072231.

27. Sarkar SN, Peters KL, Elco CP, Sakamoto S, Pal S, Sen GC. Novel roles of TLR3 tyrosine phosphorylation and PI3 kinase in double-stranded RNA signaling. Nat Struct Mol Biol 2004; 11:1060-7; PMID:15502848; http://dx.doi.org/10.1038/nsmb847.

28. Sarkar SN, Elco CP, Peters KL, Chattopadhyay S, Sen GC. Two tyrosine residues of Toll-like receptor 3 trigger different steps of NF-kappa B activation. J Biol Chem 2007; 282:3423-7; PMID:17178723; http://dx.doi.org/10.1074/jbc.C600226200.

29. Johnsen IB, Nguyen TT, Ringdal M, Tryggestad AM, Bakke O, Lien E, et al. Toll-like receptor 3 associates with c-Src tyrosine kinase on endosomes to initiate antiviral signaling. EMBO J 2006; 25:3335-46; PMID:16858407; http://dx.doi.org/10.1038/sj.emboj.7601222.

30. Weber A, Kirejczyk Z, Besch R, Potthoff S, Leverkus M, Hacker G. Proapoptotic signalling through Toll-like receptor-3 involves TRIF-dependent activation of caspase-8 and is under the control of inhibitor of apoptosis proteins in melanoma cells. Cell Death Differ 2010; 17:942-51; PMID:20019748; http://dx.doi.org/10.1038/cdd.2009.190.

31. Salaun B, Coste I, Rissoan MC, Lebecque SJ, Renno T. TLR3 can directly trigger apoptosis in human cancer cells. J Immunol 2006; 176:4894-901; PMID:16585585.

32. Kaiser WJ, Kaufman JL, Offermann MK. IFN-alpha sensitizes human umbilical vein endothelial cells to apoptosis induced by double-stranded RNA. J Immunol 2004; 172:1699-710; PMID:14734752.

33. Sun R, Zhang Y, Lv Q, Liu B, Jin M, Zhang W, et al. Toll-like receptor 3 (TLR3) induces apoptosis via death receptors and mitochondria by up-regulating the transactivating p63 isoform alpha (TAP63alpha). J Biol Chem 2011; 286:15918-28; PMID:21367858; http://dx.doi.org/10.1074/jbc.M110.178798.

34. Shiose S, Chen Y, Okano K, Roy S, Kohno H, Tang J, et al. Toll-like receptor 3 is required for development of retinopathy caused by impaired all-trans-retinal clearance in mice. J Biol Chem 2011; 286:15543-55; PMID:21383019; http://dx.doi.org/10.1074/jbc.M111.228551.

35. Lin Q, Fang D, Fang J, Ren X, Yang X, Wen F, et al. Impaired wound healing with defective expression of chemokines and recruitment of myeloid cells in TLR3-deficient mice. J Immunol 2011; 186:3710-7; PMID:21317384; http://dx.doi.org/10.4049/jimmunol.1003007.

36. Salaun B, Zitvogel L, Asselin-Paturel C, Morel Y, Chemin K, Dubois C, et al. TLR3 as a biomarker for the therapeutic efficacy of double-stranded RNA in breast cancer. Cancer Res 2011; 71:1607-14; PMID:21343393; http://dx.doi.org/10.1158/0008-5472.CAN-10-3490.

37. Kumar H, Koyama S, Ishii KJ, Kawai T, Akira S. Cutting edge: cooperation of IPS-1- and TRIF-dependent pathways in poly IC-enhanced antibody production and cytotoxic T cell responses. J Immunol 2008; 180:683-7; PMID:18178804.

38. Schulz O, Diebold SS, Chen M, Naslund TI, Nolte MA, Alexopoulou L, et al. Toll-like receptor 3 promotes cross-priming to virus-infected cells. Nature 2005; 433:887-92; PMID:15711573; http://dx.doi.org/10.1038/nature03326.

39. Zhang SY, Jouanguy E, Ugolini S, Smahi A, Elain G, Romero P, et al. TLR3 deficiency in patients with herpes simplex encephalitis. Science 2007; 317:1522-7; PMID:17872438; http://dx.doi.org/10.1126/science.1139522.

40. Gowen BB, Hoopes JD, Wong MH, Jung KH, Isakson KC, Alexopoulou L, et al. TLR3 deletion limits mortality and disease severity due to Phlebovirus infection. J Immunol 2006; 177:6301-7; PMID:17056560.

41. Hutchens M, Luker KE, Sottile P, Sonstein J, Lukacs NW, Nunez G, et al. TLR3 increases disease morbidity and mortality from vaccinia infection. J Immunol 2008; 180:483-91; PMID:18097050.

42. Wang T, Town T, Alexopoulou L, Anderson JF, Fikrig E, Flavell RA. Toll-like receptor 3 mediates West Nile virus entry into the brain causing lethal encephalitis. Nat Med 2004; 10:1366-73; PMID:15558055; http://dx.doi.org/10.1038/nm1140.

43. Bouma G, Strober W. The immunological and genetic basis of inflammatory bowel disease. Nat Rev Immunol 2003; 3:521-33; PMID:12876555; http://dx.doi.org/10.1038/nri1132.

44. Vijay-Kumar M, Wu H, Aitken J, Kolachala VL, Neish AS, Sitaraman SV, et al. Activation of toll-like receptor 3 protects against DSS-induced acute colitis. Inflamm Bowel Dis 2007; 13:856-64; PMID:17393379; http://dx.doi.org/10.1002/ibd.20142.

45. Allikmets R, Bergen AA, Dean M, Guymer RH, Hageman GS, Klaver CC, et al. Geographic atrophy in age-related macular degeneration and TLR3. N Engl J Med 2009; 360:2252-4, author reply 5-6; PMID:19469038.

46. Kleinman ME, Yamada K, Takeda A, Chandrasekaran V, Nozaki M, Baffi JZ, et al. Sequence- and target-independent angiogenesis suppression by siRNA via TLR3. Nature 2008; 452:591-7; PMID:18368052; http://dx.doi.org/10.1038/nature06765.

47. Reich SJ, Fosnot J, Kuroki A, Tang W, Yang X, Maguire AM, et al. Small interfering RNA (siRNA) targeting VEGF effectively inhibits ocular neovascularization in a mouse model. Mol Vis 2003; 9:210-6; PMID:12789138.

48. Rosenfeld PJ, Brown DM, Heier JS, Boyer DS, Kaiser PK, Chung CY, et al. Ranibizumab for neovascular age-related macular degeneration. N Engl J Med 2006; 355:1419-31; PMID:17021318; http://dx.doi.org/10.1056/NEJMoa054481.

49. Zimmer S, Steinmetz M, Asdonk T, Motz I, Coch C, Hartmann E, et al. Activation of endothelial toll-like receptor 3 impairs endothelial function. Circ Res 2011; 108:1358-66; PMID:21493895; http://dx.doi.org/10.1161/CIRCRESAHA.111.243246.

50. Castaño L, Eisenbarth GS. Type-I diabetes: a chronic autoimmune disease of human, mouse, and rat. Annu Rev Immunol 1990; 8:647-79; PMID:2188676; http://dx.doi.org/10.1146/annurev.iy.08.040190.003243.

51. Yoon JW, Austin M, Onodera T, Notkins AL. Isolation of a virus from the pancreas of a child with diabetic ketoacidosis. N Engl J Med 1979; 300:1173-9; PMID:219345; http://dx.doi.org/10.1056/NEJM197905243002102.

52. Oldstone MB, Nerenberg M, Southern P, Price J, Lewicki H. Virus infection triggers insulin-dependent diabetes mellitus in a transgenic model: role of anti-self (virus) immune response. Cell 1991; 65:319-31; PMID:1901765; http://dx.doi.org/10.1016/0092-8674(91)90165-U.

53. Cerutis DR, Bruner RH, Thomas DC, Giron DJ. Tropism and histopathology of the D, B, K, and MM variants of encephalomyocarditis virus. J Med Virol 1989; 29:63-9; PMID:2555446; http://dx.doi.org/10.1002/jmv.1890290112.

54. McCartney SA, Vermi W, Lonardi S, Rossini C, Otero K, Calderon B, et al. RNA sensor-induced type I IFN prevents diabetes caused by a beta cell-tropic virus in mice. J Clin Invest 2011; 121:1497-507; PMID:21403398; http://dx.doi.org/10.1172/JCI44005.

55. Loo YM, Gale M Jr. Immune signaling by RIG-I-like receptors. Immunity 2011; 34:680-92; PMID:21616437; http://dx.doi.org/10.1016/j.immuni.2011.05.003.

56. Kato H, Takeuchi O, Mikamo-Satoh E, Hirai R, Kawai T, Matsushita K, et al. Length-dependent recognition of double-stranded ribonucleic acids by retinoic acid-inducible gene-I and melanoma differentiation-associated gene 5. J Exp Med 2008; 205:1601-10; PMID:18591409; http://dx.doi.org/10.1084/jem.20080091.

57. Seth RB, Sun L, Ea CK, Chen ZJ. Identification and characterization of MAVS, a mitochondrial antiviral signaling protein that activates NF-kappaB and IRF 3. Cell 2005; 122:669-82; PMID:16125763; http://dx.doi.org/10.1016/j.cell.2005.08.012.

58. Peters K, Chattopadhyay S, Sen GC. IRF-3 activation by sendai virus infection is required for cellular apoptosis and avoidance of persistence. J Virol 2008; 82:3500-8; PMID:18216110; http://dx.doi.org/10.1128/JVI.02536-07.

59. Chattopadhyay S, Marques JT, Yamashita M, Peters KL, Smith K, Desai A, et al. Viral apoptosis is induced by IRF-3-mediated activation of Bax. EMBO J 2010; 29:1762-73; PMID:20360684; http://dx.doi.org/10.1038/emboj.2010.50.

60. Chattopadhyay S, Sen GC. IRF-3 and Bax: A deadly affair. Cell Cycle 2010; 9:2479-80; PMID:21483234; http://dx.doi.org/10.4161/cc.9.13.12237.

61. Chattopadhyay S, Yamashita M, Zhang Y, Sen GC. The IRF-3/Bax-mediated apoptotic pathway, activated by viral cytoplasmic RNA and DNA, inhibits virus replication. J Virol 2011; 85:3708-16; PMID:21307205; http://dx.doi.org/10.1128/JVI.02133-10.

62. White CL, Chattopadhyay S, Sen GC. Phosphatidylinositol 3-kinase signaling delays sendai virus-induced apoptosis by preventing XIAP degradation. J Virol 2011; 85:5224-7; PMID:21367892; http://dx.doi.org/10.1128/JVI.00053-11.

63. Besch R, Poeck H, Hohenauer T, Senft D, Hacker G, Berking C, et al. Proapoptotic signaling induced by RIG-I and MDA-5 results in type I interferon-independent apoptosis in human melanoma cells. J Clin Invest 2009; 119:2399-411; PMID:19620789.

64. Lallemand C, Blanchard B, Palmieri M, Lebon P, May E, Tovey MG. Single-stranded RNA viruses inactivate the transcriptional activity of p53 but induce NOXA-dependent apoptosis via post-translational modifications of IRF-1, IRF-3 and CREB. Oncogene 2007; 26:328-38; PMID:16832344; http://dx.doi.org/10.1038/sj.onc.1209795.

65. Garcia M, Dogusan Z, Moore F, Sato S, Hartmann G, Eizirik DL, et al. Regulation and function of the cytosolic viral RNA sensor RIG-I in pancreatic beta cells. Biochimica et biophysica acta 2009; 1793:1768-75.

66. Rintahaka J, Lietzen N, Ohman T, Nyman TA, Matikainen S. Recognition of cytoplasmic RNA results in cathepsin-dependent inflammasome activation and apoptosis in human macrophages. J Immunol 2011; 186:3085-92; PMID:21257972; http://dx.doi.org/10.4049/jimmunol.1002051.

67. Rintahaka J, Wiik D, Kovanen PE, Alenius H, Matikainen S. Cytosolic antiviral RNA recognition pathway activates caspases 1 and 3. J Immunol 2008; 180:1749-57; PMID:18209072.

68. Iordanov MS, Kirsch JD, Ryabinina OP, Wong J, Spitz PN, Korcheva VB, et al. Recruitment of TRADD, FADD, and caspase 8 to double-stranded RNA-triggered death inducing signaling complexes (dsRNA-DISCs). Apoptosis 2005; 10:167-76; PMID:15711932; http://dx.doi.org/10.1007/s10495-005-6071-x.

69. Pan M, Geng S, Xiao S, Ren J, Liu Y, Li X, et al. Apoptosis induced by synthetic retinoic acid CD437 on human melanoma A375 cells involves RIG-I pathway. Arch Dermatol Res 2009; 301:15-20; PMID:18936944; http://dx.doi.org/10.1007/s00403-008-0902-x.

70. Wang P, Arjona A, Zhang Y, Sultana H, Dai J, Yang L, et al. Caspase-12 controls West Nile virus infection via the viral RNA receptor RIG-I. Nat Immunol 2010; 11:912-9; PMID:20818395; http://dx.doi.org/10.1038/ni.1933.

71. Poeck H, Bscheider M, Gross O, Finger K, Roth S, Rebsamen M, et al. Recognition of RNA virus by RIG-I results in activation of CARD9 and inflammasome signaling for interleukin 1 beta production. Nat Immunol 2010; 11:63-9; PMID:19915568; http://dx.doi.org/10.1038/ni.1824.

72. Tormo D, Checinska A, Alonso-Curbelo D, Perez-Guijarro E, Canon E, Riveiro-Falkenbach E, et al. Targeted activation of innate immunity for therapeutic induction of autophagy and apoptosis in melanoma cells. Cancer Cell 2009; 16:103-14; PMID:19647221; http://dx.doi.org/10.1016/j.ccr.2009.07.004.

73. Zhang Z, Kim T, Bao M, Facchinetti V, Jung SY, Ghaffari AA, et al. DDX1, DDX21, and DHX36 helicases form a complex with the adaptor molecule TRIF to sense dsRNA in dendritic cells. Immunity 2011; 34:866-78; PMID:21703541; http://dx.doi.org/10.1016/j.immuni.2011.03.027.

74. Sadler AJ, Williams BR. Structure and function of the protein kinase R. Curr Top Microbiol Immunol 2007; 316:253-92; PMID:17969452; http://dx.doi.org/10.1007/978-3-540-71329-6_13.

75. Sadler AJ, Latchoumanin O, Hawkes D, Mak J, Williams BR. An antiviral response directed by PKR phosphorylation of the RNA helicase A. PLoS Pathog 2009; 5:e1000311; PMID:19229320; http://dx.doi.org/10.1371/journal.ppat.1000311.

76. Harashima A, Guettouche T, Barber GN. Phosphorylation of the NFAR proteins by the dsRNA-dependent protein kinase PKR constitutes a novel mechanism of translational regulation and cellular defense. Genes Dev 2010; 24:2640-53; PMID:21123651; http://dx.doi.org/10.1101/gad.1965010.

77. Patel RC, Sen GC. PACT, a protein activator of the interferon-induced protein kinase, PKR. EMBO J 1998; 17:4379-90; PMID:9687506; http://dx.doi.org/10.1093/emboj/17.15.4379.

78. Peters GA, Li S, Sen GC. Phosphorylation of specific serine residues in the PKR activation domain of PACT is essential for its ability to mediate apoptosis. J Biol Chem 2006; 281:35129-36; PMID:16982605; http://dx.doi.org/10.1074/jbc.M607714200.

79. Kok KH, Lui PY, Ng MH, Siu KL, Au SW, Jin DY. The double-stranded RNA-binding protein PACT functions as a cellular activator of RIG-I to facilitate innate antiviral response. Cell Host Microbe 2011; 9:299-309; PMID:21501829; http://dx.doi.org/10.1016/j.chom.2011.03.007.

80. Garcíia MA, Gil J, Ventoso I, Guerra S, Domingo E, Rivas C, et al. Impact of protein kinase PKR in cell biology: from antiviral to antiproliferative action. Microbiol Mol Biol Rev 2006; 70:1032-60; PMID:17158706; http://dx.doi.org/10.1128/MMBR.00027-06.

81. Gil J, Esteban M. The interferon-induced protein kinase (PKR), triggers apoptosis through FADD-mediated activation of caspase 8 in a manner independent of Fas and TNF-alpha receptors. Oncogene 2000; 19:3665-74; PMID:10951573; http://dx.doi.org/10.1038/sj.onc.1203710.

82. Cuddihy AR, Wong AH, Tam NW, Li S, Koromilas AE. The double-stranded RNA activated protein kinase PKR physically associates with the tumor suppressor p53 protein and phosphorylates human p53 on serine 392 in vitro. Oncogene 1999; 18:2690-702; PMID:10348343; http://dx.doi.org/10.1038/sj.onc.1202620.

83. Sen A, Pruijssers AJ, Dermody TS, Garcia-Sastre A, Greenberg HB. The early interferon response to rotavirus is regulated by PKR and depends on MAVS/IPS-1, RIG-I, MDA-5, and IRF3. J Virol 2011; 85:3717-32; PMID:21307186; http://dx.doi.org/10.1128/JVI.02634-10.

84. McAllister CS, Samuel CE. The RNA-activated protein kinase enhances the induction of interferon-beta and apoptosis mediated by cytoplasmic RNA sensors. J Biol Chem 2009; 284:1644-51; PMID:19028691; http://dx.doi.org/10.1074/jbc.M807888200.

85. Samuel CE. Antiviral actions of interferons. [table of contents.]. Clin Microbiol Rev 2001; 14:778-809; PMID:11585785; http://dx.doi.org/10.1128/CMR.14.4.778-809.2001.

86. Haller O, Kochs G, Weber F. The interferon response circuit: induction and suppression by pathogenic viruses. Virology 2006; 344:119-30; PMID:16364743; http://dx.doi.org/10.1016/j.virol.2005.09.024.

87. Vyas J, Elia A, Clemens MJ. Inhibition of the protein kinase PKR by the internal ribosome entry site of hepatitis C virus genomic RNA. RNA 2003; 9:858-70; PMID:12810919; http://dx.doi.org/10.1261/rna.5330503.

88. Katze MG, He Y, Gale M Jr. Viruses and interferon: a fight for supremacy. Nat Rev Immunol 2002; 2:675-87; PMID:12209136; http://dx.doi.org/10.1038/nri888.

89. Hovanessian AG. Interferon-induced and double-stranded RNA-activated enzymes: a specific protein kinase and 2',5'-oligoadenylate synthetases. J Interferon Res 1991; 11:199-205; PMID:1717615; http://dx.doi.org/10.1089/jir.1991.11.199.

90. Sen GC, Sarkar SN. The interferon-stimulated genes: targets of direct signaling by interferons, double-stranded RNA, and viruses. Curr Top Microbiol Immunol 2007; 316:233-50; PMID:17969451; http://dx.doi.org/10.1007/978-3-540-71329-6_12.

91. Sarkar SN, Bandyopadhyay S, Ghosh A, Sen GC. Enzymatic characteristics of recombinant medium isozyme of 2'-5' oligoadenylate synthetase. J Biol Chem 1999; 274:1848-55; PMID:9880569; http://dx.doi.org/10.1074/jbc.274.3.1848.

92. Hartmann R, Olsen HS, Widder S, Jorgensen R, Justesen J. p59OASL, a 2'-5' oligoadenylate synthetase like protein: a novel human gene related to the 2'-5' oligoadenylate synthetase family. Nucleic Acids Res 1998; 26:4121-8; PMID:9722630; http://dx.doi.org/10.1093/nar/26.18.4121.

93. Sarkar SN, Pal S, Sen GC. Crisscross enzymatic reaction between the two molecules in the active dimeric P69 form of the 2'-5' oligoadenylate synthetase. J Biol Chem 2002; 277:44760-4; PMID:12223486; http://dx.doi.org/10.1074/jbc.M207126200.

94. Ghosh A, Sarkar SN, Rowe TM, Sen GC. A specific isozyme of 2'-5' oligoadenylate synthetase is a dual function proapoptotic protein of the Bcl-2 family. J Biol Chem 2001; 276:25447-55; PMID:11323417; http://dx.doi.org/10.1074/jbc.M100496200.

95. Ghosh A, Sarkar SN, Sen GC. Cell growth regulatory and antiviral effects of the P69 isozyme of 2-5 (A) synthetase. Virology 2000; 266:319-28; PMID:10639318; http://dx.doi.org/10.1006/viro.1999.0085.

96. Bréhin AC, Casademont I, Frenkiel MP, Julier C, Sakuntabhai A, Despres P. The large form of human 2',5'-Oligoadenylate Synthetase (OAS3) exerts antiviral effect against Chikungunya virus. Virology 2009; 384:216-22; PMID:19056102; http://dx.doi.org/10.1016/j.virol.2008.10.021.

97. Marques J, Anwar J, Eskildsen-Larsen S, Rebouillat D, Paludan SR, Sen G, et al. The p59 oligoadenylate synthetase-like protein possesses antiviral activity that requires the C-terminal ubiquitin-like domain. J Gen Virol 2008; 89:2767-72; PMID:18931074; http://dx.doi.org/10.1099/vir.0.2008/003558-0.

98. Lim JK, Lisco A, McDermott DH, Huynh L, Ward JM, Johnson B, et al. Genetic variation in OAS1 is a risk factor for initial infection with West Nile virus in man. PLoS Pathog 2009; 5:e1000321; PMID:19247438; http://dx.doi.org/10.1371/journal.ppat.1000321.

99. Knapp S, Yee LJ, Frodsham AJ, Hennig BJ, Hellier S, Zhang L, et al. Polymorphisms in interferon-induced genes and the outcome of hepatitis C virus infection: roles of MxA, OAS-1 and PKR. Genes Immun 2003; 4:411-9; PMID:12944978; http://dx.doi.org/10.1038/sj.gene.6363984.

100. He J, Feng D, de Vlas SJ, Wang H, Fontanet A, Zhang P, et al. Association of SARS susceptibility with single nucleic acid polymorphisms of OAS1 and MxA genes: a case-control study. BMC Infect Dis 2006; 6:106; PMID:16824203; http://dx.doi.org/10.1186/1471-2334-6-106.

101. Tan JC, Avdic S, Cao JZ, Mocarski ES, White KL, Abendroth A, et al. Inhibition of 2',5'-oligoadenylate synthetase expression and function by the human cytomegalovirus ORF94 gene product. J Virol 2011; 85:5696-700; PMID:21450824; http://dx.doi.org/10.1128/JVI.02463-10.

102. Hale BG, Randall RE, Ortin J, Jackson D. The multifunctional NS1 protein of influenza A viruses. J Gen Virol 2008; 89:2359-76; PMID:18796704; http://dx.doi.org/10.1099/vir.0.2008/004606-0.

103. Samuel CE. ADARs: Viruses and Innate Immunity. Curr Top Microbiol Immunol 2011.

104. Higuchi M, Single FN, Kohler M, Sommer B, Sprengel R, Seeburg PH. RNA editing of AMPA receptor subunit GluR-B: a base-paired intron-exon structure determines position and efficiency. Cell 1993; 75:1361-70; PMID:8269514; http://dx.doi.org/10.1016/0092-8674(93)90622-W.

105. Stefl R, Xu M, Skrisovska L, Emeson RB, Allain FH. Structure and specific RNA binding of ADAR2 double-stranded RNA binding motifs. Structure 2006; 14:345-55; PMID:16472753; http://dx.doi.org/10.1016/j.str.2005.11.013.

106. George CX, Gan Z, Liu Y, Samuel CE. Adenosine deaminases acting on RNA, RNA editing, and interferon action. J Interferon Cytokine Res 2011; 31:99-117; PMID:21182352; http://dx.doi.org/10.1089/jir.2010.0097.

107. Hartner JC, Walkley CR, Lu J, Orkin SH. ADAR1 is essential for the maintenance of hematopoiesis and suppression of interferon signaling. Nat Immunol 2009; 10:109-15; PMID:19060901; http://dx.doi.org/10.1038/ni.1680.

108. Higuchi M, Maas S, Single FN, Hartner J, Rozov A, Burnashev N, et al. Point mutation in an AMPA receptor gene rescues lethality in mice deficient in the RNA-editing enzyme ADAR2. Nature 2000; 406:78-81; PMID:10894545; http://dx.doi.org/10.1038/35017558.

109. Ward SV, George CX, Welch MJ, Liou LY, Hahm B, Lewicki H, et al. RNA editing enzyme adenosine deaminase is a restriction factor for controlling measles virus replication that also is required for embryogenesis. Proc Natl Acad Sci USA 2011; 108:331-6; PMID:21173229; http://dx.doi.org/10.1073/pnas.1017241108.

110. Vitali P, Scadden AD. Double-stranded RNAs containing multiple IU pairs are sufficient to suppress interferon induction and apoptosis. Nat Struct Mol Biol 2010; 17:1043-50; PMID:20694008; http://dx.doi.org/10.1038/nsmb.1864.

111. Lee HK, Dunzendorfer S, Soldau K, Tobias PS. Double-stranded RNA-mediated TLR3 activation is enhanced by CD14. Immunity 2006; 24:153-63; PMID:16473828; http://dx.doi.org/10.1016/j.immuni.2005.12.012.

112. Brown MS, Goldstein JL. Lipoprotein metabolism in the macrophage: implications for cholesterol deposition in atherosclerosis. Annu Rev Biochem 1983; 52:223-61; PMID:6311077; http://dx.doi.org/10.1146/annurev.bi.52.070183.001255.

113. DeWitte-Orr SJ, Collins SE, Bauer CM, Bowdish DM, Mossman KL. An accessory to the 'Trinity': SR-As are essential pathogen sensors of extracellular dsRNA, mediating entry and leading to subsequent type I IFN responses. PLoS Pathog 2010; 6:e1000829; PMID:20360967; http://dx.doi.org/10.1371/journal.ppat.1000829.

114. Yanai H, Ban T, Wang Z, Choi MK, Kawamura T, Negishi H, et al. HMGB proteins function as universal sentinels for nucleic-acid-mediated innate immune responses. Nature 2009; 462:99-103; PMID:19890330; http://dx.doi.org/10.1038/nature08512.

115. Miyashita M, Oshiumi H, Matsumoto M, Seya T. DDX60, a DEXD/H Box Helicase, Is a Novel Antiviral Factor Promoting RIG-I-Like Receptor-Mediated Signaling. Mol Cell Biol 2011; 31:3802-19; PMID:21791617; http://dx.doi.org/10.1128/MCB.01368-10.

CHAPTER 15

Ligands of Pathogen Sensors as Antiviral Agents

Priya Ranjan, Victoria Jeisy-Scott, William G. Davis, Neetu Singh,
J. Bradford Bowzard, Monika Chadwick, Shivaprakash Gangappa
and Suryaprakash Sambhara*

Abstract

Currently used antiviral agents act by inhibiting viral entry, replication, or release of viral progeny. However, recent emergence of drug-resistant viruses has become a major public health concern as it is limiting our ability to prevent and treat viral diseases. Furthermore, very few antiviral agents with novel modes of action are currently in development. It is well established that the innate immune system is the first line of defense against invading pathogens. The recognition of diverse pathogen-associated molecular patterns (PAMPs) is accomplished by several classes of pattern recognition receptors (PRRs) and the ligand/receptor interactions trigger an effective innate antiviral response. In the past several years, remarkable progress has been made toward understanding both the structural and functional nature of PAMPs and PRRs. As a result of their indispensable role in virus infection, these ligands have become potential pharmacological agents against viral infection. Since their pathways of action are evolutionarily conserved, the likelihood of viruses developing resistance to PRR activation is diminished. In this chapter, we will discuss the recent developments investigating the potential utility of the ligands of innate immune receptors as antiviral agents.

Introduction

The advent of antibiotics and antivirals that target key components of molecules necessary for microbial entry, replication and virulence has allowed mankind to control and prevent microbial infections. However, overuse of antimicrobial agents, the selection pressure of these agents on the microbes and the ability of microbes to evolve genetically have resulted in the emergence of drug-resistant pathogens. In the case of influenza, currently, two classes of antiviral drugs are available to treat influenza infections: the M2 ion-channel blockers amantadine and rimantadine for influenza A viruses and the NA inhibitors oseltamivir and zanamivir for both influenza A and B viruses. However, the emergence of human seasonal as well as highly virulent H5N1 influenza viruses that are resistant to one or both the classes of drugs underscores the need for development of new generation drugs as well as other novel preventive and therapeutic strategies. For example, the worldwide circulation of adamantane-resistant influenza A viruses increased from about 0.4% in 1994–95 to almost 92% by the 2004–05 season.[1] Currently circulating H3N2 and 2009 pandemic H1N1 viruses are resistant to adamantanes, thereby leaving us with the neuraminidase inhibitors as the drug of choice for prophylactic and therapeutic use against influenza.[1] Furthermore, the recent emergence of NA inhibitor

*Influenza Division, National Center for Immunization and Respiratory Diseases, Centers for Disease Control and Prevention, Atlanta, Georgia, USA.
Corresponding Author: Suryaprakash Sambhara—Email: ssambhara@cdc.gov

Nucleic Acid Sensors and Antiviral Immunity, edited by Suryaprakash Sambhara and Takashi Fujita.
©2013 Landes Bioscience.

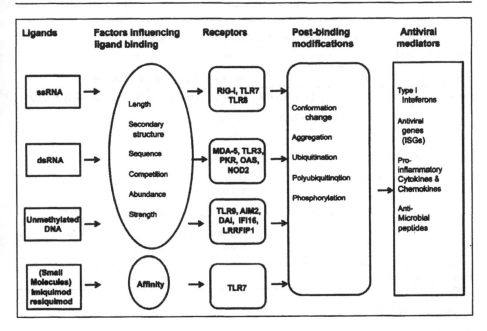

Figure 1. Ligands of nucleic acid sensors and their outcomes. The nature of authentic ligands of nucleic acid sensors and small molecules that can activate nucleic acid sensor receptors and lead to desired outcomes is currently an area of intense investigation. Several factors influence the binding of these ligands resulting in post-ligand binding modifications that initiate downstream signal transduction pathways.

(oseltamivir) resistance among human seasonal H1N1 and 2009 pandemic H1N1 viruses circulating in several countries in Europe and North America, as well as in some highly virulent avian H5N1 viruses, has been reported.[2-4] Similarly, after the introduction of lamivudine, adefovir, entecavir, and telbivudine, the antiviral drugs against Hepatitis B virus in 1998, 2002, 2005 and 2006 respectively, as many as 30–60% of Hepatitis B viruses became resistant.[5-7] Similarly, rapid generation of resistant viruses following treatment of patients with hepatitis C virus with protease inhibitors has been reported.[8-11] Cross-resistance to other drugs of choice within the same class of drugs has also limited our ability to develop new classes of drugs. Hence, there is an urgent need for development of new generation antiviral drugs as well as other novel preventive and therapeutic strategies. Given the limitations with targeting the virus due to the emergence of resistant viruses, focusing on stimulating host innate antiviral defenses has become an attractive alternate approach, as it is now well recognized that the innate immune system is crucial to the survival of species (Fig. 1).

As microbial pathogens differ in their habitats, metabolic requirements, and tropisms, host pathogen sensors or pattern recognition receptors (PRRs) that recognize pathogen associated molecular patterns (PAMPs) evolved and localized in various cellular compartments to protect the host against infectious agents.[12-17] In this chapter, we primarily focus on the nucleic acid sensors and their ligands that activate innate antiviral responses (Table 1); other antiviral approaches utilizing siRNA and microRNA against viral and host factors will not be considered here.[18-22]

Recognition of nucleic acids by host innate immune sensors results in conformational change in PRRs followed by a series of well-defined signal transduction events. The outcome of nucleic acid PAMPs-PRRs interaction is a rapid induction of type 1 interferon and interferon stimulated genes (ISGs) that promote an antiviral state and initiate an inflammatory response. We will discuss below individual pathogen sensor families, their ligands, and their potential utility as antiviral agents. The structure, function and activation cascades of these families are covered in detail in other chapters and hence, we will discuss them only briefly.

Table 1. Pathogen sensors and their ligands in antiviral immunity

PRRs		Natural/Synthetic Agonists	Viruses Used in Antiviral Studies
RLRs	RIG-I	5'PPP-ssRNA, short dsRNA	IAV,[43] HCV,[45] SeV,[48] NDV,[24] Ebola,[44] RSV,[47] VSV[49]
	MDA5	Poly (I:C), Long dsRNA	ECMV[53]
2'5'-OAS		dsRNA	HIV[74,75]
NLRs	NOD2	ssRNA	RSV, IAV and VSV[57]
TLRs	TLR3	dsRNA, poly (I:C),	Dengue,[156] Influenza,[29,109,157] HIV,[158] HSV-2,[159,160] Rift Valley virus,[106] RSV[161]
	TLR7/8	ssRNA, Imiquimod	Influenza,[162] Dengue,[163] HCV,[119] HSV[164,165]
	TLR9	CpGDNA	Vaccinia,[135] RSV,[136] Tacoribe Arena Virus,[137] HSV2,[166-169] FMDV,[138] influenza[134]

Some of the examples of ligands of PRRs that are utilized in proof-of-concept studies to demonstrate their antiviral activity in vitro and in vivo.

Cytosolic RNA Sensors

Retinoic Acid Inducible Gene-I Like Receptor (RLR) Agonists

The RLR family of cytoplasmic sensors includes retinoic acid-inducible gene 1 protein (RIG-I), Melanoma Differentiation-Associated protein 5 (MDA5) and laboratory of genetics and physiology-2 (LGP-2) which are specialized to recognize and provide protection against RNA viruses.[23-26] These sensors are characterized by a centrally located DExH-box helicase motif and all three members contain a C-terminal repressor domain. Both RIG-I and MDA5, which are critical for host protection against a number of RNA viruses, also contain two N-terminal caspase activation and recruitment domains that link ligand binding to downstream signaling. RIG-I has been shown to trigger antiviral responses against both negative- or positive-sense strands of RNA viruses such as influenza A and B, Japanese encephalitis virus (JEV), Sendai virus, Vesicular Stomatitis Virus (VSV), Hepatitis C virus (HCV), Respiratory syncytial virus (RSV), and Newcastle Disease Virus (NDV) while MDA5 has been shown to detect picornaviruses.[27-36] The ability of these sensors to detect non-overlapping subsets of viruses suggests that RIG-I and MDA5 specifically recognize nucleic acid motifs present in viral genomes, replication intermediates and transcripts.[37,38] RIG-I ligands have been the most well studied and include both short dsRNA and ssRNA containing a 5'PPP- group or with secondary structural motifs and/or poly-U motifs.[30,39-42] MDA5 has been found to detect long dsRNA while very little is known about LGP2 ligands and their role in viral infection.

Recent advances in understanding the molecular details of the activation of RLRs have prompted increased interest in the potential use of their ligands as prophylactic and therapeutic agents against viral infection. In vitro transcribed ssRNA with a 5'PPP group (5'PPP-RNA) significantly inhibited in vitro growth (in primary and transformed lung epithelial cells) not only of wild-type influenza A and influenza B viruses but also of various drug-resistant strains[43] including human seasonal H1N1 and H3N2, the 1918 and 2009 pandemic, and highly pathogenic avian H5N1 strains.[43] These findings suggest that irrespective of type or subtypes, drug-susceptibility status, or in vivo virulence, the replication of influenza viruses was inhibited by 5'PPP-RNA. Moreover, 5'PPP-RNA treatment also prevented 2009 H1N1 virus replication in an in vivo mouse model.

Prior treatment of A549 cells either with RIG-I ligand, 5'PPP-RNA or constitutively active N-terminal RIG-I domain delivered as a plasmid construct or in an adenoviral vector, induced IFN β and RIG-I and suppressed the expression of Ebola virus virulence factor vp35 and significantly inhibited the replication of Ebola virus in vitro.[44] Similarly, activation of the RIG-I pathway with poly U/UC RNA induced a hepatic innate antiviral immune response as measured by type 1 IFN in serum and RIG-I, ISG 54 and ISG 56 expression in hepatic cells in vivo in wild-type but not in RIG-I KO mice. Furthermore, RIG-I activation in human hepatocarcinoma cells (huh-7) with poly U/UC RNA triggered interferon and ISG expression that reduced HCV RNA in vitro indicating that HCV is susceptible to RIG-I-induced antiviral responses.[45] RIG-I activation has also shown to inhibit the replication of NDV, FeV, RSV and VSV[46-49] (Table 1).

Another member of RIG-I family, MDA-5 has been shown to play a critical role in protection against NDV, VSV and ECMV (Encephalomyocarditis virus) in vitro as well as in vivo using gene knockout mice.[50,51] While the nature of the ligand is not known, dsRNA longer than 180 bp without 5' modifications unlike RIG-I appears to activate MDA-5.[52] Direct inhibition of ECMV replication in response to MDA5 ligand poly I:C has been documented recently.[53]

The ongoing emergence of seasonal as well as pandemic influenza viruses that are resistant to one or both classes of currently approved influenza antiviral drugs, the emergence of drug-resistant strains of HBV, HCV and other viruses during the course of treatment, and lack of effective antiviral drugs against highly contagious and pathogenic viruses such as Ebola underscore the importance of developing novel strategies to prevent, control and treat viral infections. Developing small molecules that activate the RIG-I pathway certainly offer a broad spectrum approach as they will have broader utility against several viral diseases independent of the genetic makeup, pathogenicity and drug-sensitivity status. Since RIG-I sensing of viral ligands is evolutionarily conserved, generation of resistant viruses is less likely.

Innate immune response triggered by RLR agonists provides an optimal microenvironment to initiate adaptive immune responses against viral infection. Hence, RLR agonists also have potential application as vaccine adjuvants. H5N1 DNA vaccines co-expressing H5N1 influenza virus HA antigen and various RIG-I agonists from RNA polymerase III promoters showed enhanced humoral immune responses in mice.[54] These studies clearly demonstrate the potential utility of activating the RIG-I pathway for broad spectrum antiviral activity as well as molecular adjuvants to vaccines.

NOD-Like Receptor Ligands

NOD-like receptors (NLRs) are another group of cytosolic PRRs that contain a C-terminal Leucine-rich repeats (LRR) domain that senses pathogen components, a centrally located NACHT domain responsible for self-oligomerization, and an N-terminal effector domain that mediates protein-protein interactions for initiating downstream signaling.[55] Activation of these receptors induces the formation of inflammasomes and production of pro-inflammatory cytokines.[56] Although a majority of NLRs recognize bacterial protein or carbohydrate components, NOD2 has been shown to bind ssRNA in vitro and induce type 1 IFN via the inflammasome pathway. Viral RNA has been proposed to be a ligand for NLRP3.[57] While NLRC5 has been shown to function as both positive as well as negative regulator, NLRX1 has been shown to be a negative regulator of type 1 IFN.[58-64] The precise nature of the natural viral ligands, if any, that activate NOD2, NLRC5 and NLRX1 is not known.

RNA-Dependent Protein Kinase (PKR) Ligands

The IFN-inducible, double-stranded (ds) RNA-dependent protein kinase R (PKR) is one of the key sensors of the cellular antiviral response. PKR contains two N-terminal dsRNA binding motifs (dsRBM), a linker domain, and a C-terminal kinase domain.[65] Upon binding viral or synthetic dsRNA, PKR undergoes a conformational change thereby exposing its C-terminal kinase domain. This active conformation then binds and phosphorylates the serine at position 51 of eukaryotic initiation factor 2α (eIF2α) which inhibits the initiation of translation and induces apoptosis.[66]

PKR ligands can either activate or inhibit the kinase domain. The VA$_1$ RNA of adenovirus and small synthetic RNAs have been shown to be PKR kinase-inhibiting ligands. The inhibitory ligands bind to only one of the dsRBMs suggesting that kinase activation requires simultaneous binding of both dsRBMs.[67] PKR has also been shown to be activated by many non-RNA molecules such as heparin, dextran sulfate, and poly-L-glutamate, tumor necrosis factor (TNF)-α, interleukin (IL)-1β, IFN-γ and the bacterial product lipopolysaccharide (LPS).[68,69] In the case of RNA ligands, requirement for a 5' triphosphate (5' PPP) RNA for PKR activation depends on structure. For dsRNA molecules that contain a 5'PPP, a minimum of 33 bp are required for induction while approximately 80 bp are required for optimal induction by unphosphorylated RNAs. Smaller RNAs can activate PKR as long as they contain at least 16 bp and a 5'PPP.[70] PKR can detect a wide range of viral RNA ligands and most likely there is overlap in the detection of PKR ligands with other PRRs, namely RIG-I, MDA5, TLR3, and 2'-5'OAS as they are also known to bind dsRNA. The precise nature of the ligands that specifically bind and activate PKR but not other PRRs is unknown. Hence, antiviral responses induced by dsRNA such as poly I:C cannot be totally attributed to the activation of PKR.

2'-5' Oligoadenylate Synthetase (2'-5'OAS)/RNase L Ligands

The OAS/RNase system has evolved to recognize viral dsRNAs and degrade them, thereby preventing the replication of viral genomes and synthesis of viral proteins.[71] OAS/RNase degradation of dsRNAs generate small duplex RNA species that are sensed by other PRRs leading to the induction of IFN. OAS family consists of at least 10 members encoded by three genes. The expression of 2'-5' oligoadenylate synthetase (2'-5'OAS) family members is further induced by IFN. The potential RNAs that are recognized by OAS/RNase L system include dsRNA genomes, dsRNA intermediaries, annealed ssRNAs or ssRNAs that form stem structures. The main function of OAS is to bind RNase L which leads to dimerization and activation of RNase L. Activated RNase L degrades both cellular and viral RNAs in the cytoplasm thus inhibiting viral replication.[72,73]

The ligands for 2'-5'OAS are dsRNA and the same ligands that have been reported to be recognized by the PRRs TLR3, MDA5 and RIG-I. Interestingly, several studies have looked also at the use of more stable and nuclease resistant derivatives of 2–5A as antivirals that specifically target the 2'-5'OAS pathway. Phosphorothioate/ phosphodiester 2–5A derivates have been used to specifically target RNase L and reduce HIV replication in T cells.[74] The synthetic compound, 2–5A[N6B], which is also stable and nuclease resistant, has also been shown to reduce HIV replication and have less cytotoxicity.[75] While theses 2–5A derivatives have been shown to reduce HIV titers it is quite possible for these compounds to also mediate an antiviral effect for other viruses. Since OAS expression is enhanced by IFN, microbial PAMPS or synthetic compounds that activate PRRs to induce IFN, can also activate OAS.[76-78]

Cytosolic DNA Sensors

Unlike RNA sensors, cytosolic receptors that recognize DNA have only recently been described. DAI (also called DLM-1) was the first DNA cytosolic sensor reported to induce type 1 interferon in response to dsDNA when overexpressed in cells.[79] However, DAI deficiency did not affect type 1 interferon induction.[80] The second DNA sensor present in the cytosol was identified as AIM2 (absent in melanoma 2) which can be activated by DNA from various sources. Activation follows interaction with apoptosis-associated speck-like protein containing a CARD (ASC), a component of inflammasomes, and leads to induction of proinflammatory cytokines.[81-84] In addition to AIM2, another PYHIN family protein, IFI16 was identified as DNA sensor also present in cytoplasm.[85] However, unlike AIM2 activation, which results in pro-inflammatory cytokine production via an inflammasome pathway, IFI16 recognition of viral DNA motifs results in interferon induction. LRRFIP1 is a recently identified nucleic acid binding protein present in cytosol that recognizes an AT-rich B-form of dsDNA,GC-rich Z-form dsDNA.[86] DNA recognition triggers a β-Catenin-dependent type 1 interferon induction. Despite the discovery of these cytosolic DNA sensors and their ligands, their precise role in host antiviral innate defenses have yet to be elucidated.

Endosomal Nucleic Acid Sensors

In addition to the cytosolic nucleic acid sensing PRRs, pathogen sensing is performed by PRRs that are located in the endosomal compartments. These PRRs, namely TLRs 3, 7/8 and 9, recognize dsRNA, ssRNA, and unmethylated DNA respectively.[87-92] The transmembrane protein UNC93B1 transports these TLRs from the ER to the endosomes where they become activated by proteolytic cleavage.[93-97]

TLR3 was the first nucleic acid-recognizing endosomal nucleic acid sensor found to be involved in virus recognition.[98] Although it is present predominantly on endosomal membranes in various subsets of dendritic cells and macrophages, plasma membrane expression has also been demonstrated in fibroblasts, astrocytes and epithelial cells following virus infection.[99-104] TLR3 has been shown to sense and bind to dsRNA generated during replication of many RNA and DNA viruses.[98,105] TLR3 agonists, such as poly I:C have shown promise in providing protection against infections by a number of viruses including HSV2, HIV, Dengue and Rift Valley fever virus, rabies virus, Venezuelan equine encephalomyelitis virus, RSV, and influenza virus in prophylactic and therapeutic settings.[106-108] For example, pre-treatment of mice with poly I:C completely protected them against lethal challenge with influenza A H3N2 and laboratory-adapted H1N1 virsues and therapeutic efficacy of poly(I:C) was evaluated against highly virulent influenza viruses.[109-112] These studies clearly show that TLR3 activation is effective against several different viruses. In addition, topical application of TLR3 ligands for the treatment of genital warts and actinic keratosis, a premalignant condition of the skin, is also being pursued.

TLR7 is upregulated during inflammation and is highly expressed in plasmacytoid dendritic cells (pDCs), which are major IFNα/β producers. TLR7 ligands, either natural or synthetic small molecule agonists have become attractive immunomodulatory and antiviral candidates for the treatment of not only viral infections, but also other diseases.[113-118]

Activation of TLR7 with ligands has been previously shown to reduce HCV titers in cell lines in vitro, inhibition of influenza A virus replication in a chicken macrophage cell line, reduced persistence, clearance of herpes simplex virus (HSV), cutaneous leishmaniasis, Rift Valley Fever virus and vesiculostomatitis virus in preclinical studies. Resolution of papilloma virus-induced warts, Hepatitis C and Dengue virus and improved disease progression were observed once treated with TLR7 ligands.[119-122] Since TLR7 signaling plays an important role in the shaping of the adaptive immune response,[123-126] TLR7 ligands have been used as vaccine adjuvants in a number of preclinical studies. TLR7 ligands have been used in several studies to modulate immune responses when combined with influenza and HIV vaccines to generate both cellular and humoral immunity.[114,123,124,127-130]

TLR9 is predominantly present in plasmacytoid dentritic cells (pDCs) and B cells and detects viral or bacterial DNA that contains non-methylated CpG motifs.[131,132] Such motifs are absent or suppressed in eukaryotes. Detection of CpG motifs by TLR9 triggers IFN-dependent host defense. Prophylactic treatment with CpG oligodeoxynucleotides (CpG-ODN) protected mice against lethal challenge with vaccinia virus, RSVherpes simplex virus type-2 (HSV-2) and influenza virus.[133-136] Similarly, CpG-ODN protected newborn mice from a lethal challenge of neurotropic Tacaribe arena virus and has also been used to treat acute retroviral infection with Friend retrovirus.[137,138] CpG-ODN treatment 4 d after infection resulted in significant recovery (up to 74%) with reduced virus load in blood and spleen of treated mice. These studies suggest that TLR9 ligands have a great potential to be used as broad spectrum clinical immunomodulator against a number of infectious agents. Apart from direct antiviral activity, TLR9 ligands, have also been used in vaccination strategies either as a part of a DNA vaccine or combined with protein antigens to improve their immunogenicity as CpG-ODN upregulate costimulatory molecules, Th1 response as well as IFN-induced genes to prime adaptive immune system, thus exhibiting strong adjuvant and immunomodulatory properties.[139-144]

Non-Nucleic Acid Binding PRRs in Antiviral Immunity

Activation of PRRs is a prerequisite for early antiviral defense. While endosomal TLRs 3, 7, 8 and 9 and cytosolic PRRs, RLRs, and NLRs play pivotal roles in detecting nucleic acids produced during viral infections, several other PRRs are known to recognize non-nucleic acids and activate antiviral responses such as TLR4 that recognizes RSV F protein.[145,146] Likewise, administration of TLR4 ligands is known to inhibit the replication of Hepatitis B virus in a type 1 interferon-dependent manner in Hepatitis B transgenic mice suggesting its potential utility as an antiviral strategy, although the precise mechanism of viral clearance is not clear. The antiviral effects may be through the secretion of antimicrobial peptides such as defensins that have been shown to possess antiviral functions through direct lysis of the virus.[12,147-154] Pro-thymosin α (a small acidic protein produced and released by CD8+ T cells) acts as a ligand for TLR4 and can potently inhibit HIV-1 via TLR4-mediated type 1 interferon induction.[155] Since the majority of membrane bound PRRs, TLRs 2, 4, 5 and 6 and lectin receptors on recognition of PAMPs induce proinflammatory cytokines and chemokines, they are being explored extensively for their potential use as adjuvants for vaccines.

Conclusion

Triggering an immediate response following recognition of different structural components of invading microbes is the primary function of innate immunity. The presence of PRRs in various cellular and subcellular compartments endows the host with the ability to protect the structural and functional integrity of self. With the discoveries of the nature and roles of these PRRs over the last two decades, the understanding of ligand recognition can now be used to help design next generation antiviral agents and immunomodulators.

Acknowledgments

The authors thank Drs. Jacqueline M. Katz and Nancy J. Cox of the Influenza Division for their support. The findings and conclusions in this report are those of the authors and do not necessarily represent the views of the funding agency or Centers for Disease Control and Prevention.

About the Authors

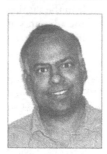

Priya Ranjan, PhD is an Associate Service Fellow in the Immunology section of Immunology and Pathology Branch of the Influenza Division, at the Centers for Disease Control and Prevention in Atlanta. He received his PhD in 2000 from The Banaras Hindu University, India, where he studied the mechanism of macrophage-mediated apoptosis in tumor cells. During 2000–2003, he worked as a postdoctoral fellow in University of Vermont, Burlington, Vermont on DNA damage and cell-cycle regulation. From 2003–2006, he worked as a postdoctoral fellow in Emory University to study transcriptional regulation of MnSOD gene at Microbiology and Immunology Department. His current research interest in Sambhara's group at CDC, Atlanta is understanding the molecular nature of Antiviral Innate Immune defenses and develop novel antiviral strategies.

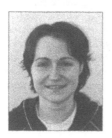

Victoria Jeisy Scott is an Emory University graduate student from the Immunology and Molecular Pathogenesis Program. She is completing her dissertation work with the Immunology section of Immunology and Pathology Branch of the Influenza Division, at the Centers for Disease Control and Prevention in Atlanta. She plans to graduate with her PhD in the spring of 2012 upon completion of her dissertation project focusing on the effect TLR7 has on influenza A infection and vaccination. She received her BS in 2006 from the University of Illinois, Urbana-Champaign.

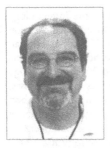

William G. Davis, PhD is an ORISE fellow working in the Immunology section of Immunology and Pathogenesis Branch of the Influenza Division at the Centers for Disease Control and Prevention in Atlanta. He earned his doctoral degree from Georgia State University investigating the role of host cellular in the replication of flaviviruses. His current studies are focused on how the cellular innate immune system is essential for the clearance of influenza viral infections.

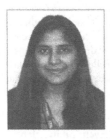

Neetu Singh is a Post-doctoral research associate in the department of Anesthesiology at SUNY, Buffalo. She is working as a guest researcher in Immunology section of Immunology and Pathology Branch of the Influenza Division, at the Centers for Disease Control and Prevention in Atlanta. She did her DVM from College of Veterinary Medicine, Pantnagar, India. She received her PhD from Purdue University in 2010 where her work was focused on development of Adenoviral vector based influenza vaccine. Soon after her PhD, she joined Dr. Sambhara's group at CDC, Atlanta (from August 2010-to date) and is working on a collaborative project (SUNY, Buffalo) investigating the mechanisms of action of ligands of Retinoic Acid Induced Gene-I (RIG-I) and their delivery with nanoparticles to stimulate antiviral defenses.

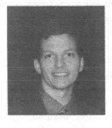

J. Bradford Bowzard, PhD is a Biologist in the Division of Preparedness and Emerging Infections at the Centers for Disease Control and Prevention in Atlanta, GA. His previous studies, in the Immunology section of the Immunology and Pathogenesis Branch of the Influenza Division, focused on understanding the mechanisms of activation of the innate immune system in response to influenza virus infection. He earned his doctoral degree from The Pennsylvania State University for work on the assembly of retroviruses and herpesviruses and completed postdoctoral work in the Department of Biochemistry at Emory University, where he was the recipient of an individual NIH NRSA for the purification and identification of the first Arl2 GTPase activating protein.

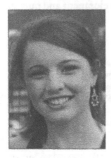

Monika Chadwick is an Honor's Program student at the Georgia Institute of Technology in Atlanta, Georgia. She was a Guest Researcher at the Centers for Disease Control and Prevention on the immunology team of the influenza division during spring of 2011. While at the CDC, she contributed to research related to the innate immune defense to influenza infection. Monika anticipates receiving her Bachelor of Science in biology from Georgia Tech in December 2012 and hopes to pursue a master's degree in public health.

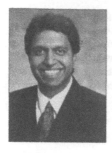

Shivaprakash Gangappa is a Senior Service Fellow in the Immunology Section of Immunology and Pathogenesis Branch of the Influenza Division at the Centers for Disease Control and Prevention (CDC) and has an adjunct faculty appointment at the Emory University School of Medicine in Atlanta, Georgia, USA. Shiva received his PhD in Viral Immunology (1994-1999) from Dr. Barry Rouse's lab at the University of Tennessee, Knoxville, Tennessee, USA. During postdoctoral fellowship in Dr. Herbert Virgin's laboratory (1999-2002) at Washington University School of Medicine, Saint Louis, Missouri, Shiva worked on viral pathogenesis. During his American Society of Microbiology fellowship (2002-2003), Shiva worked on the pathogenic mechanisms of avian influenza A viruses in Dr. Jackie Katz's laboratory at the CDC. He moved to Emory University School of Medicine (2003-2007) as an Assistant Professor where he pursued basic as well as preclinical research focusing on immune monitoring and protective immunity to viral infections in healthy and immunocompromised hosts. Currently, he is working at the CDC as a Senior Service Fellow (2007-present) on novel strategies to improve prophylactic and therapeutic measures to deal with seasonal and pandemic influenza.

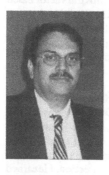

Suryaprakash Sambhara is Chief of Immunology section, Influenza Division at the Centers for Disease Control and Prevention in Atlanta, Georgia, USA. He is also an adjunct faculty member at Georgia State University and Purdue University and a member of Scientific Advisory Board, PATH for Influenza Vaccines. Prakash received his DVM (BVSc) in 1977 and MVSc in 1980 from the College of Veterinary Science, AP Agrl. University, MS in 1986 from the University of Wyoming, and a PhD in immunology from the University of Toronto. He pursued his PhD thesis work in Rick Miller's laboratory working on peripheral T-cell tolerance mechanisms. After obtaining his PhD, Prakash joined Sanofi Pasteur in 1992 as a research scientist and Section Head, Immunology at their Research and Development division in Toronto, Canada. During 1992-2000 he focused on improving influenza vaccine, developing RSV vaccine (subunit and DNA), therapeutic vaccines for melanoma and colorectal cancer, setting up human immunology platform and developing animal models of human disease. After about 9 years at Sanofi Pasteur, managing several research scientists, technologists, and programs, Prakash moved to CDC in 2000 and his research interests include Immunobiology of aging, vaccine development, adjuvants and formulations, innate and adaptive immunity to influenza, antiviral development and human immunology programs.

References

1. CDC. Update: Influenza Activity—United States, September 30, 2007–February 9, 2008. 2008. [cited 2011 November 3]; Available from: http://www.cdc.gov/mmwr/preview/mmwrhtml/mm5707a4.htm
2. de Jong MD, Tran TT, Truong HK, Vo MH, Smith GJ, Nguyen VC, et al. Oseltamivir resistance during treatment of influenza A (H5N1) infection. N Engl J Med 2005; 353:2667-72; PMID:16371632; http://dx.doi.org/10.1056/NEJMoa054512.
3. ECDC. Resistance to oseltamivir (Tamiflu) found in some European influenza virus samples. 2008 [cited 2009 July 14]; Available from: http://www.eiss.org/index.cgi
4. Baz M, Abed Y, Papenburg J, Bouhy X, Hamelin ME, Boivin G. Emergence of oseltamivir-resistant pandemic H1N1 virus during prophylaxis. N Engl J Med 2009; 361:2296-7; PMID:19907034; http://dx.doi.org/10.1056/NEJMc0910060.
5. Dienstag JL. Hepatitis B virus infection. N Engl J Med 2008; 359:1486-500; PMID:18832247; http://dx.doi.org/10.1056/NEJMra0801644.
6. Ayoub WS, Keeffe EB. Review article: current antiviral therapy of chronic hepatitis B. Aliment Pharmacol Ther 2011; 34:1145-58; PMID:21978243; http://dx.doi.org/10.1111/j.1365-2036.2011.04869.x.

7. Deng L, Tang H. Hepatitis B virus drug resistance to current nucleos(t)ide analogs: Mechanisms and mutation sites. Hepatol Res 2011; 41:1017-24; PMID:21917087; http://dx.doi.org/10.1111/j.1872-034X.2011.00873.x.

8. Rong L, Dahari H, Ribeiro RM, Perelson AS. Rapid emergence of protease inhibitor resistance in hepatitis C virus. Sci Transl Med. 2010; 2(30): 30ra2.

9. Delang L, Froeyen M, Herdewijn P, Neyts J. Identification of a novel resistance mutation for benzimidazole inhibitors of the HCV RNA-dependent RNA polymerase. Antiviral Res 2012; 93:30-8; PMID:22033247.

10. Delang L, Vliegen I, Froeyen M, Neyts J. Comparative study of the genetic barriers and pathways towards resistance of selective inhibitors of hepatitis C virus replication. Antimicrob Agents Chemother 2011; 55:4103-13; PMID:21709100; http://dx.doi.org/10.1128/AAC.00294-11.

11. Pawlotsky JM. Treatment failure and resistance with direct-acting antiviral drugs against hepatitis C virus. Hepatology 2011; 53:1742-51; PMID:21374691; http://dx.doi.org/10.1002/hep.24262.

12. Sambhara S, Lehrer RI. The innate immune system: a repository for future drugs? Expert Rev Anti Infect Ther 2007; 5:1-5; PMID:17266447; http://dx.doi.org/10.1586/14787210.5.1.1.

13. Ranjan P, Bowzard JB, Schwerzmann JW, Jeisy-Scott V, Fujita T, Sambhara S. Cytoplasmic nucleic acid sensors in antiviral immunity. Trends Mol Med 2009; 15:359-68; PMID:19665430; http://dx.doi.org/10.1016/j.molmed.2009.06.003.

14. Akira S. Innate immunity to pathogens: diversity in receptors for microbial recognition. Immunol Rev 2009; 227:5-8; PMID:19120470; http://dx.doi.org/10.1111/j.1600-065X.2008.00739.x.

15. Kawai T, Akira S. Toll-like receptors and their crosstalk with other innate receptors in infection and immunity. Immunity 2011; 34:637-50; PMID:21616434; http://dx.doi.org/10.1016/j.immuni.2011.05.006.

16. Philpott DJ, Girardin SE. Nod-like receptors: sentinels at host membranes. Curr Opin Immunol 2010; 22:428-34; PMID:20605429; http://dx.doi.org/10.1016/j.coi.2010.04.010.

17. Barber GN. Innate immune DNA sensing pathways: STING, AIMII and the regulation of interferon production and inflammatory responses. Curr Opin Immunol 2011; 23:10-20; PMID:21239155; http://dx.doi.org/10.1016/j.coi.2010.12.015.

18. Santhakumar D, Forster T, Laqtom NN, Fragkoudis R, Dickinson P, Abreu-Goodger C, et al. Combined agonist-antagonist genome-wide functional screening identifies broadly active antiviral microRNAs. Proc Natl Acad Sci U S A 2010; 107:13830-5; PMID:20643939; http://dx.doi.org/10.1073/pnas.1008861107.

19. Song L, Liu H, Gao S, Jiang W, Huang W. Cellular microRNAs inhibit replication of the H1N1 influenza A virus in infected cells. J Virol 2010; 84:8849-60; PMID:20554777; http://dx.doi.org/10.1128/JVI.00456-10.

20. Song L, Gao S, Jiang W, Chen S, Liu Y, Zhou L, et al. Silencing suppressors: viral weapons for countering host cell defenses. Protein Cell 2011; 2:273-81; PMID:21528352; http://dx.doi.org/10.1007/s13238-011-1037-y.

21. Ashfaq UA, Yousaf MZ, Aslam M, Ejaz R, Jahan S, Ullah O. siRNAs: potential therapeutic agents against hepatitis C virus. Virol J 2011; 8:276; PMID:21645341; http://dx.doi.org/10.1186/1743-422X-8-276.

22. Huang DD. The potential of RNA interference-based therapies for viral infections. Curr HIV/AIDS Rep 2008; 5:33-9; PMID:18417033; http://dx.doi.org/10.1007/s11904-008-0006-4.

23. Ramos HJ, Gale M Jr. RIG-I Like Receptors and Their Signaling Crosstalk in the Regulation of Antiviral Immunity. Curr Opin Virol 2011; 1:167-76; PMID:21949557; http://dx.doi.org/10.1016/j.coviro.2011.04.004.

24. Yoneyama M, Kikuchi M, Natsukawa T, Shinobu N, Imaizumi T, Miyagishi M, et al. The RNA helicase RIG-I has an essential function in double-stranded RNA-induced innate antiviral responses. Nat Immunol 2004; 5:730-7; PMID:15208624; http://dx.doi.org/10.1038/ni1087.

25. Satoh T, Kato H, Kumagai Y, Yoneyama M, Sato S, Matsushita K, et al. LGP2 is a positive regulator of RIG-I- and MDA5-mediated antiviral responses. Proc Natl Acad Sci U S A 2010; 107:1512-7; PMID:20080593; http://dx.doi.org/10.1073/pnas.0912986107.

26. Takeuchi O, Akira S. MDA5/RIG-I and virus recognition. Curr Opin Immunol 2008; 20:17-22; PMID:18272355; http://dx.doi.org/10.1016/j.coi.2008.01.002.

27. Kato H, Takeuchi O, Sato S, Yoneyama M, Yamamoto M, Matsui K, et al. Differential roles of MDA5 and RIG-I helicases in the recognition of RNA viruses. Nature 2006; 441:101-5; PMID:16625202; http://dx.doi.org/10.1038/nature04734.

28. Mibayashi M, Martínez-Sobrido L, Loo YM, Cárdenas WB, Gale M Jr., García-Sastre A. Inhibition of retinoic acid-inducible gene I-mediated induction of beta interferon by the NS1 protein of influenza A virus. J Virol 2007; 81:514-24; PMID:17079289; http://dx.doi.org/10.1128/JVI.01265-06.

29. Guo Z, Chen LM, Zeng H, Gomez JA, Plowden J, Fujita T, et al. NS1 protein of influenza A virus inhibits the function of intracytoplasmic pathogen sensor, RIG-I. Am J Respir Cell Mol Biol 2007; 36:263-9; PMID:17053203; http://dx.doi.org/10.1165/rcmb.2006-0283RC.
30. Pichlmair A, Schulz O, Tan CP, Näslund TI, Liljeström P, Weber F, et al. RIG-I-mediated antiviral responses to single-stranded RNA bearing 5'-phosphates. Science 2006; 314:997-1001; PMID:17038589; http://dx.doi.org/10.1126/science.1132998.
31. Opitz B, Rejaibi A, Dauber B, Eckhard J, Vinzing M, Schmeck B, et al. IFNbeta induction by influenza A virus is mediated by RIG-I which is regulated by the viral NS1 protein. Cell Microbiol 2007; 9:930-8; PMID:17140406; http://dx.doi.org/10.1111/j.1462-5822.2006.00841.x.
32. Breiman A, Grandvaux N, Lin R, Ottone C, Akira S, Yoneyama M, et al. Inhibition of RIG-I-dependent signaling to the interferon pathway during hepatitis C virus expression and restoration of signaling by IKKepsilon. J Virol 2005; 79:3969-78; PMID:15767399; http://dx.doi.org/10.1128/JVI.79.7.3969-3978.2005.
33. Foy E, Li K, Sumpter R Jr., Loo YM, Johnson CL, Wang C, et al. Control of antiviral defenses through hepatitis C virus disruption of retinoic acid-inducible gene-I signaling. Proc Natl Acad Sci U S A 2005; 102:2986-91; PMID:15710892; http://dx.doi.org/10.1073/pnas.0408707102.
34. Chang TH, Liao CL, Lin YL. Flavivirus induces interferon-beta gene expression through a pathway involving RIG-I-dependent IRF-3 and PI3K-dependent NF-kappaB activation. Microbes Infect 2006; 8:157-71; PMID:16182584; http://dx.doi.org/10.1016/j.micinf.2005.06.014.
35. Melchjorsen J, Jensen SB, Malmgaard L, Rasmussen SB, Weber F, Bowie AG, et al. Activation of innate defense against a paramyxovirus is mediated by RIG-I and TLR7 and TLR8 in a cell-type-specific manner. J Virol 2005; 79:12944-51; PMID:16188996; http://dx.doi.org/10.1128/JVI.79.20.12944-12951.2005.
36. Liu P, Jamaluddin M, Li K, Garofalo RP, Casola A, Brasier AR. Retinoic acid-inducible gene I mediates early antiviral response and Toll-like receptor 3 expression in respiratory syncytial virus-infected airway epithelial cells. J Virol 2007; 81:1401-11; PMID:17108032; http://dx.doi.org/10.1128/JVI.01740-06.
37. Baum A, Sachidanandam R, García-Sastre A. Preference of RIG-I for short viral RNA molecules in infected cells revealed by next-generation sequencing. Proc Natl Acad Sci U S A 2010; 107:16303-8; PMID:20805493; http://dx.doi.org/10.1073/pnas.1005077107.
38. Rehwinkel J, Tan CP, Goubau D, Schulz O, Pichlmair A, Bier K, et al. RIG-I detects viral genomic RNA during negative-strand RNA virus infection. Cell 2010; 140:397-408; PMID:20144762; http://dx.doi.org/10.1016/j.cell.2010.01.020.
39. Schlee M, Hartmann G. The chase for the RIG-I ligand--recent advances. Mol Ther 2010; 18:1254-62; PMID:20461060; http://dx.doi.org/10.1038/mt.2010.90.
40. Hornung V, Ellegast J, Kim S, Brzózka K, Jung A, Kato H, et al. 5'-Triphosphate RNA is the ligand for RIG-I. Science 2006; 314:994-7; PMID:17038590; http://dx.doi.org/10.1126/science.1132505.
41. Kowalinski E, Lunardi T, McCarthy AA, Louber J, Brunel J, Grigorov B, et al. Structural basis for the activation of innate immune pattern-recognition receptor RIG-I by viral RNA. Cell 2011; 147:423-35; PMID:22000019; http://dx.doi.org/10.1016/j.cell.2011.09.039.
42. Luo D, Ding SC, Vela A, Kohlway A, Lindenbach BD, Pyle AM. Structural insights into RNA recognition by RIG-I. Cell 2011; 147:409-22; PMID:22000018; http://dx.doi.org/10.1016/j.cell.2011.09.023.
43. Ranjan P, Jayashankar L, Deyde V, Zeng H, Davis WG, Pearce MB, et al. 5'PPP-RNA induced RIG-I activation inhibits drug-resistant avian H5N1 as well as 1918 and 2009 pandemic influenza virus replication. Virol J 2010; 7:102; PMID:20492658; http://dx.doi.org/10.1186/1743-422X-7-102.
44. Spiropoulou CF, Ranjan P, Pearce MB, Sealy TK, Albariño CG, Gangappa S, et al. RIG-I activation inhibits ebolavirus replication. Virology 2009; 392:11-5; PMID:19628240; http://dx.doi.org/10.1016/j.virol.2009.06.032.
45. Saito T, Owen DM, Jiang F, Marcotrigiano J, Gale M Jr. Innate immunity induced by composition-dependent RIG-I recognition of hepatitis C virus RNA. Nature 2008; 454:523-7; PMID:18548002; http://dx.doi.org/10.1038/nature07106.
46. Yoneyama M, Fujita T. Cytoplasmic double-stranded DNA sensor. Nat Immunol 2007; 8:907-8; PMID:17712341; http://dx.doi.org/10.1038/ni0907-907.
47. Loo YM, Fornek J, Crochet N, Bajwa G, Perwitasari O, Martinez-Sobrido L, et al. Distinct RIG-I and MDA5 signaling by RNA viruses in innate immunity. J Virol 2008; 82:335-45; PMID:17942531; http://dx.doi.org/10.1128/JVI.01080-07.
48. Kato H, Sato S, Yoneyama M, Yamamoto M, Uematsu S, Matsui K, et al. Cell type-specific involvement of RIG-I in antiviral response. Immunity 2005; 23:19-28; PMID:16039576; http://dx.doi.org/10.1016/j.immuni.2005.04.010.
49. Hwang SY, Sun HY, Lee KH, Oh BH, Cha YJ, Kim BH, et al. 5'-Triphosphate-RNA-independent activation of RIG-I via RNA aptamer with enhanced antiviral activity. Nucleic Acids Res 2011, Epub ahead of print; PMID:22127865; http://dx.doi.org/10.1093/nar/gkr1098.

50. Yoneyama M, Kikuchi M, Matsumoto K, Imaizumi T, Miyagishi M, Taira K, et al. Shared and unique functions of the DExD/H-box helicases RIG-I, MDA5, and LGP2 in antiviral innate immunity. J Immunol 2005; 175:2851-8; PMID:16116171.

51. Andrejeva J, Poole E, Young DF, Goodbourn S, Randall RE. The p127 subunit (DDB1) of the UV-DNA damage repair binding protein is essential for the targeted degradation of STAT1 by the V protein of the paramyxovirus simian virus 5. J Virol 2002; 76:11379-86; PMID:12388698; http://dx.doi.org/10.1128/JVI.76.22.11379-11386.2002.

52. Kato H, Takeuchi O, Mikamo-Satoh E, Hirai R, Kawai T, Matsushita K, et al. Length-dependent recognition of double-stranded ribonucleic acids by retinoic acid-inducible gene-I and melanoma differentiation-associated gene 5. J Exp Med 2008; 205:1601-10; PMID:18591409; http://dx.doi.org/10.1084/jem.20080091.

53. Gitlin L, Barchet W, Gilfillan S, Cella M, Beutler B, Flavell RA, et al. Essential role of mda-5 in type I IFN responses to polyriboinosinic:polyribocytidylic acid and encephalomyocarditis picornavirus. Proc Natl Acad Sci U S A 2006; 103:8459-64; PMID:16714379; http://dx.doi.org/10.1073/pnas.0603082103.

54. Luke JM, Simon GG, Söderholm J, Errett JS, August JT, Gale M Jr., et al. Coexpressed RIG-I agonist enhances humoral immune response to influenza virus DNA vaccine. J Virol 2011; 85:1370-83; PMID:21106745; http://dx.doi.org/10.1128/JVI.01250-10.

55. Harton JA, Linhoff MW, Zhang J, Ting JP. Cutting edge: CATERPILLER: a large family of mammalian genes containing CARD, pyrin, nucleotide-binding, and leucine-rich repeat domains. J Immunol 2002; 169:4088-93; PMID:12370334.

56. Kanneganti TD. Central roles of NLRs and inflammasomes in viral infection. Nat Rev Immunol 2010; 10:688-98; PMID:20847744; http://dx.doi.org/10.1038/nri2851.

57. Sabbah A, Chang TH, Harnack R, Frohlich V, Tominaga K, Dube PH, et al. Activation of innate immune antiviral responses by Nod2. Nat Immunol 2009; 10:1073-80; PMID:19701189; http://dx.doi.org/10.1038/ni.1782.

58. Cui J, Zhu L, Xia X, Wang HY, Legras X, Hong J, et al. NLRC5 negatively regulates the NF-kappaB and type I interferon signaling pathways. Cell 2010; 141:483-96; PMID:20434986; http://dx.doi.org/10.1016/j.cell.2010.03.040.

59. Neerincx A, Lautz K, Menning M, Kremmer E, Zigrino P, Hösel M, et al. A role for the human nucleotide-binding domain, leucine-rich repeat-containing family member NLRC5 in antiviral responses. J Biol Chem 2010; 285:26223-32; PMID:20538593; http://dx.doi.org/10.1074/jbc.M110.109736.

60. Rebsamen M, Vazquez J, Tardivel A, Guarda G, Curran J, Tschopp J. NLRX1/NOD5 deficiency does not affect MAVS signalling. Cell Death Differ 2011; 18:1387; PMID:21617692; http://dx.doi.org/10.1038/cdd.2011.64.

61. Parvatiyar K, Cheng G. NOD so fast: NLRX1 puts the brake on inflammation. Immunity 2011; 34:821-2; PMID:21703534; http://dx.doi.org/10.1016/j.immuni.2011.06.006.

62. Moore CB, Bergstralh DT, Duncan JA, Lei Y, Morrison TE, Zimmermann AG, et al. NLRX1 is a regulator of mitochondrial antiviral immunity. Nature 2008; 451:573-7; PMID:18200010; http://dx.doi.org/10.1038/nature06501.

63. Meylan E, Tschopp J. NLRX1: friend or foe? EMBO Rep 2008; 9:243-5; PMID:18311173; http://dx.doi.org/10.1038/embor.2008.23.

64. Allen IC, Moore CB, Schneider M, Lei Y, Davis BK, Scull MA, et al. NLRX1 protein attenuates inflammatory responses to infection by interfering with the RIG-I-MAVS and TRAF6-NF-κB signaling pathways. Immunity 2011; 34:854-65; PMID:21703540; http://dx.doi.org/10.1016/j.immuni.2011.03.026.

65. Clemens MJ, Elia A. The double-stranded RNA-dependent protein kinase PKR: structure and function. Journal of interferon & cytokine research: the official journal of the International Society for Interferon and Cytokine Research. 1997; 17(9): 503-24.

66. Hovanessian AG. On the discovery of interferon-inducible, double-stranded RNA activated enzymes: the 2'-5'oligoadenylate synthetases and the protein kinase PKR. Cytokine Growth Factor Rev 2007; 18:351-61; PMID:17681872; http://dx.doi.org/10.1016/j.cytogfr.2007.06.003.

67. Spanggord RJ, Vuyisich M, Beal PA. Identification of binding sites for both dsRBMs of PKR on kinase-activating and kinase-inhibiting RNA ligands. Biochemistry 2002; 41:4511-20; PMID:11926812; http://dx.doi.org/10.1021/bi0120594.

68. Hovanessian AG, Galabru J. The double-stranded RNA-dependent protein kinase is also activated by heparin. Eur J Biochem 1987; 167:467-73; PMID:3653103; http://dx.doi.org/10.1111/j.1432-1033.1987.tb13360.x.

69. Fasciano S, Hutchins B, Handy I, Patel RC. Identification of the heparin-binding domains of the interferon-induced protein kinase, PKR. FEBS J 2005; 272:1425-39; PMID:15752359; http://dx.doi.org/10.1111/j.1742-4658.2005.04575.x.

70. Nallagatla SR, Hwang J, Toroney R, Zheng X, Cameron CE, Bevilacqua PC. 5'-triphosphate-dependent activation of PKR by RNAs with short stem-loops. Science 2007; 318:1455-8; PMID:18048689; http://dx.doi.org/10.1126/science.1147347.

71. Silverman RH. Viral encounters with 2',5'-oligoadenylate synthetase and RNase L during the interferon antiviral response. J Virol 2007; 81:12720-9; PMID:17804500; http://dx.doi.org/10.1128/JVI.01471-07.

72. Hovanessian AG. Interferon-induced and double-stranded RNA-activated enzymes: a specific protein kinase and 2',5'-oligoadenylate synthetases. J Interferon Res 1991; 11:199-205; PMID:1717615; http://dx.doi.org/10.1089/jir.1991.11.199.

73. Lengyel P. Double-stranded RNA and interferon action. J Interferon Res 1987; 7:511-9; PMID:2445849; http://dx.doi.org/10.1089/jir.1987.7.511.

74. Sobol RW, Henderson EE, Kon N, Shao J, Hitzges P, Mordechai E, et al. Inhibition of HIV-1 replication and activation of RNase L by phosphorothioate/phosphodiester 2',5'-oligoadenylate derivatives. J Biol Chem 1995; 270:5963-78; PMID:7890727; http://dx.doi.org/10.1074/jbc.270.11.5963.

75. Dimitrova DI, Reichenbach NL, Yang X, Pfleiderer W, Charubala R, Gaughan JP, et al. Inhibition of HIV type 1 replication in CD4+ and CD14+ cells purified from HIV type 1-infected individuals by the 2-5A agonist immunomodulator, 2-5A(N6B). AIDS Res Hum Retroviruses 2007; 23:123-34; PMID:17263642; http://dx.doi.org/10.1089/aid.2005.0091.*

76. Li XL, Ezelle HJ, Hsi TY, Hassel BA. A central role for RNA in the induction and biological activities of type 1 interferons. Wiley Interdiscip Rev RNA 2011; 2:58-78; PMID:21956969; http://dx.doi.org/10.1002/wrna.32.

77. Horsmans Y, Berg T, Desager JP, Mueller T, Schott E, Fletcher SP, et al. Isatoribine, an agonist of TLR7, reduces plasma virus concentration in chronic hepatitis C infection. Hepatology 2005; 42:724-31; PMID:16116638; http://dx.doi.org/10.1002/hep.20839.

78. Schaefer TM, Fahey JV, Wright JA, Wira CR. Innate immunity in the human female reproductive tract: antiviral response of uterine epithelial cells to the TLR3 agonist poly(I:C). J Immunol 2005; 174:992-1002; PMID:15634923.

79. Takaoka A, Wang Z, Choi MK, Yanai H, Negishi H, Ban T, et al. DAI (DLM-1/ZBP1) is a cytosolic DNA sensor and an activator of innate immune response. Nature 2007; 448:501-5; PMID:17618271; http://dx.doi.org/10.1038/nature06013.

80. Ishii KJ, Kawagoe T, Koyama S, Matsui K, Kumar H, Kawai T, et al. TANK-binding kinase-1 delineates innate and adaptive immune responses to DNA vaccines. Nature 2008; 451:725-9; PMID:18256672; http://dx.doi.org/10.1038/nature06537.

81. Hornung V, Ablasser A, Charrel-Dennis M, Bauernfeind F, Horvath G, Caffrey DR, et al. AIM2 recognizes cytosolic dsDNA and forms a caspase-1-activating inflammasome with ASC. Nature 2009; 458:514-8; PMID:19158675; http://dx.doi.org/10.1038/nature07725.

82. Bürckstümmer T, Baumann C, Blüml S, Dixit E, Dürnberger G, Jahn H, et al. An orthogonal proteomic-genomic screen identifies AIM2 as a cytoplasmic DNA sensor for the inflammasome. Nat Immunol 2009; 10:266-72; PMID:19158679; http://dx.doi.org/10.1038/ni.1702.

83. Fernandes-Alnemri T, Yu JW, Datta P, Wu J, Alnemri ES. AIM2 activates the inflammasome and cell death in response to cytoplasmic DNA. Nature 2009; 458:509-13; PMID:19158676; http://dx.doi.org/10.1038/nature07710.

84. Jones JW, Kayagaki N, Broz P, Henry T, Newton K, O'Rourke K, et al. Absent in melanoma 2 is required for innate immune recognition of Francisella tularensis. Proc Natl Acad Sci U S A 2010; 107:9771-6; PMID:20457908; http://dx.doi.org/10.1073/pnas.1003738107.

85. Unterholzner L, Keating SE, Baran M, Horan KA, Jensen SB, Sharma S, et al. IFI16 is an innate immune sensor for intracellular DNA. Nat Immunol 2010; 11:997-1004; PMID:20890285; http://dx.doi.org/10.1038/ni.1932.

86. Yang P, An H, Liu X, Wen M, Zheng Y, Rui Y, et al. The cytosolic nucleic acid sensor LRRFIP1 mediates the production of type I interferon via a beta-catenin-dependent pathway. Nat Immunol 2010; 11:487-94; PMID:20453844; http://dx.doi.org/10.1038/ni.1876.

87. Diebold SS, Kaisho T, Hemmi H, Akira S, Reis e Sousa C. Innate antiviral responses by means of TLR7-mediated recognition of single-stranded RNA. Science 2004; 303(5663):1529-31. PMID:14976261.

88. Heil F, Hemmi H, Hochrein H, Ampenberger F, Kirschning C, Akira S, et al. Species-specific recognition of single-stranded RNA via toll-like receptor 7 and 8. Science 2004; 303(5663):1526-9. PMID:14976262.

89. Lund JM, Alexopoulou L, Sato A, Karow M, Adams NC, Gale NW, et al. Recognition of single-stranded RNA viruses by Toll-like receptor 7. Proc Natl Acad Sci U S A 2004; 101:5598-603; PMID:15034168; http://dx.doi.org/10.1073/pnas.0400937101.

90. Lee MS, Kim YJ. Signaling pathways downstream of pattern-recognition receptors and their cross talk. Annu Rev Biochem 2007; 76:447-80; PMID:17328678; http://dx.doi.org/10.1146/annurev.biochem.76.060605.122847.

91. Saitoh S, Miyake K. Regulatory molecules required for nucleotide-sensing Toll-like receptors. Immunol Rev 2009; 227:32-43; PMID:19120473; http://dx.doi.org/10.1111/j.1600-065X.2008.00729.x.

92. Sanjuan MA, Milasta S, Green DR. Toll-like receptor signaling in the lysosomal pathways. Immunol Rev 2009; 227:203-20; PMID:19120486; http://dx.doi.org/10.1111/j.1600-065X.2008.00732.x.

93. Akashi-Takamura S, Miyake K. TLR accessory molecules. Curr Opin Immunol 2008; 20:420-5; PMID:18625310; http://dx.doi.org/10.1016/j.coi.2008.07.001.

94. Brinkmann MM, Spooner E, Hoebe K, Beutler B, Ploegh HL, Kim YM. The interaction between the ER membrane protein UNC93B and TLR3, 7, and 9 is crucial for TLR signaling. J Cell Biol 2007; 177:265-75; PMID:17452530; http://dx.doi.org/10.1083/jcb.200612056.

95. Fukui R, Saitoh S, Kanno A, Onji M, Shibata T, Ito A, et al. Unc93B1 restricts systemic lethal inflammation by orchestrating Toll-like receptor 7 and 9 trafficking. Immunity 2011; 35:69-81; PMID:21683627; http://dx.doi.org/10.1016/j.immuni.2011.05.010.

96. Sasai M, Iwasaki A. Love triangle between Unc93B1, TLR7, and TLR9 prevents fatal attraction. Immunity 2011; 35:3-5; PMID:21777792; http://dx.doi.org/10.1016/j.immuni.2011.07.006.

97. Kim YM, Brinkmann MM, Paquet ME, Ploegh HL. UNC93B1 delivers nucleotide-sensing toll-like receptors to endolysosomes. Nature 2008; 452:234-8; PMID:18305481; http://dx.doi.org/10.1038/nature06726.

98. Alexopoulou L, Holt AC, Medzhitov R, Flavell RA. Recognition of double-stranded RNA and activation of NF-kappaB by Toll-like receptor 3. Nature 2001; 413:732-8; PMID:11607032; http://dx.doi.org/10.1038/35099560.

99. Lee HK, Dunzendorfer S, Soldau K, Tobias PS. Double-stranded RNA-mediated TLR3 activation is enhanced by CD14. Immunity 2006; 24:153-63; PMID:16473828; http://dx.doi.org/10.1016/j.immuni.2005.12.012.

100. Nishiya T, Kajita E, Miwa S, Defranco AL. TLR3 and TLR7 are targeted to the same intracellular compartments by distinct regulatory elements. J Biol Chem 2005; 280:37107-17; PMID:16105838; http://dx.doi.org/10.1074/jbc.M504951200.

101. Jack CS, Arbour N, Manusow J, Montgrain V, Blain M, McCrea E, et al. TLR signaling tailors innate immune responses in human microglia and astrocytes. J Immunol 2005; 175:4320-30; PMID:16177072.

102. Matsumoto M, Kikkawa S, Kohase M, Miyake K, Seya T. Establishment of a monoclonal antibody against human Toll-like receptor 3 that blocks double-stranded RNA-mediated signaling. Biochem Biophys Res Commun 2002; 293:1364-9; PMID:12054664; http://dx.doi.org/10.1016/S0006-291X(02)00380-7.

103. Groskreutz DJ, Monick MM, Powers LS, Yarovinsky TO, Look DC, Hunninghake GW. Respiratory syncytial virus induces TLR3 protein and protein kinase R, leading to increased double-stranded RNA responsiveness in airway epithelial cells. J Immunol 2006; 176:1733-40; PMID:16424203.

104. Hewson CA, Jardine A, Edwards MR, Laza-Stanca V, Johnston SL. Toll-like receptor 3 is induced by and mediates antiviral activity against rhinovirus infection of human bronchial epithelial cells. J Virol 2005; 79:12273-9; PMID:16160153; http://dx.doi.org/10.1128/JVI.79.19.12273-12279.2005.

105. Weber F, Wagner V, Rasmussen SB, Hartmann R, Paludan SR. Double-stranded RNA is produced by positive-strand RNA viruses and DNA viruses but not in detectable amounts by negative-strand RNA viruses. J Virol 2006; 80:5059-64; PMID:16641297; http://dx.doi.org/10.1128/JVI.80.10.5059-5064.2006.

106. Kende M. Prophylactic and therapeutic efficacy of poly(I,C)-LC against Rift Valley fever virus infection in mice. J Biol Response Mod 1985; 4:503-11; PMID:2416883.

107. Stephen EL, Hilmas DE, Levy HB, Spertzel RO. Protective and toxic effects of a nuclease-resistant derivative of polyriboinosinic-polyribocytidylic acid on Venezuelan equine encephalomyelitis virus in rhesus monkeys. J Infect Dis 1979; 139:267-72; PMID:109544; http://dx.doi.org/10.1093/infdis/139.3.267.

108. Guerrero-Plata A, Baron S, Poast JS, Adegboyega PA, Casola A, Garofalo RP. Activity and regulation of alpha interferon in respiratory syncytial virus and human metapneumovirus experimental infections. J Virol 2005; 79:10190-9; PMID:16051812; http://dx.doi.org/10.1128/JVI.79.16.10190-10199.2005.

109. Wong JP, Christopher ME, Viswanathan S, Karpoff N, Dai X, Das D, et al. Activation of toll-like receptor signaling pathway for protection against influenza virus infection. Vaccine 2009; 27:3481-3; PMID:19200852; http://dx.doi.org/10.1016/j.vaccine.2009.01.048.

110. Wong JP, Nagata LP, Christopher ME, Salazar AM, Dale RM. Prophylaxis of acute respiratory virus infections using nucleic acid-based drugs. Vaccine 2005; 23:2266-8; PMID:15755608; http://dx.doi.org/10.1016/j.vaccine.2005.01.037.

111. Wong JP, Saravolac EG, Sabuda D, Levy HB, Kende M. Prophylactic and therapeutic efficacies of poly(IC.LC) against respiratory influenza A virus infection in mice. Antimicrob Agents Chemother 1995; 39:2574-6; PMID:8585749.

112. Wong JP, Yang H, Nagata L, Kende M, Levy H, Schnell G, et al. Liposome-mediated immunotherapy against respiratory influenza virus infection using double-stranded RNA poly ICLC. Vaccine 1999; 17:1788-95; PMID:10194841; http://dx.doi.org/10.1016/S0264-410X(98)00439-3.

113. Xagorari A, Chlichlia K. Toll-like receptors and viruses: induction of innate antiviral immune responses. Open Microbiol J 2008; 2:49-59; PMID:19088911; http://dx.doi.org/10.2174/1874285800802010049.

114. Ichinohe T. Respective roles of TLR, RIG-I and NLRP3 in influenza virus infection and immunity: impact on vaccine design. Expert Rev Vaccines 2010; 9:1315-24; PMID:21087109; http://dx.doi.org/10.1586/erv.10.118.

115. Hiraguchi Y, Tanida H, Hosoki K, Nagao M, Tokuda R, Fujisawa T. Inhibition of eosinophil activation mediated by a Toll-like receptor 7 ligand with a combination of procaterol and budesonide. Int Arch Allergy Immunol 2011; 155(Suppl 1):85-9; PMID:21646801; http://dx.doi.org/10.1159/000327438.

116. Van LP, Bardel E, Gregoire S, Vanoirbeek J, Schneider E, Dy M, et al. Treatment with the TLR7 agonist R848 induces regulatory T-cell-mediated suppression of established asthma symptoms. Eur J Immunol 2011; 41:1992-9; PMID:21480211; http://dx.doi.org/10.1002/eji.201040914.

117. Fotin-Mleczek M, Duchardt KM, Lorenz C, Pfeiffer R, Ojkić-Zrna S, Probst J, et al. Messenger RNA-based vaccines with dual activity induce balanced TLR-7 dependent adaptive immune responses and provide antitumor activity. J Immunother 2011; 34:1-15; PMID:21150709; http://dx.doi.org/10.1097/CJI.0b013e3181f7dbe8.

118. Hayashi T, Chan M, Norton JT, Wu CC, Yao S, Cottam HB, et al. Additive melanoma suppression with intralesional phospholipid-conjugated TLR7 agonists and systemic IL-2. Melanoma Res 2010; Epub ahead of print; PMID:21030882.

119. Lee J, Wu CC, Lee KJ, Chuang TH, Katakura K, Liu YT, et al. Activation of anti-hepatitis C virus responses via Toll-like receptor 7. Proc Natl Acad Sci U S A 2006; 103:1828-33; PMID:16446426; http://dx.doi.org/10.1073/pnas.0510801103.

120. Stewart CR, Bagnaud-Baule A, Karpala AJ, Lowther S, Mohr PG, Wise TG, et al. Toll-like receptor 7 ligands inhibit influenza a infection in chickens. J Interferon Cytokine Res 2012; 32:46-51; PMID:21929369.

121. Slade HB, Owens ML, Tomai MA, Miller RL. Imiquimod 5% cream (Aldara). Expert Opin Investig Drugs 1998; 7:437-49; PMID:15991984; http://dx.doi.org/10.1517/13543784.7.3.437.

122. Averett DR, Fletcher SP, Li W, Webber SE, Appleman JR. The pharmacology of endosomal TLR agonists in viral disease. Biochem Soc Trans 2007; 35:1468-72; PMID:18031247; http://dx.doi.org/10.1042/BST0351468.

123. Koyama S, Ishii KJ, Kumar H, Tanimoto T, Coban C, Uematsu S, et al. Differential role of TLR- and RLR-signaling in the immune responses to influenza A virus infection and vaccination. J Immunol 2007; 179:4711-20; PMID:17878370.

124. Ichinohe T, Iwasaki A, Hasegawa H. Innate sensors of influenza virus: clues to developing better intranasal vaccines. Expert Rev Vaccines 2008; 7:1435-45; PMID:18980544; http://dx.doi.org/10.1586/14760584.7.9.1435.

125. Ehrhardt C, Seyer R, Hrincius ER, Eierhoff T, Wolff T, Ludwig S. Interplay between influenza A virus and the innate immune signaling. Microbes Infect 2010; 12:81-7; PMID:19782761; http://dx.doi.org/10.1016/j.micinf.2009.09.007.

126. Seo SU, Kwon HJ, Song JH, Byun YH, Seong BL, Kawai T, et al. MyD88 signaling is indispensable for primary influenza A virus infection but dispensable for secondary infection. J Virol 2010; 84:12713-22; PMID:20943980; http://dx.doi.org/10.1128/JVI.01675-10.

127. Geeraedts F, Goutagny N, Hornung V, Severa M, de Haan A, Pool J, et al. Superior immunogenicity of inactivated whole virus H5N1 influenza vaccine is primarily controlled by Toll-like receptor signalling. PLoS Pathog 2008; 4:e1000138; PMID:18769719; http://dx.doi.org/10.1371/journal.ppat.1000138.

128. Hammerbeck DM, Burleson GR, Schuller CJ, Vasilakos JP, Tomai M, Egging E, et al. Administration of a dual toll-like receptor 7 and toll-like receptor 8 agonist protects against influenza in rats. Antiviral Res 2007; 73:1-11; PMID:16959331; http://dx.doi.org/10.1016/j.antiviral.2006.07.011.

129. Wille-Reece U, Flynn BJ, Loré K, Koup RA, Kedl RM, Mattapallil JJ, et al. HIV Gag protein conjugated to a Toll-like receptor 7/8 agonist improves the magnitude and quality of Th1 and CD8+ T cell responses in nonhuman primates. Proc Natl Acad Sci U S A 2005; 102:15190-4; PMID:16219698; http://dx.doi.org/10.1073/pnas.0507484102.

130. Wille-Reece U, Flynn BJ, Loré K, Koup RA, Miles AP, Saul A, et al. Toll-like receptor agonists influence the magnitude and quality of memory T cell responses after prime-boost immunization in nonhuman primates. J Exp Med 2006; 203:1249-58; PMID:16636134; http://dx.doi.org/10.1084/jem.20052433.

131. Liu YJ. IPC: professional type 1 interferon-producing cells and plasmacytoid dendritic cell precursors. Annu Rev Immunol 2005; 23:275-306; PMID:15771572; http://dx.doi.org/10.1146/annurev.immunol.23.021704.115633.

132. Hemmi H, Takeuchi O, Kawai T, Kaisho T, Sato S, Sanjo H, et al. A Toll-like receptor recognizes bacterial DNA. Nature 2000; 408:740-5; PMID:11130078; http://dx.doi.org/10.1038/35047123.

133. Harandi AM, Holmgren J. CpG DNA as a potent inducer of mucosal immunity: implications for immunoprophylaxis and immunotherapy of mucosal infections. Curr Opin Investig Drugs 2004; 5:141-5; PMID:15043387.

134. Dong L, Mori I, Hossain MJ, Liu B, Kimura Y. An immunostimulatory oligodeoxynucleotide containing a cytidine-guanosine motif protects senescence-accelerated mice from lethal influenza virus by augmenting the T helper type 1 response. J Gen Virol 2003; 84:1623-8; PMID:12771433; http://dx.doi.org/10.1099/vir.0.19029-0.

135. Rees DG, Gates AJ, Green M, Eastaugh L, Lukaszewski RA, Griffin KF, et al. CpG-DNA protects against a lethal orthopoxvirus infection in a murine model. Antiviral Res 2005; 65:87-95; PMID:15708635; http://dx.doi.org/10.1016/j.antiviral.2004.10.004.

136. Cho JY, Miller M, Baek KJ, Castaneda D, Nayar J, Roman M, et al. Immunostimulatory DNA sequences inhibit respiratory syncytial viral load, airway inflammation, and mucus secretion. J Allergy Clin Immunol 2001; 108:697-702; PMID:11692091; http://dx.doi.org/10.1067/mai.2001.119918.

137. Pedras-Vasconcelos JA, Goucher D, Puig M, Tonelli LH, Wang V, Ito S, et al. CpG oligodeoxynucleotides protect newborn mice from a lethal challenge with the neurotropic Tacaribe arenavirus. J Immunol 2006; 176:4940-9; PMID:16585590.

138. Olbrich AR, Schimmer S, Heeg K, Schepers K, Schumacher TN, Dittmer U. Effective postexposure treatment of retrovirus-induced disease with immunostimulatory DNA containing CpG motifs. J Virol 2002; 76:11397-404; PMID:12388700; http://dx.doi.org/10.1128/JVI.76.22.11397-11404.2002.

139. Loré K, Betts MR, Brenchley JM, Kuruppu J, Khojasteh S, Perfetto S, et al. Toll-like receptor ligands modulate dendritic cells to augment cytomegalovirus- and HIV-1-specific T cell responses. J Immunol 2003; 171:4320-8; PMID:14530357.

140. Krieg AM. Antitumor applications of stimulating toll-like receptor 9 with CpG oligodeoxynucleotides. Curr Oncol Rep 2004; 6:88-95; PMID:14751085; http://dx.doi.org/10.1007/s11912-004-0019-0.

141. Weeratna RD, Makinen SR, McCluskie MJ, Davis HL. TLR agonists as vaccine adjuvants: comparison of CpG ODN and Resiquimod (R-848). Vaccine 2005; 23:5263-70; PMID:16081189; http://dx.doi.org/10.1016/j.vaccine.2005.06.024.

142. Hayashi T, Raz E. TLR9-based immunotherapy for allergic disease. Am J Med. 2006; 119(10): 897 e1-6.

143. McCluskie MJ, Krieg AM. Enhancement of infectious disease vaccines through TLR9-dependent recognition of CpG DNA. Curr Top Microbiol Immunol 2006; 311:155-78; PMID:17048708; http://dx.doi.org/10.1007/3-540-32636-7_6.

144. Kwissa M, Amara RR, Robinson HL, Moss B, Alkan S, Jabbar A, et al. Adjuvanting a DNA vaccine with a TLR9 ligand plus Flt3 ligand results in enhanced cellular immunity against the simian immunodeficiency virus. J Exp Med 2007; 204:2733-46; PMID:17954572; http://dx.doi.org/10.1084/jem.20071211.

145. Kurt-Jones EA, Popova L, Kwinn L, Haynes LM, Jones LP, Tripp RA, et al. Pattern recognition receptors TLR4 and CD14 mediate response to respiratory syncytial virus. Nat Immunol 2000; 1:398-401; PMID:11062499; http://dx.doi.org/10.1038/80833.

146. Haynes LM, Moore DD, Kurt-Jones EA, Finberg RW, Anderson LJ, Tripp RA. Involvement of toll-like receptor 4 in innate immunity to respiratory syncytial virus. J Virol 2001; 75:10730-7; PMID:11602714; http://dx.doi.org/10.1128/JVI.75.22.10730-10737.2001.

147. Bastian A, Schäfer H. Human alpha-defensin 1 (HNP-1) inhibits adenoviral infection in vitro. Regul Pept 2001; 101:157-61; PMID:11495691; http://dx.doi.org/10.1016/S0167-0115(01)00282-8.

148. Zhang L, Yu W, He T, Yu J, Caffrey RE, Dalmasso EA, et al. Contribution of human alpha-defensin 1, 2, and 3 to the anti-HIV-1 activity of CD8 antiviral factor. Science 2002; 298:995-1000; PMID:12351674; http://dx.doi.org/10.1126/science.1076185.

149. Sinha S, Cheshenko N, Lehrer RI, Herold BC. NP-1, a rabbit alpha-defensin, prevents the entry and intercellular spread of herpes simplex virus type 1. Antimicrob Agents Chemother 2003; 47:494-500; PMID:12543649; http://dx.doi.org/10.1128/AAC.47.2.494-500.2003.

150. Klotman ME, Chang TL. Defensins in innate antiviral immunity. Nat Rev Immunol 2006; 6:447-56; PMID:16724099; http://dx.doi.org/10.1038/nri1860.

151. Howell MD, Streib JE, Leung DY. Antiviral activity of human beta-defensin 3 against vaccinia virus. J Allergy Clin Immunol 2007; 119:1022-5; PMID:17353034; http://dx.doi.org/10.1016/j.jaci.2007.01.044.

152. Barlow PG, Svoboda P, Mackellar A, Nash AA, York IA, Pohl J, et al. Antiviral activity and increased host defense against influenza infection elicited by the human cathelicidin LL-37. PLoS One 2011; 6:e25333; PMID:22031815; http://dx.doi.org/10.1371/journal.pone.0025333.

153. Vareille M, Kieninger E, Edwards MR, Regamey N. The airway epithelium: soldier in the fight against respiratory viruses. Clin Microbiol Rev 2011; 24:210-29; PMID:21233513; http://dx.doi.org/10.1128/CMR.00014-10.

154. Isogawa M, Robek MD, Furuichi Y, Chisari FV. Toll-like receptor signaling inhibits hepatitis B virus replication in vivo. J Virol 2005; 79:7269-72; PMID:15890966; http://dx.doi.org/10.1128/JVI.79.11.7269-7272.2005.
155. Mosoian A, Teixeira A, Burns CS, Sander LE, Gusella GL, He C, et al. Prothymosin-alpha inhibits HIV-1 via Toll-like receptor 4-mediated type I interferon induction. Proc Natl Acad Sci U S A 2010; 107:10178-83; PMID:20479248; http://dx.doi.org/10.1073/pnas.0914870107.
156. Liang Z, Wu S, Li Y, He L, Wu M, Jiang L, et al. Activation of Toll-like receptor 3 impairs the dengue virus serotype 2 replication through induction of IFN-β in cultured hepatoma cells. PLoS One 2011; 6:e23346; PMID:21829730; http://dx.doi.org/10.1371/journal.pone.0023346.
157. Lau YF, Tang LH, Ooi EEA. A TLR3 ligand that exhibits potent inhibition of influenza virus replication and has strong adjuvant activity has the potential for dual applications in an influenza pandemic. Vaccine 2009; 27:1354-64; PMID:19150474; http://dx.doi.org/10.1016/j.vaccine.2008.12.048.
158. Zhou Y, Wang X, Liu M, Hu Q, Song L, Ye L, et al. A critical function of toll-like receptor-3 in the induction of anti-human immunodeficiency virus activities in macrophages. Immunology 2010; 131:40-9; PMID:20636339.
159. MacDonald EM, Savoy A, Gillgrass A, Fernandez S, Smieja M, Rosenthal KL, et al. Susceptibility of human female primary genital epithelial cells to herpes simplex virus, type-2 and the effect of TLR3 ligand and sex hormones on infection. Biol Reprod 2007; 77:1049-59; PMID:17881767; http://dx.doi.org/10.1095/biolreprod.107.063933.
160. Nazli A, Yao XD, Smieja M, Rosenthal KL, Ashkar AA, Kaushic C. Differential induction of innate anti-viral responses by TLR ligands against Herpes simplex virus, type 2, infection in primary genital epithelium of women. Antiviral Res 2009; 81:103-12; PMID:19013198; http://dx.doi.org/10.1016/j.antiviral.2008.10.005.
161. Boukhvalova MS, Sotomayor TB, Point RC, Pletneva LM, Prince GA, Blanco JC. Activation of interferon response through toll-like receptor 3 impacts viral pathogenesis and pulmonary toll-like receptor expression during respiratory syncytial virus and influenza infections in the cotton rat Sigmodon hispidus model. Journal of interferon & cytokine research: the official journal of the International Society for Interferon and Cytokine Research. 2010; 30(4): 229-42.
162. Stewart CR, Bagnaud-Baule A, Karpala AJ, Lowther S, Mohr PG, Wise TG, et al. Toll-like receptor 7 ligands inhibit influenza a infection in chickens. Journal of interferon & cytokine research: the official journal of the International Society for Interferon and Cytokine Research. 2012; 32(1): 46-51.
163. Sariol CA, Martínez MI, Rivera F, Rodríguez IV, Pantoja P, Abel K, et al. Decreased dengue replication and an increased anti-viral humoral response with the use of combined Toll-like receptor 3 and 7/8 agonists in macaques. PLoS One 2011; 6:e19323; PMID:21559444; http://dx.doi.org/10.1371/journal.pone.0019323.
164. Miller RL, Meng TC, Tomai MA. The antiviral activity of Toll-like receptor 7 and 7/8 agonists. Drug News Perspect 2008; 21:69-87; PMID:18389099; http://dx.doi.org/10.1358/dnp.2008.21.2.1188193.
165. Mark KE, Corey L, Meng TC, Magaret AS, Huang ML, Selke S, et al. Topical resiquimod 0.01% gel decreases herpes simplex virus type 2 genital shedding: a randomized, controlled trial. J Infect Dis 2007; 195:1324-31; PMID:17397003; http://dx.doi.org/10.1086/513276.
166. Svensson A, Bellner L, Magnusson M, Eriksson K. Role of IFN-alpha/beta signaling in the prevention of genital herpes virus type 2 infection. J Reprod Immunol 2007; 74:114-23; PMID:17092567; http://dx.doi.org/10.1016/j.jri.2006.09.002.
167. McCluskie MJ, Cartier JL, Patrick AJ, Sajic D, Weeratna RD, Rosenthal KL, et al. Treatment of intravaginal HSV-2 infection in mice: a comparison of CpG oligodeoxynucleotides and resiquimod (R-848). Antiviral Res 2006; 69:77-85; PMID:16377001; http://dx.doi.org/10.1016/j.antiviral.2005.10.007.
168. Gill N, Deacon PM, Lichty B, Mossman KL, Ashkar AA. Induction of innate immunity against herpes simplex virus type 2 infection via local delivery of Toll-like receptor ligands correlates with beta interferon production. J Virol 2006; 80:9943-50; PMID:17005672; http://dx.doi.org/10.1128/JVI.01036-06.
169. Lund J, Sato A, Akira S, Medzhitov R, Iwasaki A. Toll-like receptor 9-mediated recognition of Herpes simplex virus-2 by plasmacytoid dendritic cells. J Exp Med 2003; 198:513-20; PMID:12900525; http://dx.doi.org/10.1084/jem.20030162.

Index

Symbols

2',5'-oligoadenylate synthetase (OAS) 86, 153, 170, 218, 229-231, 242, 244
5,6-dimethylxanthenone-4-acetic acid (DMXAA) 119-121
5'-triphosphate RNA (5'-pppRNA) 77, 98, 99, 200-203, 205-208, 211, 212, 221, 242, 244

A

A20 76, 103, 104
A46 132, 134, 135
A52 132, 134-136
Absent in melanoma 2 (AIM2) 100, 122-124, 244
Adaptive immune response 10, 20, 30, 31, 114, 131, 154, 155, 159, 167, 170, 191, 197, 210, 218, 243, 245
Adenine nucleotide translocator 3 (ANT3) 171
Adenylate-uridylate (AU) 58, 60, 62, 207
Adenylate-uridylate-rich element (ARE) 58, 62, 63
AIP4 103, 104
Antigen presentation 179, 181, 183, 184, 187, 188, 190
Antiviral immunity 1, 5, 7, 9, 10, 12, 13, 151, 156, 178-180, 190, 197, 242, 246
Apoptosis 1-4, 7, 8, 12, 97, 101, 107, 119, 122, 134-136, 140, 171, 187-189, 220, 223, 225-230, 232, 233, 243, 244, 246
Argonaute 5, 59, 62
Arthropod 1
Atg5-Atg12 conjugate 103-105, 178-180, 185
Autoimmunity 19, 32, 62, 64, 114, 124, 125, 224
Autophagy 8, 49, 97, 99, 103-107, 178-191

B

B8 132, 134, 135, 137
B14 132, 134,-136
B18 132, 134, 135, 137

C

C3H/HeJ 20-22, 33
C6 6, 132, 134-136, 231
C7 132, 134, 135, 138-140
C57BL/10ScCr 20, 21, 33
Caspase 2-4, 71, 85, 98, 100, 101, 107, 121-123, 125, 151, 168, 197, 223-225, 227, 229, 242
Cellular cleavage and polyadenylation specific factor 30 (CPSF30) 170
Cephalochordate 9, 10
Chronic infection 148, 149, 151, 187
Cnidarian 9-11
Co-infection 148, 149
Cyclic di – adenosine monophosphate and cyclic di-guanosine monophosphate (Ci-di-A/GMP) 120
Cytosolic sensing 8, 43, 71, 73, 99-102, 105, 114-120, 122, 124, 125, 131, 158, 179-181, 183-185, 187, 190, 208, 211, 219, 225-227, 229, 233, 243-246

D

Death domain (DD) 10, 11, 27, 29, 44, 48, 60, 71, 119, 135, 168
DExD/H box helicase 1, 8-12, 71, 85-87, 118
DHX9 100, 118-120
DHX36 100, 118-120, 227
Dicer 1, 5, 6, 8-12, 62, 87
DNA-dependent activator of IFN-regulatory factor (DAI) 91, 99, 116, 117, 119, 120, 139, 244
DNA sensor 99, 100, 114-116, 119, 124, 125, 181, 185, 244
Double-stranded RNA (dsRNA) 1, 5-12, 19, 20, 23, 24, 41, 63, 72-74, 77-79, 85-92, 98, 102, 106, 107, 115, 122, 132, 134, 135, 138, 140, 168, 170, 197-203, 205-210, 218-234, 242-245
Drug resistance 119, 149, 240, 242, 243
DUBA 76, 104

E

E3   4, 30, 76, 92, 101, 132, 134, 135,
     138-140, 168, 181, 231
Ebola virus   197, 242, 243
Echinoderm   10

H

H1   132, 134, 135, 138, 140
Helicase   1, 8-12, 71, 73, 77-79, 85-87,
     89-92, 98, 100, 107, 115, 117-119, 136,
     168, 197, 198, 202, 206, 218, 219, 224,
     227, 228, 233, 242
Hepatitis C virus (HCV)   72, 74, 75, 86,
     106, 107, 148-153, 156, 158-160, 200,
     205, 207, 229, 231, 232, 241-243, 245
Herpes   41, 42, 48, 64, 98, 101, 116, 122,
     182, 184, 186-188, 191, 223, 232, 245
Histone tail   170
HMGB1   25, 27, 100, 118
Host defense   33, 51, 92, 148, 157, 232
Human immunodeficiency virus (HIV)   62,
     124, 148-150, 153-160, 183, 187-189,
     199, 228, 229, 242, 244-246

I

IFI16   91, 100, 119, 120, 122-125, 244
IκB kinase-ε (IKKε)   29, 30, 63, 72, 76, 86,
     116, 135, 136, 168, 222, 225
IMD pathway   7, 8, 181
Immune evasion   132, 141, 148, 157, 167
Inflammasome   100, 103, 121-124, 227, 243,
     244
Influenza   10, 41, 42, 72, 73, 85-88, 90, 92,
     98, 99, 102, 106, 119, 122, 167, 169,
     170, 172, 189, 191, 200, 208, 209, 229,
     231, 232, 240, 242; 243, 245-248
Inhibitors of apoptosis protein (IAP)   3, 4,
     223
Innate   1, 6, 10, 12, 13, 19, 20, 23, 30-33, 40,
     45, 48, 50, 51, 58-60, 64, 71, 76, 79, 80,
     85, 92, 97, 98, 100, 101, 105, 107, 108,
     114-116, 121, 124, 126, 131, 136, 140,
     148, 149, 151-160, 167, 170-172, 178,
     179, 181-183, 185, 190, 191, 197, 198,
     208, 210, 218, 221, 223, 225-227, 229,
     233, 240, 241, 243, 244, 246-248

immune signaling   32, 115, 140, 151,
     156-160, 181
immunity   1, 10, 12, 13, 19, 23, 40, 45,
     50, 51, 71, 79, 80, 97, 101, 105, 108,
     114, 116, 124, 126, 136, 149, 151,
     159, 160, 233, 246
Interferon (IFN)   4, 6, 9, 10, 12, 19, 27, 29,
     30, 41, 42, 44, 46-51, 63, 64, 71-73,
     75-77, 79, 80, 85-92, 97-103, 105-108,
     114-122, 124-126, 131, 132, 134-140,
     149, 151, 153-160, 167-172, 181, 183,
     185, 186, 188, 190, 197-200, 202,
     203, 206-209, 212, 218-221, 223-225,
     227-232, 234, 241-246
  IFN-α   42, 48, 86, 100, 103, 116-119,
     131, 132, 134, 135, 137, 138,
     154-156, 167, 170, 221, 223, 232,
     245
  IFN-β   44, 48, 63, 71, 80, 86, 88-91, 98,
     101, 102, 116-120, 124, 125, 131,
     132, 134, 135, 137, 138, 151, 167,
     170, 171, 220, 228, 231, 242
  IFN-γ   102, 119, 121, 122, 131, 132,
     134-137, 140, 181, 232, 244
  IFN-λ   131
Interferon-stimulated gene (ISG)   63, 100,
     101, 134, 138, 140, 149, 151, 153,
     155-159, 168, 170, 188, 241, 243
Interleukin (IL)   7, 21, 22, 29, 30, 43, 44,
     48-50, 60, 62-64, 88, 98, 100, 101,
     121-123, 125, 131, 132, 134-137, 140,
     153, 185, 197, 221, 222, 227, 244
  IL-1 receptor associated kinase (IRAK)
     29, 30, 44-46, 60, 118, 135, 221
  IL-18   21, 22, 30, 44, 100, 101, 121, 122
     125, 131, 132, 134-137, 140
     binding protein (IL-18BP)   132, 136
     137
Intracellular signaling pathway   87, 89, 126
IRAK1   29, 30, 45-50, 60, 61, 64, 65, 118
IRF   19, 48, 72, 76, 80, 86, 87, 89, 97, 98,
     116, 120, 131, 132, 135, 136, 140, 151,
     152, 156, 158, 160, 183, 185, 202, 203,
     220-229, 232, 233
  IRF-3   72, 76, 80, 151, 152, 156, 158,
     160, 202, 203, 220-227, 229, 232,
     233

J

JAK/STAT pathway 7, 8, 170

K

K1 132, 134-136, 138-140
K3 132, 134, 135, 138-140
K7 132, 134-136

L

Lipopolysaccharide (LPS) 19-24, 26, 27,
29-31, 33, 43, 44, 46, 61, 62, 64, 103,
115, 118, 119, 244
LPS-refractory mice 20
LRRFIP1 91, 100, 118, 124, 244
Lysosome 27, 49, 50, 105, 124, 125,
178-180, 182, 183, 189, 190

M

M2 132, 134-136, 189, 240
Macroautophagy 178
MAVS 10, 71, 86, 99-107, 117-119, 124,
151, 168, 171, 180, 185, 198, 207, 208
MicroRNA (miRNA) 5, 10, 58-65, 80, 87,
233, 241
miR-146a 64, 65
miR-155 63-65
Mitochondria 4, 71, 75, 76, 79, 86, 97,
99-102, 104-108, 152, 168, 171, 185,
225-227, 259
Mitochondrial immune signaling complex
(MISC) 97, 99, 107, 108
mRNA 19, 58-65, 86, 88, 91, 100, 102, 122,
158, 170, 171, 187, 199, 208-210, 219,
220, 229, 232
MyD88 24-27, 29-31, 42-48, 60, 61, 63,
118, 119, 132, 134, 135, 153, 156, 181,
221
dependent pathway 27, 29, 30, 43, 45,
47, 221
independent pathway 27, 29, 44, 135,
221

N

N1 132, 134-136, 199, 206
Negative strand RNA virus (ssRNA(-)) 72,
73

Nematode 1, 2, 9, 10, 45
NLRC5 76, 102-104, 243
NLRP3 102, 122, 123, 243
NLRX1 75, 102-104, 243
NOD2 102, 104, 181, 242, 243
NOD-like receptor (NLR) 20, 31, 75, 76,
101, 102, 108, 114, 121-123, 131, 148,
181, 191, 242, 243, 246
NS1 106, 167, 168, 170-172, 229, 231
Nuclear factor-κB (NF-κB) 7, 19, 22, 23, 29,
30, 44-47, 60, 64, 72, 75-77, 80, 87, 89,
97, 99-103, 105, 107, 116-121, 123, 131,
132, 134, 135, 138, 140, 157, 158, 168,
170, 183, 185, 220, 222-225, 227-229,
233
Nucleic acid 8-12, 19, 23, 27, 29, 31, 32,
40-43, 47-50, 63, 64, 97, 98, 100, 102,
114, 115, 118, 131, 148, 156, 157, 183,
197, 200, 211, 212, 221, 233, 241, 242,
244-246

O

Orthomyxovirus 225

P

Panhandle 74, 75, 86, 208-210
Pathogen 1, 2, 7, 22, 23, 40, 51, 71, 93,
97, 98, 114-116, 121, 122, 125, 126,
131, 132, 148, 159, 167, 168, 172, 178,
180-189, 208, 211, 240-243, 245
associated molecular pattern (PAMP)
40, 42, 71, 97, 98, 101, 105, 114,
115, 120, 126, 131, 132, 135, 148,
150-152, 155-160, 168, 180, 183,
190, 240, 241, 246
recognition receptor (PRR) 51, 93, 98,
100, 102, 103, 107, 114-117, 120,
121, 126, 131, 132, 135, 140, 148,
149, 151, 152, 154-158, 160, 168,
180, 181, 197, 240-246
Pattern recognition 22, 85, 98, 114, 134,
180, 197, 218, 240, 241
PB1-F2 167, 168, 170, 171
PCBP2 103, 104
Phosphatidylinositol-3-kinase (PI3K) 48,
171, 178, 180, 186, 223, 226
Phylogeny 9
Piwi-interacting RNA (piRNA) 5, 6

Polyadenylation binding protein II (PABPII)
    170
Polymerase 6, 10, 73, 91, 92, 98, 99, 106,
    117-119, 138, 167, 168, 170, 171, 199,
    200, 202, 205, 207-211, 219, 225, 226,
    243
Polyubiquitination 45, 47, 76, 106
Porifera 10
Positional cloning of the *Lps* locus 21
Post-transcriptional regulation 58-60, 65
Poxvirus 2, 3, 72, 123, 131, 132, 135-141
Pro-inflammatory cytokine 27, 30, 40-43,
    47, 49, 50, 60, 64, 72, 76, 87, 100, 115,
    120-123, 125, 126, 131, 136, 138, 149,
    159, 168, 185, 227, 232, 243, 244, 246
Protein kinase R (PKR) 86, 132, 134, 135,
    138-140, 151, 153, 157, 170, 184, 186,
    188, 209, 218, 220, 228, 229, 243, 244
Protein trafficking 48
PSMA7 103, 104

R

Retrovirus 141, 153, 156, 157, 182, 245, 247
RIG-I 1, 8-12, 20, 64, 71-80, 85-92, 98-103,
    105-107, 114, 115, 117, 118, 120, 124,
    131, 148, 151, 152, 158, 159, 168, 170,
    181, 185, 197-212, 218-221, 224-228,
    232, 233, 242-244, 247
    like receptor (RLR) 8-12, 20, 31, 71-80,
        85-92, 98, 99, 101-107, 114, 115,
        118, 131, 132, 134, 135, 138, 140,
        148, 151, 158, 159, 168, 180, 181,
        185, 197, 198, 210, 211, 218, 224,
        225, 227, 233, 242, 243, 246
Ring finger protein 5 (RNF5) 76, 101, 103,
    104
RNA
    binding protein (RBP) 58, 59, 61-63,
        229
    interference 1, 5-9, 12, 87, 99, 103, 190,
        212
    polymerase III 99, 117-119, 138, 207,
        219, 225, 226, 243
    virus 4-6, 10, 12, 72, 73, 79, 85-92, 98,
        101, 103, 115, 149, 159, 160, 167,
        172, 190, 191, 197, 200, 207, 210,
        224, 225, 229, 232, 242

S

Short interfering RNA (siRNA) 5, 6, 10,
    12, 79, 87, 100, 102, 103, 116, 118, 119,
    124, 182, 183, 185, 187, 199, 200, 208,
    212, 224, 241
Sindbis virus (SINV) 6-8, 102, 103, 182,
    186, 229, 231
Single nucleotide polymorphism 61
Single-stranded RNA (ssRNA) 19, 24, 41,
    42, 63, 72-74, 90, 98, 102, 115, 122,
    124, 198-203, 205-210, 219, 221, 227,
    242-245
Splice variant 58, 60-62, 65, 103, 222
Stimulator of interferon gene (STING) 76,
    99, 100-103, 107, 116, 117, 119-121,
    124, 180, 185

T

TANK-binding kinase 1 (TBK1) 29, 30,
    46-48, 61, 72, 76, 79, 86, 99, 100, 103,
    116, 117, 119-121, 124, 132, 134-136,
    153, 168, 180, 185, 198, 222, 225
Tirap 24, 27, 29, 43, 44, 221
Toll 7-9, 13, 19-23, 33, 40, 43, 44, 50, 51,
    58, 60, 85, 92, 93, 98, 114, 115, 117,
    124, 131, 135, 148, 153, 168, 181, 183,
    191, 197, 218, 221, 222, 233
Toll/IL-1 receptor homology domain (TIR)
    21-23, 27, 29, 43, 44, 60, 98, 119, 132,
    134, 135, 221-223
Toll-like receptor (TLR) 9, 10, 19-27, 29-33,
    40-46, 48-51, 58-65, 85, 92, 93, 98, 105,
    114-121, 124, 131, 132, 134, 135, 148,
    151-153, 155, 156, 158, 168, 181, 183,
    185, 187, 188, 191, 197, 200, 211, 212,
    218, 221, 225, 233, 242, 245, 246
    TLR3 9, 23, 24, 27, 29, 30, 32, 40-44,
        47, 61, 63, 64, 98, 100, 115, 135, 151,
        153, 168, 183, 197, 218-224, 227,
        232, 233, 242, 244, 245
    TLR7 9, 10, 24, 27, 29, 30, 32, 40-44,
        47-50, 60, 63, 64, 98, 100, 105, 156,
        159, 181, 183, 197, 199, 200, 212,
        221, 222, 242, 245, 246
    TLR9 9, 24, 25, 27, 29, 30, 32, 40-44,
        47-50, 60, 63, 98, 100, 115, 116, 118,
        119, 124, 183, 200, 207, 212, 221,
        222, 242, 245

TLR accessory protein 26, 27
TLR adaptor 153
TLR ligand 26, 42, 153, 183
TLR signaling 27, 29-33, 40, 43, 44, 46,
    50, 58, 60-65, 98, 132, 151, 156, 181,
    185, 187, 188
TLR signaling in plasmacytoid dendritic
    cell 27
Toll pathway 8, 23
TRAM adaptor with GOLD domain (TAG)
    61
Transcription 7, 19, 30, 44, 48, 58, 71, 73,
    86, 87, 89, 91, 100, 102, 116-124, 131,
    132, 135, 137, 138, 140, 148, 150,
    151, 153, 154, 158, 168, 170, 188,
    189, 198-200, 202, 203, 205, 207, 208,
    218-222, 225, 226
Translocase 76, 90, 91
TRIF 24, 27, 29-31, 41, 43-47, 61, 63, 77,
    103, 132, 134, 135, 153, 181, 221-223,
    227
TRIM25 76, 92, 104, 168, 170
Tristetraprolin (TTP) 62, 63
Tumor necrosis factor (TNF) 25, 29-33,
    60-64, 79, 86, 100, 168, 181, 185, 220,
    221, 224, 244
Type 1 interferon 27, 30, 42, 48-51, 63, 64,
    71, 72, 85-89, 91, 92, 97-103, 105-108,
    114-122, 124-126, 131, 132, 134, 135,
    137-139, 149, 151, 167, 168, 170, 183,
    185, 186, 190, 197-200, 202, 203,
    206-209, 212, 219-221, 223-225, 227,
    241, 243, 244, 246

U

Untranslated region (UTR) 58-64, 171
Urochordate 9, 10

V

Vaccinia 72, 75, 92, 119, 122, 132, 134, 141,
    223, 229, 231, 242, 245
Virus 1-10, 12, 19, 24, 25, 31, 32, 40-43,
    45, 49, 50, 63, 64, 71-73, 75, 76, 79,
    80, 85-92, 98, 99, 101-103, 106, 107,
    114-116, 119, 122-124, 126, 131,
    132, 134, 136, 137, 139-141, 148,
    149, 152-154, 156-160, 167, 169-172,
    180-191, 197-200, 203, 205-211,
    218-221, 223-233, 240-248
    evasion 136, 187, 190
    infection 1-8, 10-12, 19, 31, 42, 71-73,
        87, 98, 101, 102, 116, 122, 123, 140,
        148, 149, 151, 154, 155, 160, 179,
        180, 182, 183, 188, 203, 210, 212,
        219, 223, 224, 226, 227, 229, 232,
        240, 242, 243, 245-248
    inhibition 132, 188
    recognition 49, 85, 183, 185, 191, 225
    RNA 4-6, 8-10, 11, 71, 73, 74, 77, 79, 80,
        91, 149, 151, 153, 168, 185, 197-199,
        202, 208-210, 232, 243, 244
    subversion 190
    suppressors of apoptosis 1, 3
    suppressors of RNAi (VSR) 6-8
Voltage-dependent anion channel
    1(VDAC1) 171

Milton Keynes UK
Ingram Content Group UK Ltd.
UKHW020024071024
449327UK00032B/2921